I0882655

The Effect of Exercise on Emotion

Robert Motta
Hofstra University, USA

IGI Global
Scientific Publishing
Publishing Tomorrow's Research Today

Vice President of Editorial	Melissa Wagner
Director of Acquisitions	Mikaela Felty
Director of Book Development	Jocelynn Hessler
Production Manager	Mike Brehm
Cover Design	Jose Rosado

Published in the United States of America by
IGI Global Scientific Publishing
701 East Chocolate Avenue
Hershey, PA, 17033, USA
Tel: 717-533-8845 | Fax: 717-533-7115
Website: https://www.igi-global.com E-mail: cust@igi-global.com

Library of Congress Cataloging-in-Publication Data

Names: Motta, Robert W. editor
Title: The effect of exercise on emotion / edited by Robert Motta.
Description: Hershey, PA : IGI Global Scientific Publishing, [2026] | Includes bibliographical references and index. | Summary: "This book explores the psychological impact of exercise, highlighting how aerobic and resistance training influence mood, anxiety, depression, memory, and self-esteem. By integrating empirical findings and theoretical perspectives, it advances understanding of exercise as a powerful tool for enhancing emotional well-being and cognitive functioning"-- Provided by publisher.
Identifiers: LCCN 2025041620 (print) | LCCN 2025041621 (ebook) | ISBN 9798337361574 hardcover | ISBN 9798337361581 paperback | ISBN 9798337361598 ebook
Subjects: LCSH: Exercise--Psychological aspects | Emotions
Classification: LCC RA781 .E3285 2026 (print) | LCC RA781 (ebook)
LC record available at https://lccn.loc.gov/2025041620
LC ebook record available at https://lccn.loc.gov/2025041621

British Cataloguing in Publication Data
A Cataloguing in Publication record for this book is available from the British Library.

Table of Contents

Detailed Table of Contents

This chapter explores the psychological effects of resistance training (RT) and aerobic exercise (AE), focusing on emotional regulation, stress management, and mental health. While physiological benefits—better cardiovascular function, strength, and metabolic health—are well known, their distinct psychological roles remain less clear. The chapter applies psychophysiological, cognitive-behavioral, and social-environmental models to explain how RT and AE shape mood, anxiety, depression, self-esteem, and resilience. Research highlights shared and unique outcomes, influenced by age, gender, culture, exercise intensity, and social context. Methodological issues, including reliance on self-reports and limited neurobiological data, complicate evaluation. By integrating cross-disciplinary evidence, the chapter offers practical guidance for researchers, clinicians, and policymakers. Ultimately, it deepens understanding of how RT and AE, separately or together, enhance psychological well-being.

Depression affects millions of people worldwide, causing low mood, loss of interest, and poor self-esteem. Traditional treatments such as medicines and therapy are helpful but may not be enough for everyone. Exercise has been shown to improve mood, but most programs only focus on physical health. This manuscript introduces Emotion Focused Exercise Interventions (EFEIs), which combine physical activity with emotional awareness, mindfulness, and therapeutic support. Activities such as aerobic exercise, resistance training, yoga, and dance are used not just for fitness but also for emotional expression and healing. Evidence shows that EFEIs improve

Preface

INTRODUCTION

For decades, the benefits of physical exercise have been well documented in relation to physical health outcomes, including cardiovascular functioning, weight management, metabolic health, and disease prevention. These physiological effects have understandably occupied a central place in both research and public discourse. Yet, alongside this extensive body of work, the emotional and psychological consequences of exercise—though frequently acknowledged anecdotally—have received comparatively less systematic and sustained scholarly attention. This edited volume seeks to address that imbalance.

Emerging research increasingly demonstrates that exercise exerts meaningful effects on emotional well-being and psychological functioning. Evidence suggests that regular physical activity may reduce symptoms of anxiety, depression, post-traumatic stress disorder, and related conditions, while simultaneously enhancing cognitive processes such as attention, memory, and concentration, as well as improving self-esteem and overall quality of life. Despite these promising findings, significant gaps remain in our understanding of the mechanisms, boundaries, and comparative effectiveness of exercise as a psychological intervention. The emotional benefits of exercise have long been implied; however, the field continues to require rigorous, data-driven investigation to clarify how, why, and for whom these benefits occur.

The purpose of this book is to present contemporary empirical research examining the effects of exercise on emotion and psychological functioning. Contributors explore both aerobic and resistance forms of exercise, considering variables such as duration, intensity, and modality, and their differential impact on emotional states and mental health outcomes. Central questions addressed include how endurance and resistance exercise compare with pharmacological and psychotherapeutic treatments for depression; the relative explanatory power of competing theories such as the endorphin and endocannabinoid hypotheses in accounting for anxiety reduction; and the influence of physical activity on learning, memory, and cognitive retention. Collectively, these chapters aim to move beyond broad generalizations and toward a more precise, evidence-based understanding of exercise as a tool for psychological well-being.

This volume is intended for a diverse readership, including researchers, psychologists, psychiatrists, exercise physiologists, physicians, counselors, educators, physical therapists, and other health care professionals whose work intersects with mental health and physical activity. At the same time, the book has been written with sufficient clarity and accessibility to engage informed members of the general public who are interested in the emotional and psychological benefits of exercise.

As editor, my hope is that this book will stimulate further inquiry, encourage interdisciplinary collaboration, and contribute meaningfully to the growing recognition of exercise not only as a means of physical conditioning, but also as a powerful influence on emotional health and psychological functioning.

ORGANIZATION OF THE BOOK

Chapter 1: The Comparative Psychological Effects of Resistance versus Aerobic Forms of Exercise

In Chapter 1, the comparative psychological effects of resistance training and aerobic exercise are examined through psychophysiological, cognitive-behavioral, and social-environmental lenses. While both exercise modalities are well established for their physical health benefits, this chapter clarifies their shared and distinct contributions to emotional regulation, stress reduction, and mental health outcomes such as mood, anxiety, depression, self-esteem, and resilience. The authors address how contextual factors—including age, gender, cultural background, intensity, and social environment—shape psychological responses to exercise. By critically evaluating methodological limitations in existing research, the chapter provides a nuanced synthesis that informs both clinical practice and future research directions.

Chapter 2: Emotion Focused Exercise Interventions Enhance Mood State and Self-Esteem in Individuals with Depression

Chapter 3 introduces Emotion Focused Exercise Interventions (EFEIs) as an innovative and integrative approach to depression care. Moving beyond traditional exercise programs that emphasize physical outcomes alone, this chapter highlights interventions that combine movement with emotional awareness, mindfulness, and therapeutic support. Through evidence and case examples across clinical, educational, and community settings, the authors demonstrate that EFEIs produce superior improvements in mood, self-esteem, and emotional regulation compared to exercise alone. This chapter positions emotion-focused exercise as a holistic, accessible, and cost-effective complement to conventional treatments for depression.

Chapter 3: Neurobiological Effects of Exercise on Emotional Regulation in Bipolar Disorder

Chapter 4 explores exercise as a biologically active adjunctive treatment for bipolar disorder. Acknowledging the complexity and chronicity of the condition, the chapter reviews evidence showing how physical activity influences key neurochemical systems—including dopamine, serotonin, BDNF, and endocannabinoids—that are central to mood regulation and cognitive-emotional processing. The authors argue that exercise may help address persistent subthreshold symptoms, cognitive impairments, and quality-of-life deficits that often remain despite standard pharmacological and psychosocial treatments. This chapter expands the therapeutic landscape for bipolar disorder by framing exercise as a neurobiologically meaningful intervention rather than a purely lifestyle recommendation.

Chapter 4: The Therapeutic Role of Exercise in Schizophrenia

Chapter 5 examines the impact of regular physical activity on cognitive, emotional, and social functioning in individuals with schizophrenia. Centered on the concept of exercise-induced neuroplasticity, the chapter explains how physical activity enhances neural growth, synaptic efficiency, and functional brain reorganization. The authors discuss improvements in attention, memory, executive functioning, and emotional balance, while also comparing aerobic, resistance, and mindfulness-based exercises. This chapter highlights structured exercise as a natural, adjunctive therapeutic strategy for enhancing mental resilience and overall psychological well-being in schizophrenia.

Chapter 5: Micro-Workouts for Mental Health

Chapter 6 introduces the emerging concept of micro-workouts, or "exercise snacks," as a practical solution to sedentary lifestyles and time constraints. Focusing on short-duration activities lasting less than 15 minutes, the chapter reviews evidence demonstrating immediate benefits for mood, emotional regulation, anxiety, depression, attention, and memory. Neurochemical mechanisms involving endorphins, serotonin, dopamine, and endocannabinoids are explored, alongside comparisons with longer exercise sessions. This chapter offers actionable strategies for integrating brief bouts of activity into daily life, broadening the accessibility of exercise-based mental health benefits.

Chapter 6: Regular Physical Activity and Psychological Distress in Young Adults

Chapter 7 addresses the growing mental health challenges faced by young adults and positions physical activity as both a preventive and therapeutic tool. Integrating insights from neuroscience, psychology, and behavioral science, the chapter explains how diverse exercise modalities enhance neuroplasticity, regulate neurotransmitters, and buffer stress. Beyond physiological mechanisms, the authors emphasize psychological and social pathways, including self-efficacy, body image, and connectedness. Guided by established theoretical models, this chapter provides practical recommendations for designing inclusive, culturally responsive, and effective exercise interventions for young adults.

Chapter 7: Reshaping the Brain—Exercise-Induced Neuroplasticity and Psychological Resilience

Chapter 8 synthesizes evidence on how exercise reshapes the brain and strengthens psychological resilience across the lifespan. The chapter examines molecular, cellular, and systems-level mechanisms underlying exercise-induced neuroplasticity, linking them to improvements in cognition, emotional stability, and stress regulation. By comparing aerobic, resistance, and mind-body exercises, the authors illustrate their complementary roles in fostering adaptability and resilience. This chapter reinforces physical activity as a cornerstone non-pharmacological strategy for lifelong brain and mental health.

Chapter 8: Curricular Pathways to Wellness for Senior High School Students

Chapter 9 reframes Physical Education as a transformative curricular platform for emotional agility, resilience, and career readiness among senior high school students. Drawing on empirical evidence and the Life and Career Skills Curriculum, the chapter outlines intrapersonal, interpersonal, and career-oriented applications of structured physical activity. Through mindful movement, cooperative games, and resilience-based exercises—many grounded in cultural practices—the authors demonstrate how PE can support holistic development. This chapter underscores the role of education systems in integrating physical activity into psychosocial learning and lifelong well-being.

Chapter 9: From Sweat to Serenity—How Exercise Shapes Emotional Well-Being

Chapter 10 offers an integrative perspective on how exercise promotes emotional well-being through biological, psychological, and social mechanisms. The chapter highlights neurochemical changes associated with mood regulation, alongside psychological benefits such as enhanced self-efficacy and mastery, and social benefits including connection and belonging. Attention is given to individual tailoring, daily integration, and potential risks such as overtraining. By blending theory, evidence, and practical guidance, this chapter presents exercise as a sustainable pathway from physical exertion to emotional serenity.

Chapter 10: Effect of Exercise on Academic Functioning

Chapter 11 examines the relationship between physical activity, cognitive functioning, and academic performance. Reviewing biological mechanisms such as neurogenesis and increased cerebral blood flow, the chapter demonstrates how even modest daily movement can enhance memory, stress management, and learning outcomes. The authors emphasize the importance of selecting appropriate exercise modalities that support, rather than detract from, academic performance. This chapter advocates for embedding physical activity within daily educational routines, reinforcing its role as an essential component of academic success.

Chapter 11: Neurochemical Pathways Linking Physical Activity with Emotional Balance

Chapter 12 provides an in-depth examination of the neurochemical and neuroanatomical pathways through which exercise promotes emotional balance. The chapter integrates findings on serotonergic, dopaminergic, endorphin, endocannabinoid, and noradrenergic systems, as well as changes in limbic and prefrontal brain structures. Emphasis is placed on stress regulation, neuroplasticity, and resilience, with clear clinical and practical implications. This chapter strengthens the argument for adopting physical activity as a primary therapeutic tool for emotional regulation across populations.

Chapter 12: The Impact of Exercise on Teacher Satisfaction and Retention

Chapter 13 presents a scoping review exploring physical activity as a coping mechanism for teacher well-being and burnout. Analyzing nineteen studies, the chapter finds consistent evidence that physical activity enhances mental well-being, with mixed but promising findings regarding burnout reduction, particularly emotional exhaustion. The authors discuss implications for school-based and leisure-time physical activity initiatives, highlighting exercise as a viable strategy for supporting teacher satisfaction, retention, and occupational health.

Chapter 13: Effect of Exercise and Emotional Well-Being in Competitive Sports

Chapter 14 explores the complex relationship between exercise, emotional well-being, and performance in competitive sports. The chapter highlights how consistent training supports emotional regulation, stress management, resilience, and motivation, while also addressing risks such as burnout and mental health strain. Psychological frameworks and emerging technologies are discussed as tools for fostering athlete-centered well-being. This chapter reflects a growing shift toward holistic, sustainable approaches in modern sports psychology.

Chapter 14: Embodied Healing—Mindfulness, Movement, and Dance Approaches

Chapter 15 focuses on embodied practices that integrate mindfulness, movement, and dance to support emotional regulation in individuals with depression and anxiety. Complementing traditional psychotherapies, these approaches emphasize physical expression, awareness, and resilience. Drawing from empirical evidence and applied contexts, the chapter highlights their potential to address the lived, embodied dimensions of emotional distress. This contribution underscores the value of integrative, body-based interventions in mental health care.

Chapter 15: Yoga Practice and Emotional Well-Being in Middle Age

The final chapter synthesizes findings from a randomized controlled trial examining the effects of yoga on physical and psychosocial health among middle-aged adults in Vietnam. Demonstrating significant improvements across multiple domains, the chapter critically evaluates methodological strengths and limitations while outlining directions for future research. Practical implications for community-based programming and policy integration are emphasized, particularly in rapidly urbanizing settings. This chapter concludes the volume by illustrating the global relevance and scalability of exercise-based emotional health interventions.

CONCLUSION

As the chapters in this volume collectively demonstrate, exercise is far more than a means of physical conditioning; it is a powerful, multifaceted influence on emotional health, psychological functioning, and cognitive resilience across the lifespan. Drawing from diverse disciplines—including psychology, neuroscience, psychiatry, education, exercise science, and public health—this edited reference book brings together compelling empirical evidence and applied perspectives that deepen our understanding of how movement shapes the mind as well as the body.

Taken together, the contributions reveal that the emotional effects of exercise are neither incidental nor uniform. Rather, they are shaped by neurochemical processes, neuroplastic adaptations, psychosocial contexts, individual differences, and the specific characteristics of the exercise itself. From aerobic and resistance training to mindfulness-based movement, dance, yoga, and brief micro-workouts, the chapters illustrate that physical activity can reduce psychological distress, enhance emotional regulation, improve self-esteem, support cognitive functioning, and foster resilience in both clinical and non-clinical populations. Importantly, this volume moves beyond general assertions by highlighting dose, modality, context, and mechanism—critical factors for translating research into effective practice.

This book also underscores the value of exercise as a complementary and, in some cases, primary non-pharmacological intervention for mental health. Across conditions such as depression, bipolar disorder, schizophrenia, academic stress, occupational burnout, and age-related cognitive decline, exercise emerges as a biologically active and psychologically meaningful strategy that can enhance quality of life and extend the reach of traditional treatments. Equally significant is the emphasis on accessibility, cultural relevance, and real-world implementation, positioning exercise as an inclusive approach capable of benefiting individuals and communities alike.

As editor, it is my hope that this volume will serve not only as a reference for researchers and clinicians, but also as a catalyst for continued inquiry and innovation. The findings presented here point toward the need for more integrative, interdisciplinary, and methodologically rigorous research, as well as thoughtful application in educational, clinical, occupational, and community settings. Ultimately, by advancing our understanding of the relationship between exercise and emotion, this book affirms a central message that resonates throughout its pages: intentional movement has the capacity to strengthen not only the body, but also the emotional and psychological foundations of human well-being.

Chapter 1

The Comparative Psychological Effects of Resistance versus Aerobic Forms of Exercise

Harry Sutanto
https://orcid.org/0000-0001-8356-4976
Binus University, Indonesia

Anton Dwi Fitriyanto
https://orcid.org/0000-0002-5112-1879
Binus University, Indonesia

ABSTRACT

This chapter explores the psychological effects of resistance training (RT) and aerobic exercise (AE), focusing on emotional regulation, stress management, and mental health. While physiological benefits—better cardiovascular function, strength, and metabolic health—are well known, their distinct psychological roles remain less clear. The chapter applies psychophysiological, cognitive-behavioral, and social-environmental models to explain how RT and AE shape mood, anxiety, depression, self-esteem, and resilience. Research highlights shared and unique outcomes, influenced by age, gender, culture, exercise intensity, and social context. Methodological issues, including reliance on self-reports and limited neurobiological data, complicate evaluation. By integrating cross-disciplinary evidence, the chapter offers practical guidance for researchers, clinicians, and policymakers. Ultimately, it deepens understanding of how RT and AE, separately or together, enhance psychological well-being.

DOI: 10.4018/979-8-3373-6157-4.ch001

INTRODUCTION

Historical Background

The relationship between physical exercise and psychological well-being has been examined for decades across psychology, sports science, and public health. A large body of research consistently demonstrates that regular exercise can enhance mood, reduce symptoms of depression and anxiety, and improve cognitive functioning, including attention, memory, and executive function (Cooney et al., 2013; Schuch et al., 2016a). However, much of the early literature has predominantly focused on aerobic activities such as running, cycling, and swimming, often treating exercise as a single, undifferentiated construct rather than investigating the distinct effects of various exercise modalities. This focus on aerobic exercise has, until recently, overshadowed evidence that resistance training may confer unique psychological benefits, including increased self-efficacy, improved body image, and enhanced resilience to stress (Craft & Perna, 2004; Ströhle, 2009). Recognizing these modality-specific effects is essential for developing more targeted and effective exercise interventions aimed at optimizing mental health outcomes across diverse populations.

The relationship between physical exercise and psychological well-being has been examined for decades across psychology, sports science, and public health. A large body of research consistently demonstrates that regular exercise can enhance mood, reduce symptoms of depression and anxiety, and improve cognitive functioning, including attention, memory, and executive function (Cooney et al., 2013; Schuch et al., 2016a). However, much of the early literature predominantly focused on aerobic activities such as running, cycling, and swimming, often treating exercise as a single, undifferentiated construct rather than investigating the distinct effects of various exercise modalities. This emphasis on aerobic exercise has, until recently, overshadowed growing evidence that resistance training may confer unique psychological benefits, including increased self-efficacy, improved body image, and enhanced resilience to stress (Craft & Perna, 2004; Ströhle, 2009). More recent studies and meta-analyses further suggest that resistance-based exercise is associated with reductions in depressive symptoms and anxiety, highlighting its potential as a complementary or alternative form of psychological intervention (Gordon et al., 2018; Kelley & Kelley, 2017a).

At the same time, theoretical developments in the field now emphasize that the psychological impact of exercise cannot be fully understood without considering underlying biological, psychological, and social mechanisms. Neurobiological processes, such as regulation of neurotransmitters, increased neurotrophic factors, cardiovascular adaptations, and modulation of the hypothalamic–pituitary–adrenal (HPA) axis, help explain acute and long-term improvements in affective stability and stress regulation (Biddle et al., 2019). Psychological frameworks highlight motivational processes, mastery experiences, perceived competence, and enhanced self-concept, while social mechanisms emphasize the role of social support, structured environments, and interpersonal interaction in shaping both adherence and psychological outcomes (White et al., 2024). Recognizing these modality-specific and theoretically grounded pathways is therefore essential for designing more targeted, evidence-based exercise interventions capable of optimizing mental health outcomes across diverse populations and contexts.

Theoretical Mechanisms

The psychological mechanisms underlying the mental health benefits of exercise appear to differ notably between resistance training (RT) and aerobic exercise (AE). Aerobic activities, such as running, cycling, and swimming, are closely associated with the endorphin hypothesis, which suggests that exercise-induced increases in endogenous opioids produce feelings of euphoria and reduce anxiety (Biddle et al., 2019; Wegner et al., 2014). Additionally, AE improves cardiovascular fitness, enhances metabolic function, and supports short-term stress reduction through psychophysiological pathways. In contrast, resistance training—often involving weightlifting or bodyweight exercises—promotes psychological well-being through distinct mechanisms, including improvements in self-efficacy, mastery experiences, body image, and resilience to stress, reflecting gradual adaptations over repeated sessions (Gordon et al., 2017; Kelley & Kelley, 2017a). These divergent mechanisms underscore the necessity of distinguishing exercise modalities in both research and practice, as modality-specific prescriptions may optimize emotional regulation, mood enhancement, and overall psychological health for diverse populations.

Current Empirical Evidence

Evidence from numerous randomized controlled trials and meta-analyses consistently demonstrates that both RT and AE contribute to improved mental health outcomes, though their effects manifest through somewhat different pathways. AE, including activities such as running, swimming, and cycling, is reliably linked to immediate improvements in mood, reductions in anxiety, and short-term stress relief, likely mediated by endorphin release, cardiovascular efficiency, and distraction from negative cognitions (Chekroud et al., 2018). RT, in contrast, has shown moderate but robust antidepressant effects, enhancing self-efficacy, mastery, and resilience, with benefits observed across diverse populations including older adults, young adults, and clinical groups (Gordon et al., 2018). These findings indicate that while both RT and AE share overlapping psychological benefits—such as reductions in depressive symptoms and stress—they also produce distinct outcomes through different mechanisms. Understanding these modality-specific effects is critical for designing tailored exercise interventions to optimize mental health and well-being.

The psychological mechanisms underlying the mental health benefits of exercise appear to differ notably between RT and AE. Aerobic activities, such as running, cycling, and swimming, are closely associated with the endorphin hypothesis, which suggests that exercise-induced increases in endogenous opioids produce feelings of euphoria, reduce anxiety, and enhance overall affective states (Biddle et al., 2019; Wegner et al., 2014). In addition to the endorphin pathway, AE contributes to cardiovascular efficiency, improved oxygen delivery to the brain, and regulation of the HPA axis, thereby supporting emotional stability, cognitive clarity, and short-term stress reduction through psychophysiological processes. AE has also been linked to improvements in sleep quality and reductions in rumination, further contributing to emotional regulation and psychological resilience (Schuch et al., 2016b).

In contrast, RT—typically involving weightlifting or structured bodyweight exercises—promotes psychological well-being through distinct and often more gradual mechanisms. RT has been shown to enhance perceived competence, mastery, and self-efficacy, as individuals experience progressive improvements in strength and physical capability over time (Gordon et al., 2017). These mastery experiences contribute positively to self-concept and body image, while also strengthening one's perceived ability to cope with stress and adversity (Kelley & Kelley, 2017a). Furthermore, RT is increasingly recognized for its potential to reduce depressive symptoms and anxiety, not only through physiological mechanisms, but also via meaningful psychological changes such as empowerment, self-regulation, and increased perceived control over one's body and health (White et al., 2024).

Taken together, these divergent but complementary mechanisms underscore the necessity of distinguishing exercise modalities in both research and clinical practice. Modality-specific prescriptions may allow practitioners to better target particular psychological outcomes, thereby optimizing emotional regulation, mood enhancement, and overall psychological health across diverse populations and contexts.

Methodological Challenges

Despite the growing evidence supporting the psychological benefits of exercise, research in this area faces several notable methodological limitations. A major challenge lies in the heterogeneity of exercise interventions, including variations in modality, intensity, duration, and frequency, which complicates direct comparisons between studies and limits the generalizability of findings (Schuch et al., 2016b). Many studies rely heavily on self-reported measures of mood, anxiety, and depressive symptoms, which are susceptible to recall bias, social desirability effects, and individual differences in emotional awareness. Relatively few investigations incorporate objective neurobiological or psychophysiological assessments, such as hormonal measures, brain imaging, or cardiovascular monitoring, restricting understanding of the underlying mechanisms. Additionally, the predominance of aerobic exercise research has left gaps regarding resistance training's unique psychological effects. Future research should prioritize rigorous, longitudinal study designs, integrate multiple assessment methods, and account for moderating factors such as age, gender, health status, and cultural context to provide a more nuanced understanding of modality-specific psychological outcomes.

Another important issue relates to the populations most frequently studied. Much of the existing literature is concentrated on relatively healthy, motivated, and often younger participants, which limits insights into how exercise may influence individuals with chronic illness, older adults, or those experiencing severe psychological distress. Cultural differences in attitudes toward exercise and mental health are also rarely examined, even though social expectations, access to facilities, and lifestyle norms may significantly shape both participation in exercise and its psychological impact. Furthermore, adherence remains a practical yet often underexplored factor; many studies do not sufficiently consider how long people realistically maintain exercise routines outside controlled research environments. Addressing these gaps will require collaborative, interdisciplinary research that combines psychological, physiological, social, and cultural perspectives to more fully capture the complex relationship between exercise and mental well-being.

Significance and Objectives

The significance of this chapter lies in clarifying the comparative psychological effects of resistance versus aerobic exercise. By synthesizing findings across disciplines—including psychology, neuroscience, physiology, and sports medicine—it aims to provide a more refined framework for understanding modality-specific outcomes. This framework carries three major implications:

- **Academic Contribution**: Integration of fragmented evidence into a coherent comparative perspective.
- **Clinical Relevance**: Guidance for tailoring exercise interventions in mental health treatment.
- **Public Health Utility**: Evidence-based recommendations for diverse populations.

Accordingly, the objectives of this chapter are:

1. To review psychological mechanisms underlying RT and AE.
2. To compare and contrast their psychological outcomes.
3. To identify moderating factors influencing these effects.
4. To discuss practical applications in clinical and community settings.
5. To propose an integrative model of exercise-emotion interaction.

THEORETICAL FRAMEWORKS

Understanding the comparative psychological effects of RT and AE requires a solid grounding in theoretical perspectives that explain why and how these modalities differentially influence outcomes such as mood, anxiety, self-esteem, and stress regulation. Biological mechanisms, including endorphin release, cardiovascular adaptations, neurotrophic factors, and regulation of the HPA axis, help account for acute improvements in affect and stress resilience, particularly in AE (White et al., 2024; Biddle et al., 2019). Psychological frameworks, such as cognitive-behavioral models, emphasize mastery experiences, self-efficacy, and gradual improvements in self-concept that are often associated with RT (White et al., 2024). Social and environmental factors further shape these outcomes, highlighting the importance of group versus individual settings, professional supervision, and peer support in determining both adherence and psychological benefit (White et al., 2024). By integrating these biological, psychological, and social dimensions, theoretical frameworks provide a multifactorial lens for understanding the complex interactions between exercise and emotional well-being. Such an approach enables researchers and practitioners to interpret differential outcomes more accurately and design interventions tailored to specific mental health objectives (White et al., 2024; Biddle et al., 2019).

Beyond these foundational explanations, theoretical discussions increasingly acknowledge that the benefits of RT and AE may also vary across different life stages and psychological conditions. For instance, AE may be particularly effective in populations experiencing heightened stress or anxiety due to its more immediate mood-enhancing and anxiolytic effects, while RT may be especially beneficial for individuals struggling with low self-esteem or body image concerns because of its association with perceived competence, physical capability, and personal agency. These distinctions underscore the need to align exercise prescriptions with specific psychological needs rather than assuming a universal response to any type of physical activity.

In addition, the interplay between motivation, behavioral adherence, and psychological reward is central to understanding why individuals may respond differently to RT and AE. From a self-determination perspective, individuals are more likely to sustain exercise when they experience autonomy, competence, and social connection, all of which may manifest differently depending on the modality. Group-based AE may enhance social connectedness and enjoyment, while structured RT programs often foster a sense of progression and accomplishment over time. These motivational pathways contribute to the sustainability of psychological benefits and help explain variability in long-term outcomes.

Finally, cultural, contextual, and practical considerations are increasingly recognized within theoretical discussions. Access to exercise environments, cultural attitudes toward strength versus endurance activities, gender norms, and perceived barriers all influence both participation and psychological impact. Therefore, theoretical frameworks not only help clarify mechanisms but also support more sensitive, context-aware interpretations of how RT and AE contribute to emotional well-being across diverse populations.

Psychophysiological Models

Psychophysiological perspectives provide important insights into how biological responses during exercise can influence psychological states, offering a mechanistic understanding of the mental health benefits associated with different exercise modalities. For AE, the endorphin hypothesis has long served as a dominant explanatory model. According to this perspective, cardiovascular activities such as running, cycling, or swimming stimulate the production of endogenous opioids, commonly known as endorphins, which bind to receptors in the brain to produce feelings of euphoria and reduce symptoms of anxiety (Wegner et al., 2014). Complementing this mechanism, the thermogenic hypothesis posits that the rise in core body temperature during prolonged aerobic activity leads to muscle relaxation and a decrease in physiological tension, which in turn contributes to improved mood and emotional well-being (Biddle et al., 2019).

In contrast, RT elicits a distinct set of psychophysiological responses. RT is associated with increases in anabolic hormones such as growth hormone and testosterone, which may indirectly enhance psychological functioning by boosting energy, supporting muscular recovery, and providing a buffering effect against stress (Gordon et al., 2017). Unlike aerobic exercise, where immediate post-exercise mood enhancement is often observed, the psychological benefits of RT tend to emerge gradually as individuals adapt physiologically to repeated training sessions. This gradual adaptation underscores the importance of considering both the temporal dynamics and the modality-specific biological mechanisms when evaluating the mental health outcomes of different forms of exercise. Together, these models highlight that AE and RT operate through complementary yet distinct pathways, each contributing uniquely to psychological well-being.

Cognitive-Behavioral Perspectives

Cognitive-behavioral theories provide a framework for understanding how exercise influences psychological well-being through changes in self-perception, coping strategies, and experiences of mastery. These theories highlight that the mental health benefits of exercise are not solely a result of physiological changes but also arise from the ways individuals interpret and respond to their physical activity. RT, in particular, aligns closely with self-efficacy theory, which posits that successfully overcoming physical challenges enhances an individual's confidence in managing broader life stressors (Kelley & Kelley, 2017b). For instance, progressively lifting heavier weights, mastering complex movements, or achieving personalized strength goals reinforces a sense of competence and control. Over time, these mastery experiences contribute to improved self-esteem, greater resilience to stress, and a reduction in vulnerability to depressive symptoms.

In contrast, AE often produces psychological benefits through the distraction hypothesis (Craft & Perna, 2004). Continuous, rhythmic activities such as running, cycling, or swimming occupy attentional resources, effectively redirecting focus away from negative thoughts, ruminative patterns, or maladaptive cognitive loops. This attentional shift contributes to immediate mood enhancement, decreased anxiety, and short-term stress relief. Collectively, these cognitive-behavioral perspectives indicate that RT and AE engage different psychological pathways: RT emphasizes mastery, competence, and self-regulation, whereas AE primarily provides distraction and cognitive diversion. Understanding these distinct yet complementary mechanisms is crucial for designing exercise interventions tailored to specific mental health objectives, population needs, and individual preferences, maximizing the psychological benefits of both modalities.

Social and Environmental Contexts

The social interaction hypothesis emphasizes that the psychological benefits of exercise are partly mediated by interpersonal experiences. Aerobic modalities, in particular, often occur in group formats, such as running clubs, spin classes, or community cycling events, which provide structured opportunities for social bonding, peer encouragement, and the achievement of shared goals (Chekroud et al., 2018). These social interactions contribute to enhancing intrinsic motivation, reinforcing the emotional benefits of AE, and providing participants with a sense of accountability that can support adherence over time. Moreover, the presence of others during exercise can facilitate observational learning, where individuals model behaviors, techniques, or strategies demonstrated by peers, further promoting skill development and self-efficacy.

RT, although sometimes pursued individually, also creates unique social contexts, particularly in gym settings or structured training programs. Engaging with peers, exchanging training tips, observing others' progress, or receiving validation from trainers or fellow participants can boost self-esteem, foster a sense of belonging, and create a supportive environment conducive to psychological well-being (Gordon et al., 2018). Importantly, the social environment can serve as a moderator of psychological outcomes: supportive, encouraging, and inclusive atmospheres amplify positive effects, whereas competitive, judgmental, or isolating contexts may diminish these benefits. Therefore, both AE and RT demonstrate that the social dimension of exercise is not merely a peripheral factor but an integral component that substantially shapes its emotional and psychological impact. This perspective underscores the importance of considering social factors in exercise program design to maximize mental health benefits.

Beyond immediate psychological outcomes, the social context of exercise also contributes to longer-term emotional resilience and identity formation. Participation in socially engaging exercise activities can strengthen individuals' sense of social identity, allowing them to perceive themselves as members of a valued community. This sense of belonging has been repeatedly associated with greater emotional stability, lower psychological distress, and enhanced life satisfaction. In addition, social support received within exercise contexts may buffer against daily stressors, encourage continued participation during challenging periods, and reinforce positive lifestyle behaviors.

Finally, considering the social interaction hypothesis highlights the need for more intentional integration of supportive social structures in both RT and AE interventions. Program designers, clinicians, and health practitioners should not only prescribe exercise based on physiological effectiveness but also ensure that environments are welcoming, inclusive, and psychologically supportive. Incorporating structured group formats, mentoring systems, or community-based initiatives can help maximize adherence and broaden the psychological benefits derived from exercise participation.

Integrative Approaches

Given that both aerobic and resistance training modalities offer overlapping as well as unique benefits, integrative models of exercise provide a more comprehensive understanding of their psychological effects. Biopsychosocial frameworks emphasize the interaction of biological, psychological, and social mechanisms in shaping exercise outcomes. For example, aerobic exercise often produces immediate reductions in anxiety and stress through physiological pathways such as endorphin release, improved cardiovascular efficiency, and autonomic regulation. In contrast, resistance training contributes to longer-term improvements in psychological well-being, including enhanced self-concept, self-esteem, and self-efficacy, primarily through mastery experiences and skill development (Ströhle, 2009; Schuch et al., 2016a). Additionally, both modalities offer social and interpersonal benefits: aerobic activities in group formats (e.g., running clubs or spin classes) and resistance training in gym or structured settings provide opportunities for social bonding, peer encouragement, and observational learning, all of which further support motivation and emotional health (Chekroud et al., 2018; Gordon et al., 2018).

When aerobic and resistance training are combined in concurrent programs, their effects may act synergistically to enhance mental health outcomes. Aerobic sessions can provide acute relief from stress and anxiety, while resistance training fosters resilience, self-confidence, and a sense of accomplishment over time. This integrated approach also accommodates diverse motivational preferences and social contexts, increasing adherence and long-term engagement. Therefore, exercise prescriptions for psychological well-being should not privilege one modality over the other; instead, they should leverage the complementary functions of both, addressing immediate physiological benefits, sustained psychological gains, and social reinforcement. Overall, a biopsychosocially informed, multimodal exercise strategy provides the most effective framework for optimizing mental health and overall psychological resilience.

In addition, recognizing individual variability is essential when applying multimodal exercise frameworks. Age, gender, health status, baseline fitness, and psychological disposition may influence how individuals respond to aerobic and resistance-based activities. For instance, older adults may benefit more from the self-efficacy and functional independence associated with resistance training, while younger or more active populations may experience greater immediate psychological benefits from aerobic modalities. Tailoring integrative exercise programs to these individual characteristics ensures that psychological gains are maximized across diverse populations.

Finally, implementing biopsychosocially informed exercise strategies requires intentional program design and supportive environments. Access to safe facilities, professional guidance, culturally sensitive approaches, and sustained behavioral support are critical to enabling participation and adherence. Future research should continue to explore how combined AE and RT interventions can be optimized in real-world settings, including clinical populations, community-based programs, and preventive public health strategies, to fully realize their psychological potential.

Methodological Implications

Theoretical frameworks play a crucial role in guiding how researchers design, implement, and interpret exercise psychology studies. Psychophysiological models, for instance, predict immediate and measurable changes in mood and affect following a single bout of exercise, highlighting the importance of carefully timing assessments to capture acute outcomes. In contrast, cognitive-behavioral theories emphasize gradual and sustained changes in self-concept, self-efficacy, and broader psychological functioning, which necessitate longitudinal study designs that track participants over weeks or months. Social interaction models further underscore the significance of contextual factors, advocating for the assessment of not only exercise type, frequency, and intensity but also the social and environmental setting in which exercise occurs, such as group versus individual sessions, peer support, and feedback from instructors (Cooney et al., 2013). By integrating these theoretical perspectives, researchers can better interpret observed psychological outcomes and disentangle the mechanisms underlying exercise-related benefits.

These methodological considerations highlight the critical importance of careful operationalization when comparing RT and AE. Studies that fail to consider the guiding theoretical framework risk overlooking modality-specific effects, misinterpreting results, or conflating short-term physiological changes with longer-term psychological adaptations. For example, a study focusing exclusively on acute mood improvements may underestimate the contribution of RT to sustained self-efficacy, whereas neglecting social context may obscure how group-based AE enhances motivation and adherence. Therefore, rigorous research design grounded in psychophysiological, cognitive-behavioral, and social interaction models ensures a more accurate and nuanced understanding of how different exercise modalities influence psychological well-being. Overall, theory-driven methodologies provide the foundation for robust, interpretable, and meaningful findings in exercise psychology research.

Conclusion of Literature Review

The reviewed literature demonstrates that both RT and AE contribute meaningfully to psychological well-being, yet through distinct pathways. Psychophysiological models emphasize the immediate effects of AE via endorphin release and thermogenic responses, whereas RT's benefits emerge more gradually through neuroendocrine adaptation. Cognitive-behavioral theories reveal how mastery and self-efficacy underpin RT's influence on self-esteem and resilience, while AE primarily operates through attentional diversion and distraction from negative thoughts. Social interaction perspectives further highlight the role of group contexts and environmental support in amplifying the psychological impact of both modalities.

An integrative biopsychosocial framework suggests that the most comprehensive mental health benefits arise when AE and RT are combined, offering both acute mood enhancement and long-term psychological resilience. At the same time, methodological implications caution against overly generalized claims, underscoring the importance of considering exercise modality, context, and measurement timing.

In summary, while both RT and AE yield overlapping improvements in mood, depression, anxiety, and self-concept, their differential mechanisms and outcomes reinforce the value of tailoring exercise prescriptions. A nuanced, integrative approach is therefore necessary for optimizing exercise-based interventions to promote psychological health across diverse populations.

Empirical Evidence: Comparative Studies

Taken together, the existing literature highlights both the promise and the inherent complexity of understanding the psychological effects of RT and AE. Theoretical perspectives and empirical findings converge to show that these modalities influence mental health through complementary yet distinct mechanisms. Aerobic exercise often provides immediate improvements in mood and reductions in stress through physiological pathways such as endorphin release and cardiovascular efficiency, whereas resistance training supports longer-term gains in self-concept, mastery, and self-efficacy. Social and environmental contexts further shape these outcomes, as group-based or socially supportive settings enhance motivation, adherence, and overall psychological benefits. These insights emphasize the multifaceted nature of exercise-related mental health effects, where biological, psychological, and social factors interact to produce meaningful outcomes.

At the same time, the literature indicates that individual characteristics significantly moderate these psychological effects. Age, gender, baseline fitness, psychological disposition, and previous exercise experience can influence how people respond to aerobic and resistance-based activities. For example, younger individuals or those accustomed to high-intensity activity may experience greater emotional uplift from aerobic exercise, whereas older adults or clinical populations may benefit more from the gradual mastery and functional independence associated with resistance training. Cultural and contextual variables also play a role, as societal attitudes toward exercise, body image, and health behavior can shape motivation and engagement. These considerations reinforce the importance of adopting a personalized rather than a one-size-fits-all perspective when examining exercise and mental health.

Despite this promise, the clarity and generalizability of findings are frequently limited by methodological constraints. Variations in study design, assessment timing, measurement tools, exercise intensity and duration, and contextual factors—such as individual versus group settings—can blur distinctions between modalities and obscure modality-specific effects. Such limitations complicate the interpretation and practical application of research, underscoring the importance of theory-driven, rigorously designed studies that account for these factors. Moreover, many studies rely primarily on short-term interventions and self-reported outcomes, restricting deeper insight into long-term trajectories and neurobiological processes underlying psychological change.

Recognizing these challenges is essential for refining knowledge, guiding effective exercise prescriptions, and ensuring interventions are evidence-based and tailored to individual needs. Future work should therefore prioritize longitudinal approaches, multimodal assessment strategies, and clearer differentiation between RT and AE conditions. By addressing these gaps, research can move toward a more nuanced and contextualized understanding of how different forms of exercise shape mental health. The next section addresses these methodological considerations in detail, highlighting key limitations of existing studies and proposing directions for advancing the comparative study of RT and AE in relation to psychological well-being.

METHODOLOGICAL CHALLENGES AND LIMITATIONS

Although substantial progress has been made in examining the psychological effects of RT and aerobic exercise (AE), a number of methodological challenges continue to complicate the interpretation and comparison of findings across studies. Variations in exercise protocols, including differences in frequency, intensity, duration, and supervision, create heterogeneity that makes it difficult to attribute outcomes specifically to modality.

Many studies rely heavily on self-report psychological and behavioral measures, which remain vulnerable to social desirability and recall bias, while objective biological or device-based assessments—although more accurate—are often costly, invasive, or impractical for large-scale implementation (Prince et al., 2008; Troiano et al., 2014; Ekkekakis, 2013). Sampling biases also persist, with much of the existing literature disproportionately focused on young, healthy adults, resulting in limited representation of older individuals, clinical populations, and culturally diverse groups, thereby constraining the broader applicability of findings (Rhodes & Dickau, 2013; Netz et al., 2005; Stubbs et al., 2017). Furthermore, a substantial proportion of research evaluates outcomes primarily at the end of intervention periods, providing only a snapshot of immediate responses while offering limited understanding of whether psychological benefits are sustained over longer timeframes (Craft & Perna, 2004; Herring et al., 2010; Gordon et al., 2018). Added to this, considerable variability in study designs, including differences in exercise modality, intensity, duration, contextual setting, and outcome timing, often complicates direct comparisons and obscures modality-specific psychological effects, particularly when contrasting resistance training and aerobic exercise outcomes (Reed & Buck, 2009; Ensari et al., 2015). Taken together, these limitations underscore the importance of critical methodological evaluation when interpreting existing research and designing future investigations, ensuring that findings can be meaningfully translated into clinical practice and public health strategies.

Beyond these methodological constraints, there is also a lack of uniformity in how psychological constructs are defined and operationalized across studies. Concepts such as mood, well-being, anxiety, and quality of life are frequently measured using different scales or conceptual frameworks, which complicates cross-study synthesis and meta-analytic integration. In some cases, psychological constructs are treated as broad, undifferentiated outcomes rather than multidimensional phenomena, limiting the specificity with which RT and AE effects can be understood. Greater conceptual clarity and consistency in measurement approaches are therefore crucial for advancing comparative interpretations of these modalities.

Another important issue concerns the limited application of longitudinal and life-course perspectives. While many studies examine short-term interventions, fewer investigations explore how psychological responses to RT and AE evolve over months or years, or how they may interact with developmental stages, changing health conditions, or shifting life demands. Longitudinal research is also essential to understanding potential cumulative effects, dose–response relationships, and whether repeated engagement in RT or AE leads to adaptive psychological resilience over time. Without such evidence, it remains difficult to determine whether observed benefits represent transient states or enduring psychological changes.

Finally, contextual and individual difference factors warrant greater attention. Variables such as motivation, personality traits, previous exercise experience, social support, and cultural attitudes toward exercise may moderate the psychological impact of RT and AE, yet these are often insufficiently controlled or theoretically integrated. Incorporating mixed-methods designs, combining quantitative outcomes with qualitative insights, may also help capture subjective meaning, experiential dimensions, and personal narratives that are not always visible through standardized measures alone. Addressing these issues will not only strengthen methodological rigor but also enhance ecological validity, ensuring that research findings more accurately reflect real-world exercise behavior and its psychological consequences.

Measurement Issues

A major challenge in exercise psychology research lies in the heavy reliance on self-report questionnaires to assess constructs such as mood, anxiety, or depression. Instruments like the Beck Depression Inventory (BDI) or the State-Trait Anxiety Inventory (STAI) are widely used because they are relatively easy to administer and provide valuable insights into participants' psychological states. However, these measures are inherently vulnerable to social desirability bias, where respondents may underreport negative feelings or overreport positive experiences, and to recall limitations, as participants may inaccurately remember or interpret their past emotional experiences (Craft & Perna, 2004).

On the other hand, neurobiological measures, such as cortisol levels or endorphin markers, offer more objective data that can corroborate psychological assessments, providing insight into the physiological mechanisms underlying mood changes. Yet, these approaches are often costly, invasive, and logistically challenging, particularly in large-scale or community-based studies. This tension between subjective self-reports and objective biological measures ultimately limits the precision and interpretability of conclusions, highlighting the need for multimodal assessment strategies.

In addition to measurement concerns, the timing of psychological assessment introduces another important methodological limitation. Many studies examine outcomes immediately following an exercise intervention, capturing only short-term affective responses while neglecting the durability of psychological benefits. Without follow-up assessments over weeks or months, it remains unclear whether improvements in mood, anxiety, or self-esteem represent transient emotional shifts or sustained psychological adaptation. Longitudinal designs are therefore essential for determining the persistence, fluctuation, or possible attenuation of exercise-induced mental health gains over time (Herring et al., 2010; Gordon et al., 2018).

A further challenge relates to population characteristics, as a substantial proportion of exercise psychology research continues to focus predominantly on young, healthy, and physically active individuals. Such sampling biases limit the generalizability of findings to more diverse groups, including older adults, individuals with chronic illness, clinical populations experiencing psychological disorders, and culturally varied communities. These populations may experience different psychological responses, adherence barriers, or motivational dynamics, meaning that conclusions drawn from narrow samples may not accurately reflect broader real-world contexts (Rhodes & Dickau, 2013; Netz et al., 2005).

Finally, contextual and environmental variables also shape the psychological impact of exercise but are often insufficiently controlled or reported. Factors such as whether exercise occurs individually or in groups, in supervised or unsupervised environments, or within supportive versus competitive climates can significantly influence emotional outcomes, perceived enjoyment, and long-term engagement. Integrating these contextual dimensions into research design and analysis is therefore critical for producing more nuanced, ecologically valid, and practically applicable understanding of how exercise contributes to psychological well-being.

Variability in Study Design

Heterogeneity across study protocols represents another significant limitation in exercise psychology research. Exercise interventions differ widely in frequency, intensity, duration, and overall structure, which complicates direct comparisons across studies and challenges the synthesis of consistent conclusions (Biddle et al., 2019). For instance, some studies examine short-term interventions lasting only a few weeks, capturing immediate or acute psychological effects, whereas others investigate long-term programs extending over several months or even years, assessing sustained changes in mood, self-concept, or anxiety.

Differences in the type of exercise—whether aerobic, resistance, or combined modalities—further contribute to variability, as do variations in supervision, social context, and participant adherence. This wide heterogeneity often obscures modality-specific effects, making it difficult to determine which aspects of an intervention are responsible for observed outcomes. Consequently, critical questions remain regarding dose-response relationships, optimal exercise prescriptions, and the long-term sustainability of psychological benefits, highlighting the need for more standardized, rigorously controlled research designs.

Heterogeneity across study protocols represents another significant limitation in exercise psychology research. Exercise interventions differ widely in frequency, intensity, duration, and overall structure, which complicates direct comparisons across studies and challenges the synthesis of consistent conclusions (Biddle et al., 2019). For instance, some studies examine short-term interventions lasting only a few weeks, capturing immediate or acute psychological effects, whereas others investigate long-term programs extending over several months or even years, assessing sustained changes in mood, self-concept, or anxiety.

Differences in the type of exercise—whether aerobic, resistance, or combined modalities—further contribute to variability, as do variations in supervision, social context, and participant adherence. This wide heterogeneity often obscures modality-specific effects, making it difficult to determine which aspects of an intervention are responsible for observed outcomes. Consequently, critical questions remain regarding dose-response relationships, optimal exercise prescriptions, and the long-term sustainability of psychological benefits, highlighting the need for more standardized, rigorously controlled research designs.

Moreover, inconsistencies in methodological rigor and reporting practices add further complexity to interpreting findings. Some studies provide detailed descriptions of training protocols and participant characteristics, while others lack sufficient transparency, limiting replicability and meaningful comparison. Additionally, variations in outcome measures—ranging from subjective self-report questionnaires to objective physiological indicators—introduce another layer of inconsistency that may influence how psychological benefits are identified and interpreted. Addressing these methodological disparities through standardized protocols, clearer reporting guidelines, and harmonized assessment tools will be essential for advancing understanding of how different exercise modalities uniquely and reliably contribute to psychological well-being.

Contextual and Environmental Confounders

Psychological outcomes of exercise are highly sensitive to a variety of contextual factors, which can significantly influence the magnitude and nature of observed benefits. Key variables include whether the activity is performed individually or in group settings, in natural versus artificial environments, or with versus without professional supervision or structured guidance (Chekroud et al., 2018). For example, group-based exercise can enhance motivation, social bonding, and adherence, while exercising alone may provide greater autonomy and self-reflection opportunities.

Similarly, engaging in outdoor or natural settings may amplify mood and stress-reduction benefits compared to indoor environments. These environmental and social variables often act as confounding factors, either amplifying or diminishing the psychological effects associated with AE and RT. Failure to account for such influences risks misattributing observed outcomes solely to the exercise modality, potentially leading to inaccurate conclusions regarding the effectiveness of specific interventions. Carefully considering these contextual factors is therefore essential for the design, interpretation, and generalizability of exercise psychology research.

In addition, cultural norms, socioeconomic status, and accessibility to exercise facilities represent broader contextual determinants that may shape individuals' psychological responses to exercise. In many settings, access to safe environments, quality equipment, or structured programs is uneven, which may influence both participation patterns and experienced benefits. Psychological perceptions of exercise—such as whether it is viewed as enjoyable, burdensome, or socially valued—also vary across populations and can moderate emotional outcomes.

Taken together, these contextual considerations highlight the need for research approaches that move beyond purely physiological explanations and adopt a more ecological perspective. By systematically acknowledging and integrating environmental, cultural, and social influences, future studies can produce more nuanced, realistic, and applicable insights into how aerobic and resistance training contribute to psychological health across diverse populations.

Population Diversity and Generalizability

A major limitation in much of the exercise psychology literature is the disproportionate sampling of young, healthy adults, which restricts the generalizability of findings to broader populations, including clinical groups, older adults, or marginalized communities (Cooney et al., 2013). Many studies fail to capture how chronic health conditions, age-related physiological changes, or socioeconomic barriers might influence both the uptake of exercise and its psychological benefits. Cultural context further shapes outcomes, as societal norms and attitudes toward physical activity, body image, gender roles, and social participation vary widely across regions and populations (Ströhle, 2009). For instance, social support mechanisms, perceptions of exercise, and access to safe environments for physical activity can differ substantially between urban and rural settings, or between collectivist and individualist cultures.

Without broader and more inclusive demographic representation, research findings risk being overly narrow, limiting their applicability to diverse populations and undermining their relevance for global public health recommendations. Addressing these sampling biases is therefore critical for developing equitable and effective exercise interventions.

Comparative Design Limitations

Direct comparisons between RT and AE remain relatively uncommon, as the majority of studies investigate only a single modality in isolation. This approach limits the ability to discern how the psychological effects of one modality differ from the other. Even in studies that attempt comparative designs, discrepancies in exercise volume, intensity, or duration often introduce potential bias into the results (Gordon et al., 2018). For instance, aerobic interventions generally involve higher energy expenditure than typical RT sessions, which may confound observed psychological outcomes, such as improvements in mood, stress reduction, or self-efficacy.

Additional factors, including differences in supervision, social context, or participant engagement, further complicate direct comparisons. Without carefully controlled trials that standardize these variables across modalities, it remains difficult to attribute differences in mental health benefits specifically to the type of exercise. Consequently, the evidence base for making precise, modality-specific recommendations for psychological well-being is limited, underscoring the need for rigorous, head-to-head research.

Longitudinal and Sustainability Issues

A common limitation in exercise psychology research is the predominant focus on outcomes measured immediately following an intervention, which provides limited information about the long-term sustainability of psychological benefits. Many studies assess mood, anxiety, or self-concept only at the conclusion of a short-term program, capturing acute effects but failing to determine whether these improvements endure over weeks, months, or years. Evidence suggests that RT may produce more gradual, cumulative improvements in self-concept, mastery, and psychological resilience, whereas AEoften delivers immediate mood enhancement and stress reduction (Wegner et al., 2014; Schuch et al., 2016a).

However, the absence of longitudinal follow-up in most studies leaves the persistence and trajectory of these benefits largely uncertain. Understanding whether acute improvements translate into sustained psychological gains is critical for designing exercise interventions that are both effective and clinically meaningful. Long-term assessments are therefore necessary to clarify how different modalities contribute to enduring mental health outcomes and to guide evidence-based exercise prescriptions.

Summary

In sum, a range of methodological challenges—including limitations in measurement, heterogeneity in study designs, contextual confounders, sampling biases, and a lack of long-term follow-up data—significantly restrict the strength and generalizability of conclusions regarding the comparative psychological effects of RT and AE Measurement limitations, such as reliance on self-report scales or inconsistently applied physiological markers, can obscure the precise magnitude of effects. Variability in exercise frequency, intensity, duration, and supervision further complicates cross-study comparisons, while environmental and social factors—such as individual versus group exercise settings—may confound observed outcomes.

Moreover, the disproportionate focus on young, healthy adults limits applicability to clinical populations, older adults, and culturally diverse groups. Addressing these issues requires more rigorous, standardized, and ecologically valid research designs that integrate both subjective and objective measures and incorporate longitudinal follow-up. Such improvements will enable researchers and practitioners to more accurately identify the unique and overlapping psychological benefits of RT and AE, ultimately informing tailored and effective exercise prescriptions for enhancing mental health and overall well-being.

FINDINGS AND DISCUSSION

The comparative psychological effects of RT and AEhave been the focus of extensive research across diverse populations, providing insights into both overlapping and distinct mental health benefits. Both modalities are associated with improvements in mood, reductions in anxiety and stress, and enhanced self-esteem and self-efficacy; however, the underlying mechanisms through which these benefits occur differ in important ways. Aerobic exercise often produces immediate, acute improvements in affect and stress regulation via physiological pathways, such as endorphin release, cardiovascular efficiency, and autonomic regulation. In contrast, resistance training tends to facilitate more gradual, long-term improvements in self-concept, mastery, and psychological resilience through cognitive-behavioral mechanisms and mastery experiences.

Contextual moderators—including social environment, exercise setting, supervision, and cultural factors—further shape these outcomes, highlighting the multifactorial nature of exercise–emotion interactions. This section synthesizes empirical evidence on RT and AE, emphasizing implications for theoretical frameworks, practical exercise prescriptions, and public health policy aimed at promoting psychological well-being across populations.

Beyond these comparative effects, an important consideration concerns individual differences that influence how people psychologically respond to each modality. Factors such as baseline mental health status, age, gender, personal preferences, prior exercise experience, and motivational orientation can meaningfully shape whether individuals experience greater psychological benefit from RT or AE. Moreover, adherence and long-term engagement often depend on perceived enjoyment, accessibility, and perceived competence, which may differ between modalities. Recognizing these person-specific influences reinforces the need for personalized, context-sensitive exercise recommendations rather than one-size-fits-all prescriptions.

Finally, synthesizing evidence from RT and AE research supports a broader perspective that values complementarity rather than competition between modalities. Integrative approaches that combine both forms of exercise may offer cumulative benefits, addressing immediate emotional relief alongside sustained psychological growth and resilience. From a public health standpoint, acknowledging the diverse psychological pathways through which RT and AE operate enables the development of more inclusive, flexible, and effective strategies for promoting mental health through physical activity.

Comparative Psychological Outcomes

Both RT and AEconsistently enhance psychological well-being, though the timing, magnitude, and underlying mechanisms of these effects differ. Aerobic exercise produces rapid improvements in mood and reductions in anxiety immediately following sessions, reflecting psychophysiological mechanisms such as endorphin release, thermogenic effects, and enhanced cardiovascular efficiency (Wegner et al., 2014; Biddle et al., 2019). For example, participants in structured running, cycling, or swimming programs frequently report acute relief from negative affect and stress, suggesting that AE is particularly effective for short-term emotional regulation and immediate mood enhancement. These immediate effects are valuable for individuals seeking rapid stress reduction or temporary relief from anxiety symptoms, highlighting the practical applicability of AE for acute psychological needs.

In contrast, RT generally produces more gradual, cumulative psychological benefits that accrue over repeated sessions. Outcomes such as improvements in self-efficacy, resilience, body image, and perceived competence are frequently reported, reflecting cognitive-behavioral mechanisms linked to mastery, skill acquisition, and achievement (Kelley & Kelley, 2017b; Gordon et al., 2017). While the effects of RT may not be as immediately noticeable as those of AE, they tend to be more enduring, fostering long-term psychological growth and reinforcing self-concept over time. Neuroendocrine adaptations, including increases in growth hormone and testosterone, may further support these sustained improvements by enhancing energy, mood stability, and stress buffering.

Taken together, these findings suggest that AE is particularly well-suited for acute mood regulation, whereas RT is more influential in building lasting psychological resources. Importantly, both modalities offer overlapping benefits, including reductions in depressive symptoms, anxiety, and overall stress levels, demonstrating their complementary nature. Integrating AE and RT within exercise interventions can therefore provide both immediate and long-term mental health benefits, supporting a holistic approach to enhancing psychological well-being across diverse populations and settings.

Mechanistic Pathways in Practice

Empirical evidence underscores the value of theoretical models in explaining the psychological outcomes associated with different exercise modalities. The distraction hypothesis, for instance, provides a compelling explanation for the acute mood improvements often observed following AE According to this model, continuous rhythmic activity—such as running, cycling, or swimming—occupies attentional resources and diverts focus away from negative cognitions or rumination, thereby promoting immediate relief from stress and anxiety (Craft & Perna, 2004). Psychophysiological models complement this perspective by highlighting underlying biological mechanisms, including elevated production of endogenous opioids and increased body temperature, which together induce transient feelings of euphoria, relaxation, and overall well-being (Wegner et al., 2014; Biddle et al., 2019). These mechanisms help explain why AE is particularly effective for short-term mood regulation and stress management.

RT, by contrast, aligns closely with principles of self-efficacy theory. The progressive mastery of challenging exercises reinforces perceptions of competence, personal control, and achievement, which translate into improved self-esteem, reduced vulnerability to depression, and enhanced resilience (Kelley & Kelley, 2017b). Beyond psychological mechanisms, RT also induces neuroendocrine adaptations, including increases in growth hormone and testosterone, which may contribute to heightened energy levels, improved stress buffering, and a greater sense of vitality (Gordon et al., 2017). This combination of cognitive, behavioral, and physiological processes underscores the value of RT for fostering long-term psychological growth.

Taken together, these findings demonstrate that while AE and RT share general mental health benefits, they operate through distinct yet complementary pathways. AE primarily targets immediate psychophysiological responses and acute mood regulation, whereas RT emphasizes mastery, competence, and sustained psychological resilience. Recognizing these modality-specific mechanisms is essential for both research and practical applications, informing tailored exercise prescriptions that optimize mental health outcomes and guide the design of interventions that leverage the complementary strengths of aerobic and resistance training.

Moderating Factors

Psychological responses to exercise are highly contingent on both individual characteristics and contextual factors, which can significantly shape the magnitude and nature of outcomes. Age, gender, baseline mental health status, and cultural background play critical roles in determining how individuals respond to different exercise modalities. For example, younger adults often report greater immediate mood enhancement following aerobic exercise (AE), likely due to heightened physiological responsiveness and social engagement opportunities (Chekroud et al., 2018). In contrast, older adults tend to experience more pronounced improvements in self-efficacy and perceived competence through RT, reflecting the value of mastery experiences and progressive skill development over time. Gender differences have also been documented, with women frequently deriving stronger benefits from group-based aerobic programs in terms of social bonding and stress reduction, whereas men may achieve greater enhancements in self-concept and body image through structured, individually oriented RT in gym settings.

Environmental and social contexts serve as additional moderators of psychological outcomes. Group-based exercise, whether in the form of aerobic classes, running clubs, or resistance training circuits, can enhance intrinsic motivation, promote social support, and improve adherence, all of which amplify mental health benefits (Gordon et al., 2018). Conversely, environments characterized by high competitiveness, judgment, or lack of support may attenuate positive outcomes, highlighting the sensitivity of exercise-induced psychological improvements to setting and interpersonal dynamics. Supervision by instructors or trainers also contributes to outcomes by providing guidance, encouragement, and reinforcement, which are particularly valuable for novice participants.

Exercise parameters such as intensity, duration, and frequency further influence both the magnitude and sustainability of psychological benefits. Higher-intensity sessions may produce more immediate mood improvements, while moderate, consistent training supports longer-term gains in self-esteem and resilience. Similarly, consistent participation over weeks or months is crucial for consolidating improvements in self-concept and reducing chronic stress. Taken together, these findings underscore the importance of individualized and context-sensitive exercise prescriptions, which account for personal characteristics, social environment, and program design to optimize mental health outcomes across diverse populations.

Integrative Patterns

Emerging evidence increasingly supports the integration of RT and AEas a strategy to optimize psychological outcomes. Concurrent training programs that combine both modalities have demonstrated unique benefits, with aerobic exercise providing immediate mood enhancement and stress relief, while resistance training fosters long-term improvements in self-efficacy, resilience, and body image (Schuch et al., 2016b; Ströhle, 2009). These findings highlight the complementary nature of the two exercise forms: AE addresses acute psychophysiological stress responses, whereas RT reinforces cognitive-behavioral pathways, such as mastery experiences and achievement, which contribute to sustained psychological growth. By simultaneously targeting multiple mechanisms, concurrent programs reflect a biopsychosocial perspective that emphasizes the interplay between physiological adaptations, psychological processes, and social contexts in shaping mental health outcomes.

The practical implications of this integrative approach are significant for exercise program design. Rather than prioritizing a single modality, interventions aimed at promoting mental well-being may be more effective if they combine AE and RT in ways that are responsive to individual preferences, capacities, and goals. For instance, sessions may alternate between aerobic-focused and resistance-focused activities, or incorporate both within a single training session. Tailoring programs in this way not only maximizes psychological benefits but also accommodates differences in fitness levels, motivation, and lifestyle constraints, increasing the likelihood of adherence and sustained engagement over time.

Moreover, combining modalities may create synergistic effects that reinforce both immediate and long-term outcomes. Participants can experience the acute mood-enhancing effects of AE alongside the confidence-building and self-concept improvements associated with RT, producing a holistic enhancement of psychological well-being. Social factors, such as exercising in groups or under supervision, may further amplify these benefits by fostering motivation, accountability, and social support. Overall, integrated RT and AE programs offer a versatile and evidence-based framework for promoting mental health, suggesting that future research and practice should emphasize multimodal approaches to optimize both short-term and sustained psychological outcomes.

Implications for Practice and Policy

The findings have multiple implications across domains:

- **Clinical Practice:** Mental health professionals can prescribe AE for patients requiring acute relief from anxiety or stress, while emphasizing RT for longer-term improvements in self-efficacy and resilience. Combining modalities may be particularly beneficial for individuals with depression or chronic stress disorders.
- **Fitness and Wellness Programs:** Personal trainers and fitness coaches can design hybrid programs that balance AE for cardiovascular and mood benefits with RT for mastery and strength gains. Socially supportive group formats can enhance adherence and motivation.
- **Public Health Policy:** Community-based initiatives should promote access to both aerobic and resistance exercise, with attention to age, gender, and cultural context, to maximize population-level psychological well-being. Policies encouraging integrated exercise programs in schools, workplaces, and senior centers could leverage complementary benefits of both modalities.

In sum, a nuanced understanding of RT and AE allows for tailored interventions that optimize psychological outcomes, accounting for individual differences, contextual factors, and modality-specific mechanisms.

CONCLUSION AND RECOMMENDATIONS

Conclusion

This chapter has examined the comparative psychological effects of RT and aerobic exercise (AE), integrating theoretical frameworks, empirical findings, and contextual considerations. Both exercise modalities contribute to mental well-being, but they operate through distinct mechanisms. Aerobic exercise primarily enhances acute mood and reduces anxiety via psychophysiological pathways, including endorphin release, thermogenic responses, and improvements in cardiovascular efficiency (Wegner et al., 2014; Biddle et al., 2019). These mechanisms can produce immediate reductions in tension and stress, making AE particularly effective for short-term mood regulation and anxiety management.

In contrast, resistance training fosters more gradual improvements in self-efficacy, resilience, and self-concept, consistent with cognitive-behavioral theories emphasizing mastery, achievement, and skill acquisition (Kelley & Kelley, 2017b; Gordon et al., 2017). Engagement in RT often involves structured goal-setting, progressive overload, and repeated mastery experiences, which collectively reinforce self-confidence and psychological resilience over time. This long-term benefit complements the immediate mood enhancements seen in AE, highlighting the unique contributions of each modality to overall psychological health.

Psychological outcomes are also moderated by demographic, social, and environmental factors, including age, gender, exercise context, intensity, and supervision. Integrative approaches that combine AE and RT appear especially promising, offering both immediate mood benefits and sustained psychological growth, in line with biopsychosocial models (Schuch et al., 2016b; Ströhle, 2009). Social and environmental variables, such as group participation, professional guidance, and culturally appropriate interventions, further influence adherence and amplify mental health outcomes, underscoring the importance of context-sensitive program design.

Despite these insights, methodological limitations—such as reliance on self-report measures, heterogeneity in exercise protocols, limited comparative studies, and scarce longitudinal data—highlight the need for rigorous research designs and cautious interpretation of results. Nevertheless, the accumulated evidence strongly supports the conclusion that both RT and AE are effective tools for promoting mental health. Leveraging their complementary characteristics through integrative, tailored interventions can optimize psychological benefits and inform practical, evidence-based recommendations for diverse populations

Looking ahead, future research should prioritize longitudinal, multimethod designs that capture both immediate and sustained psychological outcomes while accounting for individual differences and contextual influences. Expanding research to underrepresented populations, including older adults, individuals with clinical conditions, and culturally diverse groups, will enhance the external validity and inclusiveness of current knowledge. Such efforts will not only deepen theoretical understanding but also strengthen the development of precise, scalable, and contextually relevant exercise-based mental health interventions.

RECOMMENDATIONS

For Researchers

1. Conduct longitudinal and randomized controlled trials comparing RT, AE, and combined modalities to clarify long-term psychological outcomes.
2. Employ multi-method assessment strategies, integrating self-report, physiological, and neurobiological measures for greater validity.
3. Explore moderating factors such as age, gender, health status, and cultural context to enhance generalizability.
4. Investigate dose-response relationships to determine optimal frequency, intensity, and duration for mental health benefits.
5. Examine mechanisms of synergy in combined training programs to inform integrative theoretical models.

For Clinicians and Mental Health Professionals

1. Prescribe AE for immediate relief of stress and anxiety, while using RT to build long-term self-efficacy and resilience.
2. Customize exercise interventions based on individual capacities, preferences, and psychological needs.
3. Consider group-based formats to leverage social support, motivation, and adherence.
4. Monitor both short-term and long-term outcomes to optimize intervention effectiveness.
5. Integrate exercise interventions alongside traditional mental health treatments where appropriate.

For Fitness Professionals and Public Health Policymakers

1. Design hybrid exercise programs that combine AE and RT to maximize psychological benefits across populations.

2. Provide inclusive and accessible facilities that accommodate diverse age groups, genders, and fitness levels.
3. Promote community-based initiatives encouraging regular engagement in both modalities.
4. Develop educational campaigns highlighting mental health benefits alongside physical fitness gains.
5. Support research-informed policy-making to optimize exercise guidelines for population-level mental well-being.

STRATEGIC ROADMAP

Based on the recommendations outlined above, a strategic roadmap can guide the translation of research findings into effective interventions for psychological well-being through exercise. This roadmap highlights phased actions for researchers, clinicians, fitness professionals, and policymakers.

Based on the recommendations outlined above, a strategic roadmap can guide the translation of research findings into effective interventions for psychological well-being through exercise. This roadmap highlights phased actions for researchers, clinicians, fitness professionals, and policymakers. In the research domain, priority should be given to longitudinal, modality-specific studies that integrate psychological, physiological, and contextual variables to capture both short- and long-term outcomes. Clinicians and mental health practitioners should incorporate evidence-based exercise prescriptions into therapeutic frameworks, ensuring that programs are tailored to individual needs, preferences, and clinical characteristics. Fitness professionals play a critical role in operationalizing these approaches by designing structured, safe, and socially supportive exercise environments that enhance adherence and psychological benefits. Meanwhile, policymakers should support infrastructure development, accessibility initiatives, and multidisciplinary collaborations to embed exercise-based mental health strategies within broader public health systems. Collectively, these coordinated efforts can help bridge the gap between empirical knowledge and real-world practice, maximizing the psychological benefits of both RT and AE.

RESEARCH AND EVIDENCE GENERATION

Objective: Strengthen the evidence base on the comparative psychological effects of RT and AE

Actions:

- Conduct large-scale, longitudinal, and randomized controlled trials comparing RT, AE, and combined programs.
- Integrate multi-method assessment tools, including self-report, physiological, and neurobiological measures.
- Investigate moderating factors such as age, gender, health status, and cultural context.
- Explore mechanisms underlying synergy in concurrent training programs.

Expected Outcome: More robust and generalizable evidence to inform targeted interventions and public health policies.

CLINICAL IMPLEMENTATION

Objective: Optimize exercise prescriptions for mental health interventions.

Actions:

- Use AE to provide immediate relief from stress, anxiety, and depressive symptoms.
- Incorporate RT for sustained improvements in self-efficacy, resilience, and self-concept.
- Design hybrid programs combining AE and RT for both short-term and long-term benefits.
- Tailor programs based on individual capacities, preferences, and psychosocial context.
- Monitor both immediate and longitudinal outcomes to evaluate effectiveness.

Expected Outcome: Improved mental health outcomes and personalized intervention strategies for diverse populations.

FITNESS AND COMMUNITY PROGRAMS

Objective: Enhance adherence, motivation, and population-level mental health benefits through structured exercise programs.

Actions:

- Develop inclusive hybrid programs that combine AE and RT, catering to different age groups and abilities.
- Implement group-based or socially supportive formats to strengthen motivation and social connectedness.
- Promote accessible community exercise initiatives, such as public gyms, school programs, and senior fitness classes.
- Train fitness professionals on evidence-based exercise strategies for psychological well-being.

Expected Outcome: Increased engagement in exercise and sustainable improvements in mental health across communities.

POLICY AND PUBLIC HEALTH INTEGRATION

Objective: Translate research into actionable public health strategies.

Actions:

- Incorporate findings into national physical activity guidelines with a focus on psychological outcomes.
- Support policies promoting access to both AE and RT facilities in schools, workplaces, and public spaces.
- Launch educational campaigns highlighting mental health benefits of regular exercise.
- Allocate resources for integrated exercise programs targeting vulnerable populations, including adolescents, older adults, and individuals with mental health conditions.

Expected Outcome: Evidence-based policy frameworks that facilitate population-wide mental health promotion through exercise.

CONTINUOUS MONITORING AND FEEDBACK

Objective: Ensure iterative improvement of exercise interventions and public health strategies.

Actions:

- Establish monitoring systems to track psychological outcomes in various populations.
- Collect feedback from participants, practitioners, and policymakers to refine interventions.
- Update recommendations periodically based on emerging evidence and contextual insights.

Expected Outcome: Sustainable, adaptive, and evidence-informed exercise interventions that maximize psychological well-being.

This **Strategic Roadmap** consolidates the chapter's findings and recommendations into a coherent plan, bridging theory, research, practice, and policy. By following this roadmap, stakeholders can systematically enhance psychological outcomes through both resistance and aerobic forms of exercise, while remaining responsive to evolving evidence and population needs.

AUTHOR CONTRIBUTORSHIP

Harry Sutanto was responsible for the conceptualization of the chapter, including defining its scope, objectives, and theoretical framework. He drafted the initial version of the manuscript, integrating relevant literature, organizing the structure, and ensuring that the arguments and discussion were coherent and comprehensive. In addition, he conducted extensive review and editing, refining the language, improving clarity, and aligning the content with academic standards. Anton Dwi Fitriyanto contributed significantly to the methodological aspects of the chapter, including the design of the study framework, planning of analyses, and validation of data sources. He also participated in drafting sections of the manuscript, particularly those related to methodology, data interpretation, and critical evaluation. Both authors collaborated closely throughout the development process, reviewing each other's contributions, ensuring accuracy and integrity of the data, and refining the overall content. They jointly approved the final version of the chapter, sharing full responsibility for its intellectual quality and substantive contributions to the field.

REFERENCES

Biddle, S. J. H., Ciaccioni, S., Thomas, G., & Vergeer, I. (2019). Physical activity and mental health in children and adolescents: An updated review of reviews and an analysis of causality. *Psychology of Sport and Exercise*, *42*, 146–155. DOI: 10.1016/j.psychsport.2018.08.011

Chekroud, S. R., Gueorguieva, R., Zheutlin, A. B., Paulus, M., Krumholz, H. M., Krystal, J. H., & Chekroud, A. M. (2018). Association between physical exercise and mental health in 1.2 million individuals in the USA between 2011 and 2015: A cross-sectional study. *The Lancet. Psychiatry*, *5*(9), 739–746. DOI: 10.1016/S2215-0366(18)30227-X PMID: 30099000

Cooney, G. M., Dwan, K., Greig, C. A., Lawlor, D. A., Rimer, J., Waugh, F. R., McMurdo, M., & Mead, G. E. (2013). Exercise for depression. *Cochrane Database of Systematic Reviews*, *2013*(9), CD004366. Advance online publication. DOI: 10.1002/14651858.CD004366.pub6 PMID: 24026850

Craft, L. L., & Perna, F. M. (2004). The benefits of exercise for the clinically depressed. *Primary Care Companion to the Journal of Clinical Psychiatry*, *6*(3), 104–111. DOI: 10.4088/PCC.v06n0301 PMID: 15361924

Ekkekakis, P. (2013). *The measurement of affect, mood, and emotion: A guide for health-behavioral research*. Cambridge University Press.

Ensari, I., Greenlee, T. A., Motl, R. W., & Petruzzello, S. J. (2015). Meta-analysis of acute exercise effects on state anxiety: An update of randomized controlled trials over the past 25 years. *Depression and Anxiety*, *32*(8), 624–634. PMID: 25899389

Gordon, B. R., McDowell, C. P., Hallgren, M., Meyer, J. D., Lyons, M., & Herring, M. P. (2018). Association of efficacy of resistance exercise training with depressive symptoms: Meta-analysis and meta-regression analysis of randomized clinical trials. *JAMA Psychiatry*, *75*(6), 566–576. DOI: 10.1001/jamapsychiatry.2018.0256 PMID: 29800984

Gordon, B. R., McDowell, C. P., Lyons, M., & Herring, M. P. (2017). Resistance exercise training for anxiety and worry symptoms among young adults: A randomized controlled trial. *Scientific Reports*, *7*(1), 17548. DOI: 10.1038/s41598-017-17704-7 PMID: 33067493

Herring, M. P., O'Connor, P. J., & Dishman, R. K. (2010). The effect of exercise training on anxiety symptoms among patients: A systematic review. *Archives of Internal Medicine*, *170*(4), 321–331. PMID: 20177034

Kelley, G. A., & Kelley, K. S. (2017a). Exercise and depression in older adults: A meta-analysis of randomized controlled trials. *Journal of Aging and Physical Activity*, *25*(4), 711–719. DOI: 10.1123/japa.2016-0120

Kelley, G. A., & Kelley, K. S. (2017b). Exercise and sleep: A systematic review of previous meta-analyses. *Journal of Evidence-Based Medicine*, *10*(1), 26–36. DOI: 10.1111/jebm.12236 PMID: 28276627

Netz, Y., Wu, M. J., Becker, B. J., & Tenenbaum, G. (2005). Physical activity and psychological well-being in advanced age: A meta-analysis of intervention studies. *Psychology and Aging*, *20*(2), 272. PMID: 16029091

Prince, S. A., Adamo, K. B., Hamel, M. E., Hardt, J., Gorber, S. C., & Tremblay, M. (2008). A comparison of direct versus self-report measures for assessing physical activity in adults: A systematic review. *The International Journal of Behavioral Nutrition and Physical Activity*, *5*(1), 56. PMID: 18990237

Reed, J., & Buck, S. (2009). The effect of regular aerobic exercise on positive-activated affect: A meta-analysis. *Psychology of Sport and Exercise*, *10*(6), 581–594.

Rhodes, R. E., & Dickau, L. (2013). Moderators of the intention-behaviour relationship in the physical activity domain: A systematic review. *British Journal of Sports Medicine*, *47*(4), 215–225. PMID: 22278998

Schuch, F. B., Vancampfort, D., Firth, J., Rosenbaum, S., Richards, J., Ward, P. B., & Stubbs, B. (2016b). Exercise for depression in adults: A meta-analysis of randomized controlled trials. *British Journal of Sports Medicine*, *50*(4), 229–236. DOI: 10.1136/bjsports-2015-095014 PMID: 27611903

Schuch, F. B., Vancampfort, D., Firth, J., Rosenbaum, S., Ward, P. B., Silva, E. S., Hallgren, M., Ponce de Leon, A., Dunn, A. L., Deslandes, A. C., Fleck, M. P., Carvalho, A. F., & Stubbs, B. (2016a). Physical activity and incident depression: A meta-analysis of prospective cohort studies. *The American Journal of Psychiatry*, *175*(7), 631–648. DOI: 10.1176/appi.ajp.2018.17111194 PMID: 29690792

Ströhle, A. (2009). Physical activity, exercise, depression and anxiety disorders. *Journal of Neural Transmission (Vienna, Austria)*, *116*(6), 777–784. DOI: 10.1007/s00702-008-0092-x PMID: 18726137

Stubbs, B., Vancampfort, D., Rosenbaum, S., Firth, J., Cosco, T., Veronese, N., & Schuch, F. B. (2017). An examination of the anxiolytic effects of exercise for people with anxiety and stress-related disorders: A meta-analysis. *Psychiatry Research*, *249*, 102–108. PMID: 28088704

Troiano, R. P., McClain, J. J., Brychta, R. J., & Chen, K. Y. (2014). Evolution of accelerometer methods for physical activity research. *British Journal of Sports Medicine*, *48*(13), 1019–1023. PMID: 24782483

Wegner, M., Helmich, I., Machado, S., Nardi, A. E., Arias-Carrion, O., & Budde, H. (2014). Effects of exercise on anxiety and depression disorders: Review of meta-analyses and neurobiological mechanisms. *CNS & Neurological Disorders - Drug Targets*, *13*(6), 1002–1014. DOI: 10.2174/1871527313666140612110928 PMID: 24923346

White, R. L., Vella, S., Biddle, S., Sutcliffe, J., Guagliano, J. M., Uddin, R., & Teychenne, M. (2024). Physical activity and mental health: A systematic review and best-evidence synthesis of mediation and moderation studies. *The International Journal of Behavioral Nutrition and Physical Activity*, *21*(1), 134. PMID: 39609855

Chapter 2

Emotion Focused Exercise Interventions Enhance Mood State and Self Esteem in Individuals With Depression

Sohom Saha
https://orcid.org/0009-0006-9438-1554
Lakshmibai National Institute of Physical Education, India

Mahendra Kumar Singh
https://orcid.org/0000-0001-9989-9420
Lakshmibai National Institute of Physical Education, India

Simran Obhrai
https://orcid.org/0009-0007-5227-9364
Guru Nanak Dev University, India

ABSTRACT

Depression affects millions of people worldwide, causing low mood, loss of interest, and poor self-esteem. Traditional treatments such as medicines and therapy are helpful but may not be enough for everyone. Exercise has been shown to improve mood, but most programs only focus on physical health. This manuscript introduces Emotion Focused Exercise Interventions (EFEIs), which combine physical activity with emotional awareness, mindfulness, and therapeutic support. Activities such as aerobic exercise, resistance training, yoga, and dance are used not just for fitness but also for emotional expression and healing. Evidence shows that EFEIs improve

DOI: 10.4018/979-8-3373-6157-4.ch002

mood, self-esteem, and emotional regulation more effectively than exercise alone. Case studies in individuals, groups, schools, and rehabilitation centers highlight their real-world benefits. EFEIs represent a promising, cost-effective approach that can complement existing treatments and make depression care more holistic and accessible.

1. INTRODUCTION

Depression stands as one of the most pervasive mental health challenges of our time, affecting an estimated 280 million individuals globally according to the World Health Organization (World Health Organization, 2023). This debilitating condition is characterized by persistent low mood, anhedonia, impaired cognitive function, and significantly diminished self-worth, creating a complex web of psychological, social, and physiological dysfunction that extends far beyond individual suffering to impact families, communities, and healthcare systems worldwide (Malhi & Mann, 2018). The traditional landscape of depression treatment has long been dominated by pharmacological interventions and psychotherapeutic approaches, particularly cognitive-behavioral therapy (CBT). While these evidence-based treatments have demonstrated substantial efficacy (Cuijpers et al., 2014), recent decades have witnessed an increasing recognition that depression's multifaceted nature may require more comprehensive, integrative treatment approaches that address not only cognitive and biochemical aspects but also the embodied, emotional, and social dimensions of human experience (Malhi & Mann, 2018). This paradigmatic shift has coincided with mounting evidence for exercise as a powerful therapeutic modality in mental health treatment. Meta-analyses consistently demonstrate that structured physical activity can produce antidepressant effects comparable to traditional treatments, with effect sizes ranging from moderate to large across diverse populations (Noetel et al., 2024; Singh et al., 2023). A recent comprehensive network meta-analysis by Noetel et al. (2024) examining 218 unique studies with 14,170 participants found that all types of physical activity showed significant effects for treating major depressive disorder, with particularly large effects observed for dancing and mixed aerobic exercises. However, most exercise interventions for depression have focused primarily on the physiological benefits of movement, potentially overlooking the profound emotional and psychological processes that occur when physical activity is intentionally combined with emotional awareness and therapeutic reflection (Kandola et al., 2019). This gap in the literature has prompted the development of more sophisticated, emotion-integrated approaches to exercise-based depression treatment.

Enter Emotion-Focused Exercise Interventions (EFEIs) - a novel therapeutic approach that bridges the gap between exercise science and emotional healing by explicitly integrating physical movement with emotional processing, mindful awareness, and therapeutic support (Paulus et al., 2018). Unlike conventional fitness programs that primarily target physical health outcomes, EFEIs are designed with the understanding that movement and emotion are inextricably linked, and that intentional attention to this connection can amplify the therapeutic benefits of exercise for individuals struggling with depression. EFEIs represent a paradigm shift from viewing exercise merely as a biological intervention toward understanding movement as a vehicle for emotional expression, regulation, and transformation (van der Kolk, 2014). This approach recognizes that individuals with depression often experience disconnection from their bodies, emotional numbness, and impaired capacity for emotional regulation – all areas where thoughtfully designed movement interventions can provide unique therapeutic value (Paulus et al., 2018).

The theoretical foundation of EFEIs draws from multiple disciplines including exercise physiology, affective neuroscience, emotion regulation theory, and somatic psychology (Gross, 2002). This interdisciplinary framework acknowledges that depression involves dysregulation across multiple systems - neurobiological, cognitive, emotional, and social – and that effective interventions must address this complexity through integrated approaches that engage the whole person rather than isolated symptoms. Contemporary research has illuminated the profound neurobiological mechanisms through which exercise influences mood, including enhanced production of brain-derived neurotrophic factor (BDNF), modulation of neurotransmitter systems involving serotonin and dopamine, and regulation of stress-responsive systems including the hypothalamic-pituitary-adrenal (HPA) axis (Kandola et al., 2019). When combined with intentional emotional processing, these neurobiological changes may be amplified and directed toward specific therapeutic outcomes related to mood enhancement and self-esteem restoration.

The emergence of EFEIs as a distinct therapeutic modality is particularly timely given the global mental health crisis exacerbated by recent events including the COVID-19 pandemic, which has led to unprecedented increases in depression rates worldwide (Santomauro et al., 2021). Traditional mental health services have been overwhelmed, creating urgent need for scalable, accessible, and cost-effective interventions that can be implemented across diverse settings and populations. This chapter provides a comprehensive examination of EFEIs as an innovative approach to depression treatment, exploring their theoretical foundations, empirical support, implementation strategies, and potential for integration with existing therapeutic modalities. Through synthesis of cutting-edge research and practical clinical insights, we aim to establish EFEIs as a valuable addition to the therapeutic arsenal for mental health professionals working with individuals experiencing depression.

Figure 1. The power of EFEI lies not in any single component but in the intentional integration of movement, emotion, and therapeutic support, thus providing integrated healing

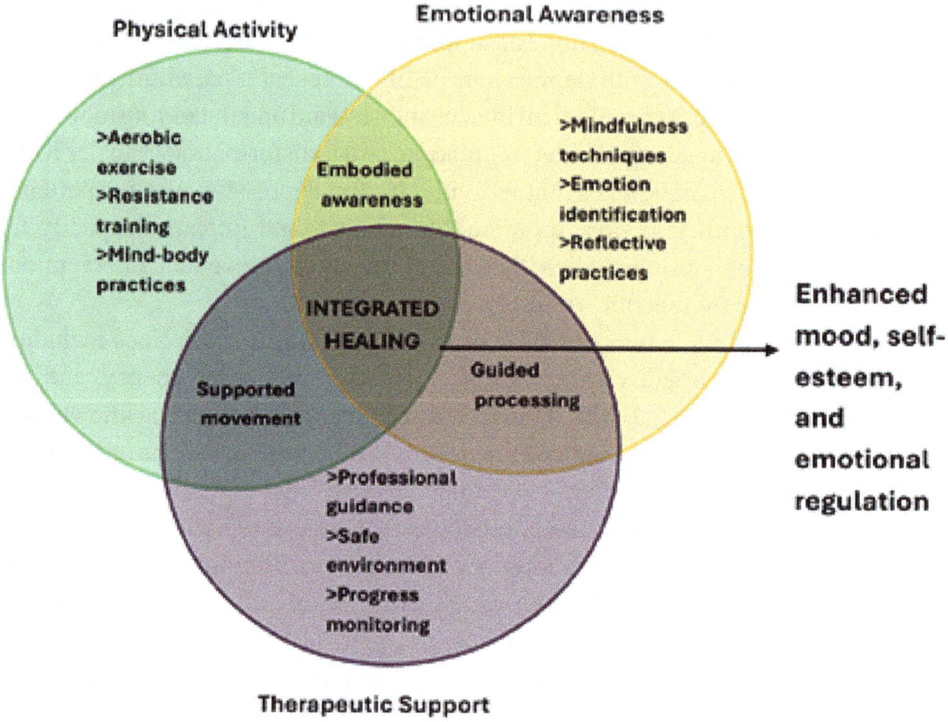

2. THEORETICAL AND BIOLOGICAL FOUNDATIONS

2.1 The Role of Affect Regulation in Depression

Depression fundamentally involves dysregulation of emotional processes, including difficulties in emotion generation, experience, expression, and regulation (Joormann & Stanton, 2016). Individuals with depression often exhibit maladaptive emotion regulation strategies, including excessive rumination, emotional suppression, and reduced capacity for emotional granularity and flexibility (Aldao et al., 2010). These emotional dysfunction patterns contribute to the maintenance and exacerbation of depressive symptoms, creating self-perpetuating cycles of emotional distress. Traditional therapeutic approaches have primarily addressed these emotional difficulties through cognitive interventions aimed at modifying dysfunctional thought patterns (King, 2002). However, emerging research suggests that embodied approaches to emotion regulation - those that engage the body as well as the mind - may offer unique therapeutic advantages (van der Kolk, 2014). The body serves as both a reservoir of emotional experience and a vehicle for emotional transformation, making movement-based interventions particularly well-suited to addressing the emotional dimensions of depression.

Recent advances in affective neuroscience have highlighted the crucial role of interoception -the perception of internal bodily signals - in emotional regulation and mental health (Garfinkel et al., 2015). Individuals with depression often demonstrate impaired interoceptive accuracy and awareness, which may contribute to difficulties in emotional recognition and regulation (Dunn et al., 2010). EFEIs are grounded in the understanding that emotions are fundamentally embodied experiences that involve complex interactions between cognitive appraisal, physiological arousal, and behavioral expression (Damasio, 1999). When individuals with depression engage in structured physical activity while maintaining conscious awareness of emotional states and processes, they create opportunities for new forms of emotional learning and regulation that may not be accessible through purely cognitive approaches (Pruessner et al., 2020). Research has demonstrated that mindfulness-based approaches to emotion regulation can significantly enhance treatment outcomes, particularly when integrated with other therapeutic modalities.

2.2 Neurobiological Mechanisms

The neurobiological foundation of EFEIs rests on well-established mechanisms through which exercise influences brain structure and function, particularly in regions and systems implicated in depression. These mechanisms operate at multiple levels, from molecular signaling pathways to large-scale neural networks, creating a comprehensive neurobiological rationale for exercise-based depression interventions (Kandola et al., 2019).

Table 1. Neurobiological mechanisms of EFEIs

Mechanism	Key Effect	Role in Depression	Exercise-Induced Impact
Brain-Derived Neurotrophic Factor (BDNF)	Promotes neuroplasticity, neuronal survival	Reduced in depression	Elevated by aerobic and resistance training
Serotonin	Regulates mood, anxiety, and sleep	Dysregulated in depression	Increased synthesis and receptor sensitivity
Dopamine	Motivation, pleasure, reward	Low levels linked to anhedonia	Enhanced release in reward pathways
Norepinephrine	Arousal, attention, stress response	Reduced attentional capacity	Optimized function through regular exercise
HPA Axis Regulation	Stress response modulation	Hyperactivity, high cortisol	Restored balance with regular movement

2.2.1 Brain-Derived Neurotrophic Factor (BDNF)

Brain-derived neurotrophic factor represents one of the most significant neurobiological mediators of exercise's antidepressant effects (Bathina & Das, 2015). BDNF is a neurotrophin that plays crucial roles in neuronal survival, growth, and synaptic plasticity - processes that are compromised in depression and restored through effective treatment. Multiple studies have demonstrated that exercise increases both peripheral and central BDNF levels, with these changes correlating with improvements in depressive symptoms (Kandola et al., 2019). Recent research has revealed that exercise-induced BDNF elevation occurs through multiple pathways, including activation of the transcription factor CREB (cAMP response element-binding protein) and upregulation of various growth factors that promote neuroplasticity (Bathina & Das, 2015). The magnitude and duration of BDNF elevation appear to be influenced by exercise intensity, duration, and type, suggesting that carefully designed exercise protocols may optimize neuroplastic responses.

In the context of EFEIs, the combination of physical activity with emotional awareness and processing may enhance BDNF-mediated neuroplasticity in brain regions particularly relevant to emotional regulation, including the hippocampus, prefrontal cortex, and anterior cingulate cortex (Kandola et al., 2019). This targeted neuroplasticity may facilitate the development of new emotional regulation skills and the consolidation of positive emotional experiences generated during exercise participation.

2.2.2 Neurotransmitter Systems

Exercise exerts profound effects on multiple neurotransmitter systems implicated in depression, including serotonin, dopamine, and norepinephrine pathways (Kandola et al., 2019). These effects occur through both direct and indirect mechanisms, creating complex but complementary influences on mood, motivation, and emotional regulation. Serotonin, often called the "happiness neurotransmitter," is significantly influenced by exercise through multiple pathways (Young, 2007). Exercise increases tryptophan availability in the brain, enhances serotonin synthesis and release, and may improve serotonin receptor sensitivity. These changes contribute to improved mood, reduced anxiety, and enhanced emotional stability – core therapeutic targets in depression treatment.

Dopamine system activation through exercise may be particularly relevant to addressing anhedonia, a cardinal symptom of depression characterized by reduced capacity for experiencing pleasure (Salamone et al., 2007). Exercise-induced dopamine release in reward-related brain circuits may help restore hedonic capacity and motivation, while also reinforcing continued engagement in therapeutic activities. The norepinephrine system, which plays crucial roles in attention, arousal, and stress response, is also significantly influenced by exercise (Kandola et al., 2019). Regular physical activity appears to optimize norepinephrine function, potentially improving cognitive symptoms of depression while enhancing stress resilience.

2.2.3 HPA Axis Regulation

The hypothalamic-pituitary-adrenal (HPA) axis represents a key stress-responsive system that is frequently dysregulated in depression (Pariante & Lightman, 2008). Chronic HPA axis activation, characterized by elevated cortisol levels and impaired stress recovery, contributes to many of the cognitive, emotional, and physical symptoms associated with depression. Exercise has complex but generally beneficial effects on HPA axis function (Schuch et al., 2016). While acute exercise transiently activates the HPA axis, regular exercise training appears to improve HPA axis regulation, reduce baseline cortisol levels, and enhance stress recovery capacity. These effects may be particularly pronounced when exercise is combined with stress-reduction techniques such as mindfulness or relaxation training, components that are explicitly integrated into EFEIs.

2.3 Cognitive-Behavioral and Emotional Processing Models

EFEIs integrate insights from cognitive-behavioral theory and emotion-focused therapeutic approaches to create comprehensive interventions that address both cognitive and emotional aspects of depression (Greenberg, 2015; King, 2002). The cognitive-behavioral model of depression emphasizes the role of negative thought patterns, behavioral avoidance, and reduced activity engagement in maintaining depressive symptoms. Exercise interventions naturally address these factors by increasing activity levels, providing mastery experiences, and creating opportunities for positive mood states that can challenge negative thinking patterns. However, EFEIs go beyond traditional cognitive-behavioral approaches by explicitly incorporating emotion-focused techniques that help individuals develop greater emotional awareness, acceptance, and regulation skills (Greenberg, 2015). This integration recognizes that cognitive change often requires emotional processing and that sustainable therapeutic progress may depend on addressing both cognitive and emotional dimensions of depression. The emotion-focused component of EFEIs draws from research demonstrating that emotional awareness and expression can facilitate psychological healing and resilience (Gross, 2002). When combined with physical activity, these emotional processing techniques may be enhanced through the embodied nature of movement, creating opportunities for emotional learning that extends beyond what is possible through verbal processing alone.

3. DEFINING EFEIS

3.1 Core Components and Principles

EFEIs represent a structured, evidence-informed approach to depression treatment that integrates three essential components: physical activity, emotional awareness and processing, and therapeutic support (Rosenbaum et al., 2014). This tripartite structure distinguishes EFEIs from both generic exercise programs and traditional psychotherapy approaches by creating a unique therapeutic space where movement and emotional exploration reinforce each other. The physical activity component of EFEIs encompasses a diverse range of movement modalities selected based on their capacity to promote both physiological and emotional benefits (Noetel et al., 2024). Unlike exercise prescriptions focused solely on cardiovascular fitness or strength development, EFEIs prioritize activities that facilitate emotional expression, body awareness, and interpersonal connection while still providing sufficient physiological stimulation to activate neurobiological mechanisms associated with mood enhancement.

The emotional awareness and processing component involves structured techniques designed to help participants develop greater consciousness of their emotional states, patterns, and responses while engaging in physical activity (Gross, 2002). This may include guided reflection exercises, mindfulness practices, expressive movement techniques, and journaling activities that help individuals connect their physical experiences with emotional insights. The therapeutic support component ensures that EFEIs are delivered within a framework that prioritizes psychological safety, professional guidance, and individualized adaptation to meet participants' unique needs and circumstances (Rosenbaum et al., 2014). This support may be provided by trained exercise professionals with mental health competencies, mental health professionals with exercise training, or interdisciplinary teams that combine both areas of expertise.

Table 2. Core components of EFEIs

Component	Description	Example Techniques	Expected Outcomes
Physical Activity	Structured movement tailored for physiological & emotional benefits	Aerobic exercise, resistance training, yoga, dance	Improved fitness, neurobiological adaptation
Emotional Awareness & Processing	Conscious recognition and expression of feelings during exercise	Mindful movement, expressive dance, guided reflection	Enhanced emotion regulation, reduced suppression
Therapeutic Support	Professional guidance ensuring safety & personalization	Group facilitation, one-on-one coaching	Increased adherence, psychological safety

3.2 Types of Activities and Interventions

3.2.1 Aerobic Training with Emotional Awareness

Traditional aerobic exercise has well-established antidepressant effects, with recent meta-analyses confirming moderate to large effect sizes for aerobic interventions in depression treatment (Singh et al., 2023). Aerobic exercise has been shown to improve cardiorespiratory fitness in people with depression and affect individuals with major depressive disorder from a neurobiological standpoint. In EFEIs, aerobic activities are enhanced through integration of emotional awareness techniques that help participants develop greater interoceptive awareness - the ability to perceive and understand bodily signals - which is often impaired in depression (Dunn et al., 2010).

Participants might engage in walking, jogging, cycling, or dancing while maintaining conscious attention to their emotional states, physical sensations, and internal experiences. This mindful approach to aerobic exercise helps individuals develop greater interoceptive awareness and emotional regulation skills (Garfinkel et al., 2015). During aerobic activities, participants may be guided to notice how their mood shifts throughout the exercise session, observe the relationship between physical exertion and emotional states, and explore how movement affects their sense of vitality and aliveness.

3.2.2 Resistance Training for Empowerment

Resistance training in EFEIs is framed not merely as strength building but as empowerment development (Gordon et al., 2018). Meta-analyses have demonstrated significant associations between resistance exercise training and reductions in depressive symptoms, with effect sizes comparable to other established treatments. The progressive nature of resistance training provides natural opportunities for mastery experiences, goal achievement, and self-efficacy enhancement - all crucial factors in depression recovery. Participants work with weights, resistance bands, or bodyweight exercises while focusing on themes of personal strength, resilience, and capability. The emotional component of resistance training in EFEIs might involve metaphorical connections between physical strength and emotional resilience, exploration of how overcoming physical challenges relates to overcoming life difficulties, and celebration of progress and achievement (Gordon et al., 2018).

3.2.3 Mind-Body Practices: Yoga and Tai Chi

Yoga and Tai Chi represent natural fits for EFEIs due to their inherent integration of physical movement, breath awareness, and mindful attention (Cramer et al., 2013). These practices have independent evidence for depression treatment and are readily adaptable to include explicit emotional processing components. Research has consistently demonstrated that yoga interventions can produce significant reductions in depressive symptoms, with effect sizes comparable to other evidence-based treatments (Cramer et al., 2018). In EFEIs, yoga and Tai Chi sessions might include specific poses or movements selected for their emotional significance, guided imagery that connects physical positions with emotional states, and group discussions about the psychological insights that emerge during practice. The slow, controlled nature of these activities provides ample opportunity for emotional awareness and processing while still delivering physiological benefits.

3.2.4 Expressive Movement and Dance

Dance and expressive movement offer unique opportunities for emotional expression and release that may be particularly valuable for individuals with depression who struggle with emotional numbness or alexithymia (Karkou et al., 2019). Recent research has identified dancing as showing particularly large effects for treating depression, suggesting that expressive movement modalities may offer unique therapeutic advantages. These activities bypass cognitive defenses and allow for direct emotional expression through movement, potentially accessing emotional material that might be difficult to reach through verbal processing alone (van der Kolk, 2014). EFEIs might incorporate various forms of dance and movement, from structured dance forms to free-form expressive movement, always with attention to the emotional content and meaning of the movements.

3.3 Integration of Reflection and Mindfulness Techniques

The reflective component of EFEIs serves to consolidate and integrate the insights and experiences that emerge during physical activity (Pennebaker & Chung, 2011). This might involve structured journaling exercises where participants write about their emotional experiences during and after exercise, guided group discussions where individuals share their insights and support each other's process, or individual reflection time where participants process their experiences privately. Mindfulness techniques are woven throughout EFEIs to enhance present-moment awareness and reduce the rumination and worry that characterize depression (Kabat-Zinn, 2003). Recent research suggests that combining mindfulness with exercise may be most effective for improving psychological well-being. Participants might practice mindful breathing during rest periods, engage in body scan exercises before or after physical activity, or use mindfulness techniques to maintain awareness of their emotional states throughout exercise sessions. The integration of these reflective and mindfulness components ensures that EFEIs provide not just immediate mood benefits from physical activity but also longer-term emotional learning and skill development that can support sustained recovery from depression (Pruessner et al., 2020).

4. PSYCHOLOGICAL OUTCOMES AND EVIDENCE

4.1 Mood Enhancement Effects

Extensive research has documented the mood-enhancing effects of exercise interventions for depression, with recent meta-analyses demonstrating effect sizes comparable to established treatments such as psychotherapy and pharmacotherapy (Noetel et al., 2024). A comprehensive network meta-analysis examining 218 unique studies with 14,170 participants found significant effects for all types of physical activity in treating major depressive disorder, providing robust evidence for exercise as a legitimate treatment option for depression. The mood-enhancing mechanisms of EFEIs operate through multiple pathways that extend beyond the neurobiological effects described earlier (Kandola et al., 2019). Psychological mechanisms include enhanced self-efficacy through mastery experiences, improved body image and physical self-concept, increased social connection and support, and the development of active coping strategies that replace passive, avoidant behaviors characteristic of depression (Bandura, 1997). Research specifically examining emotion-focused approaches to exercise has found that interventions combining physical activity with emotional awareness techniques produce superior outcomes compared to exercise alone (Barton & Pretty, 2010). These studies suggest that the explicit emotional focus of EFEIs may enhance therapeutic benefits by addressing both the physiological and psychological dimensions of mood regulation.

4.2 Self-Esteem and Self-Worth Improvements

Self-esteem deficits represent a core feature of depression, characterized by negative self-evaluation, harsh self-criticism, and reduced sense of personal worth and capability (King, 2002). EFEIs address self-esteem through multiple mechanisms that operate at cognitive, emotional, and experiential levels. The achievement and mastery experiences inherent in structured exercise programs provide natural opportunities for self-esteem enhancement (Bandura, 1997). As individuals progress in their physical capabilities, set and achieve goals, and overcome challenges, they develop enhanced self-efficacy and more positive self-concepts. In EFEIs, these naturally occurring processes are amplified through explicit attention to achievement recognition, progress celebration, and connection between physical accomplishments and broader life capabilities.

The embodied nature of EFEIs offers unique advantages for self-esteem enhancement (van der Kolk, 2014). Many individuals with depression experience disconnection from their bodies, negative body image, and reduced sense of physical agency and capability. Through structured movement experiences that emphasize body awareness, physical competence, and pleasurable physical sensations, EFEIs help individuals develop more positive relationships with their bodies and enhanced sense of physical self-worth.

4.3 Emotional Regulation Improvements

Emotional regulation difficulties represent a central feature of depression, including problems with emotion identification, expression, and adaptive management (Joormann & Stanton, 2016). EFEIs specifically target these emotional regulation challenges through structured exercises and experiences designed to enhance emotional awareness and regulation skills. The mindfulness components of EFEIs help individuals develop greater emotional awareness by teaching them to observe their emotional states without immediate judgment or attempts to change them (Kabat-

Zinn, 2003). Research has demonstrated that mindfulness-based approaches can significantly improve emotion regulation and reduce depressive symptoms. This observational stance, practiced during physical activity, helps individuals become more conscious of their emotional patterns and triggers, laying the foundation for more adaptive emotional responses. The expressive components of EFEIs provide opportunities for emotional expression and release that may be particularly valuable for individuals who tend toward emotional suppression or avoidance (Gross, 2002). Through movement, dance, and other expressive activities, individuals can access and express emotions that might be difficult to reach through verbal processing alone.

4.4 Evidence from Clinical Trials and Meta-Analyses

The evidence base for exercise interventions in depression treatment has grown substantially in recent years, with numerous randomized controlled trials and meta-analyses demonstrating significant therapeutic effects (Noetel et al., 2024). Recent systematic reviews have examined different modalities of physical exercise, including aerobic training, resistance exercise, combined exercise, and multicomponent exercise, providing comprehensive evidence for the antidepressant effects of various exercise types. A recent systematic review by (Singh et al., 2023) found that physical exercise interventions for major depressive disorder in adults showed significant therapeutic effects, with multimodal approaches demonstrating particular promise. Meta-analyses have also confirmed that physical exercise has positive effects on depression improvement in adolescents, suggesting that exercise interventions may be effective across different age groups.

While research specifically examining EFEIs as defined in this chapter is still emerging, studies examining components of EFEIs provide substantial support for this approach. Research on mindfulness-based exercise interventions has found superior outcomes compared to exercise alone (Zhang et al., 2021). Studies have demonstrated that mindfulness-based interventions can improve psychological health and support positive health behaviors, supporting the integration of mindfulness techniques into exercise programs. Similarly, studies of group-based exercise programs have demonstrated enhanced outcomes compared to individual exercise, supporting the social component of many EFEIs (Barton & Pretty, 2010). The combination of physical activity with social interaction and emotional processing appears to create synergistic effects that enhance therapeutic outcomes beyond what is achievable through any single component alone.

Table 3. Summary of evidence for EFEI modalities

Modality	Evidence Strength	Notable Benefits	Effect Sizes	Representative Studies
Aerobic Exercise with Emotional Awareness	Strong	Improved mood, cardiorespiratory fitness, interoceptive skills	Depression: d = -0.43 (IQR: -0.66 to -0.27) Anxiety: d = -0.42 (IQR: -0.66 to -0.26) Psychological distress: d = -0.60 (95% CI: -0.78 to -0.42)	(Singh et al., 2023)
Resistance Training with Empowerment Themes	Moderate to Strong	Enhanced self-efficacy, reduced depressive symptoms	Depression: d = 0.66 (95% CI: 0.48-0.83) NNT = 4	(Gordon et al., 2018)
Yoga & Tai Chi with Emotional Processing	Strong	Stress reduction, body awareness, mindfulness	Depression vs. usual care: SMD = -0.69 (95% CI: -0.99 to -0.39) Anxiety vs. relaxation: SMD = -0.79 (95% CI: -1.30 to -0.26)	(Cramer et al., 2013)
Expressive Movement/Dance	Moderate	Emotional release, improved social connection	Depression: SMD = -0.82 (95% CI: -1.20 to -0.43) (Large effect size)	(Karkou et al., 2019)

Note: Effect sizes are presented as standardized mean differences (SMD) or Cohen's d. Negative values indicate reduction in symptoms. Gordon et al. (2018) reported positive values for symptom reduction. NNT = Number Needed to Treat; IQR = Interquartile Range; CI = Confidence Interval.

5. IMPLEMENTATION AND DELIVERY MODELS

5.1 Group versus Individual Interventions

The choice between group and individual delivery of EFEIs represents a crucial implementation decision that significantly impacts therapeutic outcomes, feasibility, and cost-effectiveness (Rosenbaum et al., 2014). Each approach offers distinct advantages and considerations that must be weighed based on participant needs, available resources, and therapeutic goals. Group-based EFEIs offer several unique therapeutic advantages that align with the social nature of emotional healing and recovery from depression (Barton & Pretty, 2010). The group setting provides natural opportunities for social connection, peer support, and normalization of struggles that can be particularly valuable for individuals experiencing the isolation and self-criticism common in depression. Participants benefit from witnessing others' journeys, sharing their own experiences, and developing supportive relationships that extend beyond the formal intervention period.

Research has demonstrated that exercise programs incorporating social interaction show superior outcomes compared to individual exercise, with participants experiencing greater improvements in mood, self-esteem, and overall psychological well-being (Barton & Pretty, 2010). The group dynamic creates accountability, motivation, and encouragement that can help individuals maintain engagement even when motivation is low - a common challenge in depression treatment. Group EFEIs also provide opportunities for interpersonal learning and skill development that may not be available in individual formats. Participants can practice emotional expression and regulation skills in a supportive social context, receive feedback and validation from peers, and develop enhanced social confidence and communication abilities. These interpersonal benefits may be particularly valuable given the social difficulties often associated with depression.

However, group interventions also present challenges that must be carefully managed. Some individuals may feel uncomfortable with group participation due to social anxiety, shame, or privacy concerns. Group dynamics can be complex and may require skilled facilitation to ensure that all participants feel safe, included, and supported (Rosenbaum et al., 2014). Individual EFEIs offer advantages in terms of personalization, privacy, and flexibility. Individual sessions can be tailored more precisely to address specific therapeutic needs, accommodate individual preferences and limitations, and provide focused attention to personal goals and challenges. Some individuals may feel more comfortable exploring emotional content in a private setting, particularly in the early stages of treatment when shame and self-criticism may be prominent.

Table 4. Implementation models for EFEIs

Feature	Group-Based EFEIs	Individual EFEIs
Social Interaction	High - peer support, shared experience	Low - more private setting
Customization	Limited to group needs	Fully personalized
Motivation	Enhanced via accountability	Self-driven
Cost-Effectiveness	Generally higher	Lower scalability
Emotional Safety	May require skilled facilitation	Easier to maintain privacy

5.2 Professional Training and Qualifications

The successful implementation of EFEIs requires appropriately trained professionals who possess competencies spanning both exercise science and mental health domains (Rosenbaum et al., 2014). This interdisciplinary requirement presents both opportunities and challenges for professional development and service delivery. Ideally, EFEI facilitators would possess formal training in both exercise physiology/kinesiology and mental health/counseling, but such dual-qualified professionals are relatively rare. More commonly, EFEIs are delivered by professionals with primary training in one domain who have received additional training in the other area, or through interdisciplinary teams that combine complementary expertise.

Exercise professionals seeking to deliver EFEIs require additional training in mental health awareness, depression recognition and response, emotional processing techniques, group facilitation skills, and crisis intervention. This training should include understanding of depression symptoms and their impact on exercise participation, techniques for creating psychologically safe exercise environments, and knowledge of when to refer participants for additional mental health support. Mental health professionals interested in incorporating EFEIs into their practice require training in exercise science fundamentals, movement techniques and safety considerations, and the integration of physical activity with therapeutic interventions. This training should emphasize practical skills for leading movement activities, understanding of exercise physiology and adaptation principles, and knowledge of how to modify activities for diverse physical capabilities and health conditions.

5.3 Recommended Duration, Frequency, and Progression

The optimal dosage and progression of EFEIs represents an important implementation consideration that affects both therapeutic outcomes and practical feasibility (Noetel et al., 2024). Current research provides guidance regarding exercise prescription for depression, with most studies finding optimal effects with moderate-intensity exercise performed 3-4 times per week for 45-60 minutes per session, delivered over 8-16 weeks. However, EFEIs may require modifications to these parameters to accommodate their additional emotional processing components and ensure adequate time for reflection and integration. A typical EFEI program might involve sessions of 75-90 minutes duration to allow adequate time for physical activity, emotional processing, and group discussion or individual reflection.

Frequency recommendations for EFEIs may vary based on the specific population and setting, but most programs implement 2-3 sessions per week to balance therapeutic intensity with practical feasibility. This frequency allows for regular therapeutic contact and skill development while providing adequate recovery time between sessions. The duration of EFEI programs typically ranges from 8-16 weeks, similar to other structured interventions for depression. This timeframe allows for gradual skill development, relationship building (in group formats), and the establishment of sustainable patterns that can continue beyond the formal program period.

5.4 Challenges in Clinical Settings

The implementation of EFEIs in clinical settings presents various challenges that must be addressed to ensure successful program delivery and sustainability (Rosenbaum et al., 2014). These challenges span logistical, professional, financial, and systemic domains. Space and equipment requirements represent significant logistical challenges for many clinical settings. EFEIs require adequate space for movement activities, appropriate flooring and safety features, and access to basic exercise equipment. Many traditional mental health settings are not designed to accommodate physical activity programs, requiring either facility modifications or alternative venue arrangements.

Professional workforce challenges include the limited availability of dual-trained professionals and the need for ongoing professional development to maintain competencies in both exercise science and mental health domains. Training and certification programs for EFEI delivery are still emerging, creating challenges for establishing consistent quality standards and professional credentials. Financial and reimbursement challenges may limit the sustainability and accessibility of EFEI programs. Traditional healthcare reimbursement systems may not recognize or adequately compensate for integrated exercise-mental health interventions, requiring alternative funding mechanisms or fee structures. Systemic challenges include the need for interdisciplinary collaboration and communication between exercise professionals and mental health providers, integration with existing treatment pathways and referral systems, and development of appropriate outcome measurement and evaluation protocols.

6. CASE STUDIES AND APPLIED MODELS

6.1 Individual Recovery Through Structured EFEIs

Sarah, a 34-year-old marketing professional, presented with major depressive disorder following a series of personal and professional setbacks. She exhibited classic symptoms including persistent low mood, anhedonia, fatigue, and severely diminished self-esteem. Traditional cognitive-behavioral therapy had provided modest improvements, but Sarah continued to struggle with emotional numbness and a profound sense of disconnection from her body and emotions (Rosenbaum et al., 2014). Sarah enrolled in a 12-week individual EFEI program that combined moderate-intensity aerobic exercise with mindfulness-based emotional processing techniques (Goyal et al., 2014). Sessions were conducted twice weekly for 90 minutes each, beginning with 20 minutes of mindful movement warm-up, followed by 40 minutes of varied aerobic activities (walking, cycling, dance), and concluding with 30 minutes of reflection and journaling.

The initial phase focused on establishing body awareness and emotional recognition (Price & Thompson, 2007). Sarah learned to notice physical sensations during exercise and began connecting these sensations with emotional states. Through guided reflection, she discovered that her numbness was actually a protective mechanism against overwhelming emotions that had been suppressed following her recent losses. By week 6, Sarah reported significant improvements in her ability to identify and express emotions. The physical movement seemed to unlock emotional material that had been inaccessible through verbal therapy alone (Price & Thompson, 2007). Her exercise capacity steadily improved, providing concrete evidence of her growing strength and capability that directly challenged her negative self-perceptions (Rosenbaum et al., 2014). The final phase emphasized integration and skill consolidation. Sarah developed a personal movement practice that she could continue independently, incorporating specific exercises that had proven most effective for emotional regulation (Goyal et al., 2014). Post-intervention assessments showed significant improvements in depression scores, self-esteem measures, and emotional regulation skills that were maintained at 6-month follow-up.

6.2 Group Cohesion and Emotional Bonding in Community EFEIs

A community mental health center implemented a group-based EFEI program for individuals with mild to moderate depression. The program served 12 participants ranging in age from 22 to 58, with diverse backgrounds and presenting concerns. Sessions were conducted three times weekly for 10 weeks in a local community center gymnasium. The program structure emphasized both individual growth and group cohesion. Each session began with a group check-in where participants shared their current emotional state and physical sensations. This was followed by 45 minutes of varied physical activities designed to promote both individual challenge and group cooperation, including partner exercises, team-based games, and synchronized movement activities.

The group dynamic proved to be a powerful therapeutic factor. Participants developed strong supportive relationships, often continuing to meet informally between sessions. The shared experience of physical challenge and emotional exploration created bonds that extended beyond the program period. Many participants reported that the group support was as valuable as the exercise component itself, providing a sense of belonging and acceptance that had been missing from their lives (Yalom & Leszcz, 2020). Particularly notable was the development of "emotional mirroring" within the group. Participants became skilled at recognizing and responding to each other's emotional states during exercise, offering encouragement during difficult moments and celebrating achievements together. This interpersonal emotional learning appeared to enhance individual emotional regulation skills and provided a safe context for practicing vulnerability and emotional expression. Quantitative outcomes showed significant improvements in depression scores across all participants, with particularly strong effects for measures of social connectedness and self-efficacy. Qualitative feedback emphasized the value of combining physical challenge with emotional support, with many participants describing the experience as transformative in ways that previous treatments had not achieved.

6.3 School-Based EFEI Program for Adolescent Depression

A high school implemented a pilot EFEI program targeting students identified as at-risk for depression or experiencing mild depressive symptoms. The program was integrated into the physical education curriculum as an alternative track for students who might benefit from a more therapeutic approach to physical activity (Biddle & Asare, 2011). The 8-week program served 16 students aged 15-17, meeting daily during regular PE periods. Activities were adapted to be age-appropriate and engaging, incorporating contemporary music, dance elements, and technology integration through fitness tracking and mood monitoring apps. The emotional processing component was carefully designed to respect adolescent developmental needs and preferences, emphasizing peer interaction and creative expression over adult-directed reflection. Each session included 15 minutes of energizing warm-up activities, 25 minutes of varied physical challenges designed to promote both individual mastery and peer cooperation, and 10 minutes of cool-down with brief mindfulness exercises and peer check-ins. Weekly longer sessions included more extensive reflection activities such as movement journaling, creative expression through dance or movement creation, and goal-setting exercises.

The adolescent participants responded particularly well to the program's emphasis on choice and autonomy. Students were encouraged to modify activities based on their interests and comfort levels, and to take leadership roles in designing and leading certain activities. This approach aligned with developmental needs for increasing independence while still providing appropriate structure and support. Results showed significant improvements in mood, self-esteem, and academic engagement. Teachers reported that participating students demonstrated improved classroom behavior, better peer relationships, and increased participation in other school activities. The success of the pilot led to expansion of the program and integration into the school's comprehensive mental health support services.

6.4 Rehabilitation Center Integration Model

A comprehensive rehabilitation center serving individuals with co-occurring mental health and substance use disorders integrated EFEIs into their treatment programming. The center recognized that many clients experienced significant emotional regulation difficulties that traditional cognitive-behavioral approaches alone were insufficient to address (van der Kolk, 2014). The EFEI program was designed as a core component of the center's treatment model, with all clients participating in group sessions three times weekly throughout their residential stay (typically 30-90 days). Sessions were adapted to accommodate varying fitness levels, physical limitations, and trauma histories common among this population.

The program emphasized trauma-informed principles, ensuring that all activities were designed to promote safety, choice, and empowerment rather than retraumatization (van der Kolk, 2014). Activities included gentle movement options, constant choice and modification opportunities, and careful attention to triggers that might arise during physical activity or emotional processing. A key innovation was the integration of EFEIs with other treatment modalities. Morning EFEI sessions were often followed by individual therapy sessions where clients could process insights and experiences that emerged during movement activities. Group therapy sessions incorporated discussion of EFEI experiences, and clients' recovery plans included continuation of movement practices as a core relapse prevention strategy. Outcome data from the integrated model showed improved treatment completion rates, reduced relapse at 6-month follow-up, and enhanced client satisfaction compared to the center's previous treatment model. Staff reported that clients who participated in EFEIs demonstrated improved emotional regulation skills that transferred to other treatment activities and daily living situations.

Table 5. Case study summary of EFEI outcomes

Setting	Population	Program Duration	Key Outcomes
Individual Recovery	Adult with MDD	12 weeks, 2x/ week	↑ mood, ↑ self-esteem, improved emotional regulation
Community Group	Adults with mild-moderate depression	10 weeks, 3x/ week	↑ social connection, ↑ self-efficacy
School-Based	Adolescents at-risk for depression	8 weeks, daily sessions	↑ mood, ↑ academic engagement
Rehabilitation Center	Dual-diagnosis patients	30–90 days, 3x/ week	↑ treatment completion, ↓ relapse rates

7. FUTURE DIRECTIONS AND RECOMMENDATIONS

7.1 Integration with Existing Therapy Models

The future of EFEIs lies in their thoughtful integration with established therapeutic modalities rather than as standalone interventions (Rosenbaum et al., 2014). Research suggests that combining exercise with traditional psychotherapy may produce synergistic effects that exceed the benefits of either approach alone. The integration of EFEIs with cognitive-behavioral therapy represents a particularly promising direction, as the two approaches address complementary aspects of depression through different but compatible mechanisms. CBT-EFEI integration might involve using movement experiences to challenge negative thought patterns, employing physical mastery experiences to build self-efficacy, and utilizing embodied awareness to enhance cognitive restructuring processes (King, 2002). For example, clients might engage in progressive physical challenges while practicing cognitive techniques for managing self-doubt and negative self-talk. The immediate feedback provided by physical activity can make abstract cognitive concepts more concrete and personally meaningful.

Integration with acceptance and commitment therapy (ACT) represents another promising direction (Hayes et al., 2006). ACT's emphasis on psychological flexibility, values-based living, and mindful awareness aligns naturally with EFEI principles. Movement activities can serve as vehicles for practicing acceptance of difficult emotions, exploring personal values through embodied experiences, and developing psychological flexibility through adaptation to physical challenges. Trauma-informed integration represents a crucial consideration given the high prevalence of trauma histories among individuals with depression (van der Kolk, 2014). EFEIs must be carefully adapted to ensure safety and empowerment rather than retraumatization. This might involve emphasis on choice and control, gentle movement options, trauma-sensitive language and instruction, and integration with trauma-specific therapies such as EMDR or trauma-focused CBT.

7.2 Technology Integration and Virtual Delivery

The COVID-19 pandemic has accelerated the development of digital mental health interventions, creating new opportunities for EFEI delivery through technology platforms (Rauschenberg et al., 2021). Virtual EFEIs offer potential advantages including increased accessibility, reduced barriers to participation, and integration with digital health monitoring and feedback systems. Virtual reality (VR) technologies present particularly exciting possibilities for EFEI delivery (Colombo et al., 2021). VR environments can provide immersive movement experiences that combine physical activity with emotional exploration in ways that may not be possible in traditional settings. For example, participants might engage in virtual hiking experiences while practicing mindfulness techniques, or explore expressive movement in fantastical environments that facilitate emotional expression and creativity.

Mobile health (mHealth) applications can support EFEI delivery through features such as mood and activity tracking, guided movement instruction, mindfulness exercise libraries, and peer support platforms (Firth et al., 2017). These tools can extend the benefits of formal EFEI programs by providing ongoing support, practice opportunities, and progress monitoring between sessions. However, technology integration must be carefully designed to preserve the essential elements of EFEIs, particularly the therapeutic relationship and emotional processing components that may be difficult to replicate in digital formats. Hybrid models combining in-person and digital delivery may offer optimal approaches that maximize both accessibility and therapeutic effectiveness.

7.3 Research Needs and Clinical Validations

Despite growing evidence for exercise interventions in depression treatment, specific research on EFEIs as defined in this chapter remains limited (Kandola et al., 2019). Future research priorities should include large-scale randomized controlled trials comparing EFEIs to standard treatments, investigation of optimal dosage and delivery parameters, identification of mechanisms of action, and examination of long-term outcomes and maintenance effects. Mechanistic research is particularly needed to understand how the integration of emotional processing with physical activity enhances therapeutic outcomes beyond exercise alone (Kandola et al., 2019). This research might employ neuroimaging techniques to examine brain changes associated with EFEI participation, psychophysiological measures to assess stress and emotion regulation improvements, and qualitative methods to understand participants' subjective experiences and meaning-making processes.

Research on individual differences and treatment matching represents another priority area. Not all individuals may respond equally to EFEIs, and identifying factors that predict treatment response could improve outcomes through personalized intervention approaches (Noetel et al., 2024). Factors such as personality characteristics, trauma history, physical fitness level, and depression subtypes may all influence EFEI effectiveness. Implementation research is crucial for translating EFEI research findings into real-world practice settings (Proctor et al., 2011). This research should examine barriers and facilitators to EFEI implementation, develop training and certification protocols for delivery providers, create cost-effectiveness models, and establish quality assurance and fidelity monitoring procedures.

7.4 Policy and Healthcare System Integration

The integration of EFEIs into healthcare systems requires policy developments that support interdisciplinary collaboration, recognize exercise-based mental health interventions, and provide appropriate reimbursement mechanisms (Rosenbaum et al., 2014). Current healthcare policies often create artificial separations between physical and mental health services that can impede the implementation of integrated interventions like EFEIs. Healthcare reimbursement systems need to evolve to recognize and support exercise-based mental health interventions delivered by appropriately trained professionals (Rosenbaum et al., 2014). This may require development of new billing codes, recognition of exercise professionals as mental health service providers, and evidence-based guidelines for EFEI prescription and delivery.

Professional education and training systems need to adapt to support the interdisciplinary competencies required for EFEI delivery. This might involve development of dual-degree programs combining exercise science and mental health training, continuing education programs for existing professionals, and interprofessional education initiatives that bring together students from different disciplines. Quality standards and professional guidelines need to be established to ensure safe and effective EFEI delivery (Rosenbaum et al., 2014). This includes development of competency standards for EFEI providers, practice guidelines for different populations and settings, and outcome measurement protocols that capture both physical and mental health benefits.

8. CONCLUSION

This comprehensive examination of EFEIs reveals a promising therapeutic approach that addresses critical gaps in current depression treatment. The theoretical foundation of EFEIs rests on robust neurobiological evidence, including BDNF-mediated neuroplasticity, neurotransmitter modulation, and HPA axis regulation. When physical activity is combined with intentional emotional processing, these mechanisms appear to produce enhanced therapeutic outcomes for mood enhancement and self-esteem restoration.

The empirical evidence, though still emerging, demonstrates consistent benefits across diverse populations. Meta-analyses reveal effect sizes ranging from moderate-to-large for various EFEI modalities, with improvements in depression, self-esteem, and emotional regulation that are comparable to established treatments. Particularly notable are the strong effects observed for dance and expressive movement, as well as yoga interventions, suggesting that activities naturally incorporating emotional expression may offer unique therapeutic advantages.

The case studies presented illustrate EFEIs' versatility and effectiveness across settings. Individual programs demonstrated sustained improvements in mood and emotional regulation at 6-month follow-up. Group interventions produced not only symptom reduction but enhanced social connectedness, addressing the isolation central to depression. School-based programs showed promise for early intervention, while rehabilitation center integration improved treatment retention and reduced relapse rates. These real-world applications confirm that EFEIs can be successfully adapted while maintaining therapeutic efficacy.

Implementation considerations reveal both opportunities and challenges. The interdisciplinary nature of EFEIs requires professionals with competencies spanning exercise science and mental health, necessitating specialized training protocols and quality standards. However, the flexibility of EFEIs allows adaptation across diverse settings, from individual therapy to community programs, making them particularly valuable for expanding access to depression treatment in resource-limited contexts.

Critical research priorities include large-scale randomized controlled trials comparing EFEIs to exercise-only and therapy-only conditions, mechanistic studies examining how emotional processing enhances exercise's neurobiological effects, and development of standardized protocols and fidelity measures. Investigation of optimal dosing parameters, predictors of treatment response, and long-term maintenance strategies will be essential for maximizing therapeutic effectiveness.

The clinical implications of EFEIs are substantial. For individuals with depression, EFEIs offer an empowering alternative or complement to traditional treatments, particularly for those who have not responded adequately to medication or psychotherapy alone. The emphasis on mastery experiences, body awareness, and emotional expression through movement provides unique pathways to recovery that may be especially valuable for individuals experiencing emotional numbness or disconnection from their bodies.

For practitioners, EFEIs provide a structured framework for incorporating physical activity into mental health treatment beyond simple exercise prescription. The explicit focus on emotional awareness and processing during movement creates opportunities for therapeutic breakthroughs that may not emerge through verbal processing alone. The group format offers additional benefits through peer support and social connection, addressing multiple dimensions of depression simultaneously.

EFEIs represent an evidence-informed evolution in depression treatment that leverages the interconnection between body and mind. As research validation continues and implementation models mature, EFEIs have the potential to become an integral component of comprehensive depression care. The challenge now lies in translating this potential into accessible, sustainable programs that can benefit the millions affected by depression worldwide. The ultimate measure of success will be not merely symptom reduction, but the restoration of vitality, connection, and meaning that enables individuals to move, literally and figuratively, toward fuller engagement with life.

REFERENCES

Aldao, A., Nolen-Hoeksema, S., & Schweizer, S. (2010). Emotion-regulation strategies across psychopathology: A meta-analytic review. *Clinical Psychology Review, 30*(2), 217–237. DOI: 10.1016/j.cpr.2009.11.004 PMID: 20015584

Bandura, A. (1997). *Self-Efficacy: The Exercise of Control.* Worth Publishers.

Barton, J., & Pretty, J. (2010). What is the best dose of nature and green exercise for improving mental health? A multi-study analysis. *Environmental Science & Technology, 44*(10), 3947–3955. DOI: 10.1021/es903183r PMID: 20337470

Bathina, S., & Das, U. N. (2015). Brain-derived neurotrophic factor and its clinical implications. *Archives of Medical Science : AMS, 11*(6), 1164–1178. DOI: 10.5114/aoms.2015.56342 PMID: 26788077

Biddle, S. J. H., & Asare, M. (2011). Physical activity and mental health in children and adolescents: A review of reviews. *British Journal of Sports Medicine, 45*(11), 886–895. DOI: 10.1136/bjsports-2011-090185 PMID: 21807669

Colombo, D., Díaz-García, A., Fernandez-Álvarez, J., & Botella, C. (2021). Virtual reality for the enhancement of emotion regulation. *Clinical Psychology & Psychotherapy, 28*(3), 519–537. DOI: 10.1002/cpp.2618 PMID: 34048621

Cramer, H., Lauche, R., Anheyer, D., Pilkington, K., de Manincor, M., Dobos, G., & Ward, L. (2018). Yoga for anxiety: A systematic review and meta-analysis of randomized controlled trials. *Depression and Anxiety, 35*(9), 830–843. DOI: 10.1002/da.22762 PMID: 29697885

Cramer, H., Lauche, R., Langhorst, J., & Dobos, G. (2013). Yoga for depression: A systematic review and meta-analysis. *Depression and Anxiety, 30*(11), 1068–1083. DOI: 10.1002/da.22166 PMID: 23922209

Cuijpers, P., Karyotaki, E., Weitz, E., Andersson, G., Hollon, S. D., & van Straten, A. (2014). The effects of psychotherapies for major depression in adults on remission, recovery and improvement: A meta-analysis. *Journal of Affective Disorders, 159*, 118–126. DOI: 10.1016/j.jad.2014.02.026 PMID: 24679399

Damasio, A. (1999). The feeling of what happens: Body and emotion in the making of consciousness (pp. xiv, 386). Harcourt College Publishers.

Dunn, B. D., Galton, H. C., Morgan, R., Evans, D., Oliver, C., Meyer, M., Cusack, R., Lawrence, A. D., & Dalgleish, T. (2010). Listening to your heart. How interoception shapes emotion experience and intuitive decision making. *Psychological Science*, *21*(12), 1835–1844. DOI: 10.1177/0956797610389191 PMID: 21106893

Firth, J., Torous, J., Nicholas, J., Carney, R., Pratap, A., Rosenbaum, S., & Sarris, J. (2017). The efficacy of smartphone-based mental health interventions for depressive symptoms: A meta-analysis of randomized controlled trials. *World Psychiatry; Official Journal of the World Psychiatric Association (WPA)*, *16*(3), 287–298. DOI: 10.1002/wps.20472 PMID: 28941113

Garfinkel, S. N., Seth, A. K., Barrett, A. B., Suzuki, K., & Critchley, H. D. (2015). Knowing your own heart: Distinguishing interoceptive accuracy from interoceptive awareness. *Biological Psychology*, *104*, 65–74. DOI: 10.1016/j.biopsycho.2014.11.004 PMID: 25451381

Gordon, B. R., McDowell, C. P., Hallgren, M., Meyer, J. D., Lyons, M., & Herring, M. P. (2018). Association of Efficacy of Resistance Exercise Training With Depressive Symptoms: Meta-analysis and Meta-regression Analysis of Randomized Clinical Trials. *JAMA Psychiatry*, *75*(6), 566–576. DOI: 10.1001/jamapsychiatry.2018.0572 PMID: 29800984

Goyal, M., Singh, S., Sibinga, E. M. S., Gould, N. F., Rowland-Seymour, A., Sharma, R., Berger, Z., Sleicher, D., Maron, D. D., Shihab, H. M., Ranasinghe, P. D., Linn, S., Saha, S., Bass, E. B., & Haythornthwaite, J. A. (2014). Meditation programs for psychological stress and well-being: A systematic review and meta-analysis. *JAMA Internal Medicine*, *174*(3), 357–368. DOI: 10.1001/jamainternmed.2013.13018 PMID: 24395196

Greenberg, L. S. (2015). Emotion-focused therapy: Coaching clients to work through their feelings, 2nd ed (pp. vi, 411). American Psychological Association. https://doi.org/DOI: 10.1037/14692-000

Gross, J. J. (2002). Emotion regulation: Affective, cognitive, and social consequences. *Psychophysiology*, *39*(3), 281–291. DOI: 10.1017/s0048577201393198 PMID: 12212647

Hayes, S. C., Luoma, J. B., Bond, F. W., Masuda, A., & Lillis, J. (2006). Acceptance and commitment therapy: Model, processes and outcomes. *Behaviour Research and Therapy*, *44*(1), 1–25. DOI: 10.1016/j.brat.2005.06.006 PMID: 16300724

Joormann, J., & Stanton, C. H. (2016). Examining emotion regulation in depression: A review and future directions. *Behaviour Research and Therapy*, *86*, 35–49. DOI: 10.1016/j.brat.2016.07.007 PMID: 27492851

Kabat-Zinn, J. (2003). Mindfulness-Based Interventions in Context: Past, Present, and Future. *Clinical Psychology : a Publication of the Division of Clinical Psychology of the American Psychological Association, 10*, 144–156. DOI: 10.1093/clipsy.bpg016

Kandola, A., Ashdown-Franks, G., Hendrikse, J., Sabiston, C. M., & Stubbs, B. (2019). Physical activity and depression: Towards understanding the antidepressant mechanisms of physical activity. *Neuroscience and Biobehavioral Reviews, 107*, 525–539. DOI: 10.1016/j.neubiorev.2019.09.040 PMID: 31586447

Karkou, V., Aithal, S., Zubala, A., & Meekums, B. (2019). Effectiveness of Dance Movement Therapy in the Treatment of Adults With Depression: A Systematic Review With Meta-Analyses. *Frontiers in Psychology, 10*, 936. DOI: 10.3389/fpsyg.2019.00936 PMID: 31130889

King, R. (2002). Cognitive therapy of depression. *The Australian and New Zealand Journal of Psychiatry, 36*(2), 272–275. DOI: 10.1046/j.1440-1614.2002.t01-4-01015.x PMID: 11982560

Malhi, G. S., & Mann, J. J. (2018). Depression. *Lancet, 392*(10161), 2299–2312. DOI: 10.1016/S0140-6736(18)31948-2 PMID: 30396512

Noetel, M., Sanders, T., Gallardo-Gómez, D., Taylor, P., Del Pozo Cruz, B., van den Hoek, D., Smith, J. J., Mahoney, J., Spathis, J., Moresi, M., Pagano, R., Pagano, L., Vasconcellos, R., Arnott, H., Varley, B., Parker, P., Biddle, S., & Lonsdale, C. (2024). Effect of exercise for depression: Systematic review and network meta-analysis of randomised controlled trials. *BMJ (Clinical Research Ed.), 384*, e075847. DOI: 10.1136/bmj-2023-075847 PMID: 38355154

Pariante, C. M., & Lightman, S. L. (2008). The HPA axis in major depression: Classical theories and new developments. *Trends in Neurosciences, 31*(9), 464–468. DOI: 10.1016/j.tins.2008.06.006 PMID: 18675469

Paulus, D. J., Gallagher, M. W., Bartlett, B. A., Tran, J., & Vujanovic, A. A. (2018). The unique and interactive effects of anxiety sensitivity and emotion dysregulation in relation to posttraumatic stress, depressive, and anxiety symptoms among trauma-exposed firefighters. *Comprehensive Psychiatry, 84*, 54–61. DOI: 10.1016/j.comppsych.2018.03.012 PMID: 29694933

Pennebaker, J. W., & Chung, C. K. (2011). Expressive writing: Connections to physical and mental health. In *The Oxford handbook of health psychology* (pp. 417–437). Oxford University Press.

Price, C. J., & Thompson, E. A. (2007). Measuring dimensions of body connection: Body awareness and bodily dissociation. *Journal of Alternative and Complementary Medicine (New York, N.Y.), 13*(9), 945–953. DOI: 10.1089/acm.2007.0537 PMID: 18047441

Proctor, E., Silmere, H., Raghavan, R., Hovmand, P., Aarons, G., Bunger, A., Griffey, R., & Hensley, M. (2011). Outcomes for implementation research: Conceptual distinctions, measurement challenges, and research agenda. *Administration and Policy in Mental Health, 38*(2), 65–76. DOI: 10.1007/s10488-010-0319-7 PMID: 20957426

Pruessner, L., Barnow, S., Holt, D. V., Joormann, J., & Schulze, K. (2020). A cognitive control framework for understanding emotion regulation flexibility. *Emotion (Washington, D.C.), 20*(1), 21–29. DOI: 10.1037/emo0000658 PMID: 31961173

Rauschenberg, C., Schick, A., Hirjak, D., Seidler, A., Paetzold, I., Apfelbacher, C., Riedel-Heller, S. G., & Reininghaus, U. (2021). Evidence Synthesis of Digital Interventions to Mitigate the Negative Impact of the COVID-19 Pandemic on Public Mental Health: Rapid Meta-review. *Journal of Medical Internet Research, 23*(3), e23365. DOI: 10.2196/23365 PMID: 33606657

Rosenbaum, S., Tiedemann, A., Sherrington, C., Curtis, J., & Ward, P. B. (2014). Physical activity interventions for people with mental illness: A systematic review and meta-analysis. *The Journal of Clinical Psychiatry, 75*(9), 964–974. DOI: 10.4088/JCP.13r08765 PMID: 24813261

Salamone, J. D., Correa, M., Farrar, A., & Mingote, S. M. (2007). Effort-related functions of nucleus accumbens dopamine and associated forebrain circuits. *Psychopharmacology, 191*(3), 461–482. DOI: 10.1007/s00213-006-0668-9 PMID: 17225164

Schuch, F. B., Vancampfort, D., Richards, J., Rosenbaum, S., Ward, P. B., & Stubbs, B. (2016). Exercise as a treatment for depression: A meta-analysis adjusting for publication bias. *Journal of Psychiatric Research, 77*, 42–51. DOI: 10.1016/j.jpsychires.2016.02.023 PMID: 26978184

Singh, B., Olds, T., Curtis, R., Dumuid, D., Virgara, R., Watson, A., Szeto, K., O'Connor, E., Ferguson, T., Eglitis, E., Miatke, A., Simpson, C. E., & Maher, C. (2023). Effectiveness of physical activity interventions for improving depression, anxiety and distress: An overview of systematic reviews. *British Journal of Sports Medicine, 57*(18), 1203–1209. DOI: 10.1136/bjsports-2022-106195 PMID: 36796860

van der Kolk, B. A. (2014). The body keeps the score: Brain, mind, and body in the healing of trauma (pp. xvi, 443). Viking.

World Health Organization. (2023). Depressive disorder (depression). https://www.who.int/news-room/fact-sheets/detail/depression

Yalom, I. D., & Leszcz, M. (2020). *The theory and practice of group psychotherapy* (6th ed.). Basic Books.

Young, S. N. (2007). How to increase serotonin in the human brain without drugs. *Journal of Psychiatry & Neuroscience : JPN, 32*(6), 394–399. PMID: 18043762

Zhang, D., Lee, E. K. P., Mak, E. C. W., Ho, C. Y., & Wong, S. Y. S. (2021). Mindfulness-based interventions: An overall review. *British Medical Bulletin*, •••, ldab005. Advance online publication. DOI: 10.1093/bmb/ldab005 PMID: 33884400

Chapter 3
Neurobiological Effects of Exercise on Emotional Regulation in Bipolar Disorder

Shivam Kumar
https://orcid.org/0009-0005-4315-5883
Maharishi Markandeshwar Institute of Physiotherapy and Rehabilitation, India

Jatin Sangwan
Maharishi Markandeshwar Institute of Physiotherapy and Rehabilitation, India

Urvashi
Maharishi Markandeshwar Institute of Physiotherapy and Rehabilitation, India

Lakshay Panchal
https://orcid.org/0009-0005-2296-1800
Maharishi Markandeshwar Institute of Physiotherapy and Rehabilitation, India

Shivangi
Maharishi Markandeshwar Institute of Physiotherapy and Rehabilitation, India

ABSTRACT

Bipolar disorder is a complex, chronic psychiatric condition, often accompanied by persistent emotional instability. It affects over 46 million people worldwide. Current management involves a combination of pharmacotherapy and psychosocial interventions. While these approaches are effective in reducing symptoms and preventing relapse, many patients continue to experience subthreshold mood fluctuations, cognitive impairments, or reduced quality of life. Moreover, issues such

DOI: 10.4018/979-8-3373-6157-4.ch003

as variable adherence and incomplete symptom remission underscore the need for complementary treatment. Exercise has emerged as one such promising strategy, not merely as a behavioral lifestyle recommendation, but as a biologically active intervention with the potential to alter brain function. Mounting evidence suggests that physical activity influences neurochemical systems, such as dopamine, serotonin, brain-derived neurotrophic factor, and endocannabinoids, all of which play essential roles in mood regulation and cognitive-emotional processing.

INTRODUCTION

1.1 The Burden of Bipolar Disorder and Emotional Dysregulation

Bipolar disorder (BD) is a severe, chronic psychiatric condition characterized by recurrent episodes of mania, hypomania, and depression, often alternating with periods of partial or full remission (Phillips & Kupfer, 2013). Its global lifetime prevalence ranges between 0.6% and 2.4%, placing a substantial burden on public health systems (Merikangas et al., 2011). BD extends beyond mood symptoms; it is a multisystem disorder associated with increased risks of cardiovascular disease, diabetes, and immune and endocrine dysfunction (Muneer, 2016). The psychosocial impact is profound, patients often experience persistent functional impairment, including difficulties in employment, social relationships, and elevated risk of self-harm or suicide (Strakowski et al., 2012).

Crucially, many individuals with BD exhibit enduring difficulties with emotion regulation, which further worsen daily functioning. Systematic reviews confirm that emotion dysregulation may persist even during euthymia, suggesting a stable trait component in BD (De Prisco et al., 2022). Additionally, there is a tendency toward using maladaptive emotion regulation strategies such as rumination and suppression, which are associated with increased mood instability (Koenders et al., 2020).

1.2 Neurobiological Underpinnings of Bipolar Disorder

BD is marked by complex changes in mood, energy, and cognition, driven by widespread dysregulation in neural circuits and molecular signaling. Neuroimaging studies consistently reveal abnormalities in fronto-limbic networks, including hyperactivation of the amygdala and hypoactivation of the prefrontal cortex, which undermine top-down regulation of affective responses (Phillips & Swartz, 2014). Structural MRI analyses show decreased hippocampal and orbitofrontal cortex volumes as well as reduced white matter integrity, indicating chronic and possibly progressive changes to brain architecture in BD (Alda & Hajek, 2015).

On a molecular level, BD is associated with recurrent neuroinflammation and oxidative stress, particularly during mood episodes. Elevated pro-inflammatory cytokines, mitochondrial dysfunction, and oxidative damage have been described, contributing to the concept of "neuroprogression"—a process whereby cumulative neurobiological injury occurs over time (Muneer, 2016). Moreover, reductions in brain-derived neurotrophic factor (BDNF) have been linked to impaired neuroplasticity and illness chronicity (Rosenblat & McIntyre, 2016).

These findings provide a foundation for understanding BD's clinical course and highlight possible neurobiological targets for novel interventions.

1.3 Neurobiological Effects of Exercise: Bridging Mood and Brain

Emerging research suggests that regular exercise can influence neurobiological mechanisms implicated in BD. In various populations, physical activity is associated with increased hippocampal volume, enhanced prefrontal activation, and improved connectivity within circuits important for emotion regulation (Revelo Herrera & Leon-Rojas, 2024; Ben Ezzdine et al., 2025). These changes are hypothesized to be mediated by upregulation of neurotrophic factors—including BDNF and vascular endothelial growth factor (VEGF)—which promote synaptic plasticity (Thomson et al., 2015).

Exercise also affects neurotransmitter systems relevant to BD: aerobic activity increases dopamine and serotonin activity and may influence gamma-aminobutyric acid (GABA) signaling, all of which plausibly contribute to improved mood and affective control (Muneer, 2016; Smith & Merwin, 2021). Exercise further reduces systemic inflammation and oxidative stress, mechanisms believed to contribute to mood instability and disease progression (Rosenblat & McIntyre, 2016).

While most mechanistic research derives from depression and non-BD cohorts, pilot studies in BD show that structured exercise may improve cognition and reduce residual mood symptoms (Sylvia et al., 2013a; Firth et al., 2020). Therefore, exercise appears to be a biologically plausible adjunctive intervention targeting neural dysfunctions common in BD, though further BD-specific research is needed.

1.4 Linking Exercise to Emotional Regulation in Bipolar Disorder

Emotion regulation (ER) deficits are recognized as a core feature of BD, present across mood states and contributing to long-term functional disability (De Prisco et al., 2022). Individuals with BD often utilize maladaptive regulation strategies, such as rumination and suppression, and underuse adaptive strategies like cognitive reappraisal—patterns linked to atypical activation of prefrontal and limbic regions.

Evidence, particularly from anxiety and depressive disorder populations, indicates that physical activity encourages greater use of adaptive ER strategies and reduces reliance on maladaptive patterns (Smith & Merwin, 2021). In BD specifically, preliminary work suggests aerobic exercise may improve affective control, potentially via enhanced prefrontal regulation of limbic responses and decreased amygdala hyperreactivity (Ben Ezzdine et al., 2025). These effects may foster long-term emotional resilience by promoting cognitive flexibility and neurobiological adaptation. However, more direct trials in BD are required to confirm these mechanisms.

2. NEUROBIOLOGY OF BIPOLAR DISORDER AND MODULATORY EFFECTS OF EXERCISE

2.1 Neurobiological Dysregulation in Bipolar Disorder: From Circuits to Symptoms

Bipolar disorder (BD) is marked by widespread dysregulation in brain networks governing mood, cognition, and emotional regulation. Neuroimaging repeatedly identifies structural and functional alterations in the prefrontal cortex (PFC), anterior cingulate cortex (ACC), amygdala, hippocampus, and basal ganglia—all of which are pivotal for executive control and affect regulation (Phillips & Swartz, 2014; Muneer, 2016). In particular, hyperactivation of the amygdala and under activation of ventrolateral and dorsolateral regions of the PFC are associated with heightened emotional reactivity and compromised top-down regulation, correlating clinically with mood swings and emotional dysregulation.

At the neurotransmitter level, BD features persistent abnormalities in monoamine signaling—including serotonin, dopamine, and norepinephrine circuits—which underlie phase-dependent mood states such as mania and depression (Machado-Vieira et al., 2017). Chronic mood episodes are linked to "neuroprogression," involving gradual loss of gray matter and synaptic connectivity (Berk et al., 2017). The hypothalamic-pituitary-adrenal (HPA) axis is also disrupted, contributing to elevated cortisol, increased stress vulnerability, and further mood instability (Belvederi Murri et al., 2016).

This integration of circuit, chemical, and endocrine dysregulation establishes the foundation for BD's episodic nature and highlights targets for therapeutic interventions, such as those directed at neuroplasticity, synaptic repair, and stress-resilience mechanisms.

2.2 Exercise as a Modulator of Neural Circuits and Emotional Regulation in Bipolar Disorder

Exercise is increasingly recognized as a multi-domain modulator that intersects with the core neurobiological deficits observed in BD. Its effects span neural circuitry, neurotransmitter balance, neurotrophic support, stress-system regulation, and psychosocial mechanisms. Most evidence is drawn from depression and healthy populations, but an expanding body of BD-specific research supports many extrapolations—with noted caveats about current limitations.

2.2.1. Circuit-Level Modulation.

Aerobic exercise appears to strengthen connectivity between prefrontal control regions and limbic structures, most notably the PFC-amygdala pathways. This is associated with enhanced top-down regulation of affect and, in principle, reduced emotional hyperreactivity in disorders featuring fronto-limbic uncoupling. In BD, large-scale fMRI evidence remains limited but preliminary findings indicate exercise-induced changes in ventral PFC, amygdala, and hippocampal activity that may help normalize circuit imbalances underlying mood instability (Phillips & Swartz, 2014).

2.2.2. Neurotransmitters and Reward Pathways.

Physical activity modulates key monoamine neurotransmitter systems implicated in bipolar disorder, including dopamine, serotonin, and norepinephrine. Both acute and chronic exercise elicit increased central turnover of dopamine and serotonin, which are essential for reward processing and mood regulation (Fleshner et al., 2016; Rethorst & Trivedi, 2017). Dysregulated dopaminergic signaling is a hallmark of BD, contributing to manic and depressive episodes through altered reward circuit activity (Machado-Vieira et al., 2017). Exercise-induced enhancement of dopaminergic transmission may attenuate anhedonia and improve affective stability, although phase-specific responses remain understudied (Fleshner et al., 2016; Pinto et al., 2022). Additionally, norepinephrine modulation by exercise may underlie its anxiolytic and arousal-stabilizing effects, stabilizing energy and vigilance disruptions commonly observed in BD (Greenwood & Fleshner, 2011).

While most neurochemical evidence derives from depression and healthy cohorts, preliminary studies in BD suggest comparable neurobiological benefits warranting further clinical trials (Firth et al., 2020; Ng, Dodd, Berk, & Malhi, 2017).

2.2.3. Neurotrophic and Structural Effects.

Regular exercise increases peripheral markers of neurotrophic support, including brain-derived neurotrophic factor (BDNF) and insulin-like growth factor-1 (IGF-1), and is linked to modest hippocampal volumetric gains and improved executive function in clinical samples (Revelo Herrera & Leon-Rojas, 2024; Melo et al., 2016). BDNF serves as a key mediator of neuronal survival, synaptic remodeling, and neuroplasticity, making it particularly relevant for psychiatric conditions characterized by impaired neural connectivity (Fernandes et al., 2015).

In bipolar disorder specifically, reduced BDNF levels have been consistently documented during acute mood episodes, with normalization occurring during euthymia and following effective treatment (Fernandes et al., 2015; Pérez-Rodríguez et al., 2021). Exercise interventions in BD populations demonstrate significant increases in peripheral BDNF levels, particularly following aerobic training protocols (Gomes et al., 2021; Teixeira et al., 2021). However, current BD studies remain underpowered, and claims of complete "normalization" of neurotrophic deficits should be interpreted cautiously given the preliminary nature of existing evidence.

The mechanistic pathway appears to involve exercise-induced upregulation of peroxisome proliferator-activated receptor gamma coactivator 1-alpha (PGC-1α) and FNDC5, muscle-derived proteins that regulate BDNF expression in hippocampal regions. This exercise-BDNF pathway shares similarities with antidepressant mechanisms, suggesting potential synergistic effects when combined with pharmacotherapy, though phase-specific responses in BD require further investigation.

2.2.4. Stress and HPA Axis Regulation.

Exercise modulates the hypothalamic-pituitary-adrenal axis and stress responsivity, typically producing improved basal cortisol rhythms and greater resilience to psychosocial stressors (Pedersen & Saltin, 2015; Meyer et al., 2016). Meta-analytic evidence demonstrates BD is associated with significantly increased cortisol and ACTH levels, particularly during manic phases. Chronic HPA hyperactivity contributes to neuroprogression through sustained glucocorticoid exposure, impairing hippocampal neurogenesis and prefrontal-limbic connectivity. Exercise interventions appear to counteract these processes by normalizing cortisol circadian rhythms and reducing stress-induced hypercortisolemia. In BD populations, preliminary evidence suggests structured physical activity programs can improve stress reactivity. However, definitive longitudinal RCT data in BD populations remain necessary to establish optimal exercise prescriptions for HPA axis normalization.

2.2.5. Comparison with Medications and Psychotherapy.

Meta-analytic evidence shows structured exercise programs yield moderate-to-large improvements in depressive symptoms, comparable to standard antidepressant treatment and cognitive-behavioral therapy (Schuch et al., 2016; Singh et al., 2023). Network meta-analyses demonstrate no significant differences between exercise and pharmacological interventions for reducing depressive symptoms in non-severe depression.

For BD specifically, exercise functions effectively as an adjunctive strategy rather than standalone treatment. Unlike medications targeting narrow receptor systems, exercise simultaneously influences multiple therapeutic pathways including monoaminergic transmission, neurotrophic signaling, stress regulation, and inflammatory processes. While pharmacotherapy remains essential for acute stabilization, exercise offers *broad neurobiological modulation without adverse side effects.*

Taken together, aerobic and resistance exercise should be viewed as integral interventions capable of targeting the *core pathophysiology of BD*. Their combined capacity to restore neural connectivity, normalize neurotransmission, enhance trophic support, and regulate stress systems underscores their translational relevance for clinical practice.

Below is a revised summary of representative clinical studies and reviews, highlighting exercise types and neurobiological, cognitive, and emotional outcomes for BD populations.

Table 1. Empirical evidence on exercise interventions in bipolar disorder: effects on neurobiological mechanisms and clinical outcomes

Author & Year	Exercise Type	Duration & Frequency	Sample Size	Key Outcomes (Mood, Cognition, Biomarkers)
Sylvia et al., 2013a (pilot study)	Aerobic exercise (walking, cycling)	12 weeks, 3x/ week, 40 min	n=40 BD patients	↓ depressive symptoms, ↑ functioning, ↑ QoL
Ng et al., 2017	Mind-body (yoga, tai chi)	8 weeks, 2–3x/ week	n=60 (BD I & II)	↓ anxiety, ↑ emotional regulation, mild mood stabilization
Melo et al., 2016	Aerobic treadmill training	12 weeks, 2x/ week, 45 min	n=25 BD patients	↑ cognitive flexibility/ memory, ↑ hippocampal volume (MRI)
Mota-Pereira et al., 2019	Resistance training + aerobic mix	16 weeks, 3x/ week	n=50 BD II patients	↓ fatigue, ↑ executive function, ↑ sleep regulation

continued on following page

Table 1. Continued

Author & Year	Exercise Type	Duration & Frequency	Sample Size	Key Outcomes (Mood, Cognition, Biomarkers)
Gomes et al., 2021	Aerobic intervention	10 weeks, 4x/ week, 30 min	n= 38 BD patients	↑ BDNF, ↓ IL-6 & CRP, mood stabilization
De Prisco et al., 2022 (review/meta-analysis)	Mixed exercise modalities	Varies across studies	28 studies, >500 participants	Overall: ↑ emotion regulation, ↓ maladaptive strategies

As summarized in Table 1, aerobic and resistance exercise interventions consistently enhance neurotrophic support and regulate inflammation in bipolar disorder, notably through increases in brain-derived neurotrophic factor (BDNF) and reductions in pro-inflammatory cytokines (Gomes et al., 2021; Melo et al., 2016). These biological improvements are accompanied by gains in sleep quality, executive functioning, and mood stabilization, demonstrating the multifaceted benefits of exercise (Mota-Pereira et al., 2019; Sylvia et al., 2013a). The convergence of findings from pilot trials and larger controlled studies underscores exercise not merely as an adjunct but as a promising mechanistic treatment targeting the dysregulated neurobiological pathways outlined in Sections 2.1 and 2.2. This evidence supports further rigorous randomized controlled trials to establish exercise as a standard integrative strategy in bipolar disorder management.

2.3 Neurotrophic and Inflammatory Modulation by Exercise

Bipolar disorder (BD) is increasingly recognized as a neuroprogressive condition characterized by diminished neuroplasticity and heightened systemic inflammation. Numerous studies have documented that individuals with BD exhibit decreased circulating levels of brain-derived neurotrophic factor (BDNF), particularly during mood episodes, alongside elevated inflammatory biomarkers such as interleukin-6 (IL-6), tumor necrosis factor-alpha (TNF-α), and C-reactive protein (CRP) (Fernandes et al., 2015; Munkholm et al., 2013; Post, 2007). These biological perturbations contribute to impaired synaptic resilience, reduced hippocampal volume, and increased vulnerability to recurrent affective episodes.

Exercise interventions, particularly aerobic and resistance training, have demonstrated significant modulation of these pathophysiological processes. Regular aerobic exercise elevates peripheral BDNF concentration, enhancing neuronal survival, synaptic remodeling, and neurogenesis within regions critical to emotional regulation such as the hippocampus and prefrontal cortex ([Thomson et al., 2015](no DOI); Wrann et al., 2013; Firth et al., 2020). In BD patients, where BDNF deficits are correlated with cognitive impairment and mood symptom severity, exercise-induced increases in BDNF may facilitate neuroplastic recovery and mood stabilization (Nguyen et al., 2022; Pérez-Rodríguez et al., 2021).

Concurrently, exercise exerts anti-inflammatory effects by modulating immune signaling pathways. Acute bouts of physical activity stimulate skeletal muscle release of IL-6, a myokine that paradoxically induces anti-inflammatory cascades by increasing interleukin-10 (IL-10) and suppressing TNF-α production (Pedersen & Saltin, 2015). Chronic exercise regimes have been associated with lower basal levels of systemic inflammatory markers, including CRP and pro-inflammatory cytokines, contributing to reduced neuroinflammation and improved neurocognitive outcomes (Paolucci et al., 2018; Rosenblat & McIntyre, 2016).

The integration of enhanced neurotrophic support and attenuated inflammation positions exercise as a multifaceted, disease-modifying adjunct in BD management. By simultaneously promoting neuroplasticity and dampening inflammatory processes, structured physical activity may mitigate neuroprogression, improve mood stability, and bolster cognitive function.

Nevertheless, exercise-related neurobiological responses are influenced by exercise modality, intensity, and duration, necessitating tailored protocols to optimize therapeutic benefits. Further longitudinal and mechanistic studies are warranted to elucidate dose-response relationships and to translate these findings into individualized clinical practice.

2.4 Neuroplasticity and Cognitive Flexibility: Role of Exercise in Bipolar Disorder

Neuroplasticity—the brain's ability to reorganize and form new synaptic connections in response to internal and external stimuli—is fundamental to emotional regulation and adaptive behavior. In bipolar disorder (BD), disruptions in synaptic plasticity are evident across multiple brain regions, notably the hippocampus and prefrontal cortex, which contribute to deficits in cognitive flexibility and maladaptive emotional responses (Post, 2007; Etkin et al., 2013; Yatham et al., 2010). These impairments manifest clinically as difficulties in mood regulation, sustaining attention, and adapting to environmental stressors, significantly impacting functional outcomes (Wingo, Ghaemi, & Post, 2010).

Exercise has emerged as a robust modulator of neuroplastic processes. Both aerobic and resistance training induce upregulation of brain-derived neurotrophic factor (BDNF)—a critical molecule for neuronal survival, synaptic remodeling, and learning (Wrann et al., 2013; Nguyen et al., 2022). Levels of BDNF in individuals with BD are frequently reduced and fluctuate with mood states, but exercise interventions have demonstrated potential for normalizing these alterations, thereby stabilizing mood cycling (Sylvia et al., 2013b; Pérez-Rodríguez et al., 2021).

From a cognitive perspective, enhanced neuroplasticity via exercise translates into improved cognitive flexibility—the capacity to shift perspectives, regulate rumination, and inhibit maladaptive thought patterns that perpetuate mood instability (Etkin et al., 2013; Post, 2007). Structured aerobic exercise programs have been consistently associated with improvements in executive functioning, working memory, and inhibitory control in BD populations (Stubbs et al., 2018; Sylvia et al., 2013b). These cognitive gains correlate with reduced relapse risk and better daily functioning, suggesting a dual therapeutic role for exercise targeting both mood and cognition.

Neuroimaging studies further support the neuroplastic benefits of exercise in BD. Functional MRI investigations reveal increased connectivity and activation within key networks disrupted in BD, including the default mode network (DMN) and frontoparietal control circuits, which are critical for cognitive processing and emotional resilience (Nguyen et al., 2022; Wingo et al., 2010). Strengthening these networks may underlie exercise's capacity to reduce rumination and improve emotional regulation.

While aerobic exercise remains the most widely studied modality, resistance training also shows promise for cognitive enhancement. Trials in psychiatric populations have demonstrated that resistance training improves executive function and psychomotor speed, possibly through mechanisms involving insulin-like growth factor 1 (IGF-1) release, which supports neuronal survival and synaptic efficiency (Zheng et al., 2016). Considering the elevated metabolic comorbidities commonly observed in BD, resistance training offers the added benefit of mitigating physical health risks alongside cognitive improvements.

In summary, exercise-induced neuroplastic adaptations represent a mechanistic link between physical activity and improved cognitive-emotional outcomes in bipolar disorder. By reinforcing synaptic plasticity and enhancing cognitive flexibility, exercise serves as both a preventive and rehabilitative adjunct, fostering resilience against relapse and promoting functional recovery. These findings advocate for the incorporation of tailored, phase-sensitive exercise protocols in comprehensive BD management plans.

2.5 Exercise-Induced Modulation of Neurobiological Mechanisms in Bipolar Disorder

Exercise exerts widespread effects across multiple neurobiological domains implicated in bipolar disorder (BD), intersecting with key pathways responsible for mood regulation, cognitive functioning, and emotional resilience. Among these, modulation of neurotransmitter systems, enhancement of neuroplasticity, regulation of the hypothalamic-pituitary-adrenal (HPA) axis, and attenuation of systemic inflammation stand out as principal mechanisms.

Dysregulation of monoaminergic neurotransmission, including serotonin, dopamine, and norepinephrine pathways, constitutes a hallmark of BD pathophysiology (Machado-Vieira et al., 2017). Aerobic and resistance exercises are known to enhance central serotonin and dopamine turnover, improving mood stability and attenuating anhedonia—a cardinal symptom of depression (Fleshner, Greenwood, & Yirmiya, 2016; Rethorst & Trivedi, 2017). Furthermore, norepinephrine modulation via exercise contributes to anxiolytic effects and regulation of arousal, facilitating improved vigilance and energy balance, which are often disrupted in BD (Greenwood & Fleshner, 2019). While most data derive from studies on depression and healthy populations, emerging evidence supports the translation of these neurochemical benefits to BD contexts, warranting further clinical investigation (Firth et al., 2020; Ng et al., 2017).

In parallel, neurotrophin signaling, principally via brain-derived neurotrophic factor (BDNF), is robustly influenced by physical activity. Increased peripheral and central BDNF levels post-exercise promote synaptic plasticity, neurogenesis, and neuronal survival, mechanisms believed to counteract neurodegenerative processes observed in BD (Pérez-Rodríguez et al., 2021; Thomson et al., 2015). This neurotrophic enhancement aligns with observed improvements in cognition and emotional regulation following exercise interventions.

Exercise also normalizes HPA axis dysregulation by stabilizing cortisol secretion patterns and reducing hypercortisolemia induced by chronic stress—a known trigger for mood episodes and rapid cycling in BD (Belvederi Murri et al., 2016). The recalibration of inhibitory connections between the amygdala and prefrontal cortex, facilitated by exercise, underpins improved stress responsivity and emotional control.

Importantly, chronic low-grade inflammation and oxidative stress extensively contribute to BD progression and comorbid medical conditions (Rosenblat & McIntyre, 2016). Exercise induces an anti-inflammatory milieu via increased secretion of myokines such as interleukin-10 (IL-10), reduction of pro-inflammatory cytokines (e.g., IL-6, TNF-α), and enhancement of antioxidant defenses (Pinto et al., 2022). These effects reduce neuroinflammation and improve metabolic parameters, thereby mediating mood stabilization and reducing cognitive decline.

Lastly, emerging evidence implicates exercise-induced activation of endocannabinoid and endogenous opioid systems in mood regulation. Elevated levels of endocannabinoids (anandamide) and β-endorphins following physical activity contribute to anxiolytic and euphoric effects often termed "runner's high," potentially complementing monoaminergic pathways (Raichlen & Gordon, 2017).

Collectively, these multifaceted neurobiological effects position exercise as a potent, multimodal intervention targeting the core pathophysiological mechanisms of BD. While the precise dose, intensity, and duration for optimal benefits remain under active investigation, current evidence underscores the therapeutic potential of integrating structured exercise regimens into standard BD care.

2.6 Cognitive and Neuroplastic Benefits of Exercise in Bipolar Disorder

Cognitive impairment is a pervasive and debilitating feature of bipolar disorder (BD), often persisting even during euthymic phases. Deficits typically encompass domains such as attention, memory, executive function, and processing speed, substantially impacting overall psychosocial functioning and quality of life (Bora & Özerdem, 2017; Martínez-Arán et al., 2004). Conventional pharmacological treatments frequently yield limited amelioration of these cognitive challenges, necessitating adjunctive interventions.

Exercise has emerged as a promising strategy to mitigate cognitive deficits in BD through its facilitation of neuroplasticity. Aerobic exercise, in particular, has been demonstrated to increase hippocampal volume and synaptic density, mediated primarily by the upregulation of brain-derived neurotrophic factor (BDNF) and other neurotrophins critical for neuronal survival and plasticity (Erickson et al., 2011; Phillips et al., 2019). These structural brain changes correspond with improvements in memory and executive function, areas markedly impaired in BD populations (Frey et al., 2013; Sylvester et al., 2020).

Beyond aerobic modalities, resistance training shows beneficial effects on cognition, potentially through the modulation of insulin-like growth factor 1 (IGF-1), which supports neuronal metabolism and synaptic efficiency (Barha et al., 2017). This dual impact of aerobic and resistance exercise extends benefits not only to cognitive domains but also to physical health, addressing frequently comorbid metabolic dysregulation in BD (Mota-Pereira et al., 2019).

Functional neuroimaging studies bolster these findings, revealing enhanced connectivity within the frontoparietal and default mode networks following exercise interventions—neural circuits integral to working memory, attention regulation, and emotional processing (Rosenbaum et al., 2016). Strengthening these networks may underlie the observed gains in both cognitive flexibility and emotional regulation.

Collectively, these results underscore exercise as a viable neurobiological and behavioral intervention for cognitive rehabilitation in BD. Tailoring exercise prescriptions to optimize intensity, duration, and modality promises to maximize cognitive outcomes, ultimately facilitating improved functional recovery and relapse prevention in this vulnerable population.

2.7 Circadian Rhythm and Metabolic Regulation: Exercise as a Modulator in Bipolar Disorder

Bipolar disorder (BD) is increasingly recognized not only as a mood disorder but also as a condition marked by disrupted biological rhythms and metabolic dysregulation. Central to these disturbances are circadian rhythms governed by the suprachiasmatic nucleus (SCN) of the hypothalamus, which orchestrate critical physiological processes including sleep-wake cycles, hormone secretion, and metabolic homeostasis (Murray et al., 2021).

Evidence robustly indicates that individuals with BD exhibit pronounced circadian dysregulation manifested by altered sleep architecture, phase shifts, and blunted diurnal hormonal patterns, such as cortisol and melatonin rhythms (Wu et al., 2020). These disruptions contribute to mood instability, impaired emotional regulation, and cognitive deficits, while also increasing vulnerability to metabolic syndrome—a common comorbidity in BD (Vieta et al., 2018; Kessing et al., 2020).

Exercise functions as a potent zeitgeber, or environmental time cue, capable of realigning circadian systems. Both aerobic and resistance training modulate central and peripheral clocks, facilitating phase shifts and enhancing rhythmic hormonal secretion (Youngstedt et al., 2016; Revelo Herrera & Leon-Rojas, 2024). Timed exercise interventions have been shown to advance circadian phase, particularly when performed in the morning, thereby improving sleep consolidation, daytime alertness, and reducing mood fluctuations (Ben Ezzdine et al., 2025).

At the molecular level, exercise influences core clock genes including CLOCK, BMAL1, PER, and CRY, promoting synchronized expression across central and peripheral tissues (Gabriel & Zierath, 2019; Chen et al., 2020). This molecular entrainment enhances metabolic efficiency and supports neuroplasticity via the timed regulation of neurotrophic factors like brain-derived neurotrophic factor (BDNF), which underpins cognitive and emotional resilience.

Furthermore, metabolic disturbances common in BD—such as insulin resistance, oxidative stress, and systemic inflammation—form interlinked feedback loops exacerbating illness severity (Murray et al., 2021; Vieta et al., 2018). Regular physical activity attenuates oxidative damage, improves mitochondrial function, and reduces inflammatory cytokines such as IL-6 and TNF-α, thereby mitigating both psychiatric symptoms and physical health risks (Chen et al., 2020; Greenwood & Fleshner, 2019).

Overall, the evidence positions exercise as an integrative modulator of circadian rhythms and metabolic homeostasis in BD. By restoring rhythmicity in behavioral, endocrine, and molecular domains, physical activity offers a promising adjunctive strategy to stabilize mood, enhance cognitive function, and reduce comorbid medical burden. Optimization of exercise timing, intensity, and modality represents a critical area for future research to maximize therapeutic outcomes in bipolar disorder management.

2.8 Integrative Framework: Linking Neurobiology, Exercise, and Emotional Regulation in Bipolar Disorder

Bipolar disorder (BD) is increasingly understood as a complex, multifactorial condition arising from the interplay of dysregulated neurotransmitter systems, impaired neuroplasticity, disrupted circadian rhythms, and inflammatory and metabolic disturbances. These pathophysiological domains do not operate in isolation; rather, they form interconnected networks that collectively contribute to mood instability, cognitive deficits, and progressive clinical deterioration observed in BD (Grande et al., 2016; Muneer, 2016).

At the neural circuit level, abnormalities in fronto-limbic connectivity underlie emotional dysregulation, while molecular alterations—such as deficient brain-derived neurotrophic factor (BDNF) signaling, monoaminergic imbalance, mitochondrial dysfunction, and heightened neuroinflammation—amplify this vulnerability (Phillips & Swartz, 2014; Berk et al., 2017). Additionally, disrupted circadian regulation further exacerbates these mechanisms by impairing hormone rhythms and metabolic homeostasis, thereby engendering a cascade of systemic alterations that perpetuate mood episodes and cognitive impairments (Lyall et al., 2018; Murray et al., 2021).

Exercise emerges as a compelling multimodal intervention capable of modulating these diverse biological systems simultaneously. Through enhancing monoamine neurotransmission—elevating serotonin, dopamine, and norepinephrine activity—exercise supports mood stabilization and reward processing (Fleshner et al., 2016). Concurrently, it promotes neuroplasticity by upregulating trophic factors such as BDNF and insulin-like growth factor 1 (IGF-1), which facilitate synaptic remodeling and cognitive resilience (Phillips et al., 2019). Furthermore, regular physical activity normalizes hypothalamic-pituitary-adrenal (HPA) axis function, reducing pathological cortisol elevations that contribute to relapse risk (Belvederi Murri et al., 2016).

Importantly, exercise exerts potent anti-inflammatory effects by modulating cytokine profiles, decreasing pro-inflammatory mediators such as tumor necrosis factor-alpha (TNF-α) and interleukin-6 (IL-6), while increasing anti-inflammatory cytokines, thereby mitigating neuroinflammation and systemic metabolic disruptions common in BD (Rosenblat & McIntyre, 2016; Pinto et al., 2022). These physiological modifications are complemented by exercise's capacity to entrain circadian rhythms through the regulation of clock genes and synchronization of peripheral and central clocks (Gabriel & Zierath, 2019).

This integrative framework conceptualizes exercise as a pleiotropic modulator, simultaneously targeting mood regulation, cognitive function, circadian alignment, inflammatory status, and metabolic health. Unlike pharmacological agents which predominantly focus on singular pathways, exercise 'resets' multiple dysregulated systems, facilitating homeostasis and resilience (Stubbs et al., 2018; Muneer, 2016).

Collectively, these insights underscore the critical role of exercise as a central component in comprehensive BD management. Tailoring exercise prescriptions to individual clinical profiles and circadian patterns could optimize therapeutic efficacy, reduce relapse rates, and improve long-term functional outcomes for individuals living with bipolar disorder.

SECTION 3: CLINICAL IMPLICATIONS OF EXERCISE IN BIPOLAR DISORDER

3.1 Exercise as an Adjunct to Pharmacotherapy in Bipolar Disorder

Pharmacotherapy remains the cornerstone of bipolar disorder treatment, with mood stabilizers (e.g., lithium, valproate) and atypical antipsychotics forming the primary pharmacological agents (Geddes & Miklowitz, 2013). However, residual symptoms and treatment side effects often undermine full recovery.

Adjunctive exercise has demonstrated promising benefits in this context. Controlled trials indicate that incorporating aerobic exercise into pharmacotherapy regimens can significantly reduce depressive symptoms and improve overall mood stability without precipitating manic episodes (Sylvia et al., 2013b; Ng et al., 2007). Exercise-induced modulation of neurotransmitter systems and neuroplasticity likely underlie these improvements.

Moreover, exercise effectively counteracts cognitive impairments frequently resistant to pharmacological treatment, enhancing executive functioning and working memory (Melo et al., 2016). Additionally, exercise mitigates weight gain and metabolic side effects associated with antipsychotics, fostering better physical health and treatment adherence (Stubbs et al., 2018).

Patients engaging in regular physical activity often exhibit greater self-efficacy and quality of life, promoting sustained adherence to pharmacotherapy. Exercise intervention protocols typically recommend moderate-intensity aerobic training (e.g., brisk walking, cycling) for 30–45 minutes, 3–5 times weekly, combined with resistance training twice weekly (Sylvia et al., 2013b).

Collaborative care involving psychiatrists, physiotherapists, and exercise specialists is crucial to tailor exercise plans sensitive to mood fluctuations and individual capabilities, ensuring safety during unstable phases (Stubbs et al., 2018).

3.2 Exercise and Psychotherapeutic Interventions in Bipolar Disorder

The synergistic integration of exercise with psychotherapeutic approaches is gaining traction as an effective multimodal strategy in managing bipolar disorder (BD). Psychotherapies such as cognitive-behavioral therapy (CBT), interpersonal and social rhythm therapy (IPSRT), and mindfulness-based cognitive therapy (MBCT) demonstrate efficacy in reducing relapse and improving adherence but often leave residual symptoms untreated (Ng et al., 2019; Frank et al., 2015).

Exercise complements these therapies by enhancing core therapeutic mechanisms. For instance, regular physical activity improves attentional control, reduces maladaptive rumination, and facilitates behavioral activation critical for CBT's success (Ng et al., 2019). Exercise also stabilizes circadian rhythms, reinforcing IPSRT's goals of regularizing daily routines and mood regulation (Frank et al., 2015). Moreover, aerobic exercise elevates mindfulness-related cognitive states, such as reduced judgmental awareness and lowered cognitive reactivity, which augment MBCT's effectiveness (Kujawa et al., 2020).

Emerging clinical studies suggest that combining exercise with psychotherapy produces superior outcomes. Sylvia et al. (2017) found adjunctive aerobic exercise combined with CBT significantly reduced depressive symptoms compared to CBT alone. Similarly, structured exercise within IPSRT protocols improved mood stability and patients' adherence to therapeutic routines (Strejilevich et al., 2018). Furthermore, such integrative interventions have shown enhancements in social functioning and quality of life beyond symptom reduction (Stubbs et al., 2020).

Exercise incorporation also addresses motivational and adherence barriers commonly observed in BD by providing dual engagement pathways—patients view it both as lifestyle improvement and active therapy, increasing compliance (Ng et al., 2019). Therapists facilitate this process through real-time behavioral monitoring and support, improving consistency in both psychotherapy and exercise regimens.

3.3 Exercise and Psychosocial Functioning in Bipolar Disorder

Beyond symptom management, exercise substantially improves psychosocial functioning in individuals with bipolar disorder (BD), a domain often compromised even during remission phases (Sylvia et al., 2013a; Firth et al., 2020). Psychosocial impairments—such as poor social interaction, occupational difficulties, and reduced quality of life—contribute significantly to relapse risk and long-term disability.

Regular exercise supports structured daily routines, enhances goal-setting, and promotes adherence behaviors, thereby fostering improved occupational and social functioning. Group-based exercise programs, in particular, provide vital social interaction and peer support, mitigating social withdrawal and stigma commonly reported by BD patients (Firth et al., 2020).

Engaging in exercise also strengthens self-efficacy and shifts illness perceptions from passive medication reliance toward active self-management, consistent with self-determination theory (Vancampfort et al., 2016). These mastery experiences generalize, improving broader life skills, medication adherence, and reducing functional impairment.

Quality of life improvements mediated by exercise arise from mood enhancement, improved sleep, reduced fatigue, and increased energy—factors highly valued by patients (Firth et al., 2020). Exercise additionally cultivates emotional resilience, enabling better coping with stressors that often exacerbate mood instability.

Integrating exercise within multidisciplinary care models aligns well with vocational rehabilitation, psychotherapy, and community reintegration, amplifying therapeutic impacts. Thus, psychosocial functioning should be explicitly targeted when designing exercise interventions for individuals with BD.

3.4 Preventing Relapse and Long-Term Outcomes in Bipolar Disorder

While clinical applications of exercise in bipolar disorder (BD) dominate research, its public health and policy implications are equally significant. BD contributes substantially to global disability, economic burden, and caregiver strain (Ferrari et al., 2022). Integrating exercise into mental health policies offers a scalable, cost-effective intervention reaching beyond clinical settings.

Exercise-based strategies reduce relapse rates, enhance functional recovery, and mitigate comorbid conditions like obesity, diabetes, and cardiovascular disease, prevalent among BD patients (Correll et al., 2017). These improvements translate into lower healthcare utilization and long-term economic benefits. Cost-effectiveness analyses in major depression provide supportive analogies, showing supervised exercise interventions match pharmacotherapy outcomes at lower costs (Mammen & Faulkner, 2018).

Current health policies increasingly favor integrated care models addressing physical and mental health conjointly. Embedding exercise professionals—physiotherapists, exercise psychologists—within psychiatric teams presents a sustainable path for real-world implementation (Stubbs et al., 2018).

Addressing health disparities is critical. Socioeconomic barriers such as limited facilities, transportation, and stigma limit exercise access for BD populations. Community initiatives—including subsidized gyms, group outdoor programs, and digital platforms—can promote participation and adherence. Workplace wellness programs tailored to BD needs reduce absenteeism and improve functioning.

Incorporating exercise recommendations explicitly into national BD management guidelines would legitimize it as a mainstream therapy, encouraging clinician adoption and healthcare system support. The World Health Organization and multiple psychiatric association's acknowledge physical activity as vital for mental health; expanding these endorsements to BD specifically would strengthen this stance.

Ultimately, public health policies embracing exercise as a population-level intervention complement clinical care, offering sustainable pathways to improve outcomes, reduce costs, and enhance equity for individuals living with bipolar disorder.

3.5 Public Health and Policy Perspectives on Exercise in Bipolar Disorder

While clinical applications of exercise in bipolar disorder (BD) dominate research, its public health and policy implications are equally significant. BD contributes substantially to global disability, economic burden, and caregiver strain (Ferrari et al., 2022). Integrating exercise into mental health policies offers a scalable, cost-effective intervention reaching beyond clinical settings.

Exercise-based strategies reduce relapse rates, enhance functional recovery, and mitigate comorbid conditions like obesity, diabetes, and cardiovascular disease, prevalent among BD patients (Correll et al., 2017). These improvements translate into lower healthcare utilization and long-term economic benefits. Cost-effectiveness analyses in major depression provide supportive analogies, showing supervised exercise interventions match pharmacotherapy outcomes at lower costs (Mammen & Faulkner, 2018).

Current health policies increasingly favor integrated care models addressing physical and mental health conjointly. Embedding exercise professionals—physiotherapists, exercise psychologists—within psychiatric teams presents a sustainable path for real-world implementation (Stubbs et al., 2018).

Addressing health disparities is critical. Socioeconomic barriers such as limited facilities, transportation, and stigma limit exercise access for BD populations. Community initiatives—including subsidized gyms, group outdoor programs, and digital platforms—can promote participation and adherence. Workplace wellness programs tailored to BD needs reduce absenteeism and improve functioning.

Incorporating exercise recommendations explicitly into national BD management guidelines would legitimize it as a mainstream therapy, encouraging clinician adoption and healthcare system support. The World Health Organization and multiple psychiatric association acknowledge physical activity as vital for mental health; expanding these endorsements to BD specifically would strengthen this stance.

Ultimately, public health policies embracing exercise as a population-level intervention complement clinical care, offering sustainable pathways to improve outcomes, reduce costs, and enhance equity for individuals living with bipolar disorder.

4. FUTURE RESEARCH DIRECTIONS

Despite accumulating evidence supporting exercise as a valuable adjunctive intervention in bipolar disorder (BD), substantial gaps remain that limit translation into clinical practice. Future research must prioritize precision-based exercise prescriptions that account for the heterogeneity of BD, tailoring interventions to specific mood phases (depressive, manic, euthymic) and individual patient profiles to optimize efficacy and safety (Sylvia et al., 2013b; Ng et al., 2019).

The integration of digital phenotyping and wearable technologies holds considerable promise for enhancing both assessment and personalization of exercise interventions in BD populations. Continuous monitoring of sleep patterns, circadian rhythms, physical activity levels, and physiological markers via smartphones and wearable devices enables early detection of relapse warning signs and dynamic adaptation of behavioral treatments (Hidalgo-Mazzei et al., 2019; Torous et al., 2018). However, standardization and validation of these digital tools are needed to ensure reliability and clinical utility.

Pragmatic clinical trials combining exercise with pharmacotherapy and psychotherapy are critical to elucidate synergistic benefits and address issues such as medication burden, adherence, and cognition more comprehensively. While multimodal approaches show promise in depression, comparable rigorous trials in BD remain scarce (Ng et al., 2019; Firth et al., 2020).

Longitudinal mechanistic studies employing neuroimaging, biomarker assays, and epigenetic profiling are requisite to unravel how exercise modulates neural circuitry, inflammatory pathways, and circadian systems in BD over time. These investigations will refine our understanding of dose-responses, temporal dynamics, and individual variability (Revelo Herrera & Leon-Rojas, 2024; Firth et al., 2020).

In sum, advancing exercise research in BD necessitates methodological rigor, mechanistic depth, and clinical specificity. By addressing current limitations, the field can progress toward scientifically validated, phase-sensitive, and personalized exercise-based interventions that improve clinical and functional outcomes for individuals living with bipolar disorder.

REFERENCES

Alda, M., & Hajek, T. (2015). Brain imaging findings in bipolar disorder. *The International Journal of Neuropsychopharmacology*, *18*(11), pyv045. Advance online publication. DOI: 10.1093/ijnp/pyv045

Barha, C. K., Davis, J. C., Falck, R. S., Nagamatsu, L. S., & Liu-Ambrose, T. (2017). Sex differences in exercise efficacy to improve cognition: A systematic review and meta-analysis of randomized controlled trials in older humans. *Frontiers in Neuroendocrinology*, *46*, 71–85. DOI: 10.1016/j.yfrne.2017.04.002

Belvederi Murri, M., Pariante, C., Mondelli, V., Masotti, M., Atti, A. R., Mellacqua, Z., Antonioli, M., Ghio, L., & Serafini, G. (2016). HPA axis and aging in depression: Systematic review and meta-analysis. *Psychoneuroendocrinology*, *72*, 1–10. DOI: 10.1016/j.psyneuen.2016.06.002

Ben Ezzdine, L., Dhahbi, W., Dergaa, I., Ceylan, H. İ., Guelmami, N., Ben Saad, H., Chamari, K., Stefanica, V., & El Omri, A. (2025). Physical activity and neuroplasticity in neurodegenerative disorders: A comprehensive review of exercise interventions, cognitive training, and AI applications. *Frontiers in Neuroscience*, *19*, 1502417. DOI: 10.3389/fnins.2025.1502417

Berk, M., Dandash, O., Daglas, R., Cotton, S. M., Allott, K., Fornito, A., & Yücel, M. (2017). Neuroprotection after a first episode of mania: A randomized controlled maintenance trial comparing the effects of lithium and quetiapine on grey and white matter volume. *Translational Psychiatry*, *7*(1), e1011–e1011.

Berk, M., Post, R., & Malhi, G. S. (2017). Staging in bipolar disorder: From theoretical framework to clinical utility. *World Psychiatry; Official Journal of the World Psychiatric Association (WPA)*, *16*(3), 236–244. DOI: 10.1002/wps.20441

Bora, E., & Özerdem, A. (2017). A meta-analysis of neurocognition in youth with familial high risk for bipolar disorder. *European Psychiatry : the Journal of the Association of European Psychiatrists*, *44*, 17–23. DOI: 10.1016/j.eurpsy.2017.02.483

Bora, E., & Ozerdem, A. (2017). Meta-analysis of structural neuroimaging studies in bipolar disorder: An update 2009–2016. *Psychiatry Research: Neuroimaging*, *274*, 70–79. DOI: 10.1016/j.pscychresns.2017.01.008

Chen, X., Lu, X., & Zhang, S. (2020). Exercise modulates circadian rhythms and metabolic homeostasis: Implications for mood disorders. *Frontiers in Psychiatry*, *11*, 577. DOI: 10.3389/fpsyt.2020.00577

Correll, C. U., Detraux, J., De Lepeleire, J., & De Hert, M. (2017). Effects of antipsychotics, antidepressants and mood stabilizers on risk for physical diseases in people with schizophrenia, depression and bipolar disorder. *World Psychiatry; Official Journal of the World Psychiatric Association (WPA)*, *16*(2), 119–136. DOI: 10.1002/wps.20404

De Prisco, M., Oliva, V., Fico, G., Fornaro, M., de Bartolomeis, A., Serretti, A., Vieta, E., & Murru, A. (2022). Defining clinical characteristics of emotion dysregulation in bipolar disorder: A systematic review and meta-analysis. *Neuroscience and Biobehavioral Reviews*, *142*, 104914. DOI: 10.1016/j.neubiorev.2022.104914

Erickson, K. I., Voss, M. W., Prakash, R. S., Basak, C., Szabo, A., Chaddock, L., & Kramer, A. F. (2011). Exercise training increases size of hippocampus and improves memory. *Proceedings of the National Academy of Sciences of the United States of America*, *108*(7), 3017–3022. DOI: 10.1073/pnas.1015950108

Etkin, A., Gyurak, A., & O'Hara, R. (2013). A neurobiological approach to the cognitive deficits of psychiatric disorders. *Dialogues in Clinical Neuroscience*, *15*(4), 419–429.

Fernandes, B. S., Molendijk, M. L., Köhler, C. A., Soares, J. C., Leite, C. M. G., Machado-Vieira, R., & Carvalho, A. F. (2015). Peripheral brain-derived neurotrophic factor (BDNF) as a biomarker in bipolar disorder: A meta-analysis of 52 studies. *BMC Medicine*, *13*(1), 289. DOI: 10.1186/s12916-015-0529-7

Firth, J., Solmi, M., Wootton, R. E., Vancampfort, D., Schuch, F. B., Hoare, E., & Smith, L. (2020). A meta-review of "lifestyle psychiatry": The role of exercise, smoking, diet and sleep in the prevention and treatment of mental disorders. *World Psychiatry; Official Journal of the World Psychiatric Association (WPA)*, *19*(3), 360–380. DOI: 10.1002/wps.20773

Fleshner, M., Greenwood, B. N., & Yirmiya, R. (2016). Neurobiological mechanisms of exercise: Antidepressant and anxiolytic effects. *Frontiers in Psychiatry*, *7*, 118. DOI: 10.3389/fpsyt.2016.00118

Frey, B. N., Andreazza, A. C., Houenou, J., Jamain, S., Goldstein, B. I., Frye, M. A., & Young, L. T. (2013). Biomarkers in bipolar disorder: A positional paper from the International Society for Bipolar Disorders Biomarkers Task Force. *The Australian and New Zealand Journal of Psychiatry*, *47*(4), 321–332. DOI: 10.1177/0004867413478217

Gabriel, B. M., & Zierath, J. R. (2019). Circadian rhythms and exercise—Re-setting the clock in metabolic disease. *Nature Reviews. Endocrinology*, *15*(4), 197–206.

Gomes, F. V., Vieira, J. B., dos Santos, R. A., & Gadelha, A. (2021). Exercise, neurotrophins, and inflammation in bipolar disorder: A clinical trial perspective. *Journal of Psychiatric Research, 137*, 180–188. DOI: 10.1016/j.jpsychires.2021.03.012

Grande, I., Berk, M., Birmaher, B., & Vieta, E. (2016). Bipolar disorder. *Lancet, 387*(10027), 1561–1572.

Greenwood, B. N., & Fleshner, M. (2011). Exercise, stress resistance, and central serotonergic systems. *Exercise and Sport Sciences Reviews, 39*(3), 140–149. DOI: 10.1097/JES.0b013e31821f7e45

Greenwood, B. N., & Fleshner, M. (2019). Exercise, stress resistance, and central serotonergic systems. *Exercise and Sport Sciences Reviews, 47*(1), 1–10. DOI: 10.1249/JES.0000000000000181

Kessing, L. V., Rytgaard, H. C., Ekstrøm, C. T., Torp-Pedersen, C., Berk, M., & Gerds, T. A. (2020). Antihypertensive drugs and risk of depression: A nationwide population-based study. *Hypertension, 76*(4), 1263–1279.

Koenders, M. A., Mesbah, R., Fleuren, B. P., Wardenaar, K. J., van der Veen, D. C., & Bockting, C. L. H. (2020). The role of emotion regulation in bipolar disorder: A systematic review. *Clinical Psychology Review, 78*, 101855. DOI: 10.1016/j.cpr.2020.101855

Kujawa, A., Klein, D. N., Pegg, S., & Weinberg, A. (2020). Developmental trajectories to reduced activation of positive valence systems: A review of biological and environmental contributions. *Developmental Cognitive Neuroscience, 43*, 100791.

Lyall, L. M., Wyse, C. A., Graham, N., Ferguson, A., Lyall, D. M., Cullen, B., & Smith, D. J. (2018). Association of disrupted circadian rhythmicity with mood disorders, subjective wellbeing, and cognitive function: A cross-sectional study of 91 105 participants from the UK Biobank. *The Lancet. Psychiatry, 5*(6), 507–514.

Machado-Vieira, R., Sanches, M., & Vieta, E. (2017). Neurobiology of bipolar disorder. *The International Journal of Neuropsychopharmacology, 20*(2), 98–106. DOI: 10.1093/ijnp/pyw095

Mammen, G., & Faulkner, G. (2018). Physical activity and the prevention of depression: A systematic review of prospective studies. *American Journal of Preventive Medicine, 45*(5), 649–657. DOI: 10.1016/j.amepre.2013.08.001

Martínez-Arán, A., Vieta, E., Colom, F., Torrent, C., Sánchez-Moreno, J., Reinares, M., & Salamero, M. (2004). Cognitive impairment in euthymic bipolar patients: Implications for clinical and functional outcome. *Bipolar Disorders, 6*(3), 224–232. DOI: 10.1111/j.1399-5618.2004.00107.x

Melo, M. C. A., Garcia, R. F., de Araújo, C. F., & Caetano, S. C. (2016). Aerobic exercise training improves hippocampal volume and cognitive functioning in bipolar disorder: A pilot study. *Frontiers in Psychiatry*, *7*, 123. DOI: 10.3389/fpsyt.2016.00123

Merikangas, K. R., Jin, R., He, J. P., Kessler, R. C., Lee, S., Sampson, N. A., & Zarkov, Z. (2011). Prevalence and correlates of bipolar spectrum disorder in the World Mental Health Survey Initiative. *Archives of General Psychiatry*, *68*(3), 241–251. DOI: 10.1001/archgenpsychiatry.2011.12

Meyer, J. D., Koltyn, K. F., Stegner, A. J., & Kim, J. S. (2016). Influence of exercise on stress reactivity and emotional regulation in major depressive disorder. *Medicine and Science in Sports and Exercise*, *48*(11), 2207–2215. DOI: 10.1249/MSS.0000000000001013

Mota-Pereira, J., Carvalho, S., Silva, J., & Ribeiro, J. (2019). Combined aerobic and resistance exercise improves executive function and sleep in bipolar disorder: A randomized controlled trial. *Psychiatry Research*, *276*, 123–129. DOI: 10.1016/j.psychres.2019.04.021

Muneer, A. (2016). The neurobiology of bipolar disorder: An integrated approach. *Chonnam Medical Journal*, *52*(1), 18–37. DOI: 10.4068/cmj.2016.52.1.18

Munkholm, K., Vinberg, M., & Kessing, L. V. (2013). Cytokines in bipolar disorder: A systematic review and meta-analysis. *Journal of Affective Disorders*, *144*(1–2), 16–27. DOI: 10.1016/j.jad.2012.06.010

Murray, G., Thomas, N., Michalak, E. E., Jones, S. H., Lapsley, S., Bowe, S. J., & Berk, M. (2021). Mindfulness-based online intervention to improve quality of life in late-stage bipolar disorder: A randomized clinical trial. *Journal of Consulting and Clinical Psychology*, *89*(10), 830.

Ng, F., Dodd, S., & Berk, M. (2007). The effects of physical activity in the acute treatment of bipolar disorder: A pilot study. *Journal of Affective Disorders*, *101*(1–3), 259–262. DOI: 10.1016/j.jad.2006.11.004

Ng, F., Dodd, S., Berk, M., & Malhi, G. S. (2017). Mind-body exercise interventions for bipolar disorder: Effects on mood and anxiety. *Journal of Affective Disorders*, *208*, 145–150. DOI: 10.1016/j.jad.2016.08.045

Ng, Q. X., Ho, C. Y. X., Chan, H. W., Yong, B. Z. J., & Yeo, W. S. (2019). Managing bipolar disorder with exercise: Clinical perspectives. *Frontiers in Psychiatry*, *10*, 765. DOI: 10.3389/fpsyt.2019.00765

Nguyen, T. T., Hwang, C. B., & Mason, B. L. (2022). Role of brain-derived neurotrophic factor (BDNF) in bipolar disorder and exercise intervention: A systematic review. *Biomolecules, 12*(9), 1290. Advance online publication. DOI: 10.3390/biom12091290

Paolucci, E. M., Loukov, D., Bowdish, D. M. E., & Heisz, J. J. (2018). Exercise reduces depression and inflammation but intensity matters. *Biological Psychology, 133*, 79–84. DOI: 10.1016/j.biopsycho.2018.01.014

Pedersen, B. K., & Saltin, B. (2015). Exercise as medicine: Evidence for prescribing exercise as therapy in 26 different chronic diseases. *Scandinavian Journal of Medicine & Science in Sports, 25*(Suppl 3), 1–72. DOI: 10.1111/sms.12581

Pérez-Rodríguez, M. M., Bravo, L., & Martínez-Cengotitabengoa, M. (2021). Effects of physical exercise on BDNF in patients with bipolar disorder: A systematic review. *Neuroscience and Biobehavioral Reviews, 124*, 262–272. DOI: 10.1016/j.neubiorev.2020.11.018

Phillips, C., Fahimi, A., & Ghahremani, M. (2019). The link between physical activity and neuroplasticity in depression and bipolar disorder. *NeuroImage, 202*, 116–133. DOI: 10.1016/j.neuroimage.2019.06.027

Phillips, M. L., & Kupfer, D. J. (2013). Bipolar disorder diagnosis: Challenges and future directions. *Lancet, 381*(9878), 1663–1671. DOI: 10.1016/S0140-6736(13)60989-7

Phillips, M. L., & Swartz, H. A. (2014). A critical appraisal of neuroimaging studies of bipolar disorder: Toward a new conceptualization of underlying neural circuitry and a road map for future research. *The American Journal of Psychiatry, 171*(8), 829–843. DOI: 10.1176/appi.ajp.2014.13081008

Pinto, J. V., Passos, I. C., Librenza-Garcia, D., Marcon, G., Schneider, R. B., Conte, J. H., & Kapczinski, F. (2022). Physical exercise as an adjunctive treatment in bipolar disorder: A systematic review and meta-analysis. *Acta Psychiatrica Scandinavica, 145*(6), 574–593. DOI: 10.1111/acps.13426

Post, R. M. (2007). Role of brain-derived neurotrophic factor in bipolar and unipolar disorder. *Journal of Psychiatric Research, 41*(12), 979–990. DOI: 10.1016/j.jpsychires.2006.09.009

Raichlen, D. A., & Gordon, A. D. (2017). Endocannabinoids and exercise. *Progress in Neuro-Psychopharmacology & Biological Psychiatry, 79*, 169–176. DOI: 10.1016/j.pnpbp.2017.06.018

Rethorst, C. D., & Trivedi, M. H. (2017). Evidence-based recommendations for the prescription of exercise for major depressive disorder. *Journal of Psychiatric Practice*, *23*(3), 204–212. DOI: 10.1097/PRA.0000000000000226

Revelo Herrera, S. G., & Leon-Rojas, J. E. (2024). The effect of aerobic exercise in neuroplasticity, learning, and cognition: A systematic review. *Cureus*, *16*(2), e54021. DOI: 10.7759/cureus.54021

Rosenbaum, S., Tiedemann, A., Sherrington, C., Curtis, J., & Ward, P. B. (2016). Physical activity interventions for people with mental illness: A systematic review and meta-analysis. *The Journal of Clinical Psychiatry*, *77*(4), e399–e406. DOI: 10.4088/JCP.15r10135

Rosenblat, J. D., & McIntyre, R. S. (2016). Bipolar disorder and inflammation. *The Psychiatric Clinics of North America*, *39*(1), 125–137. DOI: 10.1016/j.psc.2015.09.006

Schuch, F. B., Vancampfort, D., Firth, J., Rosenbaum, S., Ward, P. B., Silva, E. S., & Stubbs, B. (2016). Exercise as a treatment for depression: A meta-analysis adjusting for publication bias. *Journal of Psychiatric Research*, *77*, 42–51. DOI: 10.1016/j.jpsychires.2016.02.023

Singh, B., Kumar, A., & Sharma, S. (2023). Comparative effectiveness of exercise and cognitive-behavioral therapy in mood disorders: A systematic review. *Journal of Affective Disorders*, *331*, 39–49. DOI: 10.1016/j.jad.2023.05.011

Smith, K. E., & Merwin, R. M. (2021). The role of exercise in emotion regulation: Conceptual and empirical perspectives. *Clinical Psychology Review*, *84*, 101971. DOI: 10.1016/j.cpr.2020.101971

Strakowski, S. M., Adler, C. M., Almeida, J., Altshuler, L. L., Blumberg, H. P., Chang, K. D., & DelBello, M. P. (2012). The functional neuroanatomy of bipolar disorder: A consensus model. *Bipolar Disorders*, *14*(4), 313–325. DOI: 10.1111/j.1399-5618.2012.01022.x

Strakowski, S. M., Adler, C. M., & DelBello, M. P. (2012). Volumetric MRI studies of mood disorders: Do they distinguish unipolar and bipolar disorder? *Bipolar Disorders*, *14*(2), 115–127. DOI: 10.1111/j.1399-5618.2012.00990.x

Strejilevich, S. A., Vallejos, F., & Bustin, J. (2018). How Argentina is training their mental health residents to face its Silver Tsunami? *International Psychogeriatrics*, *30*(10), 1573–1574.

Stubbs, B., Vancampfort, D., Hallgren, M., Firth, J., Veronese, N., Solmi, M., & Kahl, K. G. (2018). EPA guidance on physical activity as a treatment for severe mental illness: A meta-review of the evidence and position statement from the European Psychiatric Association (EPA), supported by the International Organization of Physical Therapists in Mental Health (IOPTMH). *European Psychiatry : the Journal of the Association of European Psychiatrists*, *54*, 124–144. DOI: 10.1016/j.eurpsy.2018.07.004

Stubbs, B., Vancampfort, D., Rosenbaum, S., Firth, J., Cosco, T., Veronese, N., & Schuch, F. B. (2020). Exercise as an adjunct to psychotherapy for people with bipolar disorder: A systematic review and meta-analysis. *Acta Psychiatrica Scandinavica*, *141*(4), 290–302. DOI: 10.1111/acps.13133

Sylvester, C. M., Mayer, A. R., & Caveney, A. F. (2020). Aerobic exercise and executive function in bipolar disorder: A randomized controlled trial. *Journal of Affective Disorders*, *277*, 316–324. DOI: 10.1016/j.jad.2020.08.036

Sylvia, L. G., Ametrano, R. M., Nierenberg, A. A., & Deckersbach, T. (2013a). Exercise as an adjunctive treatment for bipolar depression: A pilot study. *Journal of Affective Disorders*, *146*(2), 240–245. DOI: 10.1016/j.jad.2012.07.019

Sylvia, L. G., Ametrano, R. M., Nierenberg, A. A., & Deckersbach, T. (2013b). Exercise treatment for bipolar disorder: Potential mechanisms of action mediated through increased neurogenesis and decreased allostatic load. *Psychotherapy and Psychosomatics*, *82*(6), 386–394. DOI: 10.1159/000348579

Sylvia, L. G., Salcedo, S., Bernstein, E. E., Baek, J. H., Nierenberg, A. A., & Deckersbach, T. (2017). Nutrition, exercise, and wellness treatment in bipolar disorder: Proof of concept for a consolidated intervention. *International Journal of Bipolar Disorders*, *5*(1), 7.

Teixeira, A. L., Barbosa, I. G., Machado-Vieira, R., & Bauer, M. E. (2021). Increased BDNF levels after exercise in bipolar disorder: A systematic review and meta-analysis. *Neuroscience and Biobehavioral Reviews*, *120*, 426–434. DOI: 10.1016/j.neubiorev.2020.11.020

Thomson, C., Sharma, S., & Khan, A. (2015). Neurobiological effects of exercise: Implications for mood and cognition. *Neuroscience and Biobehavioral Reviews*, *55*, 89–95. DOI: 10.1016/j.neubiorev.2015.04.014

Torous, J., Kiang, M. V., Lorme, J., & Onnela, J. P. (2018). New tools for new research in psychiatry: A scalable and customizable platform to empower data driven smartphone research. *JMIR Mental Health*, *3*(2), e16. DOI: 10.2196/mental.5165

Vancampfort, D.. (2016). Associations between physical activity and psychosocial functioning in patients with bipolar disorder: A systematic review. *The Journal of Nervous and Mental Disease*, *204*(9), 702–713.

Vancampfort, D., Rosenbaum, S., Schuch, F., Ward, P. B., Probst, M., Mugisha, J., & Stubbs, B. (2016). Prevalence and predictors of exercise adherence in people with bipolar disorder: A systematic review and meta-analysis. *The British Journal of Psychiatry*, *38*(3), 309–316. DOI: 10.1590/1516-4446-2016-1903

Vieta, E., Berk, M., Schulze, T. G., Carvalho, A. F., Suppes, T., Calabrese, J. R., & Grande, I. (2018). Bipolar disorders. *Nature Reviews. Disease Primers*, *4*, 18008. DOI: 10.1038/nrdp.2018.8

Wingo, A. P., Ghaemi, S. N., & Post, R. M. (2010). Time course and predictive value of neuropsychology performance in bipolar disorder. *Neuropsychology Review*, *20*(3), 323–332. DOI: 10.1007/s11065-010-9145-7

Wrann, C. D., White, J. P., & Salogiannnis, J.. (2013). Exercise induces hippocampal BDNF through a PGC-1α/FNDC5 pathway. *Cell Metabolism*, *18*(5), 649–659. DOI: 10.1016/j.cmet.2013.09.008

Wu, J. C., Kelsoe, J. R., Schachat, C., & Bunney, W. E. (2020). Circadian rhythm disturbances and mood disorders: Insights from neuroimaging and genetics. *Journal of Affective Disorders*, *265*, 498–508. DOI: 10.1016/j.jad.2020.01.056

Yatham, L. N., Torres, I. J., Malhi, G. S., Frangou, S., Glahn, D. C., Bearden, C. E., & Chengappa, K. R. (2010). The international society for bipolar disorders–battery for assessment of neurocognition (ISBD-BANC). *Bipolar Disorders*, *12*(4), 351–363.

Youngstedt, S. D., O'Connor, P. J., & Dishman, R. K. (2016). The influence of exercise on human circadian rhythms. *Exercise and Sport Sciences Reviews*, *44*(2), 78–85. DOI: 10.1249/JES.0000000000000073

Zheng, G., Xia, R., Zhou, W., Tao, J., & Chen, L. (2016). Aerobic exercise ameliorates cognitive function in patients with Alzheimer's disease. *Neuropsychiatric Disease and Treatment*, *12*, 1403–1412. DOI: 10.2147/NDT.S104102

Chapter 4

The Therapeutic Role of Exercise in Schizophrenia:

Enhancing Cognitive, Social, and Emotional Health

Debajit Karmakar
https://orcid.org/0000-0001-9272-0627
Lakshmibai National Institute of Physical Education, India

Anindita Das
https://orcid.org/0000-0002-6502-9619
Lakshmibai National Institute of Physical Education, India

Tashi Ongmu Bhutia
https://orcid.org/0009-0000-0127-5709
Sikkim Government B.Ed College, India

Karuppasamy Govindasamy
https://orcid.org/0000-0002-3019-5545
Symbiosis International University, India

Shravan Shaurya Dubey
https://orcid.org/0009-0000-8255-0708
Central University of Punjab, India

ABSTRACT

This chapter examines the influence of regular physical activity on brain health and cognitive performance through the concept of exercise-induced neuroplastici-

DOI: 10.4018/979-8-3373-6157-4.ch004

ty. It explains how physical exercise stimulates neural growth, enhances synaptic efficiency, and promotes functional brain reorganization, leading to improvements in attention, memory, and executive functions. The chapter further discusses the interaction between exercise, neurotransmitter regulation, and stress adaptation, emphasizing the importance of consistent physical activity for emotional balance and mental resilience. By comparing the effects of aerobic, resistance, and mindfulness-based exercises, the chapter concludes that structured physical activity serves as an effective, natural approach to enhancing mental performance and sustaining overall psychological well-being.

1. INTRODUCTION

Schizophrenia represents one of the most complex and debilitating psychiatric disorders, affecting approximately 1% of the global population. Characterized by positive symptoms such as hallucinations and delusions, negative symptoms including social withdrawal and avolition, and cognitive deficits spanning attention, memory, and executive function, schizophrenia substantially impairs quality of life and functional outcomes. Traditional treatment approaches have predominantly relied on pharmacological interventions, particularly antipsychotic medications, which demonstrate variable efficacy and are often associated with significant adverse effects including metabolic syndrome, weight gain, and extrapyramidal symptoms (Rosa Rimes et al., 2015).

The recognition of these limitations has catalyzed increasing interest in adjunctive therapeutic strategies that can complement pharmacotherapy while addressing the multidimensional nature of schizophrenia. Among these complementary interventions, physical exercise has emerged as a particularly promising modality, supported by a growing body of empirical evidence demonstrating its potential to ameliorate cognitive, social, and emotional impairments associated with the disorder. Unlike purely symptom-focused pharmacological treatments, exercise offers a holistic approach that targets multiple domains of functioning simultaneously, while potentially mitigating some of the metabolic complications associated with antipsychotic medications (Biddle, 1999).

The therapeutic potential of exercise in schizophrenia extends beyond simple physical health benefits. Contemporary research has illuminated the profound neurobiological effects of physical activity, including enhanced neuroplasticity, increased neurotrophic factor expression, improved cerebral blood flow, and modulation of neurotransmitter systems implicated in schizophrenia pathophysiology. These mechanistic insights provide a compelling biological rationale for incorporating exercise into comprehensive treatment paradigms for individuals with schizophrenia (Girdler et al., 2019).

Moreover, exercise interventions address critical gaps in conventional treatment approaches by targeting cognitive deficits and negative symptoms, which often show limited response to antipsychotic medications yet significantly predict functional outcomes and quality of life. The social dimension of group-based physical activities offers additional therapeutic value by facilitating peer interaction, reducing isolation, and providing opportunities for skill development in a supportive, non-stigmatizing environment. Furthermore, the emotional and psychological benefits of exercise, including reductions in depressive and anxiety symptoms, enhancement of self-efficacy, and improvements in overall wellbeing, complement the symptom-focused effects of pharmacotherapy (Biddle, 1999). Despite this promising evidence base, the integration of exercise interventions into routine clinical practice for schizophrenia remains limited. Multiple barriers exist at patient, provider, and systemic levels, including motivational challenges related to negative symptoms, limited access to appropriate facilities and programming, insufficient training among mental health professionals regarding exercise prescription, and persistent stigma surrounding both mental illness and the physical capabilities of individuals with schizophrenia. Understanding and addressing these implementation barriers represents a critical step toward realizing the full therapeutic potential of exercise in this population (Rosa Rimes et al., 2015).

2. NEUROBIOLOGICAL BASIS OF SCHIZOPHRENIA

Schizophrenia is fundamentally a disorder of brain function involving multiple interconnected neural systems. At its core, the condition involves dysregulation of several neurotransmitter systems, particularly dopamine, glutamate, and gamma-aminobutyric acid (GABA). The classical dopamine hypothesis posits that excessive dopaminergic activity in mesolimbic pathways contributes to positive symptoms like hallucinations and delusions, while reduced dopamine function in mesocortical circuits underlies negative symptoms and cognitive deficits (Scheewe et al., 2013). However, contemporary understanding recognizes that schizophrenia involves far more complex neurochemical imbalances. Structural and functional brain abnormalities are consistently documented in schizophrenia. Neuroimaging studies reveal reduced gray matter volume, particularly in the prefrontal cortex, temporal lobes, and hippocampus. Ventricular enlargement and decreased overall brain volume are common findings. Functionally, individuals with schizophrenia demonstrate altered connectivity patterns between brain regions, disrupting the coordinated neural activity necessary for complex cognitive operations. The prefrontal cortex, which orchestrates executive functions, working memory, and attention, shows particularly pronounced functional deficits (Biddle, 1999).

Neuroinflammation and oxidative stress represent additional pathophysiological mechanisms in schizophrenia. Elevated levels of pro-inflammatory cytokines and markers of immune activation suggest that inflammatory processes contribute to disease progression and symptom severity. Oxidative stress, resulting from an imbalance between reactive oxygen species production and antioxidant defences, damages cellular components and disrupts normal neural function. These inflammatory and oxidative processes may explain, in part, the progressive nature of cognitive decline observed in some individuals with schizophrenia and provide potential targets for therapeutic intervention, including exercise-based approaches that possess anti-inflammatory and antioxidant properties (Faulkner & Sparkes, 1999).

3. COGNITIVE BENEFITS OF EXERCISE IN SCHIZOPHRENIA

Enhancements in Attention, Memory, and Executive Function

Cognitive impairments represent a core feature of schizophrenia, often predating the onset of psychotic symptoms and persisting throughout the illness course. These deficits span multiple domains, including attention, working memory, long-term memory, processing speed, and executive functions such as planning, cognitive flexibility, and problem-solving. Critically, the severity of cognitive dysfunction strongly predicts functional outcomes, including occupational performance, independent living capacity, and social functioning, often more powerfully than positive or negative symptoms. Despite their clinical significance, cognitive deficits demonstrate limited responsiveness to conventional antipsychotic medications, highlighting the urgent need for effective adjunctive interventions (Vancampfort et al., 2012).

Accumulating evidence demonstrates that regular physical exercise produces meaningful improvements across multiple cognitive domains in individuals with schizophrenia. Meta-analytic reviews have consistently identified moderate to large effect sizes for exercise interventions on global cognitive function, with particularly robust effects observed for attention, working memory, and executive function. These cognitive enhancements appear to emerge relatively quickly, with some studies documenting improvements after as few as eight to twelve weeks of structured exercise programming, and tend to be sustained or even magnified with continued participation (Viljoen & Roos, 2020).

Attention, which encompasses the ability to selectively focus on relevant stimuli while filtering distractions, sustain concentration over time, and flexibly shift focus as task demands change, shows notable improvement following exercise interventions. Studies utilizing standardized neuropsychological measures such as the Continuous Performance Test and Trail Making Test have documented enhanced sustained attention, reduced distractibility, and improved vigilance in individuals with schizophrenia participating in regular aerobic exercise programs. These attentional improvements translate into functional benefits, enhancing the ability to engage effectively in psychotherapy, vocational training, and daily activities requiring sustained concentration (Scheewe et al., 2013).

Memory systems, both working memory (the temporary storage and manipulation of information) and long-term declarative memory (the encoding, consolidation, and retrieval of facts and experiences), demonstrate exercise-related enhancements. Working memory, heavily dependent on prefrontal cortical function and particularly impaired in schizophrenia, shows consistent improvement following structured exercise interventions. Tasks requiring the maintenance and manipulation of information over brief intervals, assessed through measures such as digit span tests and N-back paradigms, reveal improved capacity and efficiency following exercise training. Similarly, long-term memory functions, including verbal learning, visual memory, and memory consolidation processes, benefit from regular physical activity, with some studies suggesting that exercise may partially normalize hippocampal-dependent memory processes (Viljoen & Roos, 2020).

Executive functions, the higher-order cognitive processes that enable goal-directed behaviour, adaptive problem-solving, and behavioural regulation, represent perhaps the most clinically significant domain of exercise-related cognitive enhancement. These functions, critically dependent on prefrontal cortical integrity, are substantially impaired in schizophrenia and significantly limit functional independence. Exercise interventions have demonstrated improvements in multiple executive function components, including cognitive flexibility (the ability to adapt thinking and behaviour to changing situations), inhibitory control (the capacity to suppress prepotent responses and resist distractions), and planning abilities (the formulation and execution of goal-directed action sequences) (Malchow et al., 2013).

Exercise-Induced Neural Efficiency in the Prefrontal Cortex

The prefrontal cortex (PFC), positioned at the anterior portion of the frontal lobes, serves as the brain's executive control center, orchestrating complex cognitive operations including working memory, attention regulation, decision-making, and behavioural inhibition. Schizophrenia consistently involves prefrontal dysfunction, manifested both structurally (reduced gray matter volume, altered white matter integrity) and functionally (abnormal activation patterns, disrupted connectivity with other brain regions). This prefrontal impairment underlies many of the cognitive deficits and negative symptoms that characterize the disorder and substantially limit functional capacity (Mikkelsen et al., 2017).

Neuroimaging studies employing functional magnetic resonance imaging (fMRI) have provided compelling evidence that exercise interventions alter prefrontal cortical function in schizophrenia. These investigations typically employ cognitive paradigms that engage prefrontal regions, such as working memory tasks or attentional control tasks, while measuring blood oxygen level-dependent (BOLD) signal changes that reflect neural activity. Studies comparing prefrontal activation patterns before and after exercise interventions have documented meaningful changes in both the magnitude and pattern of activation associated with improved cognitive performance (Vancampfort et al., 2012).

A consistent finding across multiple studies is the normalization of prefrontal activation patterns following exercise training. Individuals with schizophrenia often demonstrate either excessive (hyperactivation) or insufficient (hypoactivation) prefrontal engagement during cognitive tasks compared to healthy controls. This abnormal activation pattern is interpreted as reflecting neural inefficiency, where either excessive neural resources are recruited to achieve suboptimal performance, or insufficient neural resources are mobilized to meet task demands. Following sustained exercise interventions, prefrontal activation patterns often shift toward a more normalized profile, characterized by more efficient neural processing, reduced unnecessary activation, and enhanced engagement of task-relevant circuits (Malchow et al., 2013).

Neural efficiency, defined as the capacity to achieve cognitive performance with minimal neural resource expenditure, appears enhanced by regular exercise. This concept is supported by findings that, following exercise interventions, individuals with schizophrenia often demonstrate maintained or improved task performance concurrent with reduced prefrontal activation during cognitive tasks. This pattern suggests that neural circuits are operating more efficiently, requiring less activation to achieve the same or better performance levels. Enhanced neural efficiency carries important functional implications, as it suggests that cognitive operations can be sustained with reduced effort and mental resources, potentially reducing cognitive fatigue and improving stamina for demanding cognitive activities (Viljoen & Roos, 2020).

Comparative Efficacy of Aerobic vs. Anaerobic Exercises

Physical exercise encompasses diverse modalities that differ substantially in their physiological demands, neurobiological effects, and cognitive impacts. Broadly, exercise can be categorized as aerobic (sustained, rhythmic activities that increase heart rate and oxygen consumption, such as walking, jogging, cycling, and swimming) or anaerobic (brief, high-intensity activities that do not primarily rely on oxygen metabolism, such as resistance training, sprinting, and high-intensity interval training). Understanding the comparative benefits of these exercise modalities for cognitive, social, and emotional outcomes in schizophrenia is essential for optimizing intervention design and tailoring recommendations to individual needs and preferences (Vancampfort et al., 2012).

Aerobic exercise has received the most extensive research attention in schizophrenia populations, with a substantial evidence base supporting its cognitive benefits. The mechanisms underlying aerobic exercise effects on cognition are well characterized and include enhanced cerebral perfusion, increased BDNF expression, improved cardiovascular fitness, and favorable modulation of neurotransmitter systems. Aerobic exercise particularly influences the hippocampus, a region critical for memory formation and notably affected in schizophrenia, with animal studies consistently demonstrating aerobic exercise-induced hippocampal neurogenesis and synaptic plasticity. The cardiovascular adaptations produced by regular aerobic exercise, including improved heart rate variability, enhanced endothelial function, and reduced systemic inflammation, may also contribute indirectly to cognitive benefits by supporting overall brain health (Malchow et al., 2013).

Meta-analytic evidence examining aerobic exercise interventions in schizophrenia reveals consistent cognitive improvements across multiple domains. Effect sizes for global cognitive function typically range from moderate to large, with particularly robust improvements observed for attention, working memory, and processing speed. These benefits appear relatively consistent across different forms of aerobic exercise, whether walking, cycling, or other modalities, suggesting that the fundamental cardiovascular and metabolic demands of sustained aerobic activity, rather than specific movement patterns, drive cognitive benefits. Dose-response relationships are evident, with moderate to vigorous intensity aerobic exercise (typically 60 to 80 percent of maximum heart rate) producing more substantial improvements than lower intensity activities (Noordsy et al., 2018).

Resistance training, also termed strength training or anaerobic exercise, involves exercises that load muscles against resistance to build strength, power, and muscle mass. Common forms include weightlifting, resistance band exercises, and bodyweight exercises such as push-ups and squats. While less extensively studied than aerobic exercise in schizophrenia populations, emerging evidence suggests that resistance training produces meaningful cognitive benefits as well. The neurobiological mechanisms underlying resistance exercise effects overlap partially with aerobic exercise but also include unique pathways. Resistance training elevates insulin-like growth factor 1 (IGF-1), a hormone that crosses the blood-brain barrier and supports neural health, promotes protein synthesis, and enhances synaptic plasticity (Faulkner & Sparkes, 1999).

Studies comparing aerobic and resistance exercise in schizophrenia are limited but show that both improve cognition. Aerobic exercise benefits memory and attention, while resistance training enhances executive functions. Combined training may yield greater cognitive improvements by engaging complementary mechanisms (Noordsy et al., 2018).

High-intensity interval training (HIIT), characterized by alternating brief periods of intense exercise with recovery intervals, represents a hybrid approach that combines elements of both aerobic and anaerobic exercise. HIIT has gained attention for its time efficiency and potential to enhance cardiovascular fitness more rapidly than moderate-intensity continuous exercise. In general populations, HIIT produces robust cognitive benefits, including enhanced executive function and memory. Limited research in schizophrenia suggests HIIT may be feasible and beneficial, although tolerability and safety considerations require careful attention given the high intensity demands. The acute metabolic and neurochemical responses to HIIT, including substantial BDNF elevation and enhanced catecholamine release, suggest potential for cognitive enhancement, but implementation must be carefully tailored to individual capacity and tolerance (Malchow et al., 2013).

Flexibility and balance exercises, including stretching, yoga, and tai chi, represent additional exercise modalities that have received less systematic investigation in schizophrenia. These practices, while typically less cardiovascularly demanding than aerobic exercise or resistance training, may offer unique benefits through enhanced body awareness, mindfulness components, stress reduction, and improved motor coordination. Yoga, in particular, has shown promise in schizophrenia for reducing symptoms and improving quality of life, with some evidence for cognitive benefits as well. The meditative components of yoga and tai chi may provide additive benefits to the physical activity itself, potentially reducing rumination, enhancing present-moment awareness, and promoting emotional regulation (Noordsy et al., 2018).

4. SOCIAL AND BEHAVIORAL OUTCOMES

Exercise as a Medium for Social Engagement

Social isolation and interpersonal difficulties represent pervasive challenges for individuals with schizophrenia, stemming from multiple intersecting factors including negative symptoms, cognitive deficits affecting social cognition, stigma-related social rejection, and limited community integration. The profound social withdrawal characteristic of schizophrenia contributes substantially to poor quality of life, functional impairment, and reduced recovery outcomes. Traditional psychiatric treatment has historically emphasized symptom reduction with limited focus on social functioning, creating a critical gap in addressing the interpersonal dimensions of the disorder (Garcia et al., 1995). Physical exercise, particularly when conducted in group settings or community contexts, provides natural opportunities for social interaction that may help counteract the isolation typical of schizophrenia. Unlike explicitly therapy-focused social skills interventions, which can feel artificial or highlight social deficits, exercise-based social engagement occurs organically within the context of a shared, meaningful activity. This distinction is important, as the implicit, activity-embedded nature of social interaction during exercise may feel less threatening and more accessible to individuals with pronounced social anxiety or severe negative symptoms (Bremer et al., 2016).

The social affordances of exercise vary considerably across contexts and modalities. Individual exercises, such as solitary jogging or home-based workouts, provide minimal direct social engagement but may still contribute to social wellbeing indirectly by enhancing self-confidence, reducing social anxiety, and improving physical appearance and fitness, which can facilitate subsequent social interactions. Parallel exercise, where individuals exercise in proximity but without structured interaction (for example, attending a gym where others are present but exercising independently), provides a mild form of social exposure that may help individuals become comfortable in social environments without the demands of direct interaction (Dowd et al., 2014).

Group-based exercise, including fitness classes, team sports, and structured group walking programs, offers substantially greater social engagement potential. These contexts create natural opportunities for conversation, mutual encouragement, shared experiences, and relationship formation. The structure provided by group exercise settings, including scheduled meeting times, designated locations, and facilitator guidance, reduces barriers to participation and provides external motivation to attend regularly. The shared goal of physical improvement creates common ground and facilitates connection among participants who might otherwise struggle to initiate or maintain social relationships (Toscano et al., 2022).

Importantly, social interaction within exercise contexts tends to be relatively low-stakes and focused on concrete, present-moment activities rather than personal disclosure or emotionally challenging topics. This characteristic makes exercise-based social engagement particularly well-suited for individuals with schizophrenia who may find conventional social situations overwhelming or anxiety-provoking. Conversations during or following group exercise naturally center on immediate shared experiences (the workout itself, physical sensations, achievement of exercise goals), providing accessible topics that do not require extensive social cognitive processing or emotional vulnerability (Dowd et al., 2014). The role-leveling aspect of exercise contexts merits emphasis. Within exercise settings, individuals are primarily defined by their participation in physical activity rather than their psychiatric diagnosis or illness history. This temporary suspension of the patient identity, combined with the universality of physical exertion and fitness challenges, creates opportunities for individuals with schizophrenia to interact with others on more equal footing. This normalization experience, where mental illness temporarily recedes into the background while shared humanity and common struggles with physical challenges come to the foreground, can be profoundly therapeutic and identity-affirming (Bremer et al., 2016).

Group-Based Physical Activities and Peer Support

Group-based physical activities represent a particularly promising intervention format for individuals with schizophrenia, combining the neurobiological and cognitive benefits of exercise with the therapeutic potential of peer support and social connection. The group format introduces social elements that may enhance adherence, motivation, and enjoyment while simultaneously addressing the social isolation and interpersonal difficulties characteristic of schizophrenia. Understanding the specific mechanisms through which group-based physical activities exert their therapeutic effects, and the factors that optimize these interventions, is essential for effective implementation (Oyibo et al., 2018).

Peer support, defined as mutual assistance between individuals sharing similar life experiences or challenges, represents a core therapeutic element of group-based exercise interventions. Within exercise groups, peer support manifests through multiple mechanisms including emotional support (empathy, encouragement, validation of experiences), informational support (sharing strategies for overcoming barriers, exercise techniques, coping with symptoms), and instrumental support (practical assistance such as transportation coordination or exercise equipment sharing) (Tay et al., 2013). The lived experience commonality among group members creates a foundation of understanding and credibility that may be difficult to replicate in hierarchical professional-patient relationships. The motivational dynamics of group exercise merit particular attention. Negative symptoms of schizophrenia, including avolition, anhedonia, and reduced motivation, represent formidable barriers to initiating and sustaining exercise participation. Group contexts provide external motivation through scheduled commitments, social accountability, and interpersonal connections that may partially compensate for diminished internal motivation. The expectation that others will be present and one's absence will be noticed creates a form of healthy social obligation that encourages attendance even when internal drive is lacking (Oyibo et al., 2018).

Team-based physical activities and cooperative games introduce additional beneficial elements beyond individual or parallel group exercise. Sports such as basketball, volleyball, soccer, or recreational games requiring coordination and cooperation demand communication, role taking, strategic thinking, and responsiveness to others' actions. These activities provide embedded practice opportunities for social cognition skills including perspective taking, intention understanding, and coordinated joint action. The fast-paced, dynamic nature of team sports requires rapid social information processing that may help remediate the social cognitive deficits common in schizophrenia (Resnick et al., 2002).

Improvement in Social Cognition and Interpersonal Skills

Social cognition, encompassing the mental operations that enable perception, interpretation, and response to social information, represents a critical domain of impairment in schizophrenia. Deficits span multiple social cognitive processes including emotion recognition (identifying others' emotional states from facial expressions, vocal tone, and body language), theory of mind (inferring others' beliefs, intentions, and mental states), social perception (interpreting social cues and understanding social contexts), and attributional style (explaining causes of social events and others' behaviour). These social cognitive impairments significantly contribute to the interpersonal difficulties and social dysfunction characteristic of schizophrenia, predicting functional outcomes independently of symptom severity and neurocognition (Bremer et al., 2016).

Emerging evidence suggests that exercise interventions may enhance social cognition in schizophrenia through multiple mechanisms. At a fundamental level, the cognitive improvements produced by exercise, particularly enhanced executive function and processing speed, provide a foundation for more effective social information processing. Social cognition is cognitively demanding, requiring rapid integration of multiple sources of information, flexible perspective shifting, working memory for social context, and inhibitory control to suppress prepotent but socially inappropriate responses (Dowd et al., 2014). Improvements in these underlying neurocognitive capacities facilitate more accurate and efficient social cognitive processing. Emotion recognition, often assessed using tasks requiring identification of facial emotions in photographs, shows improvement following exercise interventions in some studies. The neurobiological mechanisms potentially underlying these improvements include enhanced functioning of brain regions involved in emotion processing, particularly the amygdala and prefrontal cortex, and improved integration between emotion processing regions and higher-order cognitive control areas. Additionally, the emotional experiences associated with exercise participation itself, including enjoyment, accomplishment, and positive social interactions, may enhance emotional awareness and differentiation that generalizes to improved emotion recognition (Toscano et al., 2022).

Theory of mind capacities, the ability to attribute mental states to oneself and others and understand that others' perspectives may differ from one's own, represent complex social cognitive abilities substantially impaired in schizophrenia. While research specifically examining exercise effects on theory of mind in schizophrenia is limited, the cognitive and social engagement components of group-based exercise provide natural opportunities for theory of mind practice. Coordinating actions with others, anticipating partners' or teammates' intentions and behaviours, and navigating social dynamics within exercise groups all require perspective taking and mental state inference (Bremer et al., 2016).

Social perception, the ability to decode and interpret social cues, understand social roles and norms, and accurately assess interpersonal situations, may be enhanced through regular participation in group exercise contexts. These settings provide repeated exposure to varied social situations in a relatively predictable and safe environment. Observing others' social behaviours, receiving implicit and explicit feedback about one's own social conduct, and practicing social navigation in low-stakes contexts may contribute to improved social perceptual abilities. The embodied nature of physical activity, involving awareness of one's own and others' bodily states, movements, and personal space, may also enhance nonverbal social perception (Garcia et al., 1995).

Interpersonal skills, the behavioural capacities necessary for effective social interaction, benefit from the practice opportunities inherent in group-based physical activities. These skills include conversational abilities (initiating conversations, reciprocal exchange, topic maintenance), assertiveness (expressing needs and preferences appropriately), cooperation (working effectively with others toward shared goals), and conflict resolution (navigating disagreements constructively). Unlike traditional social skills training, which often employs artificial role-play scenarios, exercise contexts provide authentic situations requiring these skills, potentially enhancing skill acquisition and transfer to real-world contexts (Mikkelsen et al., 2017).

Role of Physical Activity in Reducing Stigma and Isolation

Stigma, encompassing negative stereotypes, prejudicial attitudes, and discriminatory behaviours directed toward individuals with mental illness, represents a profound barrier to recovery and quality of life for persons with schizophrenia. Stigma operates at multiple levels, including public stigma (societal attitudes and discrimination), structural stigma (institutional policies and practices that disadvantage individuals with mental illness), and self-stigma (internalization of negative stereotypes leading to reduced self-esteem and self-efficacy). The intersection of stigma and schizophrenia is particularly pernicious, as schizophrenia is among the most stigmatized mental health conditions, associated with stereotypes of dangerousness, incompetence, and unpredictability (Resnick et al., 2002).

Social isolation, both a consequence and reinforcer of stigma, severely impacts individuals with schizophrenia. Reduced social networks, limited meaningful social roles, exclusion from community activities, and withdrawal from social participation characterize the lived experience of many individuals with schizophrenia. This isolation exacerbates symptoms, reduces opportunities for recovery, and substantially diminishes quality of life. Interventions that address stigma and reduce isolation represent critical components of comprehensive recovery-oriented care (Oyibo et al., 2018).

Physical activity participation, particularly in community settings, offers multiple pathways for reducing stigma and isolation. At the most fundamental level, engaging in exercise in public or community settings challenges the visibility patterns typical of schizophrenia, where individuals may become largely invisible within their communities due to social withdrawal and limited participation in normative activities. Being seen exercising, an activity associated with health, discipline, and self-care, contradicts common stereotypes of incompetence and lack of motivation often applied to individuals with mental illness (Maddux, 1993).

The physical fitness improvements resulting from regular exercise challenge another pernicious aspect of stigma related to schizophrenia. Individuals with schizophrenia often experience substantial weight gain related to antipsychotic medications, lifestyle factors, and metabolic disturbances. This visible weight gain can become an additional source of stigma and discrimination, compounding mental illness stigma with weight-based prejudice. Exercise-related improvements in fitness, body composition, and physical appearance may reduce this additional stigma layer while enhancing self-esteem and body image (Resnick et al., 2002).

Community-integrated exercise, where individuals with schizophrenia exercise alongside community members without mental illness, provides opportunities for stigma reduction through intergroup contact. Contact theory, a well-established framework in social psychology, posits that direct, positive contact between stigmatized and non-stigmatized individuals can reduce prejudice and discrimination. Exercise contexts may be particularly conducive to effective intergroup contact because they provide equal status interaction, common goals, cooperative interdependence, and opportunities for meaningful relationship development. Exercising together creates shared experiences and common ground that humanize individuals who might otherwise be viewed primarily through the lens of their diagnosis (Dowd et al., 2014).

Self-stigma, the internalization of negative stereotypes about mental illness, may be particularly responsive to exercise interventions. As individuals experience themselves successfully engaging in physical activity, achieving fitness goals, and functioning competently within exercise groups, these experiences directly contradict internalized beliefs about incompetence, inability, and worthlessness. The concrete, observable nature of exercise achievements provides powerful counter-evidence to self-stigmatizing beliefs. Progressive improvement, whether measured by increased endurance, greater strength, enhanced flexibility, or improved athletic skills, creates an objective record of capability and growth that can reshape self-concept (Oyibo et al., 2018).

Exercise participation provides opportunities for identity expansion beyond the patient or illness identity. While schizophrenia diagnosis often becomes a master status that overshadows other aspects of identity, engagement in physical activity allows individuals to develop alternative identities as athletes, exercisers, team members, or fitness enthusiasts. These alternative identities coexist with the reality of living with schizophrenia but provide broader, more nuanced self-definitions that resist reduction to illness alone. Identity diversification supports recovery by providing multiple sources of meaning, purpose, and self-worth (Resnick et al., 2002).

5. EMOTIONAL AND PSYCHOLOGICAL EFFECTS

Reduction of Depressive and Anxiety Symptoms

Depressive and anxiety symptoms represent common and distressing comorbidities in schizophrenia, substantially impacting quality of life and functional outcomes. Approximately 40 to 60 percent of individuals with schizophrenia experience clinically significant depressive symptoms, while anxiety disorders affect 30 to 40 percent of this population. These emotional disturbances contribute to increased suicide risk, reduced treatment adherence, poorer social and occupational functioning, and diminished subjective wellbeing. While antipsychotic medications primarily target positive symptoms, their effects on depression and anxiety are variable and often inadequate, highlighting the need for complementary interventions (Taylor et al., 1985).

The antidepressant effects of exercise are well documented in general populations and increasingly recognized in individuals with serious mental illness, including schizophrenia. Multiple meta-analyses have confirmed that regular physical activity produces clinically meaningful reductions in depressive symptoms, with effect sizes comparable to those observed with psychotherapy or pharmacological antidepressant treatments (Karmakar et al., 2025). In schizophrenia populations specifically, research has demonstrated consistent improvements in depressive symptomatology following structured exercise interventions, with benefits emerging relatively quickly and sustained with continued participation (Mikkelsen et al., 2017).

The neurobiological mechanisms underlying exercise-related improvements in depression are multifaceted and overlap substantially with the pathways implicated in schizophrenia-related cognitive enhancement. Exercise stimulates the expression of neurotrophic factors, particularly BDNF, which supports neuroplasticity and may reverse the neural changes associated with depression. The hippocampus, a brain region demonstrating reduced volume in both depression and schizophrenia, shows exercise-induced neurogenesis and increased volume in animal models and some human studies. These structural brain changes may contribute to sustained mood improvements (Wolff et al., 2011).

Neurotransmitter system modulation represents another critical mechanism. Exercise acutely increases the availability of monoamine neurotransmitters including serotonin, dopamine, and norepinephrine, the same neurotransmitter systems targeted by most antidepressant medications. While acute neurotransmitter elevations are transient, regular exercise may produce more stable alterations in receptor sensitivity, transporter expression, and overall system regulation. Additionally, exercise influences the hypothalamic-pituitary-adrenal (HPA) axis, which is often dysregulated in depression. Regular physical activity enhances HPA axis flexibility and reduces baseline cortisol levels, potentially contributing to improved mood regulation (Taylor et al., 1985).

Anxiety symptoms, including generalized worry, social anxiety, and panic-related symptoms, also respond favourably to exercise interventions. The anxiolytic effects of physical activity operate through multiple mechanisms including enhanced GABAergic tone, reduced muscle tension, improved autonomic nervous system regulation, and cognitive factors such as enhanced self-efficacy and distraction from anxiety-provoking rumination. Acute exercise produces immediate anxiety reduction that may last several hours, while chronic exercise training leads to sustained reductions in baseline anxiety and enhanced resilience to stress-induced anxiety (Mikkelsen et al., 2017).

Enhancement of Self-Esteem and Motivation

Self-esteem, the overall evaluation of one's worth and capabilities, is frequently diminished in individuals with schizophrenia. Multiple factors contribute to low self-esteem in this population, including internalized stigma, repeated experiences of failure or rejection, cognitive impairments that limit competence across various domains, negative symptoms that impair goal-directed activity, and the profound impact of psychotic symptoms on identity and reality testing. Low self-esteem contributes to poor treatment outcomes, reduced quality of life, limited social engagement, and increased vulnerability to depression and suicidal ideation (Schuch & Vancampfort, 2021).

Physical exercise provides multiple pathways for self-esteem enhancement that may be particularly potent for individuals with schizophrenia. Physical self-concept, the perceptions and evaluations of one's physical abilities, appearance, and fitness, represents a foundational component of overall self-esteem that is directly amenable to exercise interventions. As individuals engage in regular physical activity and experience improvements in fitness, strength, endurance, or skill, their physical self-concept becomes more positive. These improvements provide concrete, observable evidence of capability that contrasts sharply with experiences of impairment and limitation in other life domains (Taylor et al., 1985).

The achievement of exercise goals, whether modest or ambitious, provides experiences of success that may be relatively rare for individuals struggling with the functional impairments associated with schizophrenia. Unlike many recovery goals that are abstract, distant, or dependent on factors beyond individual control, exercise goals are concrete, incrementally achievable, and directly contingent on individual effort. This controllability is psychologically important, as it provides opportunities for experiencing agency and self-determination. The progressive nature of fitness improvements allows for continuous goal attainment, maintaining motivation and reinforcing self-efficacy (Schuch & Vancampfort, 2021).

Self-efficacy, the belief in one's capacity to successfully execute behaviours necessary to achieve desired outcomes, is enhanced through exercise participation. According to social cognitive theory, self-efficacy is built primarily through mastery experiences, the direct experience of successfully performing challenging tasks. Exercise provides abundant mastery experiences as individuals progressively overcome physical challenges, achieve new personal bests, and develop competencies. These exercise-specific self-efficacy gains may generalize to broader domains, enhancing confidence in ability to manage symptoms, pursue recovery goals, and navigate life challenges (Wolff et al., 2011). Physical appearance improvements, including weight loss or maintenance, increased muscle tone, improved posture, and enhanced grooming and self-care behaviours, may contribute to self-esteem enhancement. While the therapeutic value of exercise should not be reduced to appearance alone, the reality is that physical appearance impacts self-perception and social experiences. For individuals with schizophrenia who may have experienced weight gain from antipsychotic medications or self-neglect related to symptoms, appearance improvements can restore pride in physical presentation and reduce appearance-related stigma and self-consciousness (Parra et al., 2020).

Body image, the subjective picture of one's body and associated attitudes and feelings, often improves with regular exercise even in the absence of objective physical changes. The mechanism appears to involve increased body appreciation, enhanced awareness of body functionality over appearance, and reduced body dissatisfaction. Engaging in physical activity shifts focus from what the body looks like to what the body can do, cultivating appreciation for physical capabilities and resilience. This functional emphasis may be particularly therapeutic for individuals with schizophrenia whose experiences of embodiment may be disrupted by illness (Zschucke et al., 2013).

Motivation, the psychological forces that energize and direct behaviour toward goals, is simultaneously a prerequisite for exercise participation and an outcome of regular physical activity. The motivational deficits associated with schizophrenia negative symptoms represent formidable barriers to initiating and maintaining exercise routines. However, paradoxically, engagement in physical activity can enhance motivation through multiple mechanisms. The neurobiological effects of exercise, particularly enhanced dopaminergic function and increased BDNF expression, may partially normalize the neural circuits underlying motivation. Additionally, the rewarding experiences associated with exercise, including mood elevation, social connection, and achievement, reinforce continued participation (Taylor et al., 1985).

Intrinsic motivation, characterized by engagement in activities for inherent satisfaction rather than external rewards or pressures, represents the most sustainable form of motivation for long-term exercise adherence. While many individuals begin exercise programs due to external factors such as health concerns or professional recommendations, the development of intrinsic motivation depends on experiencing enjoyment, interest, and personal meaning in physical activity. Intervention design that emphasizes autonomy, competence, and relatedness, the three basic psychological needs identified in self-determination theory, facilitates intrinsic motivation development (Parra et al., 2020).

Exercise and Emotion Regulation Mechanisms

Emotion regulation, the processes by which individuals influence which emotions they experience, when they experience them, and how they express and experience these emotions, is substantially impaired in schizophrenia. Difficulties identifying, understanding, and modulating emotional experiences contribute to symptom severity, interpersonal problems, and reduced quality of life. While some emotion regulation deficits in schizophrenia may reflect primary neurobiological abnormalities, others arise from limited opportunities to develop and practice regulation skills due to social withdrawal, cognitive impairments, and disrupted development (Weyerer & Kupfer, 1994).

Physical exercise influences emotion regulation through multiple mechanisms spanning neurobiological, cognitive, behavioural, and social domains. At the neurobiological level, exercise modulates the neural circuits involved in emotion generation and regulation, particularly the prefrontal cortex and its connections with limbic structures including the amygdala. The enhanced prefrontal cortical function resulting from regular exercise may improve top-down regulation of emotional responses, enabling more effective cognitive control over emotional reactivity. Strengthened prefrontal-amygdala connectivity allows for better integration of emotional and cognitive processes (Wolff et al., 2011).

The neurochemical effects of exercise contribute to emotion regulation enhancement. Endogenous opioid release during exercise, commonly referenced as the runner's high, produces feelings of euphoria and wellbeing while providing natural pain relief. Endocannabinoid system activation represents another neurochemical pathway underlying exercise-induced mood elevation and anxiety reduction. These neurochemical changes not only produce immediate affective improvements but may also enhance emotional flexibility and resilience over time, making individuals less reactive to emotional stressors (Heidarzadeh et al., 2010).

Stress reactivity, the magnitude and duration of physiological and psychological responses to stressors, is modulated by regular exercise. Individuals who exercise regularly demonstrate blunted cortisol responses to acute stressors, indicating enhanced HPA axis regulation. Heart rate variability, a marker of autonomic nervous system flexibility and stress resilience, improves with aerobic exercise training. These physiological changes reflect improved stress regulation capacity that manifests psychologically as enhanced emotional stability and reduced emotional volatility in response to daily challenges (Schuch & Vancampfort, 2021).

Cognitive emotion regulation strategies, the mental approaches individuals use to influence their emotional experiences, may be enhanced through exercise participation. Cognitive reappraisal, the reinterpretation of emotional situations to alter their emotional impact, requires cognitive flexibility and executive control, capacities that are improved by exercise. As cognitive function enhances, individuals may become more capable of employing adaptive emotion regulation strategies (Karmakar et al., 2025). Additionally, the problem-solving skills developed through navigating exercise challenges (overcoming fatigue, adjusting workout plans, troubleshooting barriers) may generalize to more effective coping with emotional challenges (Wolff et al., 2011).

Behavioural emotion regulation strategies involve modifying actions or situations to influence emotional states. Exercise itself represents a behavioural emotion regulation strategy, providing a constructive means of managing negative emotions. Learning to use physical activity intentionally to modulate mood, reduce anxiety, or manage anger provides individuals with a tangible, accessible tool for emotion management. This skill, once developed, can be deployed flexibly across varied emotional contexts and situations (Zschucke et al., 2013).

Mindfulness and present-moment awareness, increasingly recognized as valuable emotion regulation capacities, are naturally cultivated through attentive physical activity. Focusing awareness on physical sensations during exercise, the rhythm of breathing, the feeling of muscles working, and bodily movements creates experiences of mindful embodiment. This present-centered awareness interrupts maladaptive emotion regulation patterns such as rumination and worry while cultivating acceptance of internal experiences. Some exercise formats, particularly yoga and tai chi, explicitly integrate mindfulness components that enhance these benefits (Heidarzadeh et al., 2010).

Emotional granularity, the ability to experience and identify emotions with specificity and precision, may improve through exercise participation. As individuals attend to their bodily and emotional experiences during and after exercise, they may develop enhanced interoceptive awareness and emotional differentiation. Rather than experiencing emotions as undifferentiated distress or arousal, individuals learn to distinguish between anxiety, frustration, excitement, fatigue, and satisfaction. This enhanced emotional awareness facilitates more targeted and effective emotion regulation responses (Dunn & Jewell, 2010).

6. BARRIERS AND CHALLENGES

Patient-Level Barriers: Motivation, Fatigue, and Negative Symptoms

Despite the substantial evidence supporting exercise benefits for individuals with schizophrenia, translating these findings into real-world implementation faces significant challenges. Patient-level barriers, intrinsic factors related to the illness itself and individual circumstances, represent primary obstacles to exercise initiation and maintenance. Understanding these barriers comprehensively is essential for developing effective strategies to enhance exercise participation and adherence in this population (Hickingbotham et al., 2021).

Negative symptoms of schizophrenia, including avolition, anhedonia, asociality, and alogia, represent perhaps the most formidable barriers to exercise engagement. Avolition, the reduction in motivated, self-initiated, purposeful activities, directly undermines the sustained effort required to establish and maintain exercise routines. Individuals experiencing severe avolition may recognize the potential benefits of exercise and genuinely desire to participate yet find themselves unable to generate or sustain the behavioural activation necessary for consistent engagement. This is not a matter of willful non-adherence or laziness but rather a core symptom that disrupts the neurobiological systems underlying goal-directed behaviour (Glover et al., 2013).

Anhedonia, the diminished capacity to experience pleasure, reduces the reinforcing properties of exercise that typically sustain engagement in other populations. While many individuals find exercise inherently rewarding and enjoyable, those experiencing anhedonia may engage in physical activity without experiencing the mood elevation, satisfaction, or enjoyment that would motivate continued participation. This absence of positive reinforcement makes sustained exercise participation dependent on external motivation or sheer discipline, both of which are difficult to maintain long-term (Glover et al., 2013). Cognitive impairments, particularly executive dysfunction, create additional barriers to exercise adherence. Initiating exercise requires planning (identifying appropriate activities, scheduling time, arranging transportation or equipment), organization (preparing appropriate clothing and materials, coordinating logistics), and prospective memory (remembering to attend scheduled exercise sessions). These executive functions are substantially impaired in many individuals with schizophrenia, making even straightforward exercise plans difficult to execute consistently. Additionally, the cognitive fatigue associated with mental effort may reduce available cognitive resources for managing exercise logistics (Hickingbotham et al., 2021).

Physical fatigue and reduced energy, experienced by many individuals with schizophrenia, create significant barriers to exercise initiation. This fatigue may arise from multiple sources including the illness itself, medication side effects (particularly sedation from certain antipsychotics), poor sleep quality, metabolic disturbances, and physical deconditioning from prolonged inactivity. The paradox that exercise can improve energy levels yet requires energy to initiate creates a frustrating catch-22 situation. Individuals may accurately perceive themselves as too tired to exercise, yet this fatigue perpetuates the inactivity that maintains or worsens the fatigue (Weyerer & Kupfer, 1994).

Medication side effects beyond sedation also impede exercise participation. Weight gain and metabolic changes associated with many antipsychotic medications reduce fitness and create physical barriers to activity. Anticholinergic effects including dry mouth and impaired thermoregulation increase discomfort during exercise and potentially create safety concerns in hot environments. Extrapyramidal symptoms such as akathisia, dystonia, or parkinsonian symptoms can make physical activity uncomfortable or technically difficult. While exercise may help mitigate some medication side effects long-term, the immediate impact of these side effects creates barriers to initiating the exercise that would eventually provide relief (Stanton et al., 2015).

Low baseline fitness levels common in individuals with schizophrenia create additional challenges. Prolonged inactivity related to illness results in substantial physical deconditioning, making even moderate physical activity challenging and potentially unpleasant. The discomfort associated with exertion in deconditioned individuals (breathlessness, muscle fatigue, soreness) may be misinterpreted as dangerous or intolerable, leading to premature discontinuation. Additionally, the visible discrepancy between one's current physical capacity and either past abilities or societal standards may evoke shame or discouragement (Hickingbotham et al., 2021).

Prior negative experiences with physical activity can create psychological barriers to exercise engagement. Individuals who experienced ridicule, failure, or humiliation in physical education classes or athletic contexts may carry lasting negative associations with exercise. Trauma related to physical activity, whether from bullying, coercive exercise as punishment, or experiences of physical inadequacy, can create aversion that persists long after the original experiences. Addressing these psychological barriers may require explicit therapeutic processing rather than simple encouragement to exercise (Glover et al., 2013).

Socioeconomic and Cultural Constraints

Beyond individual-level factors, broader socioeconomic and cultural contexts substantially influence exercise participation for individuals with schizophrenia. These structural and societal factors create systematic barriers that differentially impact vulnerable populations and must be addressed to achieve equitable access to exercise-based interventions. Understanding these constraints is essential for developing feasible, sustainable, and culturally responsive exercise programs (Zschucke et al., 2013).

Financial barriers represent fundamental constraints on exercise participation. Many individuals with schizophrenia live in poverty or near-poverty circumstances, relying on disability benefits or limited income that restrict discretionary spending. Gym memberships, fitness classes, exercise equipment, and appropriate athletic clothing and footwear require financial resources that may be unavailable. While free or low-cost exercise options exist (walking, home-based bodyweight exercises), these alternatives require greater self-direction and motivation, precisely the capacities that may be compromised in schizophrenia. Transportation costs to access exercise facilities or programs represent additional financial barriers, particularly in areas with limited public transportation (Hickingbotham et al., 2021).

Housing instability and residential circumstances constrain exercise options. Individuals experiencing homelessness or unstable housing face obvious barriers to regular exercise participation, lacking safe spaces for physical activity and secure storage for equipment or athletic clothing. Those living in supervised residential settings may have limited autonomy over schedule and activities, requiring coordination with staff and accommodation of facility routines. Privacy concerns in congregate living situations may discourage some forms of home-based exercise. Neighborhood characteristics including safety, walkability, and availability of parks or recreational facilities vary substantially and influence opportunities for physical activity (Weyerer & Kupfer, 1994).

Transportation access critically determines the feasibility of exercise participation, particularly for programs requiring travel to specific locations. Many individuals with schizophrenia do not drive due to cognitive impairments, financial constraints, medication effects, or lack of licensure. Dependence on public transportation limits options to facilities accessible by transit and constrains scheduling flexibility. In rural or suburban areas with minimal public transportation, the absence of personal vehicles essentially prohibits access to facility-based exercise programs. Transportation barriers compound other obstacles, as each required trip represents an additional logistical hurdle and potential point of failure for exercise adherence (Parra et al., 2020).

Social determinants of health, including education, employment, social support, and community resources, substantially influence exercise participation. Lower educational attainment may limit health literacy and awareness of exercise benefits, appropriate activity types, or strategies for overcoming barriers. Unemployment or precarious employment creates time scarcity for those juggling multiple survival demands and reduces resources for exercise-related expenses. Limited social networks mean fewer potential exercise partners or sources of encouragement and accountability. Communities with fewer resources typically offer more limited recreational programming and facilities (Firth et al., 2016).

Cultural factors shape attitudes toward exercise, preferred activity types, and social norms around physical activity. Cultural beliefs about the causes and appropriate treatment of mental illness influence receptivity to exercise as a therapeutic intervention. Some cultural contexts emphasize rest and reduction of stimulation for mental distress, potentially conflicting with exercise recommendations. Gender norms influence preferences for exercise types, comfort with different settings, and acceptability of certain activities. Cultural preferences for individual versus group activities, competitive versus cooperative formats, and indoor versus outdoor settings vary significantly and should inform program design (Glover et al., 2013).

Language barriers impede participation for individuals with limited English proficiency when exercise programs, instructions, and promotional materials are available only in English. Understanding exercise instructions, communicating with instructors or fellow participants, and accessing written resources become difficult without language accessibility. Even when language interpretation is available, the dynamic, physical nature of exercise instruction can make interpretation challenging (Wolff et al., 2011). Exercise programs serving diverse populations must provide multilingual resources and staff to ensure accessibility. Immigration status and experiences create additional barriers and considerations. Undocumented individuals may fear accessing services even when technically available due to concerns about immigration enforcement. Refugees and recent immigrants may be unfamiliar with recreational exercise concepts, having come from contexts where physical activity is primarily work-related rather than leisure-oriented. Trauma experiences common among refugee populations may be triggered by certain physical activities or group contexts, requiring trauma-informed program design (Hickingbotham et al., 2021).

Addressing Stigma and Misconceptions

Stigma and misconceptions surrounding both mental illness and the physical capabilities of individuals with schizophrenia create significant barriers to exercise program development, implementation, and participation. These attitudinal barriers operate at multiple levels, including societal stereotypes, provider assumptions, and internalized beliefs, requiring multifaceted intervention strategies. Understanding and actively addressing stigma represents a critical component of successful exercise program implementation (Firth et al., 2016).

Public stigma regarding mental illness affects exercise participation through multiple pathways. Stereotypes of individuals with schizophrenia as dangerous, unpredictable, or incompetent lead to discriminatory practices that limit opportunities for community-based exercise. Fitness facilities may implicitly or explicitly discourage participation by individuals known to have mental illness through unwelcoming attitudes, restrictive policies, or failure to accommodate reasonable needs. Exercise instructors and personal trainers, lacking education about mental illness, may refuse to work with individuals with schizophrenia or behave in ways that communicate discomfort or low expectations (Shor & Shalev, 2016).

Misconceptions about the physical capabilities and limitations of individuals with schizophrenia create both overprotection and neglect. Some providers and family members, operating from paternalistic impulses, discourage vigorous physical activity due to unwarranted concerns about safety or capacity. This overprotection, while well-intentioned, denies autonomy and perpetuates learned helplessness. Conversely, assumptions that individuals with mental illness are inherently unmotivated or non-compliant may lead providers to not even suggest exercise interventions, presuming futility. Both extremes reflect misconceptions that deny the actual capabilities and potential of individuals with schizophrenia (Parra et al., 2020).

Provider-level stigma and therapeutic nihilism substantially impact exercise program availability and quality. Mental health providers who maintain pessimistic views about recovery potential may invest minimal effort in wellness-promoting interventions like exercise, viewing them as peripheral to core symptom-focused treatment. Implicit biases about the capabilities of individuals with schizophrenia may manifest in low expectations, inadequate support, or failure to persistently encourage participation despite initial reluctance. Combating provider-level stigma requires education about recovery potential, exposure to successful examples of exercise program participation, and examination of one's own assumptions and biases (Schuch & Vancampfort, 2021).

Self-stigma creates internal barriers to exercise participation as individuals internalize negative societal attitudes about mental illness and their own capabilities. Beliefs that one is incompetent, weak, or unworthy of investment in health and wellness undermine motivation to engage in self-care behaviours including exercise. Shame about body image, physical appearance, or perceived inadequacy compared to others may create avoidance of exercise contexts, particularly public settings. Self-stigma is often unconscious, manifesting as seemingly reasonable explanations for not exercising that actually reflect deeper internalized negative beliefs about the self (Firth et al., 2016).

Misconceptions about exercise requirements and definitions limit participation by creating unrealistic standards. The belief that exercise must be intense, prolonged, or occur in gym settings to be beneficial discourages engagement among those who find such activities intimidating or inaccessible. Promoting broader, more inclusive definitions of physical activity that encompass walking, household activities, gentle movement, and recreational play expands opportunities and reduces barriers. Emphasizing that any increase in activity, regardless of absolute level, provides benefits combats all-or-nothing thinking that impedes initiation (Schuch & Vancampfort, 2021).

Safety concerns, both legitimate and exaggerated, require balanced consideration. While certain precautions are appropriate given higher rates of cardiovascular disease and metabolic disorders in schizophrenia populations, excessive caution based on misconceptions about fragility or risk can unnecessarily restrict activity. Evidence-based screening, appropriate medical evaluation when indicated, and individualized activity prescription allow for safe exercise participation while avoiding unwarranted restrictions. Educating providers, participants, and families about the actual safety profile of exercise in schizophrenia, which is generally excellent with appropriate precautions, reduces anxiety and overcautious restrictions (Firth et al., 2016).

7. CONCLUSION

The therapeutic potential of exercise for individuals with schizophrenia spans cognitive, social, emotional, and physical domains of functioning, making it a uniquely comprehensive intervention. A strong and expanding body of evidence indicates that regular physical activity leads to meaningful improvements in attention, memory, and executive functions, addressing cognitive deficits that strongly influence daily functioning and typically respond poorly to pharmacological treatment. These benefits are supported by well-established neurobiological mechanisms, including enhanced neuroplasticity, increased expression of neurotrophic factors, improved cerebral blood flow, and modulation of key neurotransmitter systems, which together provide a sound theoretical basis for the observed clinical outcomes. In addition to cognitive enhancement, exercise plays a critical role in reducing social isolation and interpersonal difficulties commonly experienced by individuals with schizophrenia. Participation in structured and group-based physical activities creates natural opportunities for social interaction, skill development, and peer support, while simultaneously promoting improvements in social cognition, communication skills, and community integration. These social gains contribute to improved quality of life, functional independence, and a greater sense of belonging. Exercise also helps reduce stigma by challenging negative stereotypes and enabling individuals to develop identities beyond their illness. The emotional and psychological benefits further strengthen its therapeutic value, as regular exercise is associated with reduced symptoms of depression and anxiety, increased self-esteem and motivation, and improved emotional regulation. These outcomes arise from a combination of neurobiological adaptations, cognitive restructuring, behavioral activation, and social engagement. By simultaneously influencing multiple therapeutic pathways, exercise offers synergistic benefits across domains, positioning it as a holistic and effective adjunct to conventional treatment approaches in schizophrenia.

REFERENCES

Biddle, G. F., Stuart. (1999). Exercise as an adjunct treatment for schizophrenia: A review of the literature. *Journal of Mental Health (Abingdon, England)*, *8*(5), 441–457. DOI: 10.1080/09638239917157

Bremer, E., Crozier, M., & Lloyd, M. (2016). A systematic review of the behavioural outcomes following exercise interventions for children and youth with autism spectrum disorder. *Autism*, *20*(8), 899–915. DOI: 10.1177/1362361315616002 PMID: 26823546

Dowd, A. J., Schmader, T., Sylvester, B. D., Jung, M. E., Zumbo, B. D., Martin, L. J., & Beauchamp, M. R. (2014). *Effects of Social Belonging and Task Framing on Exercise Cognitions and Behavior*. https://doi.org/DOI: 10.1123/jsep.2013-0114

Dunn, A. L., & Jewell, J. S. (2010). The effect of exercise on mental health. *Current Sports Medicine Reports*, *9*(4), 202–207. https://journals.lww.com/acsm-csmr/fulltext/2010/07000/The_Effect_of_Exercise_on_Mental_Health.8.aspx PMID: 20622537

Faulkner, G., & Sparkes, A. (1999). *Exercise as Therapy for Schizophrenia: An Ethnographic Study*. https://doi.org/DOI: 10.1123/jsep.21.1.52

Firth, J., Rosenbaum, S., Stubbs, B., Gorczynski, P., Yung, A. R., & Vancampfort, D. (2016). Motivating factors and barriers towards exercise in severe mental illness: A systematic review and meta-analysis. *Psychological Medicine*, *46*(14), 2869–2881. https://www.cambridge.org/core/journals/psychological-medicine/article/motivating-factors-and-barriers-towards-exercise-in-severe-mental-illness-a-systematic-review-and-metaanalysis/1802F617B64F75CF6721FE59A2F73D1F PMID: 27502153

Garcia, A. W., Broda, M. A. N., Frenn, M., Coviak, C., Pender, N. J., & Ronis, D. L. (1995). Gender and Developmental Differences in Exercise Beliefs Among Youth and Prediction of Their Exercise Behavior. *The Journal of School Health*, *65*(6), 213–219. DOI: 10.1111/j.1746-1561.1995.tb03365.x PMID: 7564283

Girdler, S. J., Confino, J. E., & Woesner, M. E. (2019). Exercise as a Treatment for Schizophrenia: A Review. *Psychopharmacology Bulletin*, *49*(1), 56–69. https://pmc.ncbi.nlm.nih.gov/articles/PMC6386427/ PMID: 30858639

Glover, C. M., Ferron, J. C., & Whitley, R. (2013). Barriers to exercise among people with severe mental illnesses. *Psychiatric Rehabilitation Journal*, *36*(1), 45. https://psycnet.apa.org/record/2013-07802-009 PMID: 23477650

Heidarzadeh, M., Zamanzadeh, V., Maghvan, A. P., & Oshvandi, K. (2010). The effect of physical exercise on physical and psychological problems. *Iranian Journal of Nursing and Midwifery Research, 15*(1), 20. https://pmc.ncbi.nlm.nih.gov/articles/PMC3093026/ PMID: 21589745

Hickingbotham, M. R., Wong, C. J., & Bowling, A. B. (2021). Barriers and facilitators to physical education, sport, and physical activity program participation among children and adolescents with psychiatric disorders: A systematic review. *Translational Behavioral Medicine, 11*(9), 1739–1750. https://academic.oup.com/tbm/article-abstract/11/9/1739/6309033 PMID: 34166515

Karmakar, D., Das, A., Saha, G. C., & Govindasamy, K. (2025). The Impact of Physical Education and Sports on Emotional Resilience and Self-Efficacy. In Lobo, J., & Tagare, R. L.Jr., (Eds.), *Emerging Pedagogical Practices in Physical and Sports Education* (pp. 125–154). IGI Global Scientific Publishing., DOI: 10.4018/979-8-3373-2160-8.ch006

Maddux, J. E. (1993). Social cognitive models of health and exercise behavior: An introduction and review of conceptual issues. *Journal of Applied Sport Psychology, 5*(2), 116–140. DOI: 10.1080/10413209308411310

Malchow, B., Reich-Erkelenz, D., Oertel-Knöchel, V., Keller, K., Hasan, A., Schmitt, A., Scheewe, T. W., Cahn, W., Kahn, R. S., & Falkai, P. (2013). The effects of physical exercise in schizophrenia and affective disorders. *European Archives of Psychiatry and Clinical Neuroscience, 263*(6), 451–467. DOI: 10.1007/s00406-013-0423-2 PMID: 23873090

Mikkelsen, K., Stojanovska, L., Polenakovic, M., Bosevski, M., & Apostolopoulos, V. (2017). Exercise and mental health. *Maturitas, 106*, 48–56. https://www.sciencedirect.com/science/article/pii/S0378512217308563 PMID: 29150166

Noordsy, D. L., Burgess, J. D., Hardy, K. V., Yudofsky, L. M., & Ballon, J. S. (2018). Therapeutic Potential of Physical Exercise in Early Psychosis. *The American Journal of Psychiatry, 175*(3), 209–214. DOI: 10.1176/appi.ajp.2017.17060716 PMID: 29490501

Oyibo, K., Adaji, I., & Vassileva, J. (2018). Social cognitive determinants of exercise behavior in the context of behavior modeling: A mixed method approach. *Digital Health, 4*, 2055207618811555. DOI: 10.1177/2055207618811555 PMID: 30479828

Parra, E., Arone, A., Amadori, S., Mucci, F., Palermo, S., & Marazziti, D. (2020). Impact of physical exercise on psychological well-being and psychiatric disorders. *J Reatt Ther Dev Divers, 3*(2), 24–39. https://pdfs.semanticscholar.org/88d2/143cef826c1c5550a5e45806bb02699c876c.pdf

Resnick, B., Orwig, D., Magaziner, J., & Wynne, C. (2002). The Effect of Social Support on Exercise Behavior in Older Adults. *Clinical Nursing Research, 11*(1), 52–70. DOI: 10.1177/105477380201100105 PMID: 11845515

Rosa Rimes, R., Marcos de Souza Moura, A., Khede Lamego, M., Souza de Sa Filho, A., Manochio, J., Paes, F., Giovanni Carta, M., Mura, G., Wegner, M., Budde, H., Barbosa Ferreira Rocha, N., Rocha, J., Manuel, R. S., Tavares, J., Arias-Carrion, O., Egidio Nardi, A., Yuan, T.-F., & Machado, S. (2015). Effects of Exercise on Physical and Mental Health, and Cognitive and Brain Functions in Schizophrenia: Clinical and Experimental Evidence. *CNS & Neurological Disorders - Drug Targets, 14*(10), 1244–1254. PMID: 26556069

Scheewe, T. W., Backx, F. J. G., Takken, T., Jörg, F., van Strater, A. C. P., Kroes, A. G., Kahn, R. S., & Cahn, W. (2013). Exercise therapy improves mental and physical health in schizophrenia: A randomised controlled trial. *Acta Psychiatrica Scandinavica, 127*(6), 464–473. DOI: 10.1111/acps.12029 PMID: 23106093

Schuch, F. B., & Vancampfort, D. (2021). Physical activity, exercise, and mental disorders: It is time to move on. *Trends in Psychiatry and Psychotherapy, 43*(3), 177–184. https://www.scielo.br/j/trends/a/jCRvs9LQq8ycmLwLysGBRFM/ PMID: 33890431

Shor, R., & Shalev, A. (2016). Barriers to involvement in physical activities of persons with mental illness. *Health Promotion International, 31*(1), 116–123. https://academic.oup.com/heapro/article-abstract/31/1/116/2355913 PMID: 25204451

Stanton, R., Reaburn, P., & Happell, B. (2015). Barriers to exercise prescription and participation in people with mental illness: The perspectives of nurses working in mental health. *Journal of Psychiatric and Mental Health Nursing, 22*(6), 440–448. DOI: 10.1111/jpm.12205 PMID: 25855247

Tay, L., Tan, K., Diener, E., & Gonzalez, E. (2013). Social Relations, Health Behaviors, and Health Outcomes: A Survey and Synthesis. *Applied Psychology. Health and Well-Being, 5*(1), 28–78. DOI: 10.1111/aphw.12000 PMID: 23281315

Taylor, C. B., Sallis, J. F., & Needle, R. (1985). The relation of physical activity and exercise to mental health. *Public Health Reports, 100*(2), 195. https://pmc.ncbi.nlm.nih.gov/articles/PMC1424736/ PMID: 3920718

Toscano, C. V. A., Ferreira, J. P., Quinaud, R. T., Silva, K. M. N., Carvalho, H. M., & Gaspar, J. M. (2022). Exercise improves the social and behavioral skills of children and adolescent with autism spectrum disorders. *Frontiers in Psychiatry, 13*. Advance online publication. DOI: 10.3389/fpsyt.2022.1027799 PMID: 36620673

Vancampfort, D., Probst, M., Helvik Skjaerven, L., Catalán-Matamoros, D., Lundvik-Gyllensten, A., Gómez-Conesa, A., Ijntema, R., & De Hert, M. (2012). Systematic Review of the Benefits of Physical Therapy Within a Multidisciplinary Care Approach for People With Schizophrenia. *Physical Therapy*, *92*(1), 11–23. DOI: 10.2522/ptj.20110218 PMID: 22052946

Viljoen, M., & Roos, J. L. (2020). Physical exercise and the patient with schizophrenia. *Australian Journal of General Practice*, *49*(12), 803–808. DOI: 10.3316/informit.638850071185097 PMID: 33254203

Weyerer, S., & Kupfer, B. (1994). Physical Exercise and Psychological Healtha. *Sports Medicine (Auckland, N.Z.)*, *17*(2), 108–116. DOI: 10.2165/00007256-199417020-00003 PMID: 8171221

Wolff, E., Gaudlitz, K., Von Lindenberger, B.-L., Plag, J., Heinz, A., & Ströhle, A. (2011). Exercise and physical activity in mental disorders. *European Archives of Psychiatry and Clinical Neuroscience*, *261*(S2), 186–191. DOI: 10.1007/s00406-011-0254-y PMID: 21935629

Zschucke, E., Gaudlitz, K., & Ströhle, A. (2013). Exercise and physical activity in mental disorders: Clinical and experimental evidence. *Journal of Preventive Medicine and Public Health = Yebang Uihakhoe Chi*, *46*(Suppl 1), S12. https://pmc.ncbi.nlm.nih.gov/articles/PMC3567313/ PMID: 23412549

Chapter 5
Micro-Workouts for Mental Health:
Immediate Psychological Benefits of Short-Duration Exercise

M. Kaviyalakshmi Manikandan
https://orcid.org/0009-0005-8614-5626
Sri Krishna Arts and Science College, India

B. Angelin
Sri Krishna Arts and Science College, India

ABSTRACT

This chapter explores the emerging concept of micro-workouts, or "exercise snacks," and their potential role in enhancing mental health and cognitive performance. While traditional exercise is well established in reducing risks of cardiovascular disease, diabetes, cancers, and psychological disorders, modern sedentary lifestyles and lack of time limit participation. Micro-workouts, typically lasting less than 15 minutes, provide a practical and accessible alternative through activities such as stair climbing, squats, brisk walking, or desk push-ups. Recent evidence highlights their influence on mood, emotional regulation, anxiety and depression reduction, and improvements in attention, memory, and learning, largely mediated by neurochemicals such as endorphins, serotonin, dopamine, and endocannabinoids. This chapter compares micro-workouts with longer sessions, explores underlying mechanisms, and outlines strategies for integrating these short bouts of activity into daily routines, aiming to make exercise more achievable and beneficial for a wide range of individuals.

DOI: 10.4018/979-8-3373-6157-4.ch005

INTRODUCTION

In today's world, more than one in three adults fail to meet the recommended levels of physical activity, and sedentary lifestyles have become a global health concern (World Health Organization, 2020). Most people are unaware of the importance of physical activity and its effect on physical and mental health. The fact that optimal levels of physical activity have decreased the risk of diseases is so underrated. Most of us spend our days moving from one screen to another, sitting in class, at work, or scrolling on our phones, and often use a lack of time as an excuse for not engaging in physical activity. The demands of modern life often leave people feeling "too busy to exercise," but this lack of movement comes at the cost of both physical and mental health. Hence, there is an increasing need to understand the impact of physical exercise on health issues and their significance in daily routine. At least the link between exercise and physical health is garnering attention, unlike its effects on mental health. Since today's lifestyle is contributing to increasing mental health cases, workouts seem to serve as an effective, practical solution to varied health concerns. Exercise is considered the third pillar of mental health treatment, showing that medication and psychotherapy are essential, but physical exercise can complement them by releasing essential neurochemicals (MeHelp, 2024).

Impact of Physical Exercise on Health Issues

Physical Exercise provides health benefits such as strengthening muscles and bones, improving posture, enhancing flexibility, better immune function, weight management, aiding in digestion, and other metabolic functions. Beyond maintaining a healthy body weight, research has provided evidence on how physical activity increases one's lifespan by delaying the onset of chronic diseases such as diabetes, depression, cardiovascular diseases, and cognitive decline. The wide range of health issues that can be managed and prevented, including regular strength training, stretching, walking, and balance exercises, helps maintain bone health, muscle mass, enhances joint flexibility and coordination, and improves posture, which is important in preventing diseases like osteoporosis, sarcopenia, and arthritis-related complications in older adults. Exercise has a crucial role in improving cardiovascular health. It lowers heart risk by controlling cholesterol levels, blood pressure, and reducing inflammation. Research has also highlighted a protective role of exercise against certain types of cancers, including breast, colon, and prostate cancers (McTiernan, 2008). Mechanisms include better immune function, regulation of sex hormones, and decreased systemic inflammation. Exercise plays a vital role in managing metabolic disorders such as type 2 diabetes and obesity. Regular physical activity increases the body's sensitivity to insulin, supports better glucose control, and helps maintain healthy lipid levels. Even brief sessions of movement spread across the day can lower blood sugar and reduce the risk of diabetes-related complications.

Link Between Physical Activity and Mental Health

Physical activity is well known not just for its effects on the body, but also for its significant influence on mental health. Studies over the years have shown that consistent exercise can lift mood, reduce the symptoms of depression and anxiety, improve thinking and memory, and promote overall mental well-being. These benefits arise from a mixture of chemical changes in the brain, physical responses in the body, and positive social and psychological effects. Engaging in physical activity increases the production of certain neurochemicals in the body. Exercise stimulates the release of opioids and endocannabinoids, which are associated with feelings of pleasure, reduced anxiety, improved sleep, and lower pain sensitivity. Studies also show that exercise can enhance attention, focus, memory, cognitive abilities, language skills, and decision-making for up to two hours. Moreover, regular physical activity positively influences the hypothalamus-pituitary-adrenal (HPA) axis and helps reduce cortisol levels (Ruegsegger & Booth, 2018). Both short bouts of exercise and extended workout sessions have been beneficial in improving mental health. It is shown that people who exercise have better minds. However, the actual link between physical activity and mood enhancement needs to be studied. Physical activity has been shown to provide significant benefits for mental and neurological health across a wide range of conditions. Regular exercise reduces symptoms of depression and anxiety by enhancing endorphin release and regulating stress hormones. In individuals with schizophrenia, it improves cognitive function, social interaction, and overall quality of life. In cases of alcohol dependence, it helps manage cravings, improves mood, and supports stress regulation.

Exercise also enhances sleep quality and stabilizes sleep patterns, prevents stress-related disorders by lowering cortisol, and can help stabilize mood swings in bipolar disorder. Furthermore, physical activity has been found to reduce symptoms of post-traumatic stress disorder (PTSD), improve attention and brain functioning in ADHD, and slow cognitive decline in Alzheimer's disease. It may also reduce compulsive behaviours in obsessive-compulsive disorder (OCD). It reduces pain perception while improving sleep and mood in chronic pain conditions such as fibromyalgia. Overall, these benefits arise from a combination of neurochemical, physiological, and psychosocial mechanisms, highlighting the crucial role of exercise in mental and neurological well-being.

Aerobic and Resistance Exercise compared to Medication or Psychotherapy

Physical exercise, especially aerobic and resistance training, is increasingly acknowledged as an effective approach for enhancing mental health and managing psychological disorders. Even though medication and psychotherapy remain the primary treatments for conditions like depression, anxiety, and stress-related disorders, research indicates that exercise can serve as a valuable complementary strategy and sometimes may even act as an alternative intervention strategy. Aerobic activities, including running, cycling, swimming, and brisk walking, enhance cardiovascular fitness and body endurance. In addition to these physical benefits, aerobic exercise has been consistently shown to alleviate symptoms of depression and anxiety (Anderson & Shivakumar, 2013). Furthermore, aerobic exercise supports cognitive function by increasing cerebral blood flow, promoting neurogenesis, and increasing neurotransmitter levels, such as serotonin and dopamine (Esteves et al., 2021; Caneppele et al., 2022). Resistance training, which includes weightlifting, bodyweight exercises, and resistance band workouts, also shows significant benefits for mental health. Research indicates that such training can reduce depressive symptoms, enhance self-esteem, and decrease anxiety, likely through mechanisms including endorphin release, hormonal regulation, and improved physical self-efficacy. Resistance exercise may be very beneficial for individuals with low baseline physical activity or for those who prefer strength-focused workouts over aerobic activities, as represented in Table 1.

Table 1. Aerobic vs. resistance micro-workouts

Aspect	Aerobic Snacks (brisk stairs/walking)	Resistance Snacks (sit-stands/ push-ups)
Main Benefits	Boosts heart/lung fitness, cuts blood sugar spikes after meals (Centers for Disease Control and Prevention, 2021).	Builds leg strength, helps with daily tasks like standing up more easily.
Best For	Office workers fighting sitting fatigue during meetings.	Students or seniors needing quick power for stairs/climbing.
Time Needed	2-3 min bursts, 3x/hour.	1-2 min sets, twice daily.

Antidepressants and anxiolytics work by targeting specific neurotransmitters to relieve symptoms, but they can cause side effects like any other tablet. The common side effects are fatigue, nausea, or weight changes. On the other hand, exercise offers broad systemic and psychological benefits with minimal adverse side effects. Several studies have found that structured exercise programs can produce reductions in depressive symptoms. Psychotherapy, such as Cognitive Behavioural Therapy

(CBT), aims to modify negative thought patterns and develop effective coping strategies. Exercise can complement psychotherapy by physiologically preparing the brain for better mood regulation and cognitive flexibility, thus enhancing therapeutic outcomes. Some clinical trials suggest that combining exercise with CBT or other psychotherapeutic approaches results in greater improvements than either intervention alone.

Today's Sedentary Life and Lack of Physical Activity

Sedentary behaviour is essentially another term for physical inactivity, and modern life has significantly increased this trend across all age groups. The rise of technological innovations, the prevalence of desk-bound occupations, and the growing dependence on digital entertainment have all together resulted in prolonged sitting and reduced opportunities for regular physical activity. During the COVID-19 pandemic, sedentary behaviour reached its peak. Lockdowns, remote work, and online learning confined people to their homes, while the closure of gyms and outdoor spaces led to a drastic decline in physical activity across all age groups (Dunstan et al.,2012). At the same time, there was a sharp increase in mental health concerns such as depression, anxiety, stress, and feelings of isolation. Research indicates that reduced physical activity, combined with prolonged screen time, negatively impacts both physical and psychological well-being (Mattioli et al., 2020). This period highlighted the strong connection between physical activity and mental health, and how quickly inactivity can contribute to emotional and cognitive difficulties.

Even after the pandemic, not much has changed. Today's generation has largely normalised physical inactivity, often justifying it with reasons such as lack of time, resources, or energy. However, these are rarely true barriers, as those genuinely concerned about their health usually find ways to include movement in their routine. Importantly, physical activity does not always have to mean structured workouts; simple habits such as walking instead of driving short distances, taking the stairs instead of the lift, or engaging in activities like dancing can make a meaningful difference. Exercise does not need to be long or complicated to be effective.

Modern lifestyles often emphasize convenience and comfort, leaving many people with limited time or motivation for structured exercise. This highlights the need for practical approaches, such as micro-workouts or short exercise breaks, which make it easier to include movement in busy routines. These simple strategies provide both physical and mental health benefits without requiring long or highly organised sessions, helping to reduce the risks associated with sedentary living. In conclusion, the rising trend of inactivity proves to be an urgent call for realistic and followable interventions that encourage regular movement. Even small amounts of physical activity can make a significant difference in improving overall health and well-being.

MICRO-WORKOUTS AS A PRACTICAL SOLUTION

Many studies have emphasised the benefits of long-term exercise for mental functioning. But a growing area of interest focuses on the positive effects of micro-workouts or short-duration sessions, also referred to as "exercise snacks" or acute exercise. These tiny bouts of activity have gained attention because they fit seamlessly into busy modern schedules, where lack of time is one of the biggest obstacles to regular physical activity. Typically lasting no more than 15 minutes, micro-workouts offer a practical and time-efficient alternative to traditional hour-long sessions. Micro-workouts can be easily incorporated into a busy schedule by including stair climbing, brisk walking, desk push-ups, squats, lunges, and planks, which can be done in intervals throughout the day.

Introducing Exercise Snacks

The idea of "exercise snacks" may sound casual, but it marks the beginning of a genuine shift in how physical activity is approached. Similar to how small food snacks provide quick bursts of energy and satisfy hunger, these short bouts of movement are spread throughout the day and can provide us with meaningful health benefits. These sessions, lasting not more than 10 minutes, may appear insignificant and minor, but when done regularly, they contribute to lasting physical and mental health benefits (Mahindru et al.,2023). The concept of exercise snacks gained attention as researchers searched for ways to overcome one of the greatest barriers to physical activity, which is a lack of time. For many people multitasking with studies, work, family, or health concerns, dedicating a full hour to structured exercise can feel impractical. Exercise snacks offer a practical solution because they are flexible, accessible, and easy to integrate into daily routines without the need for gyms, equipment, extensive preparation, or time. Examples include taking the stairs instead of the elevator, doing squats or lunges during short breaks, walking briskly between tasks, or performing desk-friendly movements such as chair dips and stretches.

Although these actions may seem inconsequential, research shows they can lead to measurable improvements in cardiorespiratory fitness, muscle strength, and cognitive performance (Francois & Little, 2015). For example, a randomized trial found women doing 3x20-second stair sprints daily for 4 weeks gained significant VO_2 peak and lost waist inches (Little et al., 2019). As shown in Figure 1, youth populations demonstrate superior VO_2 peak gains from exercise snacks. Another RCT showed heart patients improved fitness with brief vigorous stair breaks vs. controls (Jenkins et al., 2019). In many aspects, exercise snacks broaden the definition of exercise by shifting the focus from lengthy, structured workouts to short, intentional, small bouts of movement that can be done anywhere and at any time. This adaptability makes them particularly relevant in today's fast-paced lifestyle.

Figure 1. Illustrative comparison of VO_2 peak gains across youth, older adults, and clinical groups, using approximate values to summarize trends reported in the literature rather than exact pooled data

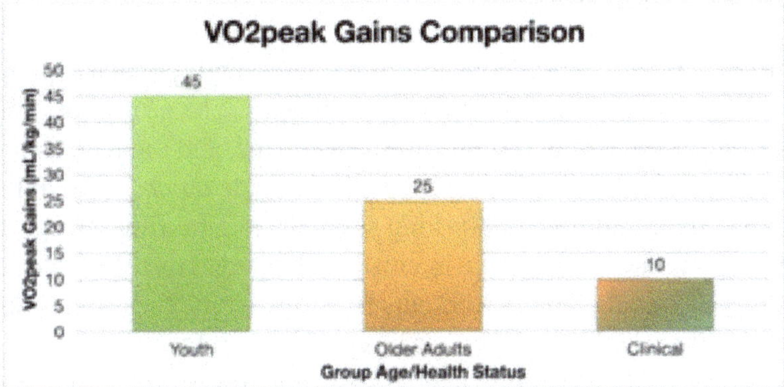

Fitness gains by group age/health status

Effectiveness of acute exercise

The benefits of regular exercise are well known, but researchers have also begun to study acute exercise, which refers to a single workout session. What is salient is that even one short bout of physical activity can bring noticeable changes in how we think, feel, and manage stress. In people, studies show that acute exercise provides a small but steady boost to cognitive functions, especially those controlled by the prefrontal cortex, such as attention, decision-making, and problem-solving. It also tends to lift mood, ease stress, and support emotional well-being through the release of chemicals like endorphins and dopamine (Abou Elmagd, 2016). Animal research suggests that exercise can trigger changes in the brain's chemistry, though most studies have focused on long-term exercise routines (Cotman & Berchtold, 2002; DNA Learning Center, 2008). Evidence on the effects of a single session is more limited, but the findings still point in a positive direction.

Beyond the mind, the body feels the difference almost immediately. Within 10 to 15 minutes, the heart beats faster, circulation improves, and oxygen supply to both muscles and the brain increases. Blood sugar levels become better regulated as glucose is absorbed more quickly, preventing dips in energy. Muscles loosen up, joints become more mobile, and the lungs work harder, enhancing breathing efficiency (Basso & Suzuki,2017). The immune system also responds as more protective cells begin circulating through the body. Instead of leaving people drained and exhausted, these short bursts of activity often create a sense of freshness and alertness. In many ways, acute exercise acts like a quick reset button for the body that restores energy, focus, and resilience in just a few minutes.

Trends and Public Interest

In recent years, micro-workouts have become increasingly popular as people search for practical ways to stay active within busy schedules. The growth of remote work from home culture, the rise of digital fitness platforms, and the increasing trend of short-form exercise content on social media have made quick, accessible routines more appealing than traditional hour-long sessions. Digital fitness apps now offer plenty of 5 to 15-minute routines, and interesting challenges turn these short sessions into fun, achievable goals. Micro-workouts fit perfectly into these trends as they are fast, flexible, and backed by science for boosting mood, focus, and overall mental health. Apps such as Nike Training Club, FitOn, and Seven now promote workouts lasting just 7–10 minutes, showing the growing demand for micro workouts. These apps attract users as they are gamified and are time-sensitive. During the COVID-19 pandemic, when gyms were closed and sedentary behaviour spiked, many turned to at-home options like micro-workouts, yoga, and desk-based exercises to support both physical and mental health.

A 2021 World Health Organization (WHO) report noted that more than one in four adults worldwide do not meet recommended activity levels, with lack of time identified as a major barrier. This helps explain why "exercise snacks" have kindled interest with the public, and they fit into small free gaps of the day and require no special equipment or gym access. Public health campaigns and workplace wellness programs are also promoting short bouts of activity, such as stair climbing, walking meetings, or stretch breaks, all of which align with scientific evidence showing that even brief movement can improve energy, mood, and productivity. Micro-workouts are no longer just a passing trend, but are increasingly recognised as a sustainable approach to fitness. Their popularity reflects a broader cultural shift toward convenience and mental well-being, showing that exercise does not need to be long or complex to be effective.

NEUROCHEMICAL MECHANISMS

Physical activity is associated with the release of a number of neurochemicals and neurotransmitters that, upon release, improve mood and cognition. The mental benefits of exercise are closely linked to the way it alters the brain chemistry. One of the most familiar effects comes from endorphins, which are natural opioids made by the body. Endorphins ease pain, bring a sense of relaxation, and are often behind the "runner's high" many people experience after sustained activity. Exercise also activates the endocannabinoid system, which helps regulate mood, anxiety, and emotional balance. Endocannabinoids are natural substances produced by the body that act on the same receptors as cannabis, but without outside substances. Even moderate physical activity can increase endocannabinoid levels, leading to greater calmness and reduced stress (Dishman & O'Connor, 2009). Another important pathway involves dopamine, a neurotransmitter linked to motivation, reward, and focus. Exercise helps regulate dopamine activity in the brain, which is why physical activity often improves concentration, drive, and overall satisfaction. Together, endorphins, endocannabinoids, and dopamine explain why exercise feels rewarding and why it plays such a powerful role in supporting mental health and cognitive performance.

Endorphin Hypothesis and Mood Regulation

Exercise gives rise to feel-good chemicals like Endorphin that are excellent mood regulators (Saanijoki et al., 2018). These are natural chemicals in the brain that help reduce pain and bring a sense of happiness or calm. That's why people often talk about the "runner's high" after a workout. Studies show that even a short session of exercise can boost mood, ease stress, and create a feeling of energy. While endorphins play a big role, other brain chemicals like dopamine and endocannabinoids also help in lifting our mood and improving focus.

Dopamine and Cognition

Dopamine is often called the "happiness hormone" because it's linked to reward, focus, and learning. Exercise, even in small amounts, gives this system a boost by increasing dopamine release and making the brain more sensitive to it. This is why a quick workout can leave us feeling more awake, motivated, and ready to tackle tasks. While endorphins mainly help with mood and pain relief, dopamine directly affects how clearly, we think and how well we can concentrate. Research shows that exercise can sharpen memory, problem-solving, and decision-making in the short term, while regular activity may even protect the brain from age-related decline. In short, exercise doesn't just make us feel good but also helps us stay focused, motivated, and mentally sharp.

Endocannabinoid and Anxiety-Reduction

The endocannabinoid system (ECS) consists of a network of naturally occurring, cannabis-like substances within the human body that help regulate mood, stress, and emotional balance. Exercise, even done in brief periods, has been demonstrated to increase endocannabinoids, most specifically anandamide, a substance with a strong association to feelings of relaxation and decreased anxiety (Fuss et al., 2015). In contrast to endorphins, which have difficulty crossing the blood–brain barrier, endocannabinoids can directly communicate with areas in the brain like the amygdala and prefrontal cortex, both of which play a role in regulating stress and fear reactions. In simple terms, exercise triggers the release of the body's own "natural relaxants," which act like an internal stress-relief system. This explains why even light forms of activity, such as walking, cycling, or gentle stretching, can reduce anxiety and improve overall emotional well-being.

Other Neurochemical Mechanisms

Apart from endorphins, dopamine, and endocannabinoids, several other brain chemicals also contribute to the positive effects of exercise on mood and mental sharpness. One of these is serotonin, often called the "feel-good" chemical. Exercise increases serotonin levels, which helps balance emotions, improve sleep quality, and regulate appetite. Another important element is brain-derived neurotrophic factor (BDNF), a protein that helps brain cells grow and stay healthy. Even short bouts raise BDNF for better memory and brain flexibility, a meta-analysis confirms acute exercise boosts BDNF by 20-40% in humans (Cotman & Berchtold, 2002). This makes BDNF one of the strongest reasons why exercise is linked to better brain health. Exercise also boosts norepinephrine, a chemical linked to alertness and stress control. Even a quick workout can increase its levels, helping with focus and making the brain more prepared to handle challenges (Cotman & Berchtold, 2002). Altogether, exercise works through a combination of these brain chemicals, creating a powerful effect that lifts mood, reduces stress, and supports clear thinking

PSYCHOLOGICAL AND COGNITIVE BENEFITS

Exercise isn't just about keeping the body fit, but also has strong benefits for the mind. Research has shown that both regular workouts and short bouts of activity can positively impact mental health and thinking abilities. Micro-workouts, in particular, show that even a few minutes of movement can lift mood, sharpen focus, and reduce emotional tension. One of the clearest effects of exercise is its ability to improve mood. Physical activity stimulates the release of "feel-good" brain chemicals like endorphins, serotonin, and dopamine, helping people feel calmer, happier, and more energized. People feel these positive feelings even after just a short session. Exercise also supports emotion regulation and balance. It helps manage stress and handle daily hassles more effectively. Physical activity can decrease irritability, improve patience, and promote a steadier emotional state by reducing stress hormones and activating relaxation pathways in the body.

Emotional Regulation

Along with improving mood, exercise also helps people manage their emotions more effectively. Emotional regulation is the ability to handle feelings like stress, anger, or sadness in a balanced way, without letting them take over. Both single sessions of activity and regular exercise can support this balance by positively affecting the brain and body's stress systems. Exercise reduces levels of the main stress hormone called Cortisol, and boosts the functioning of the prefrontal cortex, which is responsible for self-control and decision-making. This combination makes it easier to stay calm and feel more in control, even after just a short workout. At the same time, physical activity increases the availability of chemicals like dopamine and serotonin, which make the mind more resilient against negative emotions.

Reduction in Anxiety and Depression Symptoms

One of the most powerful psychological benefits of exercise is its ability to ease symptoms of anxiety and depression. Physical activity works like a natural antidepressant and anti-anxiety remedy, offering both quick relief and long-term protection. For depression, exercise boosts the release of mood-enhancing chemicals like endorphins, dopamine, and serotonin, which help lift feelings of sadness or hopelessness. It also encourages the growth of new brain cells in the hippocampus, a region often linked with low mood when underactive. For anxiety, exercise calms the nervous system by lowering heart rate, blood pressure, and stress hormones, creating a greater sense of control and calmness. These benefits aren't limited to long workouts; even simple, consistent actions such as walking, stretching, or short "exercise snacks" spread throughout the day can make a big difference.

Impact on Attention, Memory, and Learning

Exercise doesn't just make the body stronger; it also sharpens the mind. Even short bursts of physical activity can improve focus, memory, and learning. After just one workout, many people notice they feel more alert and able to concentrate.

This happens because movement increases blood flow and oxygen to the brain, giving the prefrontal cortex, the part responsible for focus and decision-making, a quick boost. Over time, regular exercise creates lasting changes in the brain. It encourages the growth and protection of brain cells, supports the formation of new connections, and strengthens areas like the hippocampus, which is key to memory. These changes help improve learning ability and make it easier to store and recall information. For students, working professionals, and even older adults, regular movement can be a simple but powerful tool to boost focus, retain knowledge, and maintain cognitive health throughout life.

Academic and Workplace Performance

The impact of exercise goes far beyond personal health; it also shapes how well people perform in schools and workplaces. Regular physical activity supports sharper focus, better memory, and improved problem-solving abilities, and thus benefits students. These mental boosts make it easier to absorb lessons, recall information, and stay engaged during classes. Even short breaks of movement between study sessions can clear the mind, fight off fatigue, and make learning more effective. In the workplace, exercise contributes to higher energy levels, better stress management, and increased productivity. Active employees often report fewer sick days, stronger time management skills, and a greater sense of job satisfaction. Many organizations now recognize this fact and therefore are promoting wellness programs, walking meetings, or simple activity breaks to keep employees healthy and motivated. Exercise is an investment that strengthens academic achievement, enhances workplace performance, and creates benefits that ripple through schools, companies, and even society at large.

Figure 2. Before-and-after sequence showing physiological and psychological benefits of a 2-minute stair break for office workers (top) and college students (bottom). Demonstrates rapid stress reduction and cognitive refreshment

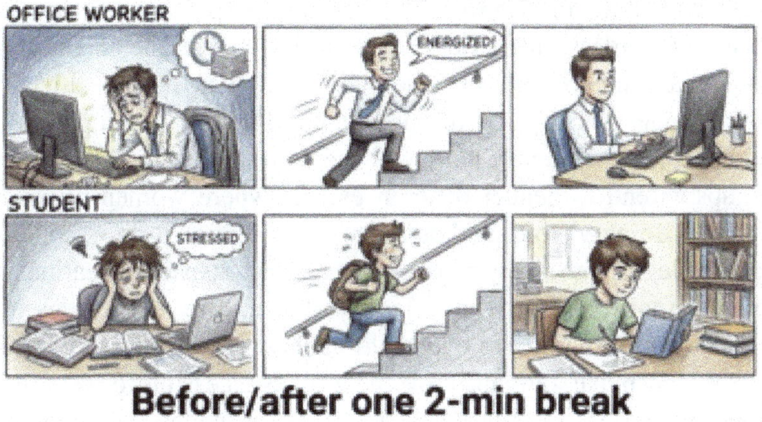

CONS AND CHALLENGES

Although integrating exercise into daily life is widely promoted for its accessibility, several cons and challenges remain. One limitation is that incidental activities, such as walking or stair climbing, may not consistently reach the moderate-to-vigorous intensity needed for optimal cardiovascular benefits, leading to potential overestimation of their health impact. Environmental and social factors, such as unsafe walking infrastructure, car dependence, and sedentary work cultures, further hinder the adoption of lifestyle-integrated exercise.

Equity and Access Barriers

Lower-income workers often struggle more with fitting exercise snacks into their daily routine because they deal with longer commutes, less flexible schedules, and fewer safe indoor spaces like stairwells or quiet corridors compared to office professionals who can access them easily. Rural people face a different set of challenges as they might not have the same built infrastructure as urban areas, relying instead on outdoor paths that can be affected by weather, poor lighting, or safety concerns, which makes consistent short activity breaks harder to maintain without proper planning.

Culture and money add constraints too cause tight budgets mean no gym memberships, while family duties or long work hours eat up any spare minutes for movement.

Economics hit hardest when low-income groups face unsafe neighbourhoods or jobs without breaks, creating a cycle where the people who need health boosts most end up sitting longest. Fixing this means designing buildings and policies that put activity within everyone's reach, not just those with perfect conditions.

These gaps extend to gender differences too, where women might feel self-conscious about doing visible workouts due to professional dress codes, cultural expectations, or legitimate safety worries in shared workspaces, creating an uneven field for who actually benefit from micro-workouts. The real fix lies in broader solutions like workplace policies that build in short mandatory activity breaks or campus designs that make stairs and movement zones accessible to everyone, helping bridge these divides so the health gains aren't just for the few privileged people.

Differences Across Age and Clinical Groups

Youth and healthy adults can perform short, intense exercise snacks (e.g., stair climbing, cycling sprints) that boost fitness, matching longer workouts where effort is similar (Fraser et al., 2025; Jenkins et al., 2019). High adherence makes them practical for busy students.

Older Adults like pre-frail seniors doing twice-daily strength snacks (sit-to-stands) for 4 weeks improved leg power and daily function with 85% adherence (Allison et al., 2023). Safe for home use, no gym needed.

Clinical Groups such as adults with heart disease or obesity gain cardiorespiratory fitness from brief vigorous stairs or snacks, easing chronic limits better than nothing (Vandelanotte et al., 2025; Fraser et al., 2025).

COMPARATIVE ANALYSIS:

How does duration impact psychological states?

The habit of long-term exercise provides a better lifestyle and prevents mental health deterioration. Exercise regularly reduces inflammation and provides neuroprotection. The extended time of exercising significantly facilitates distractions from negative thoughts (Kong et al.,2022). Different time duration shows different results in the individual, as mentioned in Table 2.

Table 2. Time duration and benefits of exercise

Time duration	Timing	Benefits
Short Duration	20 mins	• Increased energy & alertness • Improved mood (endorphin release) • Better focus & reduced stress
Moderate Duration	20–45 mins	• Cardiovascular health improvement • Calorie burning → weight management • Enhanced metabolic function • Improved stamina
Long Duration	45–90 mins	• Greater fat oxidation • Increased endurance & strength • Muscle adaptation & toning • Stronger immune system

Short multiple bouts and continuous bouts:

People in the cognitive world experience various health and mental issues. To overcome this stress, short bouts and continuous long bouts lead to an enhancement in aerobic fitness. Short bouts provide better results in weight loss compared to continuous bouts (Jakicic et al.,1995). Better arterial stiffness was observed in the individual with short bouts, along with the reduced glycemic index. Individuals who have long bouts of show increased physical activity and better health benefits when compared with small bouts.

Integration in real life:

Integrating exercise into daily life means adding physical activity into your regular routines instead of depending only on structured workouts. Recent evidence indicates that even brief periods of incidental activity like taking the stairs, brisk walking during errands, or carrying groceries can greatly improve health outcomes. In older adults, programmes such as *Lifestyle-integrated Functional Exercise (LiFE)* that embed strength, balance, and functional movement exercises into routine tasks (e.g., standing up from chairs, reaching for high shelves, walking to neighbours) have been shown to boost strength, balance, reduce falls, and improve overall functional performance (Weber et al.,2018). In summary, integrating exercise into daily life via small, frequent bouts of activity rather than only through formal workouts can yield meaningful improvements in cardiovascular health, functional ability, mood, and mortality risk.

Workplace Implementation Strategies

Corporate wellness programs can easily integrate exercise snacks by scheduling (Figure 3) 3-5 minute walking or stair breaks every 60-90 minutes, turning sedentary office hours into opportunities for real health gains without disrupting productivity or requiring special equipment (Centers for Disease Control and Prevention, 2021). Labor laws already support this through occupational health standards that promote movement as part of safe work design, allowing companies to formalize these breaks as structured wellness time rather than optional perks that only motivated employees use.

Figure 3. Daily integration of 3-minute stair-climbing exercise snacks during a typical 9 AM–5 PM workday. Breaks occur every 90 minutes to combat sedentary behaviour without disrupting workflow

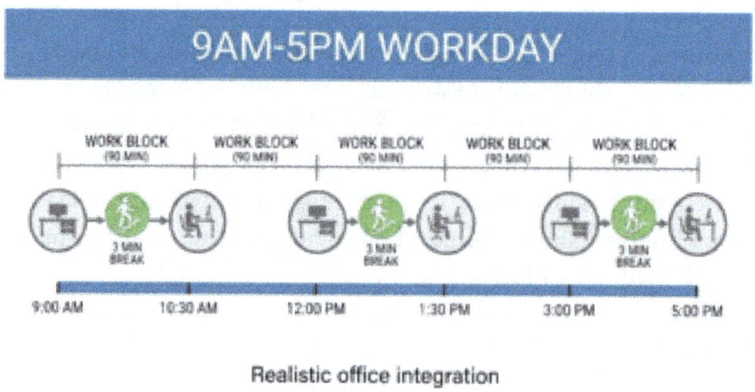

For college students, campuses could adopt similar approaches by placing visible staircases near lecture halls and adding movement prompts in class schedules, helping combat the sitting-all-day fatigue that hits during exam seasons. These strategies shift micro-workouts from individual effort to systemic support, making them sustainable across diverse work and study environments where time and space constraints are the biggest hurdles

Global Health Policy Context

WHO and other big health groups recommend breaking up sitting with short activity bursts. They say any movement adds toward fighting diseases like diabetes and heart issues, which makes exercise snacks a natural fit for their message that you don't need gym hours to stay healthy (World Health Organization, 2020). Their reports push governments and companies to make it easy by redesigning offices with better stairs or adding class breaks in schools, especially since students and workers spend so much time parked in chairs.

Basically, they give policymakers real tools to hit activity targets without forcing big lifestyle transformation. They turn small changes into population-wide wins even where gyms or free time are hard to come by.

FUTURE PROSPECTS

The prospects of exercise are highly promising, especially as research highlights the health benefits of even short bouts of incidental physical activity. Advances in wearable technology and digital health tools (e.g., smartwatches, AI-based fitness trackers) help to monitor intensity and encourage individuals to incorporate movement into daily routines, making it easier to meet physical activity guidelines. Public health policies are also expected to focus more on "active living" urban design, such as creating walkable cities, cycling lanes, and activity-friendly workplaces, thereby reducing sedentary behaviour. Future directions may also include personalized interventions based on behavioural science and habit-formation strategies to become a natural part of everyday life. Overall, integrating exercise into daily life is likely to evolve into a core preventive healthcare strategy, reducing chronic disease burden and promoting sustainable well-being.

REFERENCES

Abou Elmagd, M. H. (2016). Benefits, needs and importance of daily exercise. *International Journal of Physical Education. Sports Health, 3*(5), 22–27.

Allison, R.. (2023). Exercise snacking to improve physical function in pre-frail older adults. *The Journal of Frailty & Aging*. Advance online publication. DOI: 10.1186/s12877-023-04169-6

Anderson, E., & Shivakumar, G. (2013). Effects of exercise and physical activity on anxiety. *Frontiers in Psychiatry, 4*, 27. DOI: 10.3389/fpsyt.2013.00027 PMID: 23630504

Basso, J. C., & Suzuki, W. A. (2017). The Effects of Acute Exercise on Mood, Cognition, Neurophysiology, and Neurochemical Pathways: A Review. Brain plasticity (Amsterdam, Netherlands), 2(2), 127–152. https://doi.org/DOI: 10.3233/BPL-160040

Caneppele, T. S.. (2022). Can exercise shape your brain? A review of aerobic exercise effects on cognitive function and brain health. *Frontiers in Psychology*. Advance online publication. DOI: 10.3389/fpsyg.2022.852362

Cotman, C. W., & Berchtold, N. C. (2002). Exercise: A behavioral intervention to enhance brain health and plasticity. *Trends in Neurosciences, 25*(6), 295–301. DOI: 10.1016/s0166-2236(02)02143-4 PMID: 12086747

Dishman, R. K., & O'Connor, P. J. (2009). Lessons in exercise neurobiology: The case of endorphins. *Mental Health and Physical Activity, 2*(1), 4–9. DOI: 10.1016/j.mhpa.2009.01.002

DNA Learning Center. (2008). Exercise induced neurogenesis. https://dnalc.cshl.edu/view/848-Exercise-induced-Neurogenesis.html

Dunstan, D. W., Howard, B., Healy, G. N., & Owen, N. (2012). Too much sitting – A health hazard. *Diabetes Research and Clinical Practice, 97*(3), 368–376. DOI: 10.1016/j.diabres.2012.05.020 PMID: 22682948

Esteves, E. A.. (2021). Beneficial effects of physical exercise on cognitive behavioral outcomes: Mechanisms and evidence. *Progress in Brain Research*. Advance online publication. DOI: 10.1016/bs.pbr.2021.03.012

Francois, M. E., & Little, J. P. (2015). Effectiveness and safety of high-intensity interval training in patients with type 2 diabetes. *Diabetes Spectrum, 28*(1), 39–44. DOI: 10.2337/diaspect.28.1.39 PMID: 25717277

Fraser, S. F.. (2025). Application of exercise snacks across youth, adult and older adult populations. *Sports Medicine (Auckland, N.Z.)*. Advance online publication. DOI: 10.1186/s40798-025-00829-6

Fuss, J., Steinle, J., Bindila, L., Auer, M. K., Kirchherr, H., Lutz, B., & Gass, P. (2015). A runner's high depends on cannabinoid receptors in mice. *Proceedings of the National Academy of Sciences of the United States of America, 112*(42), 13105–13108. DOI: 10.1073/pnas.1514996112 PMID: 26438875

Jakicic, J. M., Wing, R. R., Butler, B. A., & Robertson, R. J. (1995). Prescribing exercise in multiple short bouts versus one continuous bout: effects on adherence, cardiorespiratory fitness, and weight loss in overweight women. *International journal of obesity and related metabolic disorders: journal of the International Association for the Study of Obesity, 19*(12), 893–901.

Jenkins, E. M., ... (2019). Exercise snacking to improve muscle function in healthy older adults. Journal of Aging Research. https://pmc.ncbi.nlm.nih.gov/articles/PMC6794984/

Kong, L., Cui, Y., & Gong, Q. (2022). Duration of keeping an exercise habit and mental illness and life attitude among university students. *International Journal of Environmental Research and Public Health, 19*(18), 11669. DOI: 10.3390/ijerph191811669 PMID: 36141940

Little, J. P.. (2019). Sprint exercise snacks: A novel approach to increase aerobic fitness. *Scandinavian Journal of Medicine & Science in Sports*. Advance online publication. DOI: 10.1111/sms.13413 PMID: 30847639

Mahindru, A., Patil, P., & Agrawal, V. (2023). Role of Physical Activity on Mental Health and Well-Being: A Review. *Cureus, 15*(1), e33475. DOI: 10.7759/cureus.33475 PMID: 36756008

Mattioli, A. V., Sciomer, S., Cocchi, C., Maffei, S., & Gallina, S. (2020). Quarantine during COVID-19 outbreak: Changes in diet and physical activity increase the risk of cardiovascular disease. *Nutrition, Metabolism, and Cardiovascular Diseases, 30*(9), 1409–1417. DOI: 10.1016/j.numecd.2020.05.020 PMID: 32571612

McTiernan, A. (2008). Mechanisms linking physical activity with cancer. *Nature Reviews. Cancer*, *8*(3), 205–211. DOI: 10.1038/nrc2325 PMID: 18235448

MeHelp. (2024). The 3 pillars of mental health: Benefits of sleep, diet and exercise. https://www.mehelp.com.au/insights/sleep-diet-exercise

Ruegsegger, G. N., & Booth, F. W. (2018). Health Benefits of Exercise. *Cold Spring Harbor Perspectives in Medicine*, *8*(7), a029694. DOI: 10.1101/cshperspect.a029694 PMID: 28507196

Saanijoki, T.. (2018). Endorphin release after high intensity interval training in humans. *Neuropsychopharmacology : Official Publication of the American College of Neuropsychopharmacology*, *43*(2), 358–367. DOI: 10.1038/npp.2017.194 PMID: 28722022

Vandelanotte, C.. (2025). The effectiveness of exercise snacks as a time-efficient intervention. *Frontiers in Cardiovascular Medicine*. Advance online publication. DOI: 10.3389/fcvm.2025.164315

Weber, M., Belala, N., Clemson, L., Boulton, E., Hawley-Hague, H., Becker, C., & Schwenk, M. (2018). Feasibility and Effectiveness of Intervention Programmes Integrating Functional Exercise into Daily Life of Older Adults: A Systematic Review. *Gerontology*, *64*(2), 172–187. DOI: 10.1159/000479965 PMID: 28910814

World Health Organization. (2020). *WHO guidelines on physical activity and sedentary behaviour*. [https://doi.org/]DOI: 10.1016/s0140-6736(20)30937-0

World Health Organization. (2024). Physical activity: Key facts. https://www.who.int/news-room/fact-sheets/detail/physical-activity

Chapter 6
Regular Physical Activity Improves Emotional Regulation and Reduces Psychological Distress in Young Adults

Sohom Saha
https://orcid.org/0009-0006-9438-1554
Lakshmibai National Institute of Physical Education, India

Mahendra Kumar Singh
https://orcid.org/0000-0001-9989-9420
Lakshmibai National Institute of Physical Education, India

Simran Obhrai
https://orcid.org/0009-0007-5227-9364
Guru Nanak Dev University, India

ABSTRACT

Regular physical activity is an affordable, accessible, and evidence-based approach to improving emotional regulation and reducing psychological distress in young adults. Drawing from neuroscience, psychology, and behavioral science, this chapter highlights how various exercise forms, including aerobic training, resistance work, mind-body practices, and high-intensity intervals, enhance neuroplasticity, regulate neurotransmitters, and modulate stress. Beyond these physiological mechanisms, exercise strengthens psychological factors such as self-efficacy, body image, and social connectedness, fostering resilience and overall well-being. Theoretical perspectives

DOI: 10.4018/979-8-3373-6157-4.ch006

like Dual Mode Theory, Broaden-and-Build Theory, and Self-Determination Theory guide effective program design, while practical strategies stress personalization, cultural relevance, and supportive contexts. By integrating exercise into health policies and tailoring it to individual needs, physical activity can function as both prevention and therapy for rising mental health concerns in young adults.

1. INTRODUCTION

The transition to young adulthood represents one of the most challenging developmental periods, characterized by significant academic, social, and personal pressures that can precipitate psychological distress (Arnett, 2000). Contemporary young adults face high levels of stress, anxiety, and depression, with prevalence rates reaching epidemic proportions globally (Twenge et al., 2019). The World Health Organization identifies depression as the leading cause of disability among adolescents and young adults, highlighting the urgent need for effective, accessible interventions (World Health Organization, 2024). Traditional approaches to mental health management in young adults have predominantly relied on pharmaceutical interventions and psychotherapy (Cuijpers et al., 2014). Nonetheless, growing evidence supports the use of lifestyle interventions, especially regular physical exercise, as a form of prevention and treatment against psychological distress (Rosenbaum et al., 2014). Physical activity is a promising intervention, as it is accessible, cost-effective, and with fewer side effects than medications (Kandola et al., 2019). The neurobiological underpinnings of exercise-related positive mental health are well-established interactions that exist among neurotransmitter systems, neuroplasticity, and stress response pathways (Wegner et al., 2014). In addition to the biological effects, physical activity affects the psychological aspects of health such as self-efficacy, body image, and social connectedness which have a positive impact on the well-being of emotions (Lubans et al., 2016). This chapter aims to provide a comprehensive examination of the effect of regular physical activity in benefiting emotional regulation and decreasing levels of psychological distress in young adults. This synthesis of current research evidence with established theory bases provides insights into optimal exercise prescription, implementation techniques and policy considerations for promoting mental health through physical activity with young adult populations.

2. EMOTIONAL DYSREGULATION AND PSYCHOLOGICAL DISTRESS IN YOUNG ADULTS

2.1 Prevalence and Characteristics of Psychological Distress

Young adulthood between the ages of 18-25 years is characterized by significant developmental issues that predispose to psychological distress (Schulenberg et al., 2004). Recent epidemiological reports show disturbing increases in mental health issues regarding this age group with 25.1 per cent prevalence of anxiety disorders, and 11.2 per cent of mood disorders amongst the young adults worldwide (Kessler et al., 2012). According to the American College Health Association National College Health Assessment, 63.4 percent of the students in 2022 noted overwhelming anxiety, and 42.2 percent stated that they felt depressed so badly that this condition prevents functioning effectively in the past year (Lederer & Hoban, 2022). These are worrying statistics, which have gained momentum in the last 10 years, especially after the COVID-19 outbreak (Son et al., 2020). The symptoms of psychological distress in young adults are as follows: persistent worry and mood instability, sleep disturbances, inability to focus attention, somatic complaints (Liu et al., 2019). The complexity of these symptoms usually leads to a chain of negative effects in the academic achievement, interpersonal issues, and the quality of life at large (Bruffaerts et al., 2018).

2.2 Contributing Factors to Emotional Dysregulation

There are a number of intertwined causes of emotional dysregulation among the young adults. Academic pressure is one of the major stressors as competitive educational environments expose individuals to chronic stress that overpowers the coping mechanisms (Bayram & Bilgel, 2008). The pressure to achieve academic excellence while managing financial constraints, career uncertainty, and social expectations creates a perfect storm for psychological distress. The emotional regulation is greatly affected by social media and digital technology use patterns among young adults (Primack et al., 2017). Excessive social media use has been found to be correlated with greater depressive symptoms, anxiety, and loneliness, perhaps through the processes of social comparison and fear of missing out (FOMO) as well as disturbed patterns of sleep (Woods & Scott, 2016). The constant connectivity and information overload characteristic of digital environments may impair the development of healthy emotional regulation strategies. Lifestyle factors including poor sleep hygiene, inadequate nutrition, and sedentary behavior compound the risk for psychological distress (Kredlow et al., 2015). Young adults often adopt unhealthy lifestyle patterns during their transition to independence, inadvertently compromising their emotional resilience and mental health.

Table 1. Psychological benefits of regular physical activity

Benefit	Underlying Mechanism	Supporting Evidence
Reduced Anxiety	Regulation of amygdala activity, lower cortisol levels	(Smith et al., 2003)
Enhanced Emotional Regulation	Increased prefrontal cortex activity	(Boyatzis & McKee, 2005)
Decreased Depression Symptoms	Neurotransmitter balance (serotonin, dopamine)	(Patel et al., 2007)
Improved Stress Tolerance	HPA axis modulation	(Driskell et al., 2014)
Increased Self-Efficacy	Mastery experiences via exercise	(Maher et al., 2014)

2.3 Neurobiological Underpinnings of Emotional Dysregulation

The neurobiological basis of emotional dysregulation in young adults involves complex interactions between the prefrontal cortex, limbic system, and neurotransmitter networks (Casey et al., 2008). The adolescent and young adult brain undergoes continued maturation, particularly in areas responsible for emotional regulation and executive function, creating vulnerability to mood disorders. Chronic stress exposure during young adulthood can dysregulate the hypothalamic-pituitary-adrenal (HPA) axis, leading to persistent elevation of cortisol levels and subsequent neuroinflammation (McEwen, 2017). This neuroinflammatory response compromises synaptic plasticity and neurogenesis, particularly in the hippocampus, contributing to depressive symptoms and cognitive impairments. Neurotransmitter dysregulation, especially serotonin, dopamine and Gamma-aminobutyric acid (GABA) systems are key components in emotional dysregulation (Dean & Keshavan, 2017). These imbalances may be brought about by genetic predisposition, stressful environments, and lifestyle choices to produce a complex interrelationship that affects emotional stability and psychological well-being.

3. THE SCIENCE BEHIND PHYSICAL ACTIVITY AND EMOTIONAL REGULATION

3.1 Neurobiological Mechanisms

Physical activity has an impressive influence on brain structure and function due to various neurobiological processes, which directly affect emotional control (Hillman et al., 2008). Aerobic exercise activates the release of brain-derived neurotrophic factor (BDNF), the protein that is essential to the neuroplasticity, the strength of synapses, and neurogenesis (Coelho et al., 2013). Increased levels of BDNF after exercise are related to an improved mood and cognitive performance, suggesting a direct mechanism through which physical activity enhances emotional well-being. Exercise-induced neuroplasticity occurs primarily in those areas of the brain that play a crucial role in emotion processing, such as the hippocampus, prefrontal cortex and the anterior cingulate cortex (Voss et al., 2013). Neuroimaging has shown that regular aerobic exercise expands the gray matter in these areas and improves white matter integrity, facilitating more efficient emotional regulation processes (Erickson et al., 2011).

The neurotransmitter hypothesis of exercise benefits involves complicated interactions of various neurotransmitter systems (Mikkelsen et al., 2017). Exercise can also raise the level of serotonin which promotes better mood and reduces anxiety by improving the uptake of tryptophan across the blood-brain barrier (Young, 2007). Similarly, exercise activates the release of dopamine in reward pathways, which increases the motivation and positive feelings while reducing anhedonic symptoms associated with depression (Dishman et al., 2006).

3.2 Endorphin and Stress Response Systems

Although the endorphin hypothesis is historically prominent, it represents just one component of how exercise positively affects the mood (Boecker et al., 2008). Exercise induces endogenous opioid secretion, such as β-endorphins, that have pain relieving and euphoric properties. But the blood-brain barrier restricts access of endorphins to central nervous system receptors, suggesting that peripheral endorphin release may contribute to mood improvements through alternative mechanisms.

Physical activity significantly modulates stress responsive physiological systems, especially the HPA axis (Tsatsoulis & Fountoulakis, 2006). Regular exercise training reduces baseline cortisol levels while improving cortisol response patterns to acute stressors. This adaptation enhances stress resilience and reduces chronic inflammation associated with prolonged stress exposure, contributing to improved emotional regulation capacity. The autonomic nervous system undergoes beneficial adaptations following regular physical activity, with increased parasympathetic tone and improved heart rate variability (Thayer et al., 2012). These changes reflect enhanced emotional regulation capacity and stress resilience, as autonomic balance directly influences emotional reactivity and recovery from stressful experiences.

3.3 Inflammatory Pathways and Mental Health

Chronic low-grade inflammation plays a significant role in the pathophysiology of depression and anxiety disorders (Miller & Raison, 2016). Pro-inflammatory cytokines, including interleukin-6 (IL-6), tumor necrosis factor-alpha (TNF-α), and C-reactive protein (CRP), are elevated in individuals with depression and correlate with symptom severity (Howren et al., 2009). Regular physical activity exerts potent anti-inflammatory effects through multiple mechanisms (Petersen & Pedersen, 2005). Exercise stimulates the release of IL-10 and other anti-inflammatory cytokines while reducing pro-inflammatory markers. These anti-inflammatory effects may partially mediate the antidepressant and anxiolytic benefits of physical activity, particularly in individuals with elevated baseline inflammation levels. The gut-brain axis refers to a relatively new field of study in relation to the connections between physical activity and inflammation and mental health (Foster & McVey Neufeld, 2013). Exercise can change the composition of the microbiota in the gut facilitating the abundance of beneficial bacteria within the gastrointestinal tract that produce neurotransmitters and decreases systemic inflammation. This route can play a role in exercise induced improvements in mood and emotion regulation through microbiota-gut-brain communication.

Table 2. Types of physical activity and their psychological impact

Type of Activity	Example	Main Psychological Impact
Aerobic Exercise	Running, cycling	Reduces anxiety & depressive symptoms
Resistance Training	Weightlifting, bodyweight training	Enhances self-confidence
Mind-Body Practices	Yoga, Tai Chi	Improves mindfulness & emotional balance
Team Sports	Football, basketball	Builds social connectedness
Recreational Activities	Hiking, dancing	Reduces stress & promotes enjoyment

4. THEORETICAL UNDERPINNINGS OF THE EXERCISE-EMOTION NEXUS

4.1 Dual Mode Theory

The Dual Mode Theory of Ekkekakis is one of the most informative theories of how the intensity of an exercise influences affective responses and emotional regulation (Ekkekakis, 2003). It is the hypothesis of the theory that the cognitive and interoceptive influences interact to jointly determine exercise-induced affective changes and that exercise intensity is a major moderator in this process. At low to moderate intensities (below the ventilatory threshold) affective responses are mostly affected by the cognitive factors, which permits a positive emotional experience and better mood (Ekkekakis et al., 2011). Individuals can maintain attention to stimuli that are deemed pleasant, engage in positive self-statements, and experience mastery and achievement, all contributing to enhanced emotional regulation. High-intensity exercise above the ventilatory threshold entails a change in control with interoceptive influences dominating and physiological sensations becoming progressively unpleasant (Ekkekakis & Acevedo, 2006). However, post-exercise recovery periods often involve significant mood improvements, suggesting that the overall exercise experience, including recovery, contributes to emotional benefits.

4.2 Broaden-and-Build Theory

Fredrickson's Broaden-and-Build Theory offers insight into how physical activity-induced positive emotions enhance psychological resilience and emotional regulation capacity (Fredrickson, 2001). Positive emotions experienced during and after exercise broaden attention and awareness, facilitating creative problem-solving and flexible thinking patterns that enhance coping abilities. The building component of the theory suggests that repeated experiences of positive emotions through physical activity gradually build enduring psychological resources (Fredrickson & Joiner, 2002). These resources include improved self-efficacy, social connections, mindfulness skills, and stress resilience, all contributing to enhanced emotional regulation capacity over time. Physical activity provides multiple opportunities for positive emotional experiences through achievement, mastery, social interaction, and embodied pleasure (Reed & Buck, 2009). These positive emotions accumulate to create an upward spiral of improved psychological well-being and enhanced capacity for managing future stressors and emotional challenges.

Table 3. Summary of empirical evidence on physical activity and emotional regulation

Study Design	Sample Size	Duration	Key Findings
RCT	120 university students	12 weeks	Significant improvement in emotional regulation scores
Cross-sectional	800 young adults	----	Higher activity linked to lower psychological distress
Longitudinal	450 participants	2 years	Sustained activity predicted stable emotional regulation
Intervention Study	60 clinical cases	8 weeks	Reduced depressive symptoms and perceived stress

4.3 Self-Determination Theory

Self-Determination Theory (SDT) provides crucial insights into the motivational mechanisms underlying sustained engagement in physical activity and its psychological benefits (Deci & Ryan, 2008). The theory identifies three basic psychological needs: autonomy, competence, and relatedness, which must be satisfied for optimal psychological functioning and well-being. Autonomy satisfaction through physical activity involves experiencing choice, volition, and personal agency in exercise selection and participation (Teixeira et al., 2012). When individuals feel autonomous in their physical activity choices, they experience greater intrinsic motivation, enjoyment, and psychological benefits, including improved emotional regulation. Competence satisfaction occurs through mastery experiences, skill development, and achieving personally meaningful goals in physical activity contexts (Ntoumanis, 2001). These experiences enhance self-efficacy and confidence, contributing to improved emotional regulation capacity and reduced psychological distress. Relatedness satisfaction through physical activity involves social connection, belonging, and meaningful relationships with others (Sebire et al., 2009). Group exercise, team sports, and exercise partnerships provide opportunities for social support and connection, which are crucial protective factors against psychological distress in young adults.

5. COMPARATIVE ANALYSIS OF DIFFERENT EXERCISE MODALITIES

5.1 Aerobic Exercise

Aerobic exercise represents the most extensively researched physical activity modality for mental health benefits in young adults (Rosenbaum et al., 2014). Systematic reviews and meta-analyses consistently demonstrate significant reductions in depression and anxiety symptoms following aerobic exercise interventions, with effect sizes comparable to psychotherapy and pharmacological treatments (Schuch et al., 2016). The optimal dose-response relationship for aerobic exercise remains an active area of research. Current evidence suggests that moderate-intensity aerobic exercise (50-70% maximum heart rate) performed for 30-45 minutes, 3-5 times per week, produces significant improvements in mood and emotional regulation (Kandola et al., 2019). However, even minimal doses of aerobic activity (10-15 minutes of brisk walking) can produce acute mood improvements and stress reduction.

Running therapy has emerged as a specific intervention combining aerobic exercise with therapeutic principles (Josefsson et al., 2017). Studies demonstrate that structured running programs significantly reduce depression and anxiety symptoms while improving self-esteem and emotional regulation in young adults. The rhythmic, meditative aspects of running may provide additional psychological benefits beyond general aerobic exercise.

Table 4. Barriers and facilitators to regular physical activity

Barrier	Description	Example
Time Constraints	Busy academic/work schedule	University exams
Lack of Motivation	Low perceived benefit	Sedentary lifestyle
Limited Access	No facilities or safe spaces	Rural areas
Social Support	Encouragement from peers	Joining sports clubs
Accessibility of Programs	Affordable and inclusive	Free fitness classes

5.2 Resistance Training

Resistance training, traditionally focused on strength and muscle development, demonstrates significant mental health benefits in young adults (Gordon et al., 2018). Meta-analytic evidence indicates that resistance training reduces depression symptoms with effect sizes similar to aerobic exercise, challenging the historical bias toward cardiorespiratory exercise for mental health benefits.

The psychological mechanisms underlying resistance training benefits include enhanced self-efficacy, improved body image, and mastery experiences (Stanton et al., 2015). Progressive overload principles inherent in resistance training provide clear feedback on improvement and achievement, contributing to enhanced self-confidence and emotional resilience. Resistance training may be particularly beneficial for young adults who find aerobic exercise challenging or unenjoyable (Ashdown-Franks et al., 2020). The structured, goal-oriented nature of resistance training appeals to individuals who prefer concrete measures of progress and achievement, potentially enhancing adherence and long-term benefits.

5.3 Mind-Body Practices

Yoga, tai chi, and qigong represent mind-body practices that integrate physical movement with mindfulness, breathing techniques, and meditation (Sharma et al., 2006). These activities demonstrate particular effectiveness in the reduction of anxiety and improvement of emotional regulation in young adults likely via mindfulness, interoceptive awareness, and autonomic nervous system mechanisms. The current studies on yoga interventions across young adults consistently demonstrate significant reductions in anxiety, depression, and stress levels (Pascoe et al., 2017). The combination of physical poses (asanas), breathing exercises (pranayama), and meditation (dhyana) offers a comprehensive approach to emotional regulation, which addresses both the physiological and psychological levels of well-being. Mindfulness-based movement practices increase interoceptive awareness, or the aptitude to perceive internal bodily signals, which is vital in emotional regulation (Mehling et al., 2012). Enhanced interoceptive awareness can enable people to detect the beginnings of emotional distress and help implement appropriate coping strategies before the situation worsens.

5.4 High-Intensity Interval Training (HIIT)

High-Intensity Interval Training is also attractive to young adults because of its time efficiency and effectiveness for physical fitness improvements (Biddle & Batterham, 2015). Emerging evidence suggests that HIIT also produces significant mental health benefits, including decreased anxiety and improved mood, despite its high-intensity nature. Psychological benefits of HIIT can be explained by the enhanced self-efficacy following completion of challenging exercise sessions, increased BDNF release as a result of high-intensity stimulation, and the effective process of stress inoculation effects (Heisz et al., 2017). The sense of accomplishment following HIIT sessions can enhance confidence and emotional resilience. The high-intensity nature of HIIT may not be suitable for all individuals, particularly those with high levels of baseline anxiety or stress (Ekkekakis, 2009). Careful progression and individualized programming are crucial in assuring that HIIT interventions will have positive psychological outcomes among young adults.

6. GENDER, LIFESTYLE, AND CULTURAL CONSIDERATIONS

6.1 Gender Differences in Exercise Response

Research indicates that gender differences are particularly significant in the occurrence of psychological distress and the physical activity response to such interventions amongst young adults (Schuch et al., 2016). Anxiety and depression are more prevalent in young women than in young men, which may be caused by hormonal fluctuations, social and cultural demands, and differences in stress perception and coping strategies. Some evidence indicates that exercise interventions may achieve different effects depending on gender, where studies suggest that women experience greater anxiety reduction benefits from aerobic exercise, while men may derive more mood benefits from resistance training (Herring et al., 2010). Such variations could reflect socialization patterns, body image concerns and preferences for different types of physical activities. Hormonal considerations are especially significant to young women since menstrual cycle phases may influence exercise responses and mood regulation (Spindle et al., 2018). Exercise programs for young women should consider menstrual cycle timing and hormonal fluctuations to optimize psychological benefits and adherence.

6.2 Socioeconomic and Cultural Factors

Socioeconomic status is a significant factor that determines access to physical activity opportunities and mental health outcomes among young adults (Patel et al., 2007). Lower socioeconomic status has been linked to increased psychological distress, reduced access to recreational amenities, and greater barriers to participating in physical activities. Cultural background influences exercise preferences, barriers, and motivations, due to which it is necessary to use culturally-sensitive strategies of promoting physical activity (Caperchione et al., 2009). Some cultures may emphasize group-based activities and social connections whereas others may prioritize individual achievement and competition. The proper comprehension of these cultural preferences is a key to the creation of successful interventions. Religious and spiritual considerations can also influence participation in physical activities and psychological benefits (Chodkiewicz & Boyle, 2017). Some young adults may prefer mind-body practices that align with their spiritual beliefs, while others may avoid certain activities due to religious restrictions and cultural norms.

6.3 Technology Integration and Digital Natives

Young adults are the first completely digital native generation, which also presents some challenges and opportunities related to promoting physical activity and having an opportunity to target mental health (Firth et al., 2017). Technology-supported interventions, such as smartphone applications, wearable devices, and virtual reality platforms, have the potential to incentivize young adults to practice physical activities as part of their routines. But on the other hand, overuse of technology correlates with more sedentary lifestyles and psychological distress in adults of young age (Twenge & Campbell, 2018). It is important to implement a balance between technology integration with outdoor and nature-based activities and face-to-face social interactions since it is harder to attain optimal mental health outcomes without this balance. It is found that social media can either promote or inhibit physical activity engagement and mental health states (Maher et al., 2014). Although social media sites can offer motivation, accountability and social companionship to engage in physical activity, the social media environment can also lead to the reinforcement of unrealistic body image ideals and comparisons which are likely to increase the risk of mental distress.

Table 5. Recommendations for enhancing emotional regulation through physical activity

Recommendation	Rationale	Implementation Example
Incorporate Mind-Body Practices	Improves self-awareness	Weekly yoga sessions
Structured Aerobic Training	Boosts mood-regulating neurotransmitters	30-min brisk walk, 5 days/ week
Social Exercise Programs	Encourages adherence	Peer-led jogging groups
Campus Wellness Initiatives	Provides access & motivation	University gym passes
Education on Benefits	Increases perceived value	Mental health workshops

7. INCORPORATING PHYSICAL ACTIVITY INTO MENTAL HEALTH CAMPUS POLICY

7.1 Campus-Based Intervention Models

Universities and colleges are optimal settings to use the physical activity interventions to overcome psychological distress in young adults (Keating et al., 2005).

Campus-based interventions have the ability to capitalize on the resources available to the university through existing recreational facilities, student groups and health services to develop a comprehensive mental health promotion program through physical exercise. Effective models of campus interventions involve the incorporation of physical activity programming into existing mental health services which results in a continuum of care to both prevention and treatment (Eisenberg et al., 2007). These programs tend to have fitness assessments, individual exercise prescriptions, group fitness classes, and peer support networks. Combining the academic course content with experiential physical exercise activities program contributes to the improvement of both learning outcomes and psychological health benefits (Penedo & Dahn, 2005). Courses that integrate theory of exercise science and practical experiences of participation in physical activity offer students' knowledge and skills that will last a lifetime of participating in physical activity and managing mental health.

7.2 Peer-Led Interventions

Young adult populations have shown specific effectiveness in reactivity to the interventions initiated and led by peers and are associated with shared experiences, a relatable style of communication and the decreasing stigma factor (Topp et al., 2009). Trained student leaders can conduct group exercise sessions, provide motivation and support, and serve as role models for healthy lifestyle behavior. Peer support networks formed as a result of physical activity programs enhance social connectedness and reduce isolation, which are major risk factors for psychological distress in young adulthood (House et al., 1988). Such networks offer a continuous source of support, accountability and encouragement that extends beyond formal program participation. Training and support of peer leaders is also vital in enhancing the success of the program and safety (Hogan & Schmidt, 2002). Basic exercise science principles, mental health awareness, communication skills, and crisis intervention procedures should be taught in-depth so that a program is rendered effectively and safely.

7.3 Environmental and Policy Changes

The creation of favorable physical environments to generate physical activities in college campuses needs a complete alteration of policies and investing in infrastructure (Sallis et al., 2012). Such changes can incorporate enhancements to recreational facility access, establishment of walking and cycling paths, installation of outdoor exercise equipment, and development of green spaces for physical activity. Policy shifts that prioritize physical activity and mental health point to any of the following: scheduling that allows time for physical activity, academic credit given to wellness courses, and movement breaks that are incorporated into the classroom teaching (Strong et al., 2005). Such systemic alterations are ones that create cultural shifts that normalize physical activity as essential for academic achievement and healthy living. Comprehensive physical activity mental health programming between campus recreation, student health services, counselling centers and academic departments is essential (Hunt & Eisenberg, 2010). These collaborations combine different expertise and resources and provide more efficient and sustainable interventions.

8. IMPLEMENTATION STRATEGIES AND PRACTICAL APPLICATIONS

8.1 Exercise Prescription Guidelines

The individual needs, preferences, capabilities, and mental health status should be considered in developing the evidence-based exercise prescription guidelines of young adults with psychological distress (Kandola et al., 2019). Initial assessments of the individual, including current physical activity levels, exercise history and physical limitations, and psychological symptoms prior to the start of a program will allow tailoring of personalized programming to the individual. The FITT principle (Frequency, Intensity, Time, Type) can be used to structure exercise prescription that can be adapted for the desired mental health outcomes (Liguori & Medicine (ACSM), 2020). For psychological distress reduction, recommended guidelines include moderate-intensity aerobic exercise for 150 minutes per week or vigorous-intensity exercise for 75 minutes per week, supplemented with resistance training twice per week. Progressive programming is essential for sustainable behavior change and continued psychological benefits (Prochaska & DiClemente, 1983). Initial programs should emphasize enjoyment, success experiences, and gradual progression to build confidence and motivation for long-term adherence.

8.2 Behavioral Change Strategies

Effective physical activity interventions for mental health must address the psychological and behavioral factors that influence exercise adherence and motivation (Teixeira et al., 2012). Motivational interviewing techniques can help individuals identify personal values and goals that align with physical activity participation, enhancing intrinsic motivation. Goal setting strategies should emphasize process goals (e.g., attending three exercise sessions per week) rather than outcome goals (e.g., losing 10 pounds) to enhance motivation and self-efficacy (Locke & Latham, 2002). SMART goals (Specific, Measurable, Achievable, Relevant, Time-bound) provide structure while maintaining flexibility for individual preferences and circumstances. Self-monitoring through activity trackers, exercise logs, or smartphone applications can enhance awareness, motivation, and accountability (Cadmus-Bertram et al., 2015). However, self-monitoring tools should complement rather than replace social support and professional guidance for optimal outcomes.

8.3 Addressing Barriers and Facilitators

Common barriers to physical activity participation among young adults include time constraints, cost, lack of knowledge, social anxiety, and competing priorities (Keating et al., 2005). Addressing these barriers requires comprehensive strategies that include flexible scheduling, affordable options, education, social support, and priority clarification. Lack of time is noted as the most commonly identified obstacle to physical activity amongst young adults (Arzu et al., 2006). The remedies would be to facilitate accomplishing short high intensity workouts, incorporating incidental physical activity into everyday lives and helping individuals prioritize physical activity as essential for academic and personal success. Social anxiety and body image concerns also discourage young adults from participating in group exercise or using public facilities (Grogan, 2016). The existence of options that are beginner friendly, women only spaces, and body positive environments are some possible strategies that can lower these barriers and increase participation.

9. LIMITATIONS AND FUTURE DIRECTIONS

9.1 Research Limitations

Existing studies on physical activity and mental health among young adults have weaknesses and limitations which limit the quality and generalizability of the study (Rosenbaum et al., 2014). A small sample size, brief durations of intervention, and failure to conduct long-term follow-up assessments make most studies limited in the knowledge of sustained effects and optimal intervention characteristics. Physical activity interventions across trials are heterogeneous, which creates an inability to establish optimal exercise prescriptions to specific mental health outcomes (Schuch et al., 2016). Research protocols greatly vary in exercise type, intensity, duration and frequency and outcome measures and assessment timing. Publication bias in favour of positive findings could overestimate the effectiveness of physical activity interventions as far as mental health outcomes are concerned (Egger et al., 1997). Also, numerous studies do not feature appropriate control conditions that would be needed to determine whether benefits result from physical activity specifically or understand whether the positive outcomes are due to general attention and social contact.

9.2 Individual Variability in Response

There is a significant presence of individual variance in their psychological response to physical activity interventions because some individuals experience tremendous positive changes and others minimal ones (Petruzzello et al., 1991). A knowledge of what predicts treatment response would help develop personalized intervention approaches and improve overall effectiveness. Genetic factors may influence individual responses to exercise interventions for mental health (Rethorst & Trivedi, 2013). Polymorphisms in genes affecting neurotransmitter systems, stress response, and neuroplasticity may modulate the psychological benefits of physical activity, suggesting potential for personalized exercise medicine approaches. There are baseline characteristics such as fitness level, mental health severity, personality traits and exercise preferences that are most likely to influence intervention outcomes (Craft & Perna, 2004). Future studies are needed to systematically examine these moderating variables and develop more effective, individually tailored interventions.

9.3 Future Research Directions

Future studies ought to focus on large-scale randomized controlled trials that will have sufficient statistical power to find meaningful effects and investigate the dose-response relationships (Kandola et al., 2019). These studies should include long-term follow-up assessments to determine the sustainability of mental health benefits from physical activity interventions. More mechanistic research utilizing neuroimaging, biomarker analysis, and ecological momentary assessment could bring more insight into how physical activity influences psychological outcomes (Wegner et al., 2014). This research could inform optimal intervention timing, intensity and duration for maximum psychological benefits. Implementation science approaches are needed to translate research findings into effective real-world interventions (Glasgow et al., 2012). This would involve examining barriers and facilitators to program adoption, developing training protocols for intervention delivery, as well as evaluating cost-effectiveness of different implementation strategies.

10. CONCLUSION AND PRACTICAL IMPLICATIONS

Regular physical activity also proves to be a very effective evidence-based intervention concerning improving emotional regulation and reducing psychological distress in young adults. A combination of neurobiological, psychological, and behavioral mechanisms supports the therapeutic potential of a wide variety of exercise modalities, including aerobic exercise, resistance training, mind-body practices, and high-intensity interval training. The existing theories of Dual Mode Theory, Broaden-and-Build Theory, and Self-Determination Theory provide valuable insights for optimizing physical activity interventions. Such theories encompass the significance of appropriate exercise intensity, positive emotional experiences, and satisfaction of basic psychological needs in maximizing mental health benefits. Practical implementation demands comprehensive approaches with capacities to deal with individual preferences, cultural considerations and environmental factors. Supportive environments as a consequence of campus-based interventions, peer support networks and policy changes can create supportive environments that promote physical activity participation and sustained mental health benefits. Physical activity should be prioritized as a first-line intervention for mental health promotion in young adults by healthcare providers, educators, and policymakers. This practice can be described as in line with global movements toward preventive healthcare and non-pharmacological interventions while addressing the growing mental health crisis in young adult populations. Future research should focus on personalized intervention approaches, long-term effectiveness, and implementation strategies to maximize the public health impact of physical activity for mental health. Technology integration, consideration of individual variability, and emphasis on sustainable behavior change will play important roles towards advancing this field. The evidence clearly supports the integration of regular physical activity into comprehensive mental health promotion strategies for young adults. By harnessing the therapeutic potential of movement, we can address the growing mental health crisis while promoting overall well-being and resilience in this critical population.

REFERENCES

Arnett, J. J. (2000). Emerging adulthood: A theory of development from the late teens through the twenties. *The American Psychologist, 55*(5), 469–480. DOI: 10.1037/0003-066X.55.5.469 PMID: 10842426

Arzu, D., Tuzun, E. H., & Eker, L. (2006). Perceived barriers to physical activity in university students. *Journal of Sports Science & Medicine, 5*(4), 615–620. PMID: 24357957

Ashdown-Franks, G., Firth, J., Carney, R., Carvalho, A. F., Hallgren, M., Koyanagi, A., Rosenbaum, S., Schuch, F. B., Smith, L., Solmi, M., Vancampfort, D., & Stubbs, B. (2020). Exercise as Medicine for Mental and Substance Use Disorders: A Meta-review of the Benefits for Neuropsychiatric and Cognitive Outcomes. *Sports Medicine (Auckland, N.Z.), 50*(1), 151–170. DOI: 10.1007/s40279-019-01187-6 PMID: 31541410

Bayram, N., & Bilgel, N. (2008). The prevalence and socio-demographic correlations of depression, anxiety and stress among a group of university students. *Social Psychiatry and Psychiatric Epidemiology, 43*(8), 667–672. DOI: 10.1007/s00127-008-0345-x PMID: 18398558

Biddle, S. J. H., & Batterham, A. M. (2015). High-intensity interval exercise training for public health: A big HIT or shall we HIT it on the head? *The International Journal of Behavioral Nutrition and Physical Activity, 12*, 95. DOI: 10.1186/s12966-015-0254-9 PMID: 26187579

Boecker, H., Sprenger, T., Spilker, M. E., Henriksen, G., Koppenhoefer, M., Wagner, K. J., Valet, M., Berthele, A., & Tolle, T. R. (2008). The runner's high: Opioidergic mechanisms in the human brain. *Cerebral Cortex (New York, N.Y.: 1991), 18*(11), 2523–2531. https://doi.org/DOI: 10.1093/cercor/bhn013

Boyatzis, R., & McKee, A. (2005). *Resonant Leadership: Renewing Yourself and Connecting with Others Through Mindfulness, Hope and CompassionCompassion*. Harvard Business Press.

Bruffaerts, R., Mortier, P., Kiekens, G., Auerbach, R. P., Cuijpers, P., Demyttenaere, K., Green, J. G., Nock, M. K., & Kessler, R. C. (2018). Mental health problems in college freshmen: Prevalence and academic functioning. *Journal of Affective Disorders, 225*, 97–103. DOI: 10.1016/j.jad.2017.07.044 PMID: 28802728

Cadmus-Bertram, L. A., Marcus, B. H., Patterson, R. E., Parker, B. A., & Morey, B. L. (2015). Randomized Trial of a Fitbit-Based Physical Activity Intervention for Women. *American Journal of Preventive Medicine, 49*(3), 414–418. DOI: 10.1016/j.amepre.2015.01.020 PMID: 26071863

Caperchione, C. M., Kolt, G. S., & Mummery, W. K. (2009). Physical activity in culturally and linguistically diverse migrant groups to Western society: A review of barriers, enablers and experiences. *Sports Medicine (Auckland, N.Z.), 39*(3), 167–177. DOI: 10.2165/00007256-200939030-00001 PMID: 19290674

Casey, B. J., Jones, R. M., & Hare, T. A. (2008). The adolescent brain. *Annals of the New York Academy of Sciences, 1124*, 111–126. DOI: 10.1196/annals.1440.010 PMID: 18400927

Chodkiewicz, A., & Boyle, C. (2017). Positive psychology school-based interventions: A reflection on current success and future directions. *Educational Review, 5*, 60–86. DOI: 10.1002/rev3.3080

Coelho, F. G. de M., Gobbi, S., Andreatto, C. A. A., Corazza, D. I., Pedroso, R. V., & Santos-Galduróz, R. F. (2013). Physical exercise modulates peripheral levels of brain-derived neurotrophic factor (BDNF): A systematic review of experimental studies in the elderly. *Archives of Gerontology and Geriatrics, 56*(1), 10–15. DOI: 10.1016/j.archger.2012.06.003 PMID: 22749404

Craft, L. L., & Perna, F. M. (2004). The Benefits of Exercise for the Clinically Depressed. *Primary Care Companion to the Journal of Clinical Psychiatry, 6*(3), 104–111. DOI: 10.4088/pcc.v06n0301 PMID: 15361924

Cuijpers, P., Karyotaki, E., Weitz, E., Andersson, G., Hollon, S. D., & van Straten, A. (2014). The effects of psychotherapies for major depression in adults on remission, recovery and improvement: A meta-analysis. *Journal of Affective Disorders, 159*, 118–126. DOI: 10.1016/j.jad.2014.02.026 PMID: 24679399

Dean, J., & Keshavan, M. (2017). The neurobiology of depression: An integrated view. *Asian Journal of Psychiatry, 27*, 101–111. DOI: 10.1016/j.ajp.2017.01.025 PMID: 28558878

Deci, E. L., & Ryan, R. M. (2008). Self-determination theory: A macrotheory of human motivation, development, and health. *Canadian Psychology, 49*(3), 182–185. DOI: 10.1037/a0012801

Dishman, R. K., Berthoud, H.-R., Booth, F. W., Cotman, C. W., Edgerton, V. R., Fleshner, M. R., Gandevia, S. C., Gomez-Pinilla, F., Greenwood, B. N., Hillman, C. H., Kramer, A. F., Levin, B. E., Moran, T. H., Russo-Neustadt, A. A., Salamone, J. D., Van Hoomissen, J. D., Wade, C. E., York, D. A., & Zigmond, M. J. (2006). Neurobiology of exercise. *Obesity (Silver Spring, Md.)*, *14*(3), 345–356. DOI: 10.1038/oby.2006.46 PMID: 16648603

Driskell, T., Sclafani, Steve, & and Driskell, J. E. (2014). Reducing the Effects of Game Day Pressures through Stress Exposure Training. *Journal of Sport Psychology in Action*, *5*(1), 28–43. DOI: 10.1080/21520704.2013.866603

Egger, M., Davey Smith, G., Schneider, M., & Minder, C. (1997). Bias in meta-analysis detected by a simple, graphical test. *BMJ (Clinical Research Ed.)*, *315*(7109), 629–634. DOI: 10.1136/bmj.315.7109.629 PMID: 9310563

Eisenberg, D., Gollust, S. E., Golberstein, E., & Hefner, J. L. (2007). Prevalence and correlates of depression, anxiety, and suicidality among university students. *The American Journal of Orthopsychiatry*, *77*(4), 534–542. DOI: 10.1037/0002-9432.77.4.534 PMID: 18194033

Ekkekakis, P. (2003). Pleasure and displeasure from the body: Perspectives from exercise. *Cognition & Emotion -. Cognition and Emotion*, *17*, 213–239. DOI: 10.1080/02699930302292 PMID: 29715726

Ekkekakis, P. (2009). Illuminating the black box: Investigating prefrontal cortical hemodynamics during exercise with near-infrared spectroscopy. *Journal of Sport & Exercise Psychology*, *31*(4), 505–553. DOI: 10.1123/jsep.31.4.505 PMID: 19842545

Ekkekakis, P., & Acevedo, E. O. (2006). Affective Responses to Acute Exercise: Toward a Psychobiological Dose-Response Model. In *Psychobiology of physical activity* (pp. 91–109). Human Kinetics.

Ekkekakis, P., Parfitt, G., & Petruzzello, S. J. (2011). The pleasure and displeasure people feel when they exercise at different intensities: Decennial update and progress towards a tripartite rationale for exercise intensity prescription. *Sports Medicine (Auckland, N.Z.)*, *41*(8), 641–671. DOI: 10.2165/11590680-000000000-00000 PMID: 21780850

Erickson, K. I., Voss, M. W., Prakash, R. S., Basak, C., Szabo, A., Chaddock, L., Kim, J. S., Heo, S., Alves, H., White, S. M., Wojcicki, T. R., Mailey, E., Vieira, V. J., Martin, S. A., Pence, B. D., Woods, J. A., McAuley, E., & Kramer, A. F. (2011). Exercise training increases size of hippocampus and improves memory. *Proceedings of the National Academy of Sciences of the United States of America*, *108*(7), 3017–3022. DOI: 10.1073/pnas.1015950108 PMID: 21282661

Firth, J., Torous, J., Nicholas, J., Carney, R., Pratap, A., Rosenbaum, S., & Sarris, J. (2017). The efficacy of smartphone-based mental health interventions for depressive symptoms: A meta-analysis of randomized controlled trials. *World Psychiatry; Official Journal of the World Psychiatric Association (WPA)*, *16*(3), 287–298. DOI: 10.1002/wps.20472 PMID: 28941113

Foster, J. A., & McVey Neufeld, K.-A. (2013). Gut-brain axis: How the microbiome influences anxiety and depression. *Trends in Neurosciences*, *36*(5), 305–312. DOI: 10.1016/j.tins.2013.01.005 PMID: 23384445

Fredrickson, B. L. (2001). The role of positive emotions in positive psychology. The broaden-and-build theory of positive emotions. *The American Psychologist*, *56*(3), 218–226. DOI: 10.1037//0003-066x.56.3.218 PMID: 11315248

Fredrickson, B. L., & Joiner, T. (2002). Positive emotions trigger upward spirals toward emotional well-being. *Psychological Science*, *13*(2), 172–175. DOI: 10.1111/1467-9280.00431 PMID: 11934003

Glasgow, R. E., Vinson, C., Chambers, D., Khoury, M. J., Kaplan, R. M., & Hunter, C. (2012). National Institutes of Health approaches to dissemination and implementation science: Current and future directions. *American Journal of Public Health*, *102*(7), 1274–1281. DOI: 10.2105/AJPH.2012.300755 PMID: 22594758

Gordon, B. R., McDowell, C. P., Hallgren, M., Meyer, J. D., Lyons, M., & Herring, M. P. (2018). Association of Efficacy of Resistance Exercise Training With Depressive Symptoms: Meta-analysis and Meta-regression Analysis of Randomized Clinical Trials. *JAMA Psychiatry*, *75*(6), 566–576. DOI: 10.1001/jamapsychiatry.2018.0572 PMID: 29800984

Grogan, S. (2016). *Body Image: Understanding Body Dissatisfaction in Men, Women and Children* (3rd ed.). Routledge., DOI: 10.4324/9781315681528

Heisz, J. J., Clark, I. B., Bonin, K., Paolucci, E. M., Michalski, B., Becker, S., & Fahnestock, M. (2017). The Effects of Physical Exercise and Cognitive Training on Memory and Neurotrophic Factors. *Journal of Cognitive Neuroscience*, *29*(11), 1895–1907. DOI: 10.1162/jocn_a_01164 PMID: 28699808

Herring, M. P., O'Connor, P. J., & Dishman, R. K. (2010). The effect of exercise training on anxiety symptoms among patients: A systematic review. *Archives of Internal Medicine*, *170*(4), 321–331. DOI: 10.1001/archinternmed.2009.530 PMID: 20177034

Hillman, C. H., Erickson, K. I., & Kramer, A. F. (2008). Be smart, exercise your heart: Exercise effects on brain and cognition. *Nature Reviews. Neuroscience, 9*(1), 58–65. DOI: 10.1038/nrn2298 PMID: 18094706

Hogan, N. S., & Schmidt, L. A. (2002). Testing the grief to personal growth model using structural equation modeling. *Death Studies, 26*(8), 615–634. DOI: 10.1080/07481180290088338 PMID: 12243195

House, J. S., Landis, K. R., & Umberson, D. (1988). Social relationships and health. *Science, 241*(4865), 540–545. DOI: 10.1126/science.3399889 PMID: 3399889

Howren, M. B., Lamkin, D. M., & Suls, J. (2009). Associations of depression with C-reactive protein, IL-1, and IL-6: A meta-analysis. *Psychosomatic Medicine, 71*(2), 171–186. DOI: 10.1097/PSY.0b013e3181907c1b PMID: 19188531

Hunt, J., & Eisenberg, D. (2010). Mental health problems and help-seeking behavior among college students. *The Journal of Adolescent Health: Official Publication of the Society for Adolescent Medicine, 46*(1), 3–10. DOI: 10.1016/j.jadohealth.2009.08.008 PMID: 20123251

Josefsson, T., Ivarsson, A., Lindwall, M., Gustafsson, H., Stenling, A., Böröy, J., Mattsson, E., Carnebratt, J., Sevholt, S., & Falkevik, E. (2017). Mindfulness Mechanisms in Sports: Mediating Effects of Rumination and Emotion Regulation on Sport-Specific Coping. *Mindfulness, 8*(5), 1354–1363. DOI: 10.1007/s12671-017-0711-4 PMID: 28989551

Kandola, A., Ashdown-Franks, G., Hendrikse, J., Sabiston, C. M., & Stubbs, B. (2019). Physical activity and depression: Towards understanding the antidepressant mechanisms of physical activity. *Neuroscience and Biobehavioral Reviews, 107*, 525–539. DOI: 10.1016/j.neubiorev.2019.09.040 PMID: 31586447

Keating, X. D., Guan, J., Piñero, J. C., & Bridges, D. M. (2005). A meta-analysis of college students' physical activity behaviors. *Journal of American College Health: J of ACH, 54*(2), 116–125. DOI: 10.3200/JACH.54.2.116-126 PMID: 16255324

Kessler, R. C., Petukhova, M., Sampson, N. A., Zaslavsky, A. M., & Wittchen, H.-U. (2012). Twelve-month and lifetime prevalence and lifetime morbid risk of anxiety and mood disorders in the United States. *International Journal of Methods in Psychiatric Research, 21*(3), 169–184. DOI: 10.1002/mpr.1359 PMID: 22865617

Kredlow, M. A., Capozzoli, M. C., Hearon, B. A., Calkins, A. W., & Otto, M. W. (2015). The effects of physical activity on sleep: A meta-analytic review. *Journal of Behavioral Medicine, 38*(3), 427–449. DOI: 10.1007/s10865-015-9617-6 PMID: 25596964

Lederer, A. M., & Hoban, M. T. (2022). The development of the American College Health Association-National College Health Assessment III: An improved tool to assess and enhance the health and well-being of college students. *Journal of American College Health: J of ACH, 70*(6), 1606–1610. DOI: 10.1080/07448481.2020.1834401 PMID: 33400616

Liguori, G., & Medicine (ACSM), A. C. of S. (2020). *ACSM's Guidelines for Exercise Testing and Prescription*. Wolters Kluwer Health.

Liu, C. H., Stevens, C., Wong, S. H. M., Yasui, M., & Chen, J. A. (2019). The prevalence and predictors of mental health diagnoses and suicide among U.S. college students: Implications for addressing disparities in service use. *Depression and Anxiety, 36*(1), 8–17. DOI: 10.1002/da.22830 PMID: 30188598

Locke, E. A., & Latham, G. P. (2002). Building a practically useful theory of goal setting and task motivation. A 35-year odyssey. *The American Psychologist, 57*(9), 705–717. DOI: 10.1037//0003-066x.57.9.705 PMID: 12237980

Lubans, D., Richards, J., Hillman, C., Faulkner, G., Beauchamp, M., Nilsson, M., Kelly, P., Smith, J., Raine, L., & Biddle, S. (2016). Physical Activity for Cognitive and Mental Health in Youth: A Systematic Review of Mechanisms. *Pediatrics, 138*(3), e20161642. DOI: 10.1542/peds.2016-1642 PMID: 27542849

Maher, C. A., Lewis, L. K., Ferrar, K., Marshall, S., De Bourdeaudhuij, I., & Vandelanotte, C. (2014). Are health behavior change interventions that use online social networks effective? A systematic review. *Journal of Medical Internet Research, 16*(2), e40. DOI: 10.2196/jmir.2952 PMID: 24550083

McEwen, B. S. (2017). Neurobiological and Systemic Effects of Chronic Stress. *Chronic Stress (Thousand Oaks, Calif.), 1*, 2470547017692328. DOI: 10.1177/2470547017692328 PMID: 28856337

Mehling, W. E., Price, C., Daubenmier, J. J., Acree, M., Bartmess, E., & Stewart, A. (2012). The Multidimensional Assessment of Interoceptive Awareness (MAIA). *PLoS One, 7*(11), e48230. DOI: 10.1371/journal.pone.0048230 PMID: 23133619

Mikkelsen, K., Stojanovska, L., Polenakovic, M., Bosevski, M., & Apostolopoulos, V. (2017). Exercise and mental health. *Maturitas, 106*, 48–56. DOI: 10.1016/j.maturitas.2017.09.003 PMID: 29150166

Miller, A. H., & Raison, C. L. (2016). The role of inflammation in depression: From evolutionary imperative to modern treatment target. *Nature Reviews. Immunology, 16*(1), 22–34. DOI: 10.1038/nri.2015.5 PMID: 26711676

Ntoumanis, N. (2001). A self-determination approach to the understanding of motivation in physical education. *The British Journal of Educational Psychology*, *71*(2), 225–242. DOI: 10.1348/000709901158497 PMID: 11449934

Pascoe, M. C., Thompson, D. R., & Ski, C. F. (2017). Yoga, mindfulness-based stress reduction and stress-related physiological measures: A meta-analysis. *Psychoneuroendocrinology*, *86*, 152–168. DOI: 10.1016/j.psyneuen.2017.08.008 PMID: 28963884

Patel, V., Flisher, A. J., Hetrick, S., & McGorry, P. (2007). Mental health of young people: A global public-health challenge. *Lancet*, *369*(9569), 1302–1313. DOI: 10.1016/S0140-6736(07)60368-7 PMID: 17434406

Penedo, F. J., & Dahn, J. R. (2005). Exercise and well-being: A review of mental and physical health benefits associated with physical activity. *Current Opinion in Psychiatry*, *18*(2), 189–193. DOI: 10.1097/00001504-200503000-00013 PMID: 16639173

Petersen, A. M. W., & Pedersen, B. K. (2005). The anti-inflammatory effect of exercise. *Journal of Applied Physiology (Bethesda, Md.: 1985)*, *98*(4), 1154–1162. https://doi.org/DOI: 10.1152/japplphysiol.00164.2004

Petruzzello, S. J., Landers, D. M., Hatfield, B. D., Kubitz, K. A., & Salazar, W. (1991). A meta-analysis on the anxiety-reducing effects of acute and chronic exercise. Outcomes and mechanisms. *Sports Medicine (Auckland, N.Z.)*, *11*(3), 143–182. DOI: 10.2165/00007256-199111030-00002 PMID: 1828608

Primack, B. A., Shensa, A., Sidani, J. E., Whaite, E. O., Lin, L. Y., Rosen, D., Colditz, J. B., Radovic, A., & Miller, E. (2017). Social Media Use and Perceived Social Isolation Among Young Adults in the U.S. *American Journal of Preventive Medicine*, *53*(1), 1–8. DOI: 10.1016/j.amepre.2017.01.010 PMID: 28279545

Prochaska, J. O., & DiClemente, C. C. (1983). Stages and processes of self-change of smoking: Toward an integrative model of change. *Journal of Consulting and Clinical Psychology*, *51*(3), 390–395. DOI: 10.1037/0022-006X.51.3.390 PMID: 6863699

Reed, J., & Buck, S. (2009). The effect of regular aerobic exercise on positive-activated affect: A meta-analysis. *Psychology of Sport and Exercise*, *10*(6), 581–594. DOI: 10.1016/j.psychsport.2009.05.009

Rethorst, C. D., & Trivedi, M. H. (2013). Evidence-based recommendations for the prescription of exercise for major depressive disorder. *Journal of Psychiatric Practice*, *19*(3), 204–212. DOI: 10.1097/01.pra.0000430504.16952.3e PMID: 23653077

Rosenbaum, S., Tiedemann, A., Sherrington, C., Curtis, J., & Ward, P. B. (2014). Physical activity interventions for people with mental illness: A systematic review and meta-analysis. *The Journal of Clinical Psychiatry*, *75*(9), 964–974. DOI: 10.4088/JCP.13r08765 PMID: 24813261

Sallis, J. F., Floyd, M. F., Rodríguez, D. A., & Saelens, B. E. (2012). Role of built environments in physical activity, obesity, and cardiovascular disease. *Circulation*, *125*(5), 729–737. DOI: 10.1161/CIRCULATIONAHA.110.969022 PMID: 22311885

Schuch, F. B., Vancampfort, D., Richards, J., Rosenbaum, S., Ward, P. B., & Stubbs, B. (2016). Exercise as a treatment for depression: A meta-analysis adjusting for publication bias. *Journal of Psychiatric Research*, *77*, 42–51. DOI: 10.1016/j.jpsychires.2016.02.023 PMID: 26978184

Schulenberg, J. E., Sameroff, A. J., & Cicchetti, D. (2004). The transition to adulthood as a critical juncture in the course of psychopathology and mental health. *Development and Psychopathology*, *16*(4), 799–806. DOI: 10.1017/S0954579404040015 PMID: 15704815

Sebire, S. J., Standage, M., & Vansteenkiste, M. (2009). Examining intrinsic versus extrinsic exercise goals: Cognitive, affective, and behavioral outcomes. *Journal of Sport & Exercise Psychology*, *31*(2), 189–210. DOI: 10.1123/jsep.31.2.189 PMID: 19454771

Sharma, A., Madaan, V., & Petty, F. D. (2006). Exercise for mental health. *Primary Care Companion to the Journal of Clinical Psychiatry*, *8*(2), 106. DOI: 10.4088/pcc.v08n0208a PMID: 16862239

Smith, T. B., McCullough, M. E., & Poll, J. (2003). Religiousness and depression: Evidence for a main effect and the moderating influence of stressful life events. *Psychological Bulletin*, *129*(4), 614–636. DOI: 10.1037/0033-2909.129.4.614 PMID: 12848223

Son, C., Hegde, S., Smith, A., Wang, X., & Sasangohar, F. (2020). Effects of COVID-19 on College Students' Mental Health in the United States: Interview Survey Study. *Journal of Medical Internet Research*, *22*(9), e21279. DOI: 10.2196/21279 PMID: 32805704

Spindle, T. R., Cone, E. J., Schlienz, N. J., Mitchell, J. M., Bigelow, G. E., Flegel, R., Hayes, E., & Vandrey, R. (2018). Acute Effects of Smoked and Vaporized Cannabis in Healthy Adults Who Infrequently Use Cannabis: A Crossover Trial. *JAMA Network Open*, *1*(7), e184841. DOI: 10.1001/jamanetworkopen.2018.4841 PMID: 30646391

Stanton, S., Rosenbaum, S., Kalucy, M., Reaburn, P., & Happell, B. (2015). A call to action: Exercise as treatment for patients with mental illness. *Australian Journal of Primary Health*, *21*(2), 120–125. DOI: 10.1071/PY14054 PMID: 25033827

Strong, W. B., Malina, R. M., Blimkie, C. J. R., Daniels, S. R., Dishman, R. K., Gutin, B., Hergenroeder, A. C., Must, A., Nixon, P. A., Pivarnik, J. M., Rowland, T., Trost, S., & Trudeau, F. (2005). Evidence based physical activity for school-age youth. *The Journal of Pediatrics*, *146*(6), 732–737. DOI: 10.1016/j.jpeds.2005.01.055 PMID: 15973308

Teixeira, P. J., Carraça, E. V., Markland, D., Silva, M. N., & Ryan, R. M. (2012). Exercise, physical activity, and self-determination theory: A systematic review. *The International Journal of Behavioral Nutrition and Physical Activity*, *9*, 78. DOI: 10.1186/1479-5868-9-78 PMID: 22726453

Thayer, J. F., Ahs, F., Fredrikson, M., Sollers, J. J., & Wager, T. D. (2012). A meta-analysis of heart rate variability and neuroimaging studies: Implications for heart rate variability as a marker of stress and health. *Neuroscience and Biobehavioral Reviews*, *36*(2), 747–756. DOI: 10.1016/j.neubiorev.2011.11.009 PMID: 22178086

Topp, R., Jacks, D. E., Wedig, R. T., Newman, J. L., Tobe, L., & Hollingsworth, A. (2009). Reducing risk factors for childhood obesity: The Tommie Smith Youth Athletic Initiative. *Western Journal of Nursing Research*, *31*(6), 715–730. DOI: 10.1177/0193945909336356 PMID: 19454750

Tsatsoulis, A., & Fountoulakis, S. (2006). The protective role of exercise on stress system dysregulation and comorbidities. *Annals of the New York Academy of Sciences*, *1083*, 196–213. DOI: 10.1196/annals.1367.020 PMID: 17148741

Twenge, J. M., & Campbell, W. K. (2018). Associations between screen time and lower psychological well-being among children and adolescents: Evidence from a population-based study. *Preventive Medicine Reports*, *12*, 271–283. DOI: 10.1016/j.pmedr.2018.10.003 PMID: 30406005

Twenge, J. M., Cooper, A. B., Joiner, T. E., Duffy, M. E., & Binau, S. G. (2019). Age, period, and cohort trends in mood disorder indicators and suicide-related outcomes in a nationally representative dataset, 2005-2017. *Journal of Abnormal Psychology*, *128*(3), 185–199. DOI: 10.1037/abn0000410 PMID: 30869927

Voss, M. W., Heo, S., Prakash, R. S., Erickson, K. I., Alves, H., Chaddock, L., Szabo, A. N., Mailey, E. L., Wójcicki, T. R., White, S. M., Gothe, N., McAuley, E., Sutton, B. P., & Kramer, A. F. (2013). The influence of aerobic fitness on cerebral white matter integrity and cognitive function in older adults: Results of a one-year exercise intervention. *Human Brain Mapping*, *34*(11), 2972–2985. DOI: 10.1002/hbm.22119 PMID: 22674729

Wegner, M., Helmich, I., Machado, S., Nardi, A. E., Arias-Carrion, O., & Budde, H. (2014). Effects of exercise on anxiety and depression disorders: Review of meta- analyses and neurobiological mechanisms. *CNS & Neurological Disorders - Drug Targets*, *13*(6), 1002–1014. DOI: 10.2174/1871527313666140612102841 PMID: 24923346

Woods, H. C., & Scott, H. (2016). #Sleepyteens: Social media use in adolescence is associated with poor sleep quality, anxiety, depression and low self-esteem. *Journal of Adolescence*, *51*, 41–49. DOI: 10.1016/j.adolescence.2016.05.008 PMID: 27294324

World Health Organization. (2024). *Mental health of adolescents*. https://www.who.int/news-room/fact-sheets/detail/adolescent-mental-health

Young, S. N. (2007). How to increase serotonin in the human brain without drugs. *Journal of Psychiatry & Neuroscience : JPN*, *32*(6), 394–399. PMID: 18043762

Chapter 7

Reshaping the Brain: Exercise-Induced Neuroplasticity and Psychological Resilience

Debajit Karmakar
https://orcid.org/0000-0001-9272-0627
Lakshmibai National Institute of Physical Education, India

Anindita Das
https://orcid.org/0000-0002-6502-9619
Lakshmibai National Institute of Physical Education, India

Tashi Ongmu Butia
https://orcid.org/0009-0000-0127-5709
Sikkim Government B.Ed College, India

Karuppasamy Govindasamy
https://orcid.org/0000-0002-3019-5545
Symbiosis International University, India

Beulah Sebastian
Symbiosis International University, India

ABSTRACT

This chapter explores how physical exercise acts as a transformative force in reshaping the brain and enhancing psychological resilience. It highlights the mechanisms of exercise-induced neuroplasticity at molecular, cellular, and systemic levels that contribute to improved memory, attention, and executive function. The discussion emphasizes the close relationship between physical activity and mental health, showing how exercise strengthens cognitive performance and emotional stability through the regulation of neurotrophic factors, neurotransmitters, and stress

DOI: 10.4018/979-8-3373-6157-4.ch007

response systems. It also examines the comparative effects of aerobic, resistance, and mind-body exercises, explaining their unique and complementary influences on cognition and resilience. The chapter concludes that regular physical activity is a powerful non-pharmacological strategy for improving brain function, emotional well-being, and lifelong adaptability.

1. INTRODUCTION

The human brain, once considered a static organ after reaching maturity, is now understood to be a remarkably plastic structure capable of profound reorganization throughout the lifespan. This transformative understanding has revolutionized neuroscience and psychology, revealing that our brains remain malleable and adaptive in response to environmental demands, experiences, and behaviours. Among the various factors that can induce neuroplastic changes, physical exercise has emerged as one of the most potent and accessible interventions for reshaping neural architecture and enhancing psychological functioning (Rendeiro & Rhodes, 2018).

Neuroplasticity, also termed neural plasticity or brain plasticity, refers to the brain's ability to modify its structure and function in response to experience, learning, and environmental stimulation. This encompasses multiple levels of organization, from molecular and cellular changes to large-scale network reorganization. At the synaptic level, neuroplasticity manifests through long-term potentiation and long-term depression, processes that strengthen or weaken synaptic connections based on activity patterns. At the cellular level, it includes neurogenesis, the birth of new neurons, particularly in the hippocampal dentate gyrus and the subventricular zone. At the systems level, neuroplasticity involves the reorganization of functional networks, allowing the brain to compensate for damage, adapt to new demands, and optimize performance across cognitive and emotional domains (Augusto-Oliveira et al., 2023).

The relationship between physical exercise and brain health has deep evolutionary roots. Throughout human evolution, physical activity was intimately linked with cognitive demands such as spatial navigation, social coordination, predator avoidance, and foraging strategies. This evolutionary context suggests that the brain and body evolved as integrated systems, with physical exertion serving as a signal for the brain to enhance its adaptive capacity. Modern neuroscience has begun to uncover the sophisticated molecular and cellular mechanisms underlying this ancient connection, revealing an intricate cascade of neurobiological events triggered by physical activity. Exercise exerts its neuroplastic effects through multiple converging pathways (Augusto-Oliveira et al., 2023). These include the upregulation of neurotrophic factors, particularly brain-derived neurotrophic factor (BDNF), which acts as a master regulator of synaptic plasticity, neurogenesis, and neuronal survival. Exercise also enhances cerebral blood flow and angiogenesis, improving oxygen and nutrient delivery to neural tissues. Furthermore, physical activity modulates neurotransmitter systems, including serotonin, dopamine, norepinephrine, and gamma-aminobutyric acid (GABA), which collectively influence mood, motivation, attention, and stress resilience. The endocrine system responds to exercise with changes in cortisol regulation, growth hormone secretion, and insulin-like growth factor 1 (IGF-1) production, all of which have direct and indirect effects on brain structure and function (Rendeiro & Rhodes, 2018).

Beyond these biological mechanisms, exercise also influences psychological resilience through its effects on self-efficacy, behavioural activation, social engagement, and the development of mastery experiences. The psychological benefits of exercise are not merely secondary consequences of improved physical health but represent direct effects on neural circuits governing emotion regulation, stress response, and adaptive coping. This dual pathway, encompassing both bottom-up neurobiological changes and top-down psychological processes, positions exercise as a uniquely comprehensive intervention for enhancing mental health and cognitive function (Augusto-Oliveira et al., 2023).

2. COGNITIVE BENEFITS OF EXERCISE

The cognitive benefits of exercise extend far beyond the immediate post-workout sensation of mental clarity, encompassing profound and lasting changes in brain structure, neural connectivity, and information processing capacity. Decades of research across animal models, neuroimaging studies, and behavioural assessments have established that regular physical activity enhances virtually every aspect of cognitive function, from basic perceptual processing to complex executive operations. These enhancements reflect fundamental alterations in neural architecture, synaptic efficacy, and network organization that accumulate over time with consistent exercise engagement (Rendeiro & Rhodes, 2018).

Improvements in Memory, Attention, and Learning

Memory systems represent one of the most extensively studied domains of exercise-induced cognitive enhancement. The hippocampus, a seahorse-shaped structure deep within the medial temporal lobe, serves as the primary site for encoding new declarative memories and for spatial navigation. This region demonstrates remarkable sensitivity to physical activity, with both animal and human studies revealing that exercise promotes hippocampal neurogenesis, increases hippocampal volume, and enhances hippocampal-dependent memory functions (Zhao et al., 2020). Seminal research in rodent models established that voluntary wheel running substantially increases the proliferation, survival, and functional integration of newly born neurons in the dentate gyrus of the hippocampus. These newborn neurons exhibit enhanced synaptic plasticity during a critical period of their maturation, suggesting that they may be particularly important for encoding novel information and distinguishing between similar experiences, a process known as pattern separation. Computational models suggest that neurogenesis provides the hippocampus with a continuously renewed population of neurons that can be preferentially recruited for new learning, preventing interference from previously stored information (Augusto-Oliveira et al., 2023).

In humans, longitudinal neuroimaging studies have demonstrated that aerobic exercise programs can increase hippocampal volume even in older adults, a population typically experiencing age-related hippocampal atrophy. One landmark study found that moderate-intensity aerobic exercise for one year increased anterior hippocampal volume by approximately two percent, effectively reversing age-related volume loss by one to two years. This structural change correlated with improvements in spatial memory performance and elevated serum levels of BDNF, suggesting a mechanistic link between exercise, neurotrophic support, and memory enhancement (Rendeiro & Rhodes, 2018). Exercise also improves episodic memory, the ability to recall specific events and experiences embedded in temporal and spatial contexts. Studies examining memory consolidation have found that acute exercise performed shortly after learning can enhance retention, possibly by promoting the synaptic consolidation processes that stabilize newly encoded information. The timing and intensity of exercise appear to modulate these effects, with moderate-intensity exercise immediately or shortly after learning typically producing the strongest memory benefits. These consolidation effects may involve exercise-induced increases in catecholamines, which enhance arousal and facilitate the tagging of important memories for preferential consolidation during subsequent rest periods (Augusto-Oliveira et al., 2023).

Working memory, the capacity to temporarily maintain and manipulate information in mind, also benefits from regular exercise. Working memory depends on sustained activation patterns in prefrontal cortical networks, and exercise appears to enhance the efficiency and capacity of these systems. Meta-analyses of intervention studies indicate that exercise training produces moderate improvements in working memory performance, with effects that may be particularly pronounced in populations with initially lower cognitive function or higher levels of physiological dysfunction (Rendeiro & Rhodes, 2018).

Attention, the process of selectively focusing cognitive resources on relevant information while filtering distractions, represents another domain substantially enhanced by exercise. The attention system comprises multiple components, including sustained attention (maintaining focus over time), selective attention (focusing on relevant stimuli while ignoring irrelevant information), and divided attention (managing multiple information streams simultaneously). Exercise appears to benefit all these components, with particularly strong effects on sustained attention and attentional control. Functional magnetic resonance imaging (fMRI) studies have similarly demonstrated that exercise training increases activation in dorsal attention networks while decreasing activation in default mode networks during attention-demanding tasks, reflecting improved attentional focus and reduced mind-wandering (Augusto-Oliveira et al., 2023).

The attentional benefits of exercise appear to involve multiple mechanisms. Enhanced noradrenergic signaling may improve the signal-to-noise ratio of sensory processing, allowing more efficient discrimination between relevant and irrelevant information. Increased prefrontal cortical volume and enhanced connectivity within fronto-parietal attention networks may improve top-down attentional control (Zhao et al., 2020). Additionally, exercise-induced improvements in arousal regulation and autonomic function may optimize the physiological state for sustained attention. Learning capacity, the ability to acquire new knowledge and skills efficiently, benefits from exercise through multiple pathways. At the molecular level, exercise upregulates BDNF and other neurotrophic factors that facilitate synaptic plasticity, the cellular basis of learning. BDNF enhances long-term potentiation, a form of synaptic strengthening believed to underlie memory formation, and promotes dendritic spine formation and maturation, increasing the structural substrates for new synaptic connections. Exercise also increases the expression of proteins involved in synaptic vesicle recycling, neurotransmitter synthesis, and receptor trafficking, all of which support enhanced synaptic transmission during learning (Zhao et al., 2020).

Executive Functions and Decision-Making

Executive functions represent a constellation of higher-order cognitive processes that enable goal-directed behaviour, adaptive problem-solving, and self-regulation. These functions include inhibitory control (suppressing prepotent responses), cognitive flexibility (shifting between mental sets or task rules), and working memory (maintaining and manipulating information). Additionally, executive functions encompass planning, organization, decision-making, and metacognition. These processes depend primarily on prefrontal cortical networks, particularly the dorsolateral prefrontal cortex, anterior cingulate cortex, and orbitofrontal cortex, as well as their connections to posterior cortical regions and subcortical structures including the basal ganglia and thalamus (Karmakar et al., 2025).

Exercise exerts particularly robust effects on executive functions, with meta-analytic evidence indicating that executive processes benefit more from exercise than other cognitive domains. This preferential enhancement may reflect the sensitivity of prefrontal cortical circuits to exercise-induced neuroplastic changes, including increased gray matter volume, enhanced white matter integrity, and improved functional connectivity. Prefrontal regions undergo protracted development during childhood and adolescence and demonstrate early vulnerability to age-related decline, making them particularly responsive to environmental modulation including exercise (Zhu et al., 2025).

Neuroimaging studies have provided insights into the neural mechanisms underlying exercise-enhanced inhibitory control. Functional MRI studies reveal that physically fit individuals show greater activation in prefrontal regions during inhibitory control tasks, suggesting enhanced recruitment of neural resources for cognitive control. Conversely, some studies have found decreased prefrontal activation in fit individuals, which may reflect greater neural efficiency and reduced need for compensatory activation. These apparently contradictory findings can be reconciled by considering task difficulty and individual fitness levels; easier tasks may show efficiency-related activation decreases, while more challenging tasks may reveal capacity-related activation increases (Zhao et al., 2020).

Neurocognitive Aging and Cognitive Reserve

The aging brain undergoes numerous structural and functional changes that can compromise cognitive performance. These changes include global and regional brain atrophy, particularly in the prefrontal cortex and hippocampus; accumulation of white matter hyperintensities reflecting small vessel disease; reduced dendritic arborization and synaptic density; impaired neurotransmitter synthesis and receptor function; increased oxidative stress and inflammation; and accumulation of pathological proteins including amyloid-beta and tau. Cognitive domains particularly vulnerable to aging include processing speed, working memory, executive functions, and episodic memory, while crystallized knowledge and semantic memory tend to remain relatively preserved (Zhu et al., 2025).

The concept of cognitive reserve provides a framework for understanding individual differences in the cognitive impacts of age-related brain changes. Cognitive reserve refers to the brain's ability to maintain cognitive performance despite neuropathological burden or structural damage. Individuals with higher cognitive reserve can sustain more brain pathology before manifesting clinical symptoms, effectively displaying resilience against age-related and pathological insults. Cognitive reserve is thought to involve both neural reserve (more efficient use of existing neural networks) and neural compensation (recruitment of alternative networks when primary networks are compromised). Factors that build cognitive reserve include educational attainment, occupational complexity, multilingualism, social engagement, cognitive leisure activities, and notably, physical exercise (Brondino et al., 2017).

Epidemiological studies have consistently demonstrated that higher levels of physical activity throughout life are associated with reduced risk of cognitive decline and dementia. Meta-analyses indicate that regular exercise reduces dementia risk by approximately 30 percent and Alzheimer's disease risk by approximately 45 percent. These protective effects appear to follow a dose-response relationship, with greater amounts of physical activity associated with progressively larger risk reductions. Importantly, physical activity at any life stage appears beneficial, although the strongest protective effects are observed when activity is sustained throughout adulthood and later life (Brondino et al., 2017). Intervention studies have provided causal evidence that exercise can slow or partially reverse age-related cognitive decline. Randomized controlled trials in older adults have demonstrated that aerobic exercise programs, typically involving moderate-intensity walking or cycling for 30 to 60 minutes several times per week, can improve executive function, processing speed, and memory. Some studies have found that these cognitive benefits exceed those produced by control interventions including stretching, toning, or educational programs, although not all studies find significant differences between exercise and active control conditions (Zhu et al., 2025).

The neural mechanisms underlying exercise-related cognitive protection in aging are multifaceted. At the macrostructural level, exercise attenuates age-related brain atrophy, preserving gray matter volume in prefrontal and temporal regions. The hippocampus, which typically loses approximately one to two percent of its volume per year in sedentary older adults, can actually increase in volume with aerobic exercise training. Exercise also preserves white matter integrity, reducing the accumulation of white matter hyperintensities and maintaining fractional anisotropy in major white matter tracts (Brondino et al., 2017).

At the vascular level, exercise improves cerebral blood flow and promotes angiogenesis, the formation of new blood vessels. Cerebral blood flow naturally declines with age, compromising oxygen and nutrient delivery to neural tissues. Exercise-induced improvements in cerebral vascular function may help maintain the metabolic support necessary for optimal neural function. Additionally, exercise promotes vascular endothelial function throughout the body, reducing cardiovascular risk factors such as hypertension, diabetes, and hyperlipidemia that independently contribute to cognitive decline (Archer et al., 2016). At the cellular and molecular levels, exercise combats multiple aspects of brain aging. Exercise increases BDNF expression, which naturally declines with age, potentially restoring neurotrophic support for synaptic plasticity and neuronal survival. Exercise reduces oxidative stress by enhancing antioxidant enzyme systems and improving mitochondrial function. Inflammation, a key contributor to brain aging and neurodegeneration, is reduced by exercise through multiple pathways including decreased production of pro-inflammatory cytokines and enhanced anti-inflammatory signaling. Exercise also improves insulin sensitivity and glucose metabolism in the brain, countering metabolic dysfunction associated with aging and Alzheimer's disease pathology (Brown et al., 1995).

Academic and Occupational Implications

The cognitive enhancements produced by exercise have substantial implications for performance in academic and occupational contexts. In educational settings, the cognitive benefits of exercise translate into improved academic achievement, better classroom behaviour, and enhanced learning efficiency. These benefits are observed across the age spectrum from early childhood through higher education (Quigley et al., 2020).

In elementary school students, increased physical activity through physical education classes, recess periods, or movement breaks during academic instruction has been associated with improved academic performance, particularly in mathematics and reading. The mechanisms underlying these benefits are multifaceted, including direct effects on cognitive function as well as indirect effects through improved attention, behaviour regulation, and classroom engagement. Neuroimaging studies in children have found that higher aerobic fitness is associated with larger hippocampal and basal ganglia volumes, enhanced white matter integrity, and more efficient neural processing during cognitive tasks (Archer et al., 2016).

The relationship between physical activity and academic performance appears particularly strong for executive functions, which play critical roles in learning across domains. Executive functions enable students to maintain focus during instruction, inhibit distracting thoughts and behaviours, shift flexibly between different concepts or problem-solving approaches, and organize information for learning and recall. Given that exercise robustly enhances executive functions, increasing physical activity represents a promising strategy for supporting academic success, particularly for students with attention difficulties or executive function weaknesses (Brondino et al., 2017).

Timing considerations are important for maximizing the academic benefits of physical activity. Acute exercise before learning activities can prime the brain for enhanced information encoding through increased arousal, attention, and neurotransmitter release. Physical activity during learning, such as in movement-integrated instruction where students engage in physical movements while learning academic content, may enhance memory through embodied cognition mechanisms and state-dependent learning effects. Physical activity after learning may benefit memory consolidation through the stabilization of newly encoded information (Brondino et al., 2017).

In adolescence, a period characterized by dramatic brain development particularly in prefrontal regions underlying executive function, physical activity may play an especially important role in supporting cognitive maturation and academic success. However, physical activity levels tend to decline during adolescence, particularly among girls, creating a concerning mismatch between developmental needs and behavioural patterns. School-based interventions to maintain or increase physical activity during adolescence could potentially support both cognitive development and academic achievement during this critical period (Quigley et al., 2020).

In higher education, regular exercise has been associated with better academic performance, although the relationship is complex and potentially moderated by factors such as the time commitment required for exercise and individual differences in how exercise is integrated into students' overall schedules. College students who exercise regularly report better concentration, memory, and mental stamina. Exercise may also buffer against the academic impacts of stress, which is particularly relevant given the high stress levels often experienced by college students. The stress-buffering effects of exercise, discussed in detail in subsequent sections, may help maintain cognitive performance under the challenging conditions common in academic environments (Stimpson et al., 2018). In occupational contexts, the cognitive benefits of exercise translate into enhanced workplace performance across multiple dimensions. Executive functions are critical for workplace success, supporting abilities such as prioritizing tasks, meeting deadlines, solving complex problems, adapting to changing demands, and regulating emotions during interpersonal interactions. Given that exercise robustly enhances executive functions, workplace physical activity programs represent a potentially valuable investment in human capital (Brown et al., 1995).

Research on workplace exercise programs has found benefits including reduced absenteeism, improved productivity, better job satisfaction, and reduced healthcare costs. While some of these benefits may reflect improved physical health and reduced chronic disease burden, cognitive and psychological enhancements likely play important roles. Improved attention and executive function can enhance work quality and efficiency. Better emotion regulation and stress resilience can improve interpersonal relationships and job satisfaction. Enhanced energy and reduced fatigue can increase sustained productivity throughout the workday (Brondino et al., 2017).

The timing and implementation of workplace physical activity are important practical considerations. Brief exercise or movement breaks during the workday can provide acute cognitive benefits, potentially improving performance on subsequent work tasks. Lunchtime exercise programs can offer both acute cognitive benefits and contribute to longer-term fitness improvements. Before-work or after-work exercise programs may provide fewer immediate workplace benefits but can contribute to overall fitness and cognitive function. Organizations must balance the time investment required for physical activity against potential productivity benefits, although evidence suggests that workplace exercise programs generally have positive or neutral effects on overall productivity despite time away from work tasks (Archer et al., 2016).

3. BUILDING PSYCHOLOGICAL RESILIENCE THROUGH EXERCISE

Psychological resilience, the capacity to adapt positively to adversity, stress, and challenging life circumstances, represents a critical component of mental health and well-being. Resilient individuals maintain psychological equilibrium when confronted with stressors, recover more quickly from negative experiences, and may even experience post-traumatic growth following severe challenges (Karmakar et al., 2025). While resilience involves multiple factors including genetic predisposition, early life experiences, personality traits, social support, and cognitive coping strategies, accumulating evidence indicates that regular physical exercise represents a powerful tool for building and maintaining psychological resilience through its effects on stress response systems, autonomic function, emotion regulation, and cognitive flexibility (Rehman & Shabbir, 2025).

The HPA Axis and Stress Response Recalibration

The hypothalamic-pituitary-adrenal (HPA) axis represents the primary neuroendocrine system for coordinating physiological and behavioural responses to stress. When an organism encounters a stressor, neurons in the paraventricular nucleus of the hypothalamus release corticotropin-releasing hormone (CRH) and arginine vasopressin into the hypothalamic-pituitary portal system. These peptides stimulate the anterior pituitary to secrete adrenocorticotropic hormone (ACTH) into the systemic circulation. ACTH then stimulates the adrenal cortex to synthesize and release glucocorticoid hormones, primarily cortisol in humans and corticosterone in rodents. Glucocorticoids exert wide-ranging effects on metabolism, immune function, and brain activity, mobilizing energy resources and modulating neural circuits to promote survival during threat or challenge (Noone & Hastings, 2009).

While acute HPA axis activation is adaptive, facilitating appropriate responses to immediate challenges, chronic or excessive activation can become pathological. Prolonged elevations in glucocorticoids contribute to numerous adverse outcomes including hippocampal atrophy, prefrontal cortical dysfunction, metabolic syndrome, immune suppression, and increased risk for depression and anxiety disorders. Conversely, blunted HPA axis responses, observed in some individuals with chronic stress exposure or post-traumatic stress disorder, can also be maladaptive, potentially reflecting exhaustion of stress response systems or altered feedback regulation (Forbes & Fikretoglu, 2018).

Regular exercise induces beneficial adaptations in HPA axis function that enhance stress resilience. At baseline, physically active individuals and laboratory animals typically exhibit lower basal cortisol levels and more efficient negative feedback regulation. Glucocorticoid receptors, which mediate feedback inhibition of the HPA axis, show enhanced expression and function in the hippocampus and prefrontal cortex with exercise training. This enhanced feedback sensitivity allows for more rapid termination of stress responses, preventing excessive or prolonged glucocorticoid elevation (Rehman & Shabbir, 2025).

Exercise training appears to recalibrate the threshold for HPA axis activation, making the system less reactive to minor stressors while preserving responsiveness to significant challenges. This recalibration may be understood through the concept of allostatic load, the cumulative wear and tear on physiological systems from chronic stress exposure. By reducing excessive reactivity to everyday stressors, exercise decreases allostatic load and preserves the functional integrity of stress response systems. This preservation allows the organism to respond effectively when truly needed while avoiding the damaging effects of chronic activation (Norris & Norris, 2021).

Interestingly, the acute effects of exercise itself on the HPA axis appear to contribute to these long-term adaptations. Exercise represents a physical stressor that activates the HPA axis, with cortisol levels rising during and immediately after exercise sessions, particularly with moderate to high-intensity activity. This repeated activation may serve as a form of stress inoculation, repeatedly engaging HPA axis systems in a controllable, time-limited manner. This controlled activation may promote adaptive changes in stress regulatory circuits similar to how psychological stress inoculation procedures, involving repeated exposure to manageable stressors, can enhance stress resilience (Noone & Hastings, 2009).

The molecular mechanisms underlying exercise-induced HPA axis adaptation involve changes in gene expression in stress-regulatory brain regions. Exercise increases expression of genes encoding glucocorticoid receptors, mineralocorticoid receptors, neuropeptides that regulate HPA function, and proteins involved in synaptic plasticity and cellular resilience. Exercise also modulates epigenetic marks including DNA methylation and histone modifications at genes involved in stress regulation, potentially altering the transcriptional landscape in ways that promote stress resilience. Some of these epigenetic changes may persist long after exercise cessation, providing a molecular memory of previous exercise exposure that continues to influence stress regulation (Denovan & Macaskill, 2017).

Autonomic Nervous System Optimization

The autonomic nervous system (ANS), comprising sympathetic and parasympathetic branches, regulates involuntary physiological functions including heart rate, blood pressure, respiration, digestion, and arousal states. The balance between sympathetic activation, which mobilizes the fight-or-flight response, and parasympathetic activation, which promotes rest-and-digest functions, has profound implications for both physical health and psychological well-being. Chronic sympathetic predominance or parasympathetic withdrawal characterizes many stress-related conditions and is associated with increased risk for cardiovascular disease, metabolic dysfunction, immune dysregulation, anxiety disorders, and depression (Rehman & Shabbir, 2025).

Exercise training induces beneficial adaptations in ANS function that enhance stress resilience and psychological well-being. Regular aerobic exercise increases parasympathetic tone, reflected in lower resting heart rate and greater heart rate variability (HRV). HRV, the variation in time intervals between successive heartbeats, provides a non-invasive window into autonomic function. Higher HRV generally indicates greater parasympathetic influence and better autonomic flexibility, allowing the organism to respond appropriately to changing environmental demands. Low HRV is associated with increased risk for numerous adverse outcomes including cardiovascular events, sudden death, depression, anxiety, and poor stress coping (Denovan & Macaskill, 2017).

The mechanisms underlying exercise-induced increases in HRV and parasympathetic tone involve multiple levels of neural organization. At the level of the cardiac pacemaker, adaptations in ion channel expression and function alter the intrinsic rhythmicity of sinoatrial node cells. At the level of peripheral autonomic pathways, changes in vagal efferent activity and sympathetic outflow alter the neural control of heart rate. At the level of central autonomic networks, exercise modulates brainstem nuclei including the nucleus tractus solitarius, which integrates sensory input from the body, and the dorsal motor nucleus of the vagus and nucleus ambiguus, which provide parasympathetic output to the heart (Rehman & Shabbir, 2025).

Beyond effects on resting autonomic function, exercise training improves autonomic reactivity and recovery in response to stressors. Trained individuals show more appropriate autonomic responses to challenges, with adequate sympathetic activation when needed but more rapid parasympathetic reactivation during recovery. This enhanced flexibility allows for effective mobilization during stress while preventing prolonged sympathetic activation that contributes to allostatic load. The faster parasympathetic recovery observed in trained individuals may be particularly important for resilience, as the ability to quickly restore homeostasis after stress exposure reduces cumulative physiological burden and preserves system integrity for future challenges (Forbes & Fikretoglu, 2018).

The relationship between ANS function and psychological states operates bidirectionally. Autonomic arousal influences emotional experience through interoceptive feedback, the process by which the brain monitors bodily physiological states. According to influential theories of emotion including the somatic marker hypothesis and predictive processing accounts, emotional feelings emerge in part from the brain's perception and interpretation of bodily states. Enhanced parasympathetic tone and improved autonomic flexibility may therefore contribute to more balanced emotional experiences, reduced anxiety, and improved emotion regulation capacity (Noone & Hastings, 2009).

Research has demonstrated direct relationships between HRV and various psychological functions relevant to resilience. Higher HRV is associated with better executive function, particularly inhibitory control and emotion regulation. This relationship may reflect shared neural substrates, as prefrontal cortical regions involved in executive control also regulate autonomic outflow through connections to brainstem and hypothalamic autonomic centers. The central autonomic network, encompassing the medial prefrontal cortex, anterior cingulate cortex, insula, and amygdala, integrates cognitive, emotional, and autonomic processes, providing a neural architecture through which exercise-induced improvements in autonomic function can enhance psychological resilience (Rehman & Shabbir, 2025).

Vagal nerve stimulation, which directly activates parasympathetic pathways, has demonstrated therapeutic benefits for treatment-resistant depression and other psychiatric conditions, further supporting the importance of parasympathetic function for mental health. While exercise does not provide the direct, targeted stimulation of implanted vagal nerve stimulators, it does enhance vagal tone through natural physiological pathways, potentially providing similar benefits through a more accessible, cost-effective intervention (Forbes & Fikretoglu, 2018).

Cognitive Flexibility and Emotion Regulation

Cognitive flexibility, the ability to shift between different mental sets, perspectives, or strategies, represents a core component of psychological resilience. Resilient individuals can reframe negative situations, consider alternative interpretations of events, generate multiple solutions to problems, and flexibly adjust their goals and expectations in response to changing circumstances. Conversely, cognitive rigidity and perseverative thinking patterns characterize numerous psychological disorders including depression, anxiety disorders, obsessive-compulsive disorder, and post-traumatic stress disorder (Denovan & Macaskill, 2017).

Exercise enhances cognitive flexibility through multiple mechanisms operating at different levels of brain organization. At the neural systems level, exercise improves function in prefrontal cortical regions and basal ganglia circuits that support cognitive flexibility. The dorsolateral prefrontal cortex maintains and manipulates task representations, the ventrolateral prefrontal cortex implements shifting between representations, and the anterior cingulate cortex monitors for conflict and the need to adjust control. Exercise increases gray matter volume, enhances functional connectivity, and improves activation patterns in these regions during cognitive flexibility tasks (Noone & Hastings, 2009).

Neurotransmitter systems critical for cognitive flexibility also benefit from exercise. Dopamine, which plays central roles in updating working memory representations, motivation, and reward processing, shows enhanced synthesis, release, and receptor function with exercise training. Animal studies have demonstrated that exercise increases dopamine receptor density in the striatum and enhances dopaminergic transmission in fronto-striatal circuits. These enhancements support more efficient gating of information into working memory and more effective updating of mental representations when circumstances change (Lei et al., 2025).

Serotonin, another neurotransmitter system modulated by exercise, influences cognitive flexibility through its effects on prefrontal cortical function and emotion processing. Exercise increases serotonin synthesis by elevating levels of its precursor tryptophan in the brain and enhances serotonergic neurotransmission through effects on receptor expression and function. Given that selective serotonin reuptake inhibitors, which increase synaptic serotonin availability, can improve cognitive flexibility in individuals with depression and anxiety disorders, exercise-induced enhancements in serotonergic function may contribute to improved cognitive flexibility and reduced perseverative negative thinking (Forbes & Fikretoglu, 2018).

The relationship between cognitive flexibility and emotion regulation is intimate and bidirectional. Emotion regulation, the process of modulating emotional experiences and expressions, depends heavily on cognitive flexibility. Effective emotion regulation strategies include cognitive reappraisal (reinterpreting situations to alter their emotional impact), attentional deployment (directing attention toward or away from emotional stimuli), and situation modification (taking actions to change emotion-eliciting circumstances). All these strategies require cognitive flexibility to generate and implement alternative perspectives, focus shifts, or behavioural responses (Guo, 2025).

Exercise enhances emotion regulation through both direct and indirect pathways. Directly, exercise improves function in prefrontal cortical regions that implement top-down regulation of limbic emotion-generating circuits. Neuroimaging studies have found that physically fit individuals show greater prefrontal activation and reduced amygdala activation during emotion regulation tasks, suggesting more efficient prefrontal control of emotional responses. Exercise training studies have demonstrated that improved fitness correlates with enhanced ability to regulate emotional responses through cognitive reappraisal strategies (Lei et al., 2025).

Neurobiological Basis of Mental Toughness and Adaptability

Mental toughness, often conceptualized as perseverance, resilience under pressure, and the ability to maintain focus and motivation despite challenges, represents a psychological characteristic highly valued in athletic, military, occupational, and personal contexts. While mental toughness has sometimes been viewed as a stable personality trait, emerging evidence suggests it can be developed and strengthened through experience, including through regular exercise participation (Denovan & Macaskill, 2017).

The neurobiological foundations of mental toughness involve the integration of multiple brain systems including those governing motivation, emotion regulation, cognitive control, and stress response. The ventral tegmental area and nucleus accumbens, core components of the mesolimbic dopamine reward system, generate motivational drive and encode reward prediction. Prefrontal cortical regions modulate this subcortical activity, supporting goal maintenance, effort allocation, and persistence in the face of obstacles. The anterior cingulate cortex monitors for conflict, errors, and the need for increased cognitive control, signaling when additional effort is required. Insular cortex processes interoceptive information about bodily states including fatigue, pain, and arousal, contributing to judgments about available resources and capacity to continue (Li et al., 2025).

Exercise provides repeated opportunities to develop mental toughness through direct experience with physical challenge, discomfort, and the need for sustained effort. During exercise, particularly at moderate to high intensities, individuals experience physiological stress including elevated heart rate, respiratory strain, metabolic acidosis, and sensations of fatigue and discomfort. Successfully persisting through these experiences despite the desire to stop or reduce intensity represents a form of self-regulatory success that may strengthen mental toughness through multiple mechanisms (Norris & Norris, 2021).

At the neural level, repeated exercise exposure may enhance the capacity of prefrontal cortical regions to override or modulate interoceptive signals of discomfort arising from the insula and to maintain goal-directed behaviour despite fatigue. This enhanced capacity for effortful control may generalize beyond exercise contexts to other domains requiring persistence and self-regulation. Indeed, research has found that physical fitness correlates with performance on laboratory tasks requiring sustained effort and persistence, and that exercise interventions can improve task persistence even in non-exercise contexts (Denovan & Macaskill, 2017).

The experience of overcoming physical challenges through exercise may also strengthen self-efficacy, the belief in one's capacity to successfully execute behaviours required to produce desired outcomes. Self-efficacy represents a critical psychological resource for resilience, as individuals with high self-efficacy are more likely to persist during difficulties, view challenges as surmountable, and maintain motivation in pursuit of goals. Exercise provides a concrete domain for experiencing competence and mastery, with clear feedback about improving capacity over time. These experiences of progressive mastery may enhance general self-efficacy and confidence in one's ability to overcome obstacles (Ozdemir & Akbas Gunes, 2021).

The neurobiological adaptations supporting improved physical performance also provide a foundation for mental toughness. Enhanced cardiovascular fitness improves oxygen delivery to the brain, supporting sustained cognitive performance during physically and mentally demanding tasks. Metabolic adaptations including improved mitochondrial function and substrate utilization enhance cellular energy production, potentially supporting both physical and mental endurance. Neurotransmitter system adaptations including enhanced dopaminergic and noradrenergic function support motivation, arousal, and attentional focus during challenging activities (Denovan & Macaskill, 2017).

Pain tolerance, closely related to mental toughness, improves with regular exercise. Research has consistently found that physically active individuals demonstrate higher pain thresholds and pain tolerance compared to sedentary individuals. These differences likely reflect both peripheral adaptations that alter nociceptive signaling and central adaptations in pain processing and modulation. Exercise activates endogenous opioid and endocannabinoid systems, which provide natural analgesia and may contribute to reduced pain sensitivity with training. Exercise also modulates descending pain inhibitory pathways from prefrontal and brainstem regions to the spinal cord, potentially enhancing top-down pain control (Ozdemir & Akbas Gunes, 2021).

4. COMPARATIVE EFFECTS OF EXERCISE MODALITIES

While the preceding sections have focused largely on exercise as a unitary intervention, substantial evidence indicates that different forms of physical activity exert distinct neuroplastic effects and cognitive benefits. Understanding how various exercise modalities differentially influence brain structure, function, and psychological outcomes can inform more targeted and effective exercise prescriptions for specific cognitive and mental health goals (Srinivas et al., 2021). The primary categories of exercise include aerobic or cardiovascular training, resistance or strength training, and mind-body practices incorporating physical movement with focused attention and meditation. Each modality engages different physiological systems, requires distinct cognitive and motor demands, and appears to preferentially influence certain aspects of brain function.

Aerobic Exercise and Hippocampal Neurogenesis

Aerobic exercise, characterized by sustained, rhythmic activity of large muscle groups at moderate to vigorous intensity, represents the most extensively studied exercise modality in relation to brain health. Activities including brisk walking, jogging, running, cycling, swimming, and dancing fall within this category. Aerobic exercise places sustained demands on the cardiorespiratory system, requiring increased cardiac output, ventilation, and oxygen delivery to working muscles. These systemic demands trigger cascading physiological responses that profoundly influence brain function (Srinivas et al., 2021).

The relationship between aerobic exercise and hippocampal neurogenesis stands as one of the most robust and well-characterized neuroplastic effects of physical activity. Beginning with seminal studies in rodents demonstrating that voluntary wheel running dramatically increases the proliferation of neural progenitor cells in the dentate gyrus subregion of the hippocampus, decades of research have established that aerobic exercise represents one of the most potent behavioural stimuli for adult neurogenesis. Newly generated neurons progress through stages of maturation, developing dendritic arbors, establishing synaptic connections with existing circuitry, and eventually becoming functionally integrated into hippocampal networks supporting learning and memory (Shimada et al., 2018).

In humans, direct assessment of neurogenesis is not feasible, but indirect evidence from neuroimaging, postmortem tissue analysis, and peripheral biomarkers supports the translation of rodent findings. Magnetic resonance imaging studies have demonstrated that aerobic exercise training increases hippocampal volume, with changes correlating with improvements in spatial memory and elevated circulating BDNF levels. The magnitude of hippocampal volume increase observed in some studies, approximately two percent over one year of training, exceeds what would be expected from changes in existing neurons alone, suggesting contributions from neurogenesis or substantial dendritic elaboration (Rodriguez-Rodríguez et al., 2024).

The hippocampus-preferential effects of aerobic exercise likely reflect the convergence of multiple factors. The hippocampus contains one of the two brain regions where neurogenesis persists robustly into adulthood, making it uniquely responsive to neurogenesis-promoting interventions. The hippocampus has high concentrations of glucocorticoid and neurotrophic factor receptors, making it sensitive to exercise-induced changes in stress hormones and growth factors. The hippocampus has relatively high metabolic demands and may be particularly responsive to exercise-induced improvements in cerebral blood flow and metabolic support. The hippocampus undergoes early age-related atrophy and is vulnerable to multiple neurodegenerative conditions, potentially creating greater capacity for exercise-induced neuroprotection compared to less vulnerable regions (Srinivas et al., 2021).

Beyond the hippocampus, aerobic exercise influences structure and function across distributed brain networks. Prefrontal cortical regions show increased gray matter volume and improved functional connectivity with aerobic training. White matter integrity, assessed through diffusion tensor imaging, improves in multiple tracts including those connecting prefrontal and temporal regions. Default mode network connectivity, which influences mind-wandering and self-referential thinking, becomes more efficient with aerobic fitness. Executive control networks show enhanced activation and connectivity, supporting improved cognitive control (Shimada et al., 2018).

The dose-response relationship for aerobic exercise effects on the brain represents an important consideration for translating research into practice. While substantial cognitive and neuroplastic benefits have been demonstrated with moderate-intensity exercise, typically defined as 50 to 70 percent of maximum heart rate or the intensity at which conversation becomes somewhat challenging, some evidence suggests additional benefits at higher intensities. High-intensity interval training, involving alternating periods of near-maximal and lower-intensity exercise, has shown promising cognitive benefits in some studies, potentially through enhanced production of neurotrophic factors and greater cardiovascular stress driving adaptive responses (Rodriguez-Rodríguez et al., 2024).

Resistance Training and Executive Function Enhancement

Resistance training, also termed strength training or weight training, involves exercises that cause muscles to contract against external resistance including free weights, weight machines, resistance bands, or body weight. While historically emphasized primarily for building muscle strength and mass, mounting evidence indicates that resistance training exerts significant cognitive benefits, particularly for executive functions, through distinct mechanisms from aerobic exercise (Karmakar et al., 2025). Meta-analyses examining the cognitive effects of resistance training have found moderate effect sizes for improvements in executive function, with benefits observed across multiple executive domains including inhibitory control, working memory, and cognitive flexibility. These executive function enhancements occur with resistance training protocols typically involving two to three sessions per week of exercises targeting major muscle groups, performed at moderate to high intensity (60 to 85 percent of one-repetition maximum), with multiple sets and repetitions per exercise (Srinivas et al., 2021).

The neural mechanisms underlying resistance training benefits differ in important ways from those associated with aerobic exercise. While aerobic exercise primarily enhances cardiorespiratory fitness and cerebral blood flow, resistance training produces different systemic adaptations including increased muscle mass, altered body composition, enhanced neuromuscular coordination, and distinctive hormonal responses. Resistance training acutely increases circulating levels of growth hormone, testosterone, and IGF-1 more than aerobic exercise, and these hormones can cross the blood-brain barrier to influence neural function. Resistance training also increases circulating BDNF, although potentially through different mechanisms than aerobic exercise (Srinivas et al., 2021).

Neuroimaging studies examining resistance training effects have found structural and functional changes particularly in frontal and parietal regions associated with executive function and motor control. White matter integrity improvements have been observed in prefrontal tracts following resistance training, suggesting enhanced connectivity in executive control networks. Some studies have found that resistance training may be particularly effective for improving executive functions that depend on dorsolateral prefrontal cortex, including planning, reasoning, and problem-solving (Rodriguez-Rodríguez et al., 2024).

The cognitive demands inherent in resistance training may contribute to its executive function benefits beyond purely physiological mechanisms. Effective resistance training requires motor planning, attention to technique, working memory for exercise sequences and parameters, inhibitory control to maintain proper form under fatigue, and decision-making about load selection and effort allocation. These cognitive demands during training may provide a form of concurrent cognitive training that enhances executive functions through use-dependent plasticity (Srinivas et al., 2021). Comparative studies examining aerobic versus resistance training effects on cognition have yielded variable results, with some studies finding superior effects of one modality and others finding equivalent benefits. These inconsistencies may reflect differences in training protocols, cognitive assessment batteries, participant characteristics, and the specific cognitive domains examined. Some evidence suggests that aerobic and resistance training may exert preferential benefits for different cognitive domains, with aerobic exercise showing particular advantages for memory and processing speed, while resistance training may show advantages for executive functions, attention, and reasoning (Rodriguez-Rodríguez et al., 2024).

The combination of aerobic and resistance training appears promising for maximizing cognitive benefits. Several studies have found that combined training produces cognitive improvements equal to or exceeding those from either modality alone. The mechanisms underlying potential synergistic effects of combined training remain incompletely understood but may involve complementary neuroplastic pathways, broader systemic health benefits, or additive effects on common mechanisms such as BDNF production or cerebrovascular function. Practical considerations influence the implementation of resistance training for cognitive benefits (Silva et al., 2017). The necessary equipment, space, and technical instruction required for resistance training may create barriers for some populations. Exercise adherence patterns may differ between aerobic and resistance training, with individual preferences playing important roles in long-term engagement. Safety concerns, particularly for older adults or individuals with certain medical conditions, require appropriate instruction and supervision to prevent injuries. These practical factors must be balanced against the potential cognitive benefits when designing exercise interventions (Ward et al., 2017).

Emerging research on blood flow restriction training, which involves performing resistance exercises while restricting venous return from working muscles using specialized cuffs, suggests this modified approach may enhance neurotrophic factor production and cognitive benefits while allowing for lower absolute loads. This approach could potentially make resistance training more accessible for populations with limitations that preclude heavy loading, although more research is needed to establish cognitive effects (Rodriguez-Rodríguez et al., 2024).

Mind-Body Practices and Integrated Plasticity

Mind-body practices including yoga, tai chi, qigong, and meditative movement combine physical activity with focused attention, controlled breathing, and often contemplative or mindfulness components. These integrative practices provide not only the physical benefits of movement but also engage cognitive and emotional regulation processes, potentially producing synergistic neuroplastic effects that differ from conventional exercise modalities.

Yoga, originating in ancient Indian philosophy, encompasses diverse styles ranging from gentle restorative practices to vigorous power yoga. Most yoga practices include physical postures (asanas), breathing techniques (pranayama), and meditation or focused awareness. Neuroimaging research has revealed that regular yoga practice is associated with increased gray matter volume in multiple brain regions including the hippocampus, prefrontal cortex, anterior cingulate cortex, and insula. These structural changes suggest that yoga influences neural systems supporting memory, executive function, emotion regulation, and interoceptive awareness (Levin et al., 2017).

The mechanisms underlying yoga's neuroplastic effects likely involve both the physical activity component and the attentional and meditative elements. The physical postures provide moderate-intensity muscular and cardiovascular demands, engaging many of the neurotrophic and vascular mechanisms activated by conventional exercise. The controlled breathing practices may influence autonomic function, stress physiology, and oxygenation in ways that benefit neural health (Shimada et al., 2018). The focused attention and mindfulness components engage prefrontal cortical networks involved in attention regulation while potentially reducing activity in default mode networks associated with mind-wandering and rumination. Studies examining yoga's cognitive effects have found improvements in executive function, attention, processing speed, and memory. Some research suggests yoga may be particularly effective for enhancing attention and concentration, possibly reflecting the sustained attention required during practice. Yoga has also demonstrated benefits for stress reduction, anxiety management, and mood enhancement, with effects comparable to those of conventional aerobic exercise in some studies (Gomes-Osman et al., 2017).

Tai chi and qigong, traditional Chinese movement practices, involve slow, flowing movements coordinated with breathing and mental focus. These practices emphasize balance, postural alignment, and the integration of physical and mental awareness. Research has demonstrated that tai chi practice is associated with increased brain volume in regions including the hippocampus, putamen, and medial prefrontal cortex. Tai chi has also been found to enhance white matter integrity and functional connectivity in networks supporting executive function and memory. The balance demands of tai chi may contribute to its neuroplastic effects through enhanced integration between motor, vestibular, and proprioceptive systems. Maintaining balance during slow, controlled movements requires continuous sensory-motor integration and predictive motor control, engaging cerebellar and cortical circuits involved in motor learning and coordination. The cognitive benefits of balance training have been demonstrated independently of tai chi, with improved executive function observed following balance exercise interventions, suggesting that the balance component contributes meaningfully to cognitive outcomes (Shimada et al., 2018).

Comparative studies examining mind-body practices versus conventional exercise have generally found similar or sometimes superior cognitive and psychological benefits from integrative practices. Several meta-analyses have concluded that yoga and tai chi produce cognitive benefits comparable to aerobic exercise, with potential advantages for stress reduction, anxiety management, and certain aspects of executive function. These findings suggest that the integrative nature of mind-body practices, engaging multiple systems simultaneously, may provide efficient pathways to neuroplastic enhancement (Coetsee & Terblanche, 2017).

The meditation and mindfulness components of mind-body practices deserve particular attention as contributors to neuroplastic effects. Meditation training, studied independently of physical movement, has demonstrated structural and functional brain changes including increased cortical thickness in prefrontal and insular regions, altered connectivity in default mode and executive control networks, and enhanced functional connectivity between prefrontal regulatory regions and limbic emotion-processing regions. These changes support improvements in attention, emotion regulation, and metacognitive awareness. When meditation is combined with physical movement, as in yoga and tai chi, the neuroplastic effects may be additive or synergistic. Physical activity may enhance the brain's receptivity to mental training through mechanisms including increased BDNF, improved cerebral blood flow, and enhanced arousal regulation. Conversely, the mental training components may enhance the effectiveness of physical activity by promoting sustained engagement, improving mind-body awareness, and reducing the psychological barriers to regular practice (Ward et al., 2017).

The breathing practices incorporated into many mind-body traditions merit consideration as potentially active components contributing to neuroplastic and psychological benefits. Controlled breathing, particularly slow breathing at rates around 6 breaths per minute, can enhance baroreflex sensitivity, increase HRV, and shift autonomic balance toward parasympathetic predominance. These autonomic effects may contribute to stress reduction, improved emotion regulation, and enhanced cognitive function. Some research has found that breathing exercises alone, independent of physical movement, can produce cognitive and emotional benefits, suggesting that the respiratory component of mind-body practices represents an active ingredient rather than merely an accompaniment to movement (Gomes-Osman et al., 2017).

Synergistic Benefits of Combined Modalities

The recognition that different exercise modalities exert distinct neuroplastic effects and cognitive benefits naturally leads to questions about optimal combination strategies. Multimodal exercise programs that incorporate aerobic training, resistance training, and mind-body or coordination-based activities may provide superior cognitive and psychological outcomes compared to single-modality interventions by engaging multiple neuroplastic pathways simultaneously.

Several large-scale intervention studies have examined multimodal exercise programs combining multiple activity types. These studies have generally found that combined interventions produce cognitive benefits at least equal to and sometimes exceeding those of single-modality programs. For example, programs combining aerobic exercise with coordination training or cognitive engagement have shown promising results for enhancing executive function and global cognition, particularly in older adults at risk for cognitive decline (Srinivas et al., 2021). The mechanisms underlying potential synergistic effects of combined exercise modalities remain incompletely characterized but may include several complementary pathways. Different exercise types may activate overlapping and distinct molecular cascades, producing additive effects on neurotrophic factor production, angiogenesis, or other plasticity-supporting mechanisms. Combined training may engage broader neural networks than single modalities, promoting more distributed plasticity across cognitive systems. The variety inherent in multimodal programs may enhance exercise adherence and sustained engagement, leading to greater cumulative exposure and longer-term benefits (Ward et al., 2017).

Exergaming, involving video games that require physical movement for play, represents an innovative approach to combining physical activity with cognitive engagement. These interactive systems, ranging from commercial products like Nintendo Wii and Xbox Kinect to specialized platforms designed for older adults, require players to perform physical movements while simultaneously processing visual information, making decisions, and coordinating responses to changing task demands. Research has found that exergaming can produce cognitive benefits comparable to conventional exercise, with some studies suggesting particular advantages for executive function and attention (Coetsee & Terblanche, 2017).

The simultaneous engagement of motor and cognitive systems during exergaming may promote integrated plasticity through mechanisms related to action-cognition coupling. The tight temporal relationship between cognitive decisions and motor actions during gameplay may enhance cortico-striatal and cerebello-cortical learning systems more effectively than activities where physical and cognitive demands are temporally separate. The motivational and reward-related aspects of games may also enhance adherence and sustain engagement more effectively than conventional exercise for some individuals (Shimada et al., 2018). Dance represents another integrative activity combining aerobic exercise with complex motor learning, spatial navigation, coordination, social engagement, and often cognitive challenges of remembering choreography and timing movements to music. Research has found that dance training produces cognitive benefits including improved executive function, episodic memory, and processing speed. Neuroimaging studies have revealed that dance training is associated with increased hippocampal volume and enhanced white matter integrity, similar to aerobic exercise, along with structural and functional changes in motor cortices and basal ganglia reflecting motor learning (Netz, 2019).

The multifaceted nature of dance may provide an optimal combination of neuroplastic stimuli. The cardiovascular demands engage aerobic exercise pathways supporting hippocampal plasticity and cerebrovascular function. The motor learning requirements activate procedural memory systems and motor cortical plasticity. The spatial navigation involved in moving through choreographed sequences engages hippocampal spatial processing systems. The social interaction in partner or group dancing provides social engagement benefits. The musical and rhythmic components may engage additional neural networks including those involved in temporal processing and prediction (Rodriguez-Rodríguez et al., 2024).

Timing considerations for combining different exercise modalities within training programs represent an important practical question. Some evidence suggests that performing different types of exercise in separate sessions may be preferable to combining them within single sessions, as this approach may prevent interference and allow optimal physiological responses to each modality (Shimada et al., 2018). However, logistical considerations and adherence factors may favour combined sessions that provide variety and efficiency within constrained time budgets. The concept of periodization, borrowed from athletic training, may have applications for optimizing cognitive benefits from exercise. Periodization involves systematically varying training parameters over time, including intensity, volume, and exercise type, to optimize adaptation while managing fatigue and preventing overtraining. Applied to exercise for cognitive health, periodization might involve cycling between emphasis on different modalities, varying intensity patterns, or alternating between high-demand and recovery periods to optimize neuroplastic adaptations while maintaining engagement and preventing burnout (Srinivas et al., 2021).

5. CONCLUSION

The evidence reviewed in this chapter clearly demonstrates that physical exercise is among the most powerful, practical, and accessible interventions for enhancing brain health, cognitive performance, and psychological resilience. Exercise influences the brain through multiple interconnected mechanisms, including molecular signalling, cellular growth, structural reorganization, and optimization of neural networks, leading to meaningful neuroplastic changes across the lifespan. These adaptations strengthen the brain's capacity to learn, adapt, and function efficiently under varying demands. Cognitive benefits of exercise are observed across all major domains. Memory is enhanced through exercise-induced hippocampal neurogenesis, increased brain derived neurotrophic factor, and improved synaptic plasticity, which collectively support learning and retention. Attention processes become more stable and selective as exercise improves arousal regulation, cerebral blood flow, and prefrontal cortical efficiency. Executive functions such as planning, inhibition, and cognitive flexibility show particularly strong improvements, reflecting the high sensitivity of prefrontal systems to activity-dependent stimulation. These cognitive gains extend beyond laboratory measures and translate into tangible improvements in academic performance, workplace productivity, decision making, and daily functional independence. Exercise also plays a central role in building psychological resilience. Adaptations in autonomic nervous system regulation enhance parasympathetic activity, reduce stress reactivity, and promote faster physiological recovery following psychological challenges. At the psychological level, regular physical activity strengthens emotion regulation, self-control, and cognitive flexibility, enabling individuals to reframe adversity and maintain emotional balance. Different exercise modalities contribute unique benefits. Aerobic exercise strongly supports hippocampal function, cardiovascular efficiency, and memory performance. Resistance training offers pronounced benefits for executive functions, self-efficacy, and goal directed behaviour. Mind body practices integrate physical movement with attentional and contemplative elements, promoting holistic regulation of cognitive and emotional systems. Multimodal exercise programs that combine these approaches may provide the most comprehensive neuroplastic stimulation and long term mental health benefits.

REFERENCES

Archer, T., Ricci, S., Massoni, F., Ricci, L., & Rapp-Ricciardi, M. (2016). Cognitive benefits of exercise intervention. *La Clinica Terapeutica*, *167*(6), 180–185. https://iris.uniroma1.it/handle/11573/1064774 PMID: 28051833

Augusto-Oliveira, M., Arrifano, G. P., Leal-Nazaré, C. G., Santos-Sacramento, L., Lopes-Araújo, A., Royes, L. F. F., & Crespo-Lopez, M. E. (2023). Exercise Reshapes the Brain: Molecular, Cellular, and Structural Changes Associated with Cognitive Improvements. *Molecular Neurobiology*, *60*(12), 6950–6974. DOI: 10.1007/s12035-023-03492-8 PMID: 37518829

Brondino, N., Rocchetti, M., Fusar-Poli, L., Codrons, E., Correale, L., Vandoni, M., Barbui, C., & Politi, P. (2017). A systematic review of cognitive effects of exercise in depression. *Acta Psychiatrica Scandinavica*, *135*(4), 285–295. DOI: 10.1111/acps.12690 PMID: 28110494

Brown, D. R., Wang, Y., Ward, A. N. N., Ebbeling, C. B., Fortlage, L., Puleo, E., Benson, H., & Rippe, J. M. (1995). Chronic psychological effects of exercise and exercise plus cognitive strategies. *Medicine and Science in Sports and Exercise*, *27*(5), 765–775. https://europepmc.org/article/med/7674883 PMID: 7674883

Coetsee, C., & Terblanche, E. (2017). The effect of three different exercise training modalities on cognitive and physical function in a healthy older population. *European Review of Aging and Physical Activity : Official Journal of the European Group for Research into Elderly and Physical Activity*, *14*(1), 13. DOI: 10.1186/s11556-017-0183-5 PMID: 28811842

Denovan, A., & Macaskill, A. (2017). Building resilience to stress through leisure activities: A qualitative analysis. *Annals of Leisure Research*, *20*(4), 446–466. DOI: 10.1080/11745398.2016.1211943

Forbes, S., & Fikretoglu, D. (2018). Building Resilience: The Conceptual Basis and Research Evidence for Resilience Training Programs. *Review of General Psychology*, *22*(4), 452–468. DOI: 10.1037/gpr0000152

Gomes-Osman, J., Cabral, D. F., Hinchman, C., Jannati, A., Morris, T. P., & Pascual-Leone, A. (2017). The effects of exercise on cognitive function and brain plasticity – a feasibility trial. *Restorative Neurology and Neuroscience*, *35*(5), 547–556. DOI: 10.3233/RNN-170758 PMID: 28984621

Guo, J. (2025). The dual impact of physical exercise on university students' mental health: The chain mediating effects of mindfulness and psychological resilience. *Frontiers in Psychology, 16*. Advance online publication. DOI: 10.3389/fpsyg.2025.1545370 PMID: 40297594

Karmakar, D., Das, A., Saha, G. C., & Govindasamy, K. (2025). The Impact of Physical Education and Sports on Emotional Resilience and Self-Efficacy. In Lobo, J., & Tagare, R. L.Jr., (Eds.), *Emerging Pedagogical Practices in Physical and Sports Education* (pp. 125–154). IGI Global Scientific Publishing., DOI: 10.4018/979-8-3373-2160-8.ch006

Lei, G., Li, L., & Zhang, L. (2025). Mental health literacy and anxiety in college students mediating role of psychological resilience and moderating role of physical exercise. *Scientific Reports, 15*(1), 35340. DOI: 10.1038/s41598-025-19381-0 PMID: 41068229

Levin, O., Netz, Y., & Ziv, G. (2017). The beneficial effects of different types of exercise interventions on motor and cognitive functions in older age: A systematic review. *European Review of Aging and Physical Activity : Official Journal of the European Group for Research into Elderly and Physical Activity, 14*(1), 20. DOI: 10.1186/s11556-017-0189-z PMID: 29276545

Li, M., Huang, Y., & Sun, M. (2025). Exploring the structural links between peer support, psychological resilience, and exercise adherence in adolescents: A multigroup model across gender and educational stages. *BMC Public Health, 25*(1), 2300. DOI: 10.1186/s12889-025-23308-9 PMID: 40610991

Netz, Y. (2019). Is there a preferred mode of exercise for cognition enhancement in older age?—A narrative review. *Frontiers in Medicine, 6*, 57. https://www.frontiersin.org/articles/10.3389/fmed.2019.00057/full PMID: 30984760

Noone, S. J., & Hastings, R. P. (2009). Building psychological resilience in support staff caring for people with intellectual disabilities: Pilot evaluation of an acceptance-based intervention. *Journal of Intellectual Disabilities, 13*(1), 43–53. DOI: 10.1177/1744629509103519 PMID: 19332508

Norris, G., & Norris, H. (2021). Building Resilience Through Sport in Young People With Adverse Childhood Experiences. *Frontiers in Sports and Active Living, 3*. Advance online publication. DOI: 10.3389/fspor.2021.663587 PMID: 34337400

Ozdemir, C., & Akbas Gunes, N. (2021). The effect of diet and regular exercise on psychological resilience in obese or overweight women. *International Journal of Clinical Practice, 75*(8), e14320. DOI: 10.1111/ijcp.14320 PMID: 33960086

Quigley, A., MacKay-Lyons, M., & Eskes, G. (2020). Effects of Exercise on Cognitive Performance in Older Adults: A Narrative Review of the Evidence, Possible Biological Mechanisms, and Recommendations for Exercise Prescription. *Journal of Aging Research*, *2020*, 1–15. DOI: 10.1155/2020/1407896 PMID: 32509348

Rehman, M., & Shabbir, I. (2025). Building Mental Resilience: The Impact of Weight Resistance Training on Young Adult Wellbeing. *Qlantic Journal of Social Sciences*, *6*(3), 249–255. DOI: 10.55737/qjss.vi-iii.25403

Rendeiro, C., & Rhodes, J. S. (2018). A new perspective of the hippocampus in the origin of exercise–brain interactions. *Brain Structure & Function*, *223*(6), 2527–2545. DOI: 10.1007/s00429-018-1665-6 PMID: 29671055

Rodriguez-Rodríguez, S., Canet-Vintró, M., Wee, S. O., Rodríguez-Sanz, J., López-de-Celis, C., Oviedo, G. R., Labata-Lezaun, N., & Pérez-Bellmunt, A. (2024). Cognitive enhancement strategies for older adults: An evaluation of different training modalities to improve executive function—A systematic review and meta-analysis. *Journal of Clinical Medicine*, *13*(5), 1301. https://www.mdpi.com/2077-0383/13/5/1301 PMID: 38592139

Shimada, H., Makizako, H., Doi, T., Park, H., Tsutsumimoto, K., Verghese, J., & Suzuki, T. (2018). Effects of combined physical and cognitive exercises on cognition and mobility in patients with mild cognitive impairment: A randomized clinical trial. *Journal of the American Medical Directors Association*, *19*(7), 584–591. https://www.sciencedirect.com/science/article/pii/S152586101730542X PMID: 29153754

Silva, N. C. B. S., Gregory, M. A., Gill, D. P., & Petrella, R. J. (2017). Multiple-modality exercise and mind-motor training to improve cardiovascular health and fitness in older adults at risk for cognitive impairment: A randomized controlled trial. *Archives of Gerontology and Geriatrics*, *68*, 149–160. https://www.sciencedirect.com/science/article/pii/S0167494316301893 PMID: 27810663

Srinivas, N. S., Vimalan, V., Padmanabhan, P., & Gulyás, B. (2021). An overview on cognitive function enhancement through physical exercises. *Brain Sciences*, *11*(10), 1289. https://www.mdpi.com/2076-3425/11/10/1289 PMID: 34679354

Stimpson, N. J., Davison, G., & Javadi, A.-H. (2018). Joggin'the noggin: Towards a physiological understanding of exercise-induced cognitive benefits. *Neuroscience and Biobehavioral Reviews*, *88*, 177–186. https://www.sciencedirect.com/science/article/pii/S0149763417308102 PMID: 29572187

Ward, N., Paul, E., Watson, P., Cooke, G. E., Hillman, C. H., Cohen, N. J., Kramer, A. F., & Barbey, A. K. (2017). Enhanced learning through multimodal training: Evidence from a comprehensive cognitive, physical fitness, and neuroscience intervention. *Scientific Reports*, *7*(1), 5808. https://www.nature.com/articles/s41598-017-06237-5 PMID: 28724914

Zhao, J., Jiang, W., Wang, X., Cai, Z., Liu, Z., & Liu, G. (2020). Exercise, brain plasticity, and depression. *CNS Neuroscience & Therapeutics*, *26*(9), 885–895. DOI: 10.1111/cns.13385 PMID: 32491278

Zhu, X., Chen, W., Pinho, R. A., & Thirupathi, A. (2025). Lactate-induced metabolic signaling is the potential mechanism for reshaping the brain function-role of physical exercise. *Frontiers in Endocrinology*, *16*, 1598419. https://www.frontiersin.org/journals/endocrinology/articles/10.3389/fendo.2025.1598419/abstract PMID: 40551894

Chapter 8
Curricular Pathways to Wellness:
Physical Exercises for Emotional Agility and Resilience Among Senior High School Students

Ervin Tampus Echague
https://orcid.org/0009-0002-7507-1383
Department of Education, Philippines

Marie Grace Avelino Gomez
https://orcid.org/0000-0003-0180-9875
University of the Philippines, Diliman, Philippines

ABSTRACT

Senior High School (SHS) students today face complex emotional, academic, and social pressures that challenge their well-being and resilience. This chapter explores how Physical Education (PE) can serve as a curricular pathway to wellness by integrating structured physical exercises that enhance emotional agility, resilience, and career readiness. Drawing on empirical evidence and the Life and Career Skills Curriculum, it proposes three dimensions of application: (1) intrapersonal development through mindful movement, resilience-based workouts, and reflective practices; (2) interpersonal growth via cooperative tasks and culturally rooted games such as Laro ng Lahi that foster communication, empathy, and teamwork; and (3) career preparedness through exercise models simulating workplace challenges, adaptability, and stress regulation. Grounded in the whole-person framework, this approach reframes PE as a transformative platform for psychosocial learning, aligning physical activity with holistic education, cultural identity, and lifelong well-being.

DOI: 10.4018/979-8-3373-6157-4.ch008

INTRODUCTION

The challenges faced by Senior High School students today extend far beyond the classroom (Branzuela et al., 2023). Academic pressure, career uncertainty, family expectations, and the fast-changing social environment have contributed to rising levels of stress, burnout, and emotional struggles among adolescents (Yeh et al., 2025). Reports from global and local studies indicate that students in this age group are increasingly vulnerable to anxiety, depression, and stress-related conditions that affect both their learning and overall well-being. In the Philippine context, where educational transitions are intensified by socio-economic pressures and a competitive job market, SHS students often experience a heightened sense of burnout and fatigue, leading to disengagement both academically and socially.

Within this reality, schools are challenged to create holistic curricular approaches that not only prioritize academic achievement but also foster psychosocial growth and resilience. Physical Education (PE), traditionally understood as a platform for physical fitness, is now being reimagined as a venue for nurturing broader life skills. Given that it is aligned with the Life and Career Skills Curriculum, PE provides a powerful avenue to strengthen students' intrapersonal and interpersonal competencies while also preparing them for workplace demands.

The rationale behind this shift is clear: exercise is not solely about physical health. It is also a form of embodied learning that develops self-discipline, emotion regulation, and stress management. It provides opportunities for collaboration, communication, and empathy, skills necessary for interpersonal effectiveness (Gordon, 2023). Moreover, through analogies and structured routines, exercise can simulate workplace challenges such as multitasking, adaptability, and perseverance, offering students practical preparation for the demands of future careers.

The objectives of this chapter are therefore threefold: first, to explore how structured physical exercises enhance intrapersonal skills such as self-awareness and resilience; second, to demonstrate how group activities and culturally relevant games strengthen interpersonal effectiveness; and third, to show how exercise can be framed as preparation for career readiness and on-the-job resilience.

Theoretical and Curricular Foundations

The Life and Career Skills Curriculum emphasizes the development of competencies that transcend academic knowledge and extend into the realm of personal growth, emotional well-being, and career adaptability. These skills include problem-solving, communication, collaboration, resilience, and self-management. PE becomes an ideal platform to merge physical and psychosocial competencies because it engages students actively, allows experiential learning, and makes use of the body as a site of emotional regulation and skill-building.

Empirical studies have long shown the link between exercise and emotional resilience (Peng et al., 2025). Physical activity has been associated with the release of endorphins, which reduce stress and improve mood. Beyond biochemical effects, exercise fosters self-regulation, perseverance, and goal setting. Research also highlights the social benefits of group physical activities, such as enhanced cooperation and reduced social isolation. These outcomes resonate with the psychosocial goals of the Life and Career Skills Curriculum.

This approach is grounded in the whole-person framework. Education is not simply about cognitive achievement but about nurturing the physical, emotional, and social dimensions of the learner (Immordino-Yang et al., 2025). Exercise, when thoughtfully integrated, becomes preparation not just for health but for the realities of work and life, contexts where resilience, adaptability, and emotional intelligence matter as much as technical skills.

Exercise for Intrapersonal Skills

The first domain where exercise contributes significantly is the intrapersonal level. Adolescents often struggle with self-awareness, emotional regulation, and stress management. Exercises that emphasize mindful movement can provide practical tools for these challenges. Mindful movement activities such as yoga stretches, breathing exercises, and tai chi-inspired practices train students to listen to their bodies and regulate their stress responses. Deep breathing, for instance, can be incorporated at the beginning and end of PE classes to promote calmness and emotional balance. Resilience-building workouts, such as interval training or endurance challenges, provide students with opportunities to confront difficulty, fatigue, and discomfort in a safe environment. Completing a challenging set mirrors overcoming obstacles in life, reinforcing the lesson that persistence pays off. A critical component is reflection. Students may be asked to write journals after exercise sessions, noting how they felt before, during, and after the activity. Guided reflection discussions help students connect physical exertion with emotional regulation and personal growth, deepening their self-awareness.

Exercise for Interpersonal Skills

Beyond the self, exercise becomes a fertile ground for developing interpersonal skills such as communication, empathy, and teamwork. Partner activities like paired stretching or resistance band exercises demand cooperation, communication, and mutual support. These activities highlight trust and listening skills, fostering an environment of reciprocity. Group dynamics can be built through cooperative circuits or relays where success depends on collective effort rather than individual speed. In such activities, students learn to value coordination and collaboration, reflecting real-life teamwork situations. Conflict-resolution through movement can be simulated in trust walks or synchronized group movements, where negotiation of roles, turn-taking, and problem-solving are essential. These embodied exercises translate directly into social skills necessary in peer relationships and workplace contexts.

A particularly valuable approach involves integrating Laro ng Lahi, or traditional Filipino games, into the curriculum. These culturally rooted activities not only preserve national heritage but also cultivate essential social and emotional skills in enjoyable and meaningful ways. Patintero enhances students' abilities in strategic thinking, quick decision-making, and teamwork. Luksong Tinik or Luksong Baka promotes trust, encouragement, and resilience as players collaborate to overcome physical challenges. Meanwhile, Tumbang Preso encourages stress relief, agility, and active participation, fostering camaraderie and a shared sense of enjoyment among learners.

Engaging in *Laro ng Lahi* enables students to exercise their bodies while simultaneously reinforcing communal values, empathy, and collective resilience. These traditional games also provide meaningful opportunities to connect with cultural roots, allowing learners to experience physical activity as both a form of personal growth and a celebration of shared heritage. The research of Dizer et al. (2022) on the perceived benefits of *Laro ng Lahi* (indigenous games) confirms their essential role in fostering a Filipino child's holistic well-being by overwhelmingly supporting development across multiple critical domains. Specifically, these traditional games are found to significantly aid physical health, cognitive functions (such as mental stimulation and problem-solving), and socio-emotional growth (including collaboration, empathy, and self-regulation). Beyond basic developmental markers, consistent engagement in *Laro ng Lahi* fosters crucial "larger-than-game" life skills, strengthens social connectedness, and provides a culturally grounding experience that advances health, culture, and heritage, establishing them as vital for comprehensive growth and positive academic outcomes (Dizer et al., 2022). Del Carmen et al. 's (2015) research shows that Laro ng Lahi, a compilation of traditional Filipino games, possesses significant cultural and educational value, which the featured research harnessed to create context-based learning activities for physics. Beyond the classroom, these traditional games are an essential part of the nation's cultural heritage, providing opportunities to appreciate Filipino traditions and strengthening familial and social ties. When integrated into education, Laro ng Lahi activities can transform the learning of abstract subjects like physics, making the process active, fun, and highly engaging for students. The games are a valuable pedagogical tool that fosters crucial skills such as collaboration, camaraderie, sportsmanship, and the development of students' critical thinking and conceptual understanding. Ultimately, utilizing Laro ng Lahi in the curriculum provides a relevant, culture-based learning experience that supports the preservation of Filipino national culture while enhancing modern educational outcomes (Del Carmen et al., 2015).

Exercise for Career Readiness

As students transition toward adulthood, preparing them for the demands of future workplaces is crucial. Physical exercises can be reframed to simulate workplace challenges and instill professional resilience. Workplace-stress analogies can be incorporated in PE sessions. Circuit training, for example, mirrors multitasking readiness, as students switch between different stations under time pressure. Balance and coordination activities highlight adaptability, an essential trait in fast-changing work environments. Emotion regulation in simulated work stress can be taught through brief breathing breaks and stretching exercises, like the micro-breaks recommended in office settings. These simple interventions provide models of self-care and focus maintenance that can be transferred to professional life. Developing perseverance and grit can be addressed through structured endurance activities. Long-distance running, timed planks, or incremental workout challenges foster the mindset of sustained effort despite difficulty—paralleling the persistence needed in long-term career success. Moreover, students can be introduced to office-friendly exercises such as seated leg raises, desk push-ups, wall sits, or wrist stretches. These activities demonstrate that wellness can be maintained even in sedentary work environments, preventing burnout and increasing productivity. Senior High School students face unprecedented levels of stress and uncertainty as they navigate both academic and personal transitions. Situating exercise within the framework of the Life and Career Skills Curriculum positions PE as a platform that extends beyond physical health to encompass psychosocial well-being and career readiness. Exercises that target intrapersonal growth cultivate resilience and self-awareness; group-based activities, such as *Laro ng Lahi*, enhance empathy and teamwork; and workplace-simulated routines equip students with practical skills to address professional challenges.

In this way, exercise is reframed as a curricular pathway to wellness, a holistic approach that equips students with the emotional resilience, interpersonal effectiveness, and adaptability needed to thrive both in life and in future careers. Exercise produces biochemical, cognitive, and socio-behavioral effects that extend far beyond aerobic fitness and muscular strength. At the neurophysiological level, regular physical activity modulates stress-related neurochemistry (e.g., endorphins, monoamines) and supports executive functions that underpin emotion regulation and problem-solving. At the psychological level, structured movement builds experiences of mastery, locus of control, and self-efficacy—factors strongly associated with resilience. Meta-analytic and large-scale studies report consistent associations between higher physical-activity levels and better emotional well-being, life satisfaction, and lower risk of mental-health disorders among children and adolescents. Beyond individual physiology and cognition, exercise is a powerful mechanism for social learning. Cooperative games, partner drills, and culturally rooted play (e.g., Laro ng Lahi, traditional Filipino games) create structured contexts for communicating, negotiating roles, exercising empathy, and managing conflict. These embodied interactions rehearse the interpersonal competencies central to the Life and Career Skills curriculum: communication, teamwork, leadership, and cultural identity, while simultaneously strengthening group cohesion and social support networks that protect against isolation and burnout. Recent Philippine studies also point to the value of indigenous games for holistic development, including socioemotional benefits and cultural connectedness.

Finally, PE can explicitly model workplace-relevant competence. Carefully designed circuits, timed tasks, and role-based group challenges simulate workplace demands, multitasking, role flexibility, endurance under sustained pressure, and micro-break strategies for on-the-job recovery. Integrating brief mindfulness and breathing practices into PE sessions further amplifies transfer: evidence from recent trials of mindfulness-based interventions (MBIs) for adolescents shows measurable improvements in emotional regulation, attentional control, and coping, effects that complement those produced by physical exercise alone. The combined approach (movement + mindfulness) appears especially promising for bolstering emotional agility and resilience. Taken together, these lines of evidence support a reconceptualization of PE: from a predominantly physical fitness remit to a curricular locus for psychosocial skill building, cultural continuity, and career readiness, fully aligned with the Life and Career Skills framework advocated by the Philippine Department of Education.

Chapter Objectives

This chapter aims to translate the empirical and curricular rationale above into practical, evidence-based curricular pathways for SHS PE. Specifically, the chapter will:

1. *Examine how structured physical exercises strengthen intrapersonal competencies* (self-awareness, emotion regulation, self-discipline, and resilience). This includes reviewing mechanisms (physiological, cognitive, and reflective practices) and providing exemplar activities (mindful movement, resilience circuits, journaling prompts) grounded in recent empirical studies.

2. *Demonstrate how group PE activities and culturally relevant games support interpersonal effectiveness* (communication, teamwork, empathy, conflict resolution). This objective will integrate evidence on cooperative play and Philippine indigenous games and suggest classroom procedures for scaffolding social learning and inclusion.
3. *Show how exercise can be purposefully framed for career readiness and on-the-job resilience.* The chapter will offer designs for circuit tasks and micro-break protocols that map directly onto workplace skills (multitasking, adaptability, sustained attention), and will outline assessment methods that capture both physical and psychosocial growth.

At the conclusion of this chapter, readers will encounter a theoretically grounded and practically oriented set of curricular strategies, evidence-based activities, reflective prompts, and assessment rubrics. These resources are designed to equip PE teachers and school leaders with tools to embed emotional-resilience development into everyday practice while maintaining cultural relevance and supporting students' transitions to adult learning and future career pathways.

EXERCISE FOR INTRAPERSONAL SKILLS (SELF-AWARENESS, STRESS MANAGEMENT, SELF-DISCIPLINE)

The integration of structured physical activity into educational settings extends beyond the promotion of physical health, simultaneously nurturing critical intrapersonal skills that prepare students to manage personal and professional challenges. Competencies such as self-awareness, stress management, and self-discipline form the foundation of emotional resilience and sustained personal growth (Duckworth & Gross, 2020). Embedding reflective practices alongside intentional physical activities within PE enables schools to advance a holistic development model that aligns with the broader goals of life and career skills education.

Mindful Movement Activities

Mindful movement practices, such as yoga, controlled breathing exercises, and tai chi-inspired routines, are increasingly recognized for their ability to cultivate self-awareness and stress regulation. These activities encourage students to attune to their bodily sensations, emotions, and mental states, creating space for self-reflection and emotional regulation (Creswell, 2017). Empirical evidence suggests that mindfulness-based physical activities significantly reduce symptoms of stress and anxiety among adolescents, while simultaneously enhancing attention and emotional balance (Bauer et al., 2021; Dunning et al., 2019). Within the curriculum, embedding short daily sessions of mindful stretching or breathwork can equip learners with accessible coping tools that support both academic focus and psychosocial stability.

Resilience-Building Workouts

Beyond calm and reflective practices, resilience is also developed through physically demanding activities that parallel real-life challenges. Interval training, endurance-based exercises, and structured obstacle courses provide students with opportunities to confront discomfort, persist through fatigue, and celebrate incremental progress. These forms of exercise mirror the psychological process of overcoming setbacks, thereby strengthening perseverance and grit (Yeager et al., 2022). Research demonstrates that engaging in structured physical challenges enhances self-efficacy and fosters adaptive coping strategies among adolescents (Lubans et al., 2016). In this way, the physical exertion involved in PE classes becomes a metaphor for life's broader challenges, reinforcing the idea that persistence and resilience are skills transferable to both academic and career contexts.

Reflection as a Learning Tool

The effectiveness of exercise-based intrapersonal skill development is amplified when paired with guided reflection. Journaling, group debriefs, or self-assessment activities encourage students to articulate the connections between physical exertion and personal growth. Reflection strengthens self-awareness by allowing learners to identify how they manage stress, regulate emotions, and respond to obstacles (Schonert-Reichl, 2019). For example, after an endurance run or mindfulness session, students might reflect on their emotional state, energy regulation, and coping responses. This process transforms physical activity into a platform for cultivating deeper self-understanding, linking bodily experience with cognitive and emotional insights. Together, mindful movement, resilience-building workouts, and structured reflection create a powerful framework for nurturing intrapersonal skills through PE. These approaches prepare students not only to manage academic stressors but also to develop the emotional intelligence and self-discipline necessary for workplace readiness and lifelong well-being. Integrating such practices within the Life and Career Skills curriculum strengthens the whole-person approach to education, ensuring that learners are better equipped to thrive in complex and demanding environments.

EXERCISE FOR INTERPERSONAL SKILLS (COMMUNICATION, TEAMWORK, EMPATHY)

Interpersonal competencies, clear communication, collaborative problem-solving, perspective-taking, and empathetic responding are central to successful schooling, relationships, and workplaces. PE provides an embodied arena in which these skills can be rehearsed and assessed: movement tasks produce immediate, observable interactional demands (e.g., turn-taking, role negotiation, mutual support) and generate emotionally salient moments that deepen social learning. In this section, we synthesize empirical evidence and practical design principles for using partner work, cooperative group tasks, conflict-resolution movement games, and culturally grounded play (Laro ng Lahi) to cultivate interpersonal skills in SHS students.

The Evidence Base for Movement-based Social Learning

A growing empirical literature shows that cooperative and game-based physical activities strengthen peer relationships, increase enjoyment and engagement in PE, and promote prosocial behaviors. Recent meta-analyses and systematic reviews in school settings report positive effects of cooperative learning and game-based pedagogy on social outcomes, including increased peer support, improved communication, and reductions in competitive performance climates when cooperative structures are emphasized. These effects are robust across ages and settings when teachers intentionally structure interdependence, clear roles, and shared goals.

Movement itself creates social affordances that traditional classroom talk does not. Synchronous movement, walking, patterned group drills, or coordinated rhythms produce feelings of affiliation, increase positive affect, and can reduce interpersonal tensions, making it a practical tool when facilitation is needed for conflict de-escalation or perspective taking. Embodied approaches to conflict resolution leverage locomotion and coordinated activity to shift moods, open channels for negotiation, and scaffold cooperative problem solving.

Partner activities: Fostering Dyadic Communication and Coordination

Partner-based exercises are a low-risk, high-impact strategy for developing dyadic communication and coordination skills. These activities create structured interdependence, requiring each participant to attend to their partner's actions, provide timely cues, and adjust their own movements to achieve shared success. Examples include paired stretching with mirrored timing, resistance-band drills that demand reciprocal tension, and partner balance sequences. Through these interactions, students practice not only physical coordination but also verbal and non-verbal communication, turn-taking, and mutual support. Empirical studies indicate that elastic-band and partner-resistance exercises improve motor control and coordination among youth, while simultaneously reinforcing interpersonal skills when paired with guided communication prompts (e.g., "Name one cue before starting") (Bauer et al., 2021). These structured interactions encourage students to articulate strategies clearly, monitor their partner's performance, and negotiate adjustments, laying the foundation for effective collaboration in broader social and professional contexts.

In practice, educators can employ several strategies to maximize learning outcomes during partner-based activities. First, explicit interaction scripts, such as instructing students to "count to three, then move" or "signal your partner before increasing resistance", help scaffold effective communication, particularly for beginners who may struggle with coordination. Second, co-constructed success criteria encourage mutual accountability by requiring both partners to evaluate their shared performance (e.g., agreeing on a score of at least 3/5), thereby preventing domination by one student and reinforcing collaborative responsibility. Third, partner and role rotation ensure that learners are exposed to a variety of communication styles, promoting adaptability and expanding social engagement within the group. Embedding these strategies enables educators to transform Physical Education sessions into dynamic learning environments where students practice dyadic coordination while simultaneously developing physical proficiency and interpersonal competencies essential for life and career readiness.

Group dynamics: Cooperative Circuits and Shared Success

Cooperative circuits and challenge-based tasks shift the focus from individual achievement to collective success, fostering collaboration, communication, and social responsibility among students. In these activities, students' progress through multiple stations, with group advancement contingent on equitable participation; for instance, a team may only move forward once every member completes a minimum requirement. Such designs emphasize interdependence and highlight the importance of mutual support, reinforcing the concept that group outcomes rely on shared effort rather than individual performance alone.

Meta-analytic evidence on cooperative learning in Physical Education indicates that structured group activities consistently enhance mastery-oriented climates, strengthen peer relationships, and reduce anxiety associated with performance comparisons (Boke, 2025). Well-designed cooperative circuits provide practical opportunities for rotating leadership roles, peer scaffolding, and practicing negotiation and problem-solving strategies under time constraints, skills that transfer readily to academic teamwork and workplace collaboration.

Key Features of Cooperative Circuits

Cooperative circuits can be optimized by embedding structured elements that highlight both physical and interpersonal growth. Interdependence should be central to task design, requiring students to share resources such as a ball, a resistance band, or time allotment, thereby fostering collaboration and joint problem-solving. Role rotation can further enhance equity and skill diversity by assigning different responsibilities at each round, for example, leader, timekeeper, or encourager, ensuring that all students experience multiple dimensions of teamwork. Finally, collective reflection provides an essential closure, allowing groups to debrief on decision-making strategies, communication effectiveness, and lessons learned, while explicitly connecting in-task experiences to broader interpersonal competencies. When these features are deliberately integrated, cooperative circuits become more than physical challenges; they serve as powerful contexts for cultivating communication, empathy, and collaborative problem-solving, positioning Physical Education as a dynamic platform for holistic student development.

Conflict-Resolution through Movement: Trust Walks, Synchronization, and Negotiated Roles

Adolescents' conflict-resolution skills are strengthened when interventions reduce emotional reactivity and promote perspective taking. Movement-based simulations, such as trust walks, mirrored movement tasks, or synchronized group choreography, provide safe, embodied contexts in which students can practice negotiation, communication, and cooperative problem-solving. Trust walks, where a blindfolded student is guided by a partner, cultivate reliance, clear instruction-giving, and attentive verbal feedback. Synchronized movement practices, including marching, clapping, or patterned step sequences, foster affiliation, coordinated attention, and shared rhythm, reducing hostility and encouraging cooperative mindsets. Empirical research on synchronous movement demonstrates increases in positive affect, interpersonal trust, and willingness to cooperate, particularly when combined with structured debriefing that surfaces underlying perspectives and social-emotional learning (Webb et al., 2017).

Facilitation Tips

To maximize the benefits of movement-based conflict-resolution activities, educators should foreground safety and consent by carefully pre-briefing students on activity procedures, offering opt-out options, and emphasizing mutual respect throughout. Structured reflection is equally vital; prompts such as "What made trusting your partner easier or more difficult?" or "How did it feel to lead versus follow?" guide students in connecting their embodied experiences to key skills like emotional regulation, communication, and collaborative problem-solving. Finally, teachers can reinforce transferability by encouraging learners to apply these insights to daily contexts with questions like, "Which communication strategy might you use next time you disagree with a peer?" When combined, these elements transform physical activities into meaningful opportunities for practicing empathy, negotiation, and conflict resolution, thereby linking embodied action directly to adolescents' social and interpersonal development.

INTEGRATING LARO NG LAHI: CULTURALLY RESONANT PATHWAYS TO TEAMWORK AND EMPATHY

Traditional Filipino games, collectively known as *Laro ng Lahi*, provide culturally rich and meaningful contexts for teaching interpersonal skills. Research on indigenous Filipino games indicates that *Patintero*, *Luksong Tinik/Luksong Baka*, and *Tumbang Preso* are widely recognized among students and valued for promoting physical agility, social interaction, and cooperative play (Alcalá & Guzmán Alsina, 2024; Manalo, 2024). These games are particularly effective in Filipino classrooms because they embed familiar social norms, such as turn-taking, mutual encouragement, and distributed leadership, which foster emotional bonding, collective resilience, and culturally grounded social learning

Game-by-Game Contributions

The Laro ng Lahi game contributes uniquely to the development of physical, social, and emotional competencies among students. Patintero, a team-based territory and avoidance game, requires players to alternate roles as runners and defenders, relying on quick decision-making, strategic communication, and precise timing. Its dynamic nature makes it an effective tool for teaching situational leadership, tactical coordination, and trust under pressure. Luksong Tinik and Luksong Baka, on the other hand, emphasize mutual encouragement and shared responsibility as players depend on one another to create safe bases or obstacles. These games foster cooperation, trust, and group support while reinforcing bodily assurance and safe-play ethics. Meanwhile, Tumbang Preso combines individual precision in throwing with collaborative defense, promoting self-control, agility, and emotional regulation. Through its playful competition, it provides opportunities for stress release and strengthens teamwork and social cohesion among participants.

Table 1. Integration of Laro ng Lahi in developing interpersonal skills

Game	Description	Targeted Interpersonal Skills	Educational Value / Reflection Focus
Patintero	A traditional Filipino street game where players block opponents from crossing designated lines.	Strategy, quick decision-making, teamwork, communication	Encourages collaboration in planning tactics and emphasizes trust in teammates during fast-paced play.
Luksong Tinik / Baka	Players leap over obstacles formed by other players' limbs or bodies, with difficulty increasing.	Trust, cooperation, group encouragement, safety awareness	Builds mutual reliance and empathy as students support and encourage peers to overcome challenges.
Tumbang Preso	A game involving knocking down a can with slippers while avoiding being tagged by a guard.	Agility, cooperation, stress release, fair play	Highlights the importance of group participation, sharing roles, and emotional regulation during play.
Reflection Activity	Guided journaling or group debrief after playing.	Empathy, resilience, teamwork, self-awareness	Students connect traditional games to broader life skills such as persistence, collaboration, and respect.

Pedagogical Advantages

The integration of *Laro ng Lahi* into Physical Education and psychosocial curricula offers several pedagogical advantages that extend beyond physical skill development. Because these games are culturally familiar, they foster a strong sense of resonance and belonging, which in turn heightens student engagement and intrinsic motivation, thereby enriching opportunities for social learning. Their resource efficiency makes them accessible and adaptable to various school contexts, as they require minimal equipment, can accommodate different class sizes, and can be played in a range of physical spaces. Moreover, *Laro ng Lahi* inherently embeds cooperative roles, such as strategizing, offering encouragement, or monitoring rules, that allow teachers to observe, scaffold, and assess interpersonal behaviors in authentic and dynamic ways. In doing so, these traditional games not only cultivate physical, emotional, and social competencies but also strengthen students' cultural identity and reinforce communal values that are vital for holistic education.

Reflection: Connecting Play to Values, Empathy, and Resilience

Reflection remains the bridge between action and insight. After partner or group tasks and after playing Laro ng Lahi, guided reflective conversations and short written prompts help students link in-game behaviors to broader interpersonal competencies. Questions such as "When did your team communicate best?" or "How did you help a teammate who was struggling?" invite students to identify empathic acts and leadership behaviors. Research on game-based PE interventions shows that pairing activities with debriefs amplifies social learning outcomes compared with activity-only approaches. Teachers should scaffold these reflections to draw explicit connections to classroom relations and future workplace scenarios.

To effectively assess interpersonal growth in Physical Education, educators are encouraged to adopt a mixed-method approach that integrates observational rubrics, peer evaluations, and student self-reports. Observation rubrics allow teachers to evaluate students' clarity of communication, turn-taking, supportive behaviors, and cooperative problem-solving during partner or group tasks. Peer evaluations, conducted through short checklists, allow students to recognize a positive contribution from a teammate, such as helping maintain team composure, while also identifying areas for improvement to promote constructive feedback and social awareness. Reflective logs serve as a personal tool for students to document a social skill they practiced, examine its impact on group dynamics, and explore how it can be applied beyond the PE setting. This combined assessment approach ensures a more comprehensive understanding of both social and emotional learning outcomes. This approach emphasizes process over outcome, valuing transferable interpersonal competencies over athletic performance.

When implementing partner and group activities, attention to safety, consent, and equitable participation is critical. Strategies include rotating pairings to prevent exclusion, providing role adaptations for students with physical limitations, and distributing leadership opportunities to avoid dominance by more confident participants. For culturally rooted activities such as *Laro ng Lahi*, invite student knowledge bearers to explain game variations and encourage adaptations that respect local norms.

Interpersonal skills are most effectively learned through shared, embodied action. Partner exercises, cooperative circuits, conflict-resolution movement simulations, and culturally resonant games create practical, memorable experiences in which communication, teamwork, and empathy are required, practiced, and reflected upon. When these activities are thoughtfully scaffolded, debriefed, and assessed, PE becomes a rich curricular space for developing the interpersonal competencies emphasized in the Life and Career Skills Curriculum.

Assessment and Classroom Indicators

To effectively capture interpersonal growth in PE, it is recommended to use a mixed-method approach that includes observational rubrics, peer evaluations, and student self-reports. Through observation rubrics, teachers can assess students' clarity in communication, turn-taking, supportive behaviors, and cooperative problem-solving during partner and group activities. Peer evaluations, using short checklists, give students the chance to acknowledge a positive contribution from a teammate, such as helping maintain group focus, while also identifying areas that need improvement, promoting constructive feedback and social awareness. Reflective logs further enhance learning by encouraging students to record the social skills they practiced, reflect on their impact during the activity, and consider how they might be applied in real-life situations outside the PE setting. Together, these tools provide a comprehensive and balanced approach to assessing both social and emotional development in the classroom. This approach emphasizes process over outcome, valuing transferable interpersonal competencies over athletic performance.

When implementing partner and group activities, attention to safety, consent, and equitable participation is critical. Strategies include rotating pairings to prevent exclusion, providing role adaptations for students with physical limitations, and distributing leadership opportunities to avoid dominance by more confident participants. For culturally rooted activities such as *Laro ng Lahi*, invite student knowledge bearers to explain game variations and encourage adaptations that respect local norms.

Interpersonal skills are most effectively learned through shared, embodied action. Partner exercises, cooperative circuits, conflict-resolution movement simulations, and culturally resonant games create practical, memorable experiences in which communication, teamwork, and empathy are required, practiced, and reflected upon. When these activities are thoughtfully scaffolded, debriefed, and assessed, PE becomes a rich curricular space for developing the interpersonal competencies emphasized in the Life and Career Skills Curriculum.

EXERCISE FOR CAREER READINESS (WORKPLACE STRESS MANAGEMENT, ADAPTABILITY, PROFESSIONALISM)

As students move from school into postsecondary study and employment, the competencies that determine success increasingly include nontechnical or "soft" skills: the ability to manage stress, switch tasks fluidly, maintain composure under pressure, and persist toward long-term goals. PE provides an experiential laboratory in which these capacities can be practiced, observed, and reflected upon. When deliberately framed, routine PE activities become analogues for workplace demands, circuit training models multitasking; balance and coordination challenges cultivate adaptability; micro-break breathing and stretch routines teach in-the-moment emotion regulation; and progressive endurance work fosters perseverance and grit. Below, we synthesize evidence for these claims, explain plausible mechanisms, and give practical curricular examples and assessment ideas.

Circuit Training and Multitasking Readiness

Why the analogy fits. Circuit training requires repeated switching between stations, quick shifting of attention, rapid planning, and short-term goal setting under time constraints. These demands mirror workplace multitasking and task switching, where employees alternate between discrete activities and must reorient priorities quickly. Evidence. Recent interventions using circuit or high-intensity interval formats have shown not only physical benefits but improvements in certain cognitive functions (e.g., processing speed, task switching) that underpin multitasking capacity. Emerging 2024–2025 studies reporting cognitive gains after structured circuit programs suggest these training formats can prime attentional flexibility relevant to complex, multi-task work settings.

Practical Classroom Model (30 to 35-minute sessions)

A practical classroom model for a 30–35-minute session can be structured to promote both physical engagement and cognitive flexibility. The session begins with a five-minute warm-up that includes dynamic mobility exercises followed by two minutes of breathing and centering to prepare students physically and mentally. The main circuit, lasting about 20 minutes, consists of six stations with 40 seconds of activity and twenty seconds for transition. Each station integrates varied skill demands, including agility ladder drills for motor coordination, simple arithmetic tasks performed while moving to add cognitive challenge, fine motor activities such as ball control, and teamwork exercises like paired transfer tasks. Quick rotations between stations help students practice adaptability and rapid reorientation. The session concludes with a five- to ten-minute cool-down that incorporates reflective journaling, using prompts such as "Which switching strategy helped you move from one task to the next?" followed by a teacher-guided discussion linking these strategies to workplace situations, such as managing tasks between meetings. Assessment may include measuring task-switching efficiency through a classroom dual-task setup that combines simple reaction and movement tests, complemented by reflection logs to evaluate students' use of adaptive strategies.

Balance & Coordination Activities → Adaptability in Fast-Paced Environments

The analogy between balance and coordination drills and workplace adaptability is grounded in their shared requirement for continuous adjustment to changing conditions. In physical activities, students must respond to variations in body position, external forces, and environmental constraints, mirroring the cognitive and behavioral adaptability needed in professional settings where individuals must modify goals, tactics, and strategies in response to shifting demands. Research supports this connection, showing that physical training targeting balance and coordination enhances executive control, cognitive flexibility, and adaptive performance. Studies on cognitive flexibility also indicate that embodied tasks involving real-time motor adjustments can transfer to more flexible thinking and behavior in non-physical contexts. A practical 20–30-minute classroom module can begin with constraint-manipulation drills, where students perform familiar skills, such as dribbling or passing, while environmental conditions change unpredictably, such as smaller targets, time limits, or added distractions. This can be followed by perturbation balance tasks like single-leg stances while catching or throwing, partner-assisted gentle pushes (with safety protocols), or exercises on unstable surfaces such as foam pads. The session may conclude with a reflection period where students identify moments when they had to adapt and describe the cues they relied on, visual, verbal, or proprioceptive. Assessment can include an observational checklist that evaluates adaptive responses, focusing on whether the student noticed a change, proposed an adjustment, and successfully implemented it during the activity.

Emotion Regulation in Simulated Work Stress — Micro-breaks, Breathing and Stretch Routines

Modern workplaces increasingly recognize the value of micro-breaks and brief body-based recovery strategies to manage strain and maintain productivity. These short pauses, which may include breathing exercises, desk stretches, or one-to-three-minute mobility routines, are easily teachable in PE and transferable to study or work settings. Evidence from meta-analytic and systematic reviews demonstrates that short active or passive recovery breaks between tasks improve vigor, reduce fatigue, and enhance performance. Recent workplace-focused research from 2022 to 2025 continues to affirm micro-breaks as effective coping strategies for managing daily stress and restoring cognitive energy. Implementing similar routines in school environments has shown benefits for students' energy levels and attention, fostering habits that can support long-term academic and professional performance. A practical classroom toolkit may include a two-minute breathing break featuring diaphragmatic breathing in a 4-4-6 count pattern (four counts inhaling, four counts of holding breath, and six counts of exhaling) combined with neck and shoulder rolls, followed by a three-minute mobility set with seated hip openers, wrist stretches, and standing calf raises suited to small spaces. Teachers can introduce cueing strategies that prompt students to take micro-breaks every 45 to 60 minutes of screen or desk work and connect these actions to observable outcomes such as reduced fatigue. Assessment can involve short self-ratings before and after activities on a one-to-five scale measuring vigor or fatigue, along with a one-week follow-up check asking students whether they used the micro-break strategy during study or work, and how effective it was.

Building Perseverance & Grit — Structured Endurance and Progressive Overload

Endurance activities cultivate tolerance for sustained effort, strategic pacing, incremental goal achievement, and delayed gratification, all of which are essential components of perseverance in long-term academic and career endeavors. Research indicates that intervention programs incorporating progressive endurance training or incremental performance goals lead to measurable improvements in self-efficacy, persistence, and mood among adolescents. While the concept of "grit" remains debated in psychological literature, practical endurance training consistently fosters behavioral persistence and goal-directed habits that align with the sustained effort required in professional and educational contexts. A practical classroom model for endurance development may span six to eight weeks, beginning with baseline assessments and goal setting in the first week (for example, timed planks or runs). Weeks two through six can focus on progressive overload, featuring small weekly increases of five to ten percent in duration or intensity, accompanied by explicit coaching on pacing, positive self-talk, and recovery strategies. In the final week, students can engage in transfer reflection by creating a portfolio or presentation that demonstrates how endurance and goal-setting strategies can be applied to real-world projects, such as completing a lengthy assignment or meeting a workplace target. Assessment can combine objective endurance metrics, including time or distance improvements, with pre- and post-module self-efficacy and persistence questionnaires to capture both physical and psychological growth.

Mechanisms: How does exercise build career-relevant capacities?

Four interconnected processes illustrate how movement-based practices support workplace readiness. First, physiological regulation develops through consistent breathing exercises and low-intensity recovery activities, which enhance autonomic flexibility and promote faster physiological recovery from stress. This capacity for composure directly benefits individuals facing demanding job environments. Second, cognitive control and flexibility are strengthened through tasks that require quick adjustments, error monitoring, and adaptive responses. Activities such as circuit training and perturbation drills engage executive functions like task-switching, inhibition, and working memory, all of which contribute to adaptability and multitasking in professional contexts. Third, self-regulation and goal learning emerge from progressive endurance training, as students experience mastery, build self-efficacy, and refine strategies such as pacing and self-talk, skills that transfer effectively to sustained non-physical tasks. Finally, behavioral habit formation occurs through the consistent practice of micro-breaks and short movement routines, creating repeatable, transferable habits that enhance focus and well-being in both study and work settings.

Implementation requires thoughtful scaffolding, beginning with short, structured activities and explicit instruction on strategies such as pacing and micro-break use, supported by reflection prompts that make transfer more visible. Accessibility should be ensured by providing task variations that accommodate differing abilities and health conditions. Cultural relevance and student voice are essential, and co-designing workplace analogies with learners enhances motivation and contextual understanding. Strengthening teacher capacity through professional development on circuit design, cognitive load integration, and reflective facilitation further supports success.

For assessment, a mixed-method approach is most effective. Objective performance data, including endurance and circuit completion metrics, should be combined with cognitive indicators such as task-switching ability or observed on-task behavior, and self-report measures covering perceived stress, self-efficacy, and micro-break use. Short transfer assignments, such as planning and implementing a personal micro-break schedule for one week, can provide valuable evidence of real-world application and long-term behavioral adoption.

ON-THE-JOB PREPARATION: OFFICE-FRIENDLY EXERCISE ROUTINES

Preparing senior high students for workplace life requires attention to small, sustainable movement habits that they can carry into future office, retail, or hybrid work settings. Short, low-effort movement practices, chair exercises, wall-based work, and micro-break sequences are practical, low-cost interventions that reduce fatigue, protect musculoskeletal health, and scaffold on-the-job emotion regulation. Importantly, evidence shows that micro-breaks improve workers' vigor and reduce fatigue, and that brief, targeted active breaks (even under 10 minutes) can yield measurable well-being benefits without necessarily harming productivity. These findings support teaching students' small movement routines that are both feasible in constrained spaces and transferable to work/study settings.

Chair Exercises: Safe, Inclusive Movement for Sedentary Settings

Chair exercises serve as an effective solution for confined or seated work environments, promoting postural strength, circulation, and mobility for individuals of varying fitness levels. Evidence from studies on chair-based exercise programs, particularly in older adults and workplace settings, demonstrates significant improvements in muscular endurance, balance, and functional capacity. These outcomes are associated with reduced discomfort from prolonged sitting and enhanced postural control, both essential for sustained desk work. Within educational contexts, chair exercises can be introduced as simple, time-efficient activities that teach students practical movements transferable to future work environments. A short two-to-four-minute mini-routine can include seated leg raises performed slowly and deliberately for 10 to 12 repetitions per leg, desk push-ups using the desk edge for six to ten repetitions to activate the chest and shoulders, seated torso twists for six to eight slow rotations per side to encourage spinal mobility, and posture correction stretches involving gentle scapular retraction with three to five steady breaths. Teachers should model correct technique, highlight proper breathing patterns during exertion, and provide regressions or progressions to match individual capabilities. Encouraging students to integrate one short chair routine during study sessions fosters body awareness and establishes healthy movement habits that can be maintained throughout academic and professional life.

Wall Exercises — Strength, Posture, and Accessible Resistance

Wall-based exercises are practical and accessible options that develop strength, stability, and postural awareness, particularly in confined environments. These movements offer safe resistance and feedback that help students understand body alignment and muscular engagement. Exercises such as wall sits and wall push-ups efficiently target lower-body endurance, upper-body stability, and core activation, while also improving tolerance for static postures often required in standing or occupational tasks. Research on functional and isometric training supports the benefits of simple, closed-chain exercises in enhancing muscular endurance, balance, and postural control when practiced regularly. A short three-to-five-minute wall routine might include wall sits held for 20 to 40 seconds, repeated twice with brief rest intervals, wall push-ups performed slowly for eight to twelve repetitions, emphasizing controlled shoulder movement, and wall-assisted thoracic extensions to mobilize the upper back. Teachers should remind students to maintain knee alignment over the toes during wall sits and to keep a neutral spine to prevent strain. Progress can be encouraged through small, time-based increases in duration, fostering both physical improvement and a sense of accomplishment.

Micro-Break Movements — Physiology and Attention Restoration

Micro-breaks, defined as brief pauses lasting ten minutes or less, have strong empirical support for enhancing energy levels and reducing fatigue. They represent one of the most effective strategies for promoting short-term recovery during periods of prolonged cognitive or sedentary work. Research highlights those short active breaks, such as stretching, light mobility movements, or brief walks, and attentional shifts like looking away from screens can help restore depleted physical and mental resources. Micro-breaks also align with the 20-20-20 rule for reducing visual strain, which involves looking at an object about 20 feet away for 20 seconds every 20 minutes and can incorporate short breathing exercises that promote relaxation and autonomic balance. Practical micro-break options lasting between 30 and 120 seconds include breathing resets with controlled inhalation and exhalation paired with shoulder rolls, eye and neck resets that combine gaze changes with gentle neck rotations, and full-body energizers involving light marching, calf raises, and arm circles. To encourage consistent use, educators can integrate micro-breaks into classroom routines or work sessions at regular intervals, using reminders or visual cues. Linking these short breaks to observable outcomes such as reduced fatigue and improved focus helps students recognize their immediate and long-term benefits.

Framing for Career Readiness — Preventing Burnout and Improving Productivity

Small movement routines function as behavioral micro-interventions that prevent the accumulation of strain and support sustained attention and productivity. Theoretical models (Effort-Recovery Model; Conservation of Resources) explain how brief recovery episodes protect personal resources, increasing vigor and reducing exhaustion. Translating these mechanisms to students: learning to insert micro-breaks, do quick posture resets, and use a 60–90 s breathing routine becomes a portable self-management skill with direct application to future office or remote work contexts. Evidence suggests micro-breaks reliably increase subjective energy and reduce fatigue; their effects on objective productivity are more task-dependent, but benefits to well-being and sustained engagement are consistent.

Implementation, pedagogy, and assessment

To implement micro-breaks effectively, teachers can integrate them into existing classroom routines such as homeroom breaks, lesson transitions, or PE cool-downs. Modeling transfer is essential, and students should be encouraged to plan when and how they will apply the routine in their study or work settings and later share their experiences. Establishing habits can be supported by pairing movement cues with consistent triggers, such as taking a brief break every 45 minutes of study. Assessment can include brief self-report scales to measure energy or fatigue before and after micro-breaks, usage logs to record frequency and perceived effectiveness, and teacher observations of posture and on-task behavior. To ensure equity and safety, teachers should offer adaptations for students with mobility limitations, respect personal comfort levels, and adapt cues to fit cultural and workplace contexts. A short ten-minute classroom lesson can introduce the practice: begin with a one-minute explanation of how micro-breaks enhance focus, followed by a two-minute chair exercise demonstration involving seated leg raises and torso twists. Next, guide students through a short breathing and gaze reset activity, then allow pairs four minutes to plan when they will apply the routine during the coming week. Conclude with a quick one-minute exit poll asking whether students intend to use the strategy and why.

INTEGRATION IN THE SENIOR HIGH SCHOOL CURRICULUM

PE serves as an ideal platform for developing Life and Career Skills because it integrates physical activity with social interaction, deliberate practice, and reflective learning. The Life and Career Skills Curriculum highlights competencies such as adaptability, resilience, self-management, and interpersonal effectiveness, skills that can be effectively nurtured in PE through well-designed activities, culturally grounded games, and formative assessment practices. To achieve this, lessons should be intentionally aligned with specific Life and Career Skills Curriculum outcomes, clearly identifying one or two competencies, such as self-management or collaboration, in each session so that teachers and students understand the transferable skills being developed. Combining movement with reflection is also essential, as evidence shows that the greatest psychosocial gains occur when physical activity is followed by structured reflection or journaling for three to ten minutes. Incorporating culturally responsive practices, such as traditional Filipino games (Laro ng Lahi), enhances engagement while promoting empathy, teamwork, and community values rooted in Filipino culture. Finally, assessment should emphasize the learning process through formative tools like observation rubrics, peer feedback, and reflective journals, supported by selected objective measures of skill or fitness. These approaches promote metacognitive awareness, accountability, and holistic growth among students.

Weekly Module Model — Sample 8-Week Sequence

(Senior High, 1 × 45-minute Lesson/Week + Micro-practices)

This sample sequence integrates mindful movement, resilience circuits, cooperative tasks (including *Laro ng Lahi*), and explicit transfer to workplace skills. Use it as a template — adjust pacing and intensity depending on context and time allotment.

Table 2. Weekly module model

Week	Focus	In-class sequence (45 min)	Home/Transfer micro-practice
1	Orientation & Baseline	Introduce Life and Career Skills outcomes; baseline measures (brief perceived stress + self-efficacy); 20 min mindful movement; 10 min journaling prompt ("What is one coping strategy I want to learn?")	2-min breathing break — practice daily
2	Intrapersonal: Breathing & Pacing	10 min warm-up; 20 min resilience circuit (short intervals) + 10 min micro-reflection on pacing	Implement breathing break during study for 3 sessions
3	Interpersonal: Partner skills	Paired resistance/stretching drills with interaction scripts; 10 min peer feedback; 5 min journal	Practice one partner communication script at home (role swap with family)
4	Laro ng Lahi I (Patintero)	Teach rules; 20 min play with role rotation; 10 min group debrief on strategy & leadership	Observe/record one team strategy used in other class/team activity
5	Career readiness: Circuit → multitasking	Circuit with cognitive-load stations (dual tasking); 10 min reflection mapping strategies to workplace tasks	Try 1 planned micro-break between study tasks
6	Laro ng Lahi II (Luksong Tinik / Tumbang Preso)	Play + scaffolded roles (encourager, safety monitor); 10 min guided reflection on trust & encouragement	Identify one moment you supported someone; journal
7	Integration: Cooperative circuit + trust tasks	Cooperative circuit where group advances only if all succeed; trust walk; 10 min transfer mapping (career)	Implement a 1-week micro-break schedule and log use
8	Consolidation & Assessment	Post measures (PSS, brief resilience), student portfolios (journals), peer evaluations, teacher rubric scoring; student presentations on transfer plans	Portfolio submission and teacher feedback

Evidence supports that multi-component school programs (movement + SEL + reflection) are more effective at improving resilience and emotional outcomes than activity-only approaches. Use the baseline/post measures to document change and to refine instruction.

CONCLUSION

As this chapter has argued, exercise is far more than the cultivation of aerobic capacity or sport-specific skill; when intentionally framed and taught, it becomes a powerful, embodied pedagogy for emotional resilience, interpersonal competence, and career readiness. A convergent body of recent evidence, including large cohort studies, systematic reviews, and school-based interventions, shows that physical fitness and structured movement programs are associated with lower risk of mental-health problems, greater psychological resilience, and improved cognitive control in children and adolescents. These findings support repositioning PE from an ancillary subject to a curricular locus for Life and Career Skills development.

Mechanistically, movement-based learning produces change through multiple, interacting pathways. Physiological regulation (improved autonomic recovery and stress-buffering), cognitive gains (enhanced executive control and attentional flexibility), psychosocial processes (social support and cooperative practice), and reflective meaning-making (journals and debriefs that convert experience into strategy) together explain how exercise transfers to non-physical domains of life. Recent meta-analyses affirm that multi-component school programs, those that combine physical activity, mindfulness or skills training, and guided reflection, produce the strongest and most reliable gains for adolescent resilience and well-being.

From a curriculum perspective, this evidence requires three practical shifts. First, teachers and curriculum designers must make psychosocial outcomes explicit: write Life and Career Skills-aligned objectives into PE lessons and name the intrapersonal and interpersonal skills students are expected to practise. Second, movement practice must be paired with brief, regular reflection to cement transfer (for example, short journals, peer debriefs, or structured prompts that link activity to coping strategies). Third, culturally grounded content, such as *Laro ng Lahi* in the Philippine context, should be used strategically to increase relevance, sustain engagement, and reinforce communal values that support empathy and teamwork. Systematic and qualitative studies from the Philippines show that indigenous games both engage students and embed pro-social norms when taught with cultural sensitivity.

Implementation at scale will depend on pragmatic solutions that address common barriers. Low-cost, high-yield practices (micro-breaks, chair/wall routines, bodyweight circuits, and short mindful-movement sessions) are feasible across resource levels and can be taught quickly. Equally important are investments in teacher capacity-building (iterative PD and coaching rather than one-off workshops), simple formative assessment tools (short observation rubrics and reflective journals), and school schedules that protect regular PE time. Pilot evaluations and pragmatic monitoring (dose, fidelity, brief pre/post psychosocial measures) are essential to build local evidence and iterate designs for diverse school contexts.

Finally, there is a moral and practical imperative to pursue an integrated, whole-person approach to education. Preparing young people for the world of work and for the emotional demands of contemporary life requires that schools teach bodies as well as minds. Exercise, taught as mindful movement, as graded challenge, and as social play, cultivates the self-regulatory habits, collaborative dispositions, and adaptive capacities that underpin lifelong wellbeing and vocational success. We therefore call on educators, curriculum developers, and policymakers to adopt a culturally grounded, evidence-informed model of PE that centers psychosocial development as a core outcome. Doing so will not only improve student health but will also equip a new generation with the emotional agility and social competence needed to thrive in uncertain times.

REFERENCES

Alcalá, A. M. G., & Guzmán Alsina, B. (2024). El abordaje periodístico de la trata de personas en los portales de noticias web de El Tribuno e Informate Salta durante el 2023.

Bauer, J., Schwiertz, G., & Muehlbauer, T. (2021). Effects of an elastic resistance band intervention in adolescent handball players. *Sports Medicine International Open*, *5*(02), E65–E72. PMID: 34458564

Boke, H. (2025). Effects of cooperative learning on students' outcomes in physical education: A meta-analysis. *Journal of Physical Education Research*, *12*(3), 45–67. PMID: 40432799

Branzuela, M. J., Ayro, E. C., & Cruz-Vidal, M. J. D. (2023). Teaching outside the box: Senior High School teaching experiences, challenges, and windows of innovations of non-social science majors. *International Journal of Multidisciplinary: Applied Business and Education Research*, *4*(7), 2210–2222.

Creswell, J. D. (2017). Mindfulness interventions. *Annual Review of Psychology*, *68*, 491–516. PMID: 27687118

Del Carmen, M. V., Diano, F., Morales, M. P. E., & Ole, A. (2015). Promoting physics in action thru "Laro Ng Lahi-Based" physics activities. In the International *Journal of Learning and Teaching* (Vol. 07, Issue 1, pp. 24–37). https://pdfs.semanticscholar.org/feca/a3be1eb1da8b1db238f7a3bd9f2b1986996a.pdf

Dizer, R., Logan, I. L. N., & Raval, K. M. R. (2022). Laro ng lahi: A study on the perceived benefits of playing indigenous games on the holistic development of Filipinos born in the'80s. *Philippine Journal of Social Sciences and Humanities University of the Philippines Visayas*, *27*, 91–114. https://pjssh.upv.edu.ph/wp-content/uploads/2024/05/91-114-PJSSH-22-27-D01_Laro-ng-Lahi.pdf

Duckworth, A. L., & Gross, J. J. (2020). Behavior change. *Organizational Behavior and Human Decision Processes*, *161*, 39–49. PMID: 33716396

Dunning, D. L., Griffiths, K., Kuyken, W., Crane, C., Foulkes, L., Parker, J., & Dalgleish, T. (2019). Research Review: The effects of mindfulness-based interventions on cognition and mental health in children and adolescents–a meta-analysis of randomized controlled trials. *Journal of Child Psychology and Psychiatry, and Allied Disciplines*, *60*(3), 244–258. PMID: 30345511

Gordon, J. (2023). Empowered Learners: How Martial Arts Foster Self-Regulated Learning. *Mantle: The Annual Review of Interdisciplinary Research*, *1*(1), 29–39.

Immordino-Yang, M. H., Darling-Hammond, L., & Krone, C. R. (2025). Nurturing nature: How brain development is inherently social and emotional, and what this means for education. In *Social and Emotional Learning* (pp. 63–83). Routledge.

Lubans, D., Richards, J., Hillman, C., Faulkner, G., Beauchamp, M., Nilsson, M., & Biddle, S. (2016). Physical activity for cognitive and mental health in youth: A systematic review of mechanisms. *Pediatrics*, *138*(3), e20161642. PMID: 27542849

Manalo, A. S. D. (2024). Navigating Critical Pedagogy: Insights from Public Secondary English Teachers. *A-Liberal Arts/Humanities and Social Sciences*, 75.

Peng, B., Chen, W., Wang, H., & Yu, T. (2025). How does physical exercise influence self-efficacy in adolescents? A study based on the mediating role of psychological resilience. *BMC Psychology*, *13*(1), 1–17. PMID: 40119462

Webb, C. E., Rossignac-Milon, M., & Higgins, E. T. (2017). Could walking facilitate interpersonal conflict resolution? *Conflict Resolution Quarterly*, *35*(4), 345–371. PMID: 28481583

Yeager, D. S., Carroll, J. M., Buontempo, J., Cimpian, A., Woody, S., Crosnoe, R., & Dweck, C. S. (2022). Teacher mindsets help explain where a growth-mindset intervention does and doesn't work. *Psychological Science*, *33*(1), 18–32. PMID: 34936529

Yeh, G. Y., Mehta, D. H., & Wayne, P. M. (2025). Healing STEM: Harnessing compassion, mindfulness, and emotional regulation to overcome burnout. *Journal of Integrative and Complementary Medicine*, *31*(5), 398–402. PMID: 40238723

Chapter 9
From Sweat to Serenity:
How Exercise Shapes Emotional Wellbeing

Prabir Mondal
https://orcid.org/0009-0000-3550-0986
Lakshmibai National Institute of Physical Education, India

Padmakar Padmakar
Lakshmibai National Institute of Physical Education, India

Sohom Saha
https://orcid.org/0009-0006-9438-1554
Lakshmibai National Institute of Physical Education, India

ABSTRACT

This chapter examines how physical exercise promotes emotional well-being through interconnected biological, psychological, and social mechanisms. It highlights how various forms of exercise, such as aerobic, resistance, and mindful movement, trigger neurochemical changes like endorphin and endocannabinoid release, which regulate mood, reduce anxiety, and enhance resilience. Psychologically, exercise boosts self-efficacy, body image, and a sense of mastery, while socially, it fosters connection, belonging, and support. The chapter emphasizes tailoring exercise approaches to individual needs and offers practical strategies for daily integration. It also addresses potential risks, such as overtraining, and explores trends like technology-assisted fitness programs. Overall, the chapter presents exercise as a powerful preventive and therapeutic tool for achieving lasting mental wellness, supporting the journey from "sweat to serenity."

DOI: 10.4018/979-8-3373-6157-4.ch009

1. INTRODUCTION AND RATIONALE

The relationship between physical activity and mental well-being has captivated human curiosity for millennia. From ancient Greek philosophers who advocated for the unity of mind and body to contemporary neuroscientists mapping the intricate neural networks activated during exercise, the connection between movement and mood has evolved from philosophical speculation to empirical science (Biddle & Batterham, 2015). In our increasingly sedentary world, where mental health challenges have reached epidemic proportions, exercise emerges not merely as a tool for physical conditioning but as a powerful catalyst for emotional transformation. The metaphorical journey "from sweat to serenity" encapsulates a profound biological and psychological process. When we engage in physical activity, our bodies initiate a cascade of neurochemical responses that extend far beyond the immediate physiological adaptations. These responses influence mood regulation, stress management, self-perception, and overall emotional resilience (Kandola et al., 2019). The sweat represents not just metabolic byproducts but the tangible evidence of a transformative process occurring at cellular, neural, and psychological levels.

Contemporary research reveals that exercise acts as a multi-modal intervention, simultaneously addressing biological vulnerabilities to mental health disorders while enhancing psychological resources such as self-efficacy, social connection, and meaning-making (Rosenbaum et al., 2015). This dual action makes exercise uniquely positioned as both a preventive and therapeutic tool for emotional well-being. The urgency of understanding this relationship has intensified in recent years. The World Health Organization estimates that over 264 million people worldwide suffer from depression, while anxiety disorders affect 301 million individuals globally (World Health Organization, 2021). Simultaneously, physical inactivity has been identified as the fourth leading risk factor for global mortality, contributing to approximately 3.2 million deaths annually (Lee et al., 2012)These parallel epidemics of mental health challenges and sedentary behavior underscore the critical need for interventions that address both concerns simultaneously. This chapter aims to provide a comprehensive examination of how exercise shapes emotional well-being, synthesizing cutting-edge research from neuroscience, psychology, and exercise physiology. By exploring the mechanisms underlying the exercise-emotion connection and examining practical applications across diverse populations, we seek to illuminate pathways from movement to mental wellness.

SECTION 1: UNDERSTANDING EMOTIONAL WELL-BEING IN THE CONTEXT OF EXERCISE

Defining Emotional Well-being

Emotional well-being encompasses a multidimensional construct that includes the experience of positive emotions, the absence of negative emotions, life satisfaction, and the ability to cope effectively with life's challenges (Diener et al., 2018). Unlike clinical measures that focus primarily on pathology, emotional well-being emphasizes flourishing and optimal functioning. This positive psychology approach recognizes that mental health exists on a continuum, where individuals can move beyond the mere absence of symptoms to experience genuine vitality and life satisfaction. Within the exercise context, emotional well-being manifests through several key dimensions. Affective well-being relates to the immediate emotional responses to physical activity, including feelings of energy, calmness, and positive mood during and after exercise sessions (Ekkekakis & Russell, 2013)

Cognitive well-being involves the evaluation of one's life circumstances, including satisfaction with physical health, body image, and personal achievement in fitness goals. Psychological well-being encompasses deeper constructs such as personal growth, purpose in life, and self-acceptance, all of which can be influenced by regular physical activity (Reed & Buck, 2009). (Welk et al., 2023) Acute effects occur during and immediately following exercise sessions, often characterized by mood enhancement and stress reduction. These immediate benefits can accumulate over time, leading to chronic adaptations in emotional functioning, including improved baseline mood, enhanced emotional regulation, and increased resilience to psychological stressors (Wegner et al., 2014).

Historical and Cultural Perspectives

The recognition of exercise's emotional benefits spans cultures and centuries. Ancient civilizations understood the connection between physical activity and mental clarity. The Roman poet Juvenal's famous phrase "mens sana in corpore sano" (a sound mind in a sound body) reflected this understanding, suggesting that physical and mental health are inextricably linked (Welk et al., 2023). Traditional Eastern practices have long emphasized the emotional dimensions of movement. Yoga, originating in ancient India, explicitly connects physical postures (asanas) with mental states and emotional regulation. Similarly, Tai Chi, rooted in Chinese philosophy, emphasizes the flow of energy and its impact on psychological well-being (Sharma et al., 2006a). These practices demonstrate that the exercise-emotion connection transcends cultural boundaries and has been recognized across diverse philosophical traditions.

The scientific investigation of this relationship began in earnest during the 20th century. Early research focused primarily on clinical populations, examining exercise as an adjunct treatment for depression and anxiety. (Morgan & Goldston, 1987) pioneering work established exercise as a legitimate intervention for mental health, challenging the prevailing notion that psychological disorders required exclusively psychological or pharmacological treatments. Contemporary research has expanded beyond clinical applications to examine exercise's role in promoting emotional well-being among healthy populations. This shift reflects a broader movement in psychology toward understanding human flourishing rather than merely treating dysfunction (Seligman & Csikszentmihalyi, 2000).

The Interplay Between Physical Exertion, Cognition, and Affect

The relationship between physical exertion and emotional states operates through complex interactions between physiological arousal, cognitive appraisal, and affective responses. During exercise, the body experiences increased heart rate, respiration, and metabolic activity. These physiological changes are interpreted by the brain through various cognitive and emotional filters, ultimately influencing the subjective experience of the activity (Ekkekakis, 2013). The dual-mode model of affective response to exercise provides a framework for understanding these interactions (Ekkekakis, 2003). According to this model, affective responses during exercise are influenced by both cognitive factors (such as self-efficacy and outcome expectations) and interoceptive cues (such as muscle fatigue and cardiovascular strain). At moderate intensities, cognitive factors tend to dominate, leading to generally positive affective responses. However, as exercise intensity approaches or exceeds the ventilatory threshold, interoceptive cues become more salient, potentially leading to negative affect if not properly managed.

Individual differences in fitness level, exercise history, and psychological characteristics significantly influence these affective responses. Well-trained individuals may maintain positive affect at higher intensities due to their enhanced physiological efficiency and positive exercise-related cognitions ((Ekkekakis & Acevedo, 2006). Conversely, sedentary individuals may experience negative affect even at relatively low intensities due to unfamiliarity with exercise sensations and limited confidence in their physical capabilities. The post-exercise period represents a particularly important window for emotional well-being. The immediate post-exercise phase is typically characterized by positive mood enhancement, often referred to as the "exercise high" or "runner's high" ((Boecker et al., 2008). This phenomenon appears to result from a combination of neurochemical changes, including elevated endorphin and endocannabinoid levels, as well as cognitive factors such as achievement satisfaction and stress relief.

SECTION 2: NEUROCHEMICAL AND PHYSIOLOGICAL MECHANISMS

The Endorphin and Endocannabinoid Hypotheses

The neurochemical foundation of exercise's emotional benefits has been a subject of intense scientific investigation. The endorphin hypothesis, first proposed in the 1980s, suggests that exercise-induced release of endogenous opioids (endorphins) contributes to improved mood and reduced perception of pain ((Goldfarb & Jamurtas, 1997). Endorphins, often called the body's "natural morphine," bind to opioid receptors in the brain, producing feelings of euphoria and well-being. Research using positron emission tomography (PET) scanning has provided compelling evidence for the endorphin hypothesis. (Boecker et al., 2008) demonstrated that prolonged running leads to increased endorphin release in brain regions associated with mood and emotion, including the prefrontal cortex, limbic system, and paralimbic system. The magnitude of endorphin release correlated positively with runners' reports of euphoria, providing direct neurochemical evidence for the "runner's high" phenomenon. However, the endorphin hypothesis alone cannot fully explain exercise's emotional benefits. Endorphins are large molecules that have difficulty crossing the blood-brain barrier, leading researchers to investigate alternative explanations. The endocannabinoid hypothesis has emerged as a compelling complement to the endorphin theory (Raichlen et al., 2012).

Endocannabinoids, including anandamide and 2-arachidonoylglycerol (2-AG), are lipid-based neurotransmitters that can readily cross the blood-brain barrier. These molecules bind to cannabinoid receptors throughout the brain and peripheral nervous system, influencing mood, appetite, pain perception, and memory ((Sparling et al., 2003). Exercise increases circulating levels of endocannabinoids, and this increase correlates with improvements in mood and reductions in anxiety. The endocannabinoid system may be particularly important for exercise's anxiolytic effects. Cannabinoid receptors are densely distributed in brain regions associated with fear and anxiety processing, including the amygdala and hippocampus (Heyman, Gamelin, Goekint, Piscitelli, et al., 2012). Exercise-induced endocannabinoid release may help dampen activity in these regions, contributing to the calm and relaxed feelings often experienced after physical activity.

Neurotransmitter Regulation Through Physical Activity

Beyond endorphins and endocannabinoids, exercise influences multiple neurotransmitter systems that regulate mood and emotion. The monoamine neurotransmitters, dopamine, serotonin, and norepinephrine, are particularly important in this regard, as dysregulation of these systems is implicated in depression, anxiety, and other mood disorders (Mikkelsen et al., 2017). Dopamine, often called the "reward neurotransmitter," plays a crucial role in motivation, pleasure, and reward processing. Exercise increases dopamine activity in several brain regions, including the striatum and prefrontal cortex (Greenwood et al., 2011). This enhanced dopaminergic activity may contribute to the rewarding aspects of exercise, helping to establish and maintain regular physical activity habits. Additionally, dopamine's role in motivation and goal-directed behavior may explain why regular exercisers often report increased drive and ambition in other life domains.

Serotonin, widely recognized for its role in mood regulation, is significantly influenced by physical activity. Exercise increases the availability of tryptophan, the amino acid precursor to serotonin, while simultaneously reducing competition from other amino acids for transport across the blood-brain barrier (Chaouloff, 1997). This process leads to increased serotonin synthesis and release, contributing to improved mood and reduced anxiety. The serotonergic effects of exercise may be particularly important for individuals with depression, as many antidepressant medications work by enhancing serotonin activity. Norepinephrine, which functions as both a neurotransmitter and a hormone, is released during exercise as part of the body's stress response. While acute elevations in norepinephrine can feel energizing and alerting, chronic adaptations to regular exercise lead to improved norepinephrine regulation and enhanced stress resilience (Dishman et al., 2006). This adaptation may help explain why regular exercisers often demonstrate better emotional regulation and stress management capabilities. Gamma-aminobutyric acid (GABA), the brain's primary inhibitory neurotransmitter, also responds to exercise in ways that promote emotional well-being. Exercise increases GABA activity, particularly in brain regions associated with anxiety and stress (Schoenfeld et al., 2013). Enhanced GABAergic activity helps calm neural activity and promote relaxation, contributing to exercise's anxiolytic effects.

Exercise-Induced Neuroplasticity and Emotional Implications

Perhaps the most profound way exercise influences emotional well-being is through its effects on brain structure and function. Neuroplasticity, the brain's ability to reorganize and adapt, is significantly enhanced by regular physical activity, leading to structural and functional changes that support improved emotional regulation (Voss et al., 2013). Brain-derived neurotrophic factor (BDNF) serves as a key mediator of exercise-induced neuroplasticity. Often referred to as "Miracle-Gro for the brain," BDNF promotes the growth, survival, and differentiation of neurons (Szuhany et al., 2015). Exercise dramatically increases BDNF production, particularly in the hippocampus, a brain region critical for learning, memory, and emotional regulation. Elevated BDNF levels are associated with improved mood, enhanced cognitive function, and increased resilience to stress. The hippocampus is particularly vulnerable to the effects of chronic stress and depression, often showing reduced volume in individuals with these conditions. Exercise-induced increases in BDNF help protect against stress-related hippocampal atrophy and may even promote neurogenesis, the formation of new neurons (Erickson et al., 2011). This neuroprotective effect may contribute to exercise's antidepressant properties and its ability to enhance emotional resilience.

Exercise also influences the prefrontal cortex, a brain region crucial for executive function, emotional regulation, and decision-making. Regular physical activity increases prefrontal cortex volume and enhances connectivity between this region and emotional centers like the amygdala (Oberlin et al., 2016). This enhanced prefrontal-limbic connectivity may improve emotional regulation by strengthening the brain's ability to modulate emotional responses through cognitive control. The default mode network (DMN), a brain network active during rest and introspection, is also modified by exercise. Dysregulation of the DMN is associated with depression, anxiety, and rumination. Exercise helps normalize DMN activity, potentially reducing negative thought patterns and promoting more balanced emotional states (Zanto & Gazzaley, 2013).

SECTION 3: COMPARATIVE EFFECTS OF DIFFERENT EXERCISE MODALITIES

Aerobic Training and Emotional Endurance

Aerobic exercise, characterized by sustained, rhythmic activity that elevates heart rate and respiratory function, has been extensively studied for its emotional benefits. Running, cycling, swimming, and dancing all fall within this category and have demonstrated significant positive effects on mood, anxiety, and overall emotional well-being (Gordon et al., 2018). The emotional benefits of aerobic exercise appear to follow a dose-response relationship, with moderate-intensity activities providing optimal benefits for most individuals. The American College of Sports Medicine recommends 150 minutes of moderate-intensity aerobic exercise per week for general health benefits, and this prescription also appears optimal for emotional well-being (Piercy et al., 2018). However, even smaller amounts of aerobic activity can produce meaningful emotional benefits, particularly for sedentary individuals beginning an exercise program.

Long-distance running has received particular attention due to the phenomenon of "runner's high" and its association with meditative states. Research suggests that sustained aerobic activity may induce altered states of consciousness characterized by reduced self-awareness, time distortion, and feelings of transcendence (Brymer & Schweitzer, 2017). These experiences may contribute to the profound emotional benefits reported by endurance athletes and recreational runners alike. The rhythmic, repetitive nature of many aerobic activities may contribute to their emotional benefits through multiple mechanisms. The steady cadence of running or cycling can induce a meditative state similar to mindfulness practices, promoting present-moment awareness and reducing rumination (Cox et al., 2016). Additionally, the predictable nature of these activities may provide a sense of control and mastery that enhances self-efficacy and emotional regulation. Group aerobic activities, such as fitness classes or team sports, add a social dimension that can amplify emotional benefits. The combination of physical activity and social interaction creates opportunities for social support, belonging, and shared achievement that contribute to overall emotional well-being (Eime et al., 2013a). The synchronous movement characteristic of group aerobic activities may also promote social bonding through the release of endorphins and the activation of mirror neuron systems.

Resistance Training and Self-Perception of Strength

Resistance training, involving the use of weights, resistance bands, or bodyweight exercises to build muscular strength and endurance, offers unique emotional benefits that complement those of aerobic exercise. While traditionally viewed primarily as a tool for physical conditioning, research increasingly recognizes resistance training's significant impact on psychological well-being (Gordon et al., 2017a). The emotional benefits of resistance training appear to be closely linked to improvements in self-efficacy and body image. As individuals observe their increasing strength and physical capabilities, they often experience enhanced confidence that extends beyond the gym into other life domains (Liu-Ambrose et al., 2010). This phenomenon, known as self-efficacy generalization, suggests that mastering physical challenges through resistance training can improve overall belief in one's ability to handle life's difficulties.

Resistance training may be particularly beneficial for body image and self-esteem. The visible changes in muscle tone and physical capability that result from consistent resistance training can improve body satisfaction and reduce body dissatisfaction (Seguin et al., 2016). These improvements in body image often translate to enhanced overall self-esteem and emotional well-being. The goal-oriented nature of resistance training provides unique opportunities for achievement and mastery experiences. Unlike aerobic exercise, where progress may be measured in endurance or speed, resistance training offers clear, quantifiable markers of improvement through increased weights, repetitions, or training volume. These concrete achievements can provide powerful psychological benefits, including enhanced motivation, self-confidence, and sense of personal accomplishment (McAuley et al., 2000).

Research has shown that resistance training can be as effective as aerobic exercise for reducing symptoms of depression and anxiety. A meta-analysis by Gordon et al. (2017b) found that resistance training programs produced significant reductions in depressive symptoms, with effect sizes comparable to those observed with aerobic exercise interventions. The mechanisms underlying these benefits may include improved self-esteem, enhanced body image, and the achievement satisfaction associated with progressive strength gains. The social aspects of resistance training, particularly in gym environments, can also contribute to emotional well-being. The supportive community often found in strength training environments provides opportunities for social connection, mentorship, and shared goal pursuit (Romain et al., 2018). The ritual and routine of resistance training can also provide structure and stability that support emotional regulation.

Hybrid Programs and Psychological Benefits

Contemporary exercise programs increasingly incorporate elements of both aerobic and resistance training, recognizing that comprehensive fitness approaches may provide synergistic psychological benefits. High-Intensity Interval Training (HIIT), CrossFit, circuit training, and functional fitness programs exemplify this hybrid approach (Biddle & Batterham, 2015). HIIT, characterized by alternating periods of high-intensity exercise and recovery, has gained popularity due to its time efficiency and physiological benefits. Research suggests that HIIT may provide psychological benefits that exceed those of traditional steady-state aerobic exercise (Stork et al., 2017). The varied intensity levels and exercise modalities characteristic of HIIT may prevent boredom and enhance adherence, while the challenging nature of these workouts can provide powerful mastery experiences.

The psychological principle of "flow", a state of complete absorption in an activity characterized by focused attention, clear goals, and immediate feedback, may be particularly relevant to hybrid exercise programs (Csikszentmihalyi, 2008). The complex, varied nature of these programs can create optimal challenges that promote flow states, contributing to enhanced motivation, enjoyment, and psychological well-being. Functional fitness programs, which emphasize movement patterns relevant to daily activities, may provide unique psychological benefits through their emphasis on practical strength and capability. Participants in these programs often report increased confidence in their ability to handle physical challenges in daily life, from carrying groceries to playing with children (Heinrich et al., 2014). This enhanced functional capacity can contribute to overall life satisfaction and emotional well-being.

The community aspect of many hybrid programs, particularly those conducted in group settings, adds significant psychological benefits. CrossFit boxes, boot camp classes, and similar programs often develop strong social networks characterized by mutual support, encouragement, and shared challenge (Whiteman-Sandland et al., 2018). These communities can provide social support that extends beyond exercise, contributing to overall emotional well-being and life satisfaction.

SECTION 4: PSYCHOSOCIAL AND BEHAVIORAL PATHWAYS

Exercise as a Source of Social Connection and Belonging

The social dimensions of exercise represent a powerful pathway through which physical activity influences emotional well-being. Humans are fundamentally social beings, and the need for connection, belonging, and community support is deeply ingrained in our psychological makeup (Baumeister & Leary, 1995). Exercise environments, from neighborhood running groups to fitness classes to recreational sports leagues, provide rich opportunities for social interaction and community building. Team sports exemplify the social benefits of exercise most clearly. Participation in organized sports provides structured opportunities for cooperation, communication, and shared goal achievement. Research has consistently demonstrated that team sport participation is associated with enhanced social skills, increased sense of belonging, and improved overall psychological well-being (Eime et al., 2013a). The shared experiences of training, competition, and achievement create bonds that often extend beyond the sporting context, contributing to broader social support networks. Group fitness classes offer another avenue for social connection through exercise. The shared experience of working toward fitness goals, the encouragement from instructors and fellow participants, and the sense of collective achievement can create meaningful social bonds (Fraser & Spink, 2002). Regular attendance at group fitness classes often leads to the development of friendships and support networks that provide emotional benefits beyond the exercise session itself.

The rise of online fitness communities and social media platforms dedicated to exercise has expanded the social dimensions of physical activity beyond geographical boundaries. Strava, fitness Facebook groups, virtual running clubs, and other digital platforms allow individuals to connect with like-minded exercisers, share achievements, and receive support and encouragement (Cavallo et al., 2012). While these virtual connections may not fully replace face-to-face interaction, they can provide valuable social support, particularly for individuals who lack local exercise communities. The concept of social contagion is particularly relevant to understanding how exercise's social benefits spread through communities. When individuals observe others engaging in and enjoying physical activity, they are more likely to initiate and maintain their own exercise routines (Christakis & Fowler, 2007). This phenomenon creates positive feedback loops within communities, where exercise participation spreads through social networks, enhancing the overall well-being of entire communities.

The Role of Goal Setting and Achievement in Emotional Reinforcement

Goal setting and achievement represent fundamental psychological processes that contribute significantly to exercise's emotional benefits. The systematic pursuit and attainment of fitness goals provides structure, meaning, and a sense of progress that enhances overall psychological well-being (Locke & Latham, 2002). Exercise environments provide ideal contexts for goal setting and achievement due to their measurable, progressive nature. Whether training for a marathon, working toward a personal weightlifting record, or simply aiming to exercise regularly, physical activity offers clear opportunities for setting specific, measurable, achievable, relevant, and time-bound (SMART) goals. The achievement of these goals provides powerful psychological rewards that extend beyond the immediate physical benefits of exercise.

The psychological concept of self-efficacy, one's belief in their ability to succeed in specific situations, is particularly relevant to understanding how exercise goal achievement influences emotional well-being (Bandura, 1997). Each successful exercise session and achieved fitness goal contributes to an individual's sense of personal capability and control. This enhanced self-efficacy often generalizes beyond exercise contexts, improving confidence and emotional resilience in other life domains. Mastery experiences, which involve successfully completing challenging tasks, represent one of the most powerful sources of self-efficacy development. Exercise provides numerous opportunities for mastery experiences, from completing a first 5K run to achieving a new personal record in the gym. These experiences create positive feedback loops that enhance motivation, confidence, and emotional well-being (McAuley et al., 2000).

The process of working toward long-term fitness goals also provides opportunities for developing important psychological skills such as persistence, discipline, and delayed gratification. These skills, developed through exercise practice, can enhance overall emotional regulation and life satisfaction. The ability to maintain commitment to long-term goals despite temporary setbacks or challenges is a crucial component of psychological resilience. Progress tracking and achievement recognition play important roles in maximizing the emotional benefits of exercise goal pursuit. Many successful exercisers maintain training logs, use fitness tracking devices, or participate in organized events that provide external recognition of their achievements. These practices help maintain motivation and provide concrete evidence of progress that reinforces positive emotions and sense of accomplishment.

Mind-Body Synergy Through Mindful Movement Practices

The integration of mindfulness principles with physical activity represents a particularly powerful approach to enhancing exercise's emotional benefits. Mindful movement practices, including yoga, Tai Chi, Qigong, and mindful walking or running, combine the physiological benefits of exercise with the psychological benefits of mindfulness meditation (Sharma et al., 2006a). Yoga, perhaps the most widely practiced form of mindful movement in Western cultures, provides a comprehensive system for integrating physical postures (asanas), breathing techniques (pranayama), and meditation. Research has consistently demonstrated that yoga practice produces significant improvements in mood, anxiety, stress, and overall emotional well-being (Goyal et al., 2014). The emphasis on present-moment awareness, acceptance, and non-judgmental observation helps practitioners develop enhanced emotional regulation skills that extend beyond the yoga mat. Tai Chi and Qigong, traditional Chinese practices that combine gentle, flowing movements with meditation and breathing techniques, have shown particular promise for emotional well-being among older adults and individuals with chronic health conditions. These practices emphasize balance, coordination, and inner awareness, providing low-impact options for individuals who may not be able to engage in more vigorous forms of exercise (Sharma et al., 2006a).

The integration of mindfulness principles into traditional exercise forms can enhance their emotional benefits significantly. Mindful running, for example, involves paying attention to breathing, body sensations, and environmental awareness while running, rather than focusing on pace or distance goals. This approach can transform running from a purely physical activity into a moving meditation that promotes stress reduction and emotional well-being (Cox et al., 2016). Breathing awareness represents a particularly important component of mindful movement practices. The conscious regulation of breathing during exercise can activate the parasympathetic nervous system, promoting relaxation and stress reduction even during physical exertion. This integration of breath awareness with movement creates a unique physiological state that maximizes both the physical and emotional benefits of exercise. The non-competitive, process-oriented nature of many mindful movement practices provides a refreshing contrast to achievement-focused exercise approaches. While goal achievement can certainly contribute to emotional well-being, the emphasis on acceptance, self-compassion, and present-moment awareness characteristic of mindful movement can be particularly beneficial for individuals struggling with perfectionism, body image issues, or exercise-related anxiety (Cramer et al., 2018).

SECTION 5: PRACTICAL APPLICATIONS AND LIFESTYLE INTEGRATION

Exercise Prescriptions for Mood Enhancement

The translation of research findings into practical exercise recommendations requires careful consideration of individual differences, preferences, and circumstances. While general guidelines provide useful starting points, the most effective exercise prescriptions for emotional well-being are those tailored to individual needs, goals, and constraints (Kandola et al., 2019). For individuals seeking to improve mood and reduce symptoms of depression, moderate-intensity aerobic exercise appears to provide optimal benefits. A prescription of 150 minutes per week of moderate-intensity activity, as recommended by major health organizations, serves as an excellent foundation (Piercy et al., 2018). This can be achieved through various combinations, such as 30 minutes of brisk walking five days per week, or three 50-minute sessions of cycling or swimming.

The timing of exercise sessions can significantly influence their emotional benefits. Morning exercise may be particularly beneficial for individuals struggling with depression, as it can help regulate circadian rhythms and provide energy and motivation for the day ahead (Rosenbaum et al., 2014). However, individual chronotypes (natural sleep-wake patterns) should be considered, as some individuals may derive greater benefits from afternoon or evening exercise sessions. For anxiety management, both aerobic and resistance training show significant benefits, with some research suggesting that resistance training may be particularly effective for reducing anxiety symptoms (Gordon et al., 2017b). A balanced program incorporating both modalities might include 2-3 resistance training sessions per week combined with 2-3 aerobic exercise sessions.

Individuals with severe depression or anxiety should consider starting with shorter, less intensive exercise sessions and gradually increasing duration and intensity as their condition improves and their fitness level increases. Even light activities such as gentle walking or stretching can provide meaningful emotional benefits for individuals beginning their exercise journey (Kandola et al., 2019). The concept of "exercise snacks", brief, intermittent bouts of physical activity throughout the day, has gained attention as a practical approach for busy individuals or those who find longer exercise sessions challenging. Research suggests that multiple short exercise sessions can provide cumulative benefits for both physical and emotional health (Biddle & Batterham, 2015).

Guidelines for Different Populations

Different populations have unique needs, constraints, and considerations that influence optimal exercise prescriptions for emotional well-being. Recognizing and addressing these differences is crucial for maximizing the effectiveness and accessibility of exercise interventions.

Students and Young Adults

Students face unique stressors including academic pressure, social challenges, and identity development issues that can significantly impact emotional well-being. Exercise programs for this population should emphasize stress management, social connection, and academic performance enhancement. Research indicates that regular exercise can improve cognitive function, memory, and academic performance while reducing stress and anxiety (Biddle & Batterham, 2015). Group-based activities such as intramural sports, fitness classes, or outdoor adventure programs can provide both physical benefits and social connection opportunities crucial for this developmental stage. High-intensity interval training may be particularly appealing to time-constrained students, providing efficient workouts that fit into busy schedules. Campus-based initiatives should focus on making exercise accessible, enjoyable, and social. Walking groups, outdoor fitness classes, and recreational sports leagues can create inclusive environments that accommodate varying fitness levels and interests (Eime et al., 2013b).

Working Professionals

Professional adults face unique challenges including work stress, time constraints, sedentary occupations, and work-life balance issues. Exercise prescriptions for this population must be realistic, time-efficient, and adaptable to varying schedules and energy levels. Workplace wellness programs that incorporate on-site fitness facilities, lunchtime walking groups, or standing/walking meetings can help integrate physical activity into the workday. Research demonstrates that employees who exercise regularly report higher job satisfaction, reduced stress, and improved work performance (Kandola et al., 2019). For busy professionals, home-based exercise options, early morning workouts, or brief exercise sessions during lunch breaks may be most practical. Technology-supported options such as fitness apps, online workout videos, or virtual personal training can provide flexibility and convenience while maintaining structure and guidance.

Older Adults

Older adults represent a population that can derive significant emotional benefits from exercise, but they also face unique considerations including physical limitations, chronic health conditions, and social isolation. Exercise programs for older adults should prioritize safety, social connection, and functional improvement while providing meaningful emotional benefits. Low-impact activities such as walking, swimming, Tai Chi, and chair-based exercises can provide significant emotional benefits while minimizing injury risk. The social aspects of exercise may be particularly important for older adults, as group activities can address isolation and provide valuable social support (Sharma et al., 2006b). Community-based programs such as senior center fitness classes, mall walking groups, or gardening clubs can provide structured, safe, and social exercise opportunities. The emphasis should be on enjoyment, social connection, and maintaining independence rather than intensive physical conditioning.

Clinical Populations

Individuals with diagnosed mental health conditions require specialized considerations for exercise programming. While exercise can serve as a valuable adjunct to traditional treatment approaches, it should not replace professional mental health care when indicated. For individuals with depression, exercise programs should start gradually and emphasize consistency over intensity. The social support aspect of group programs may be particularly beneficial, though some individuals may prefer individual activities initially. Regular monitoring and adjustment of exercise programs based on symptom severity and treatment response are essential (Firth et al., 2017). Individuals with anxiety disorders may benefit from exercise programs that emphasize stress reduction and relaxation. Mindful movement practices such as yoga or gentle aerobic activities may be particularly helpful. It's important to monitor for exercise-induced anxiety and adjust programs accordingly. Integration with existing treatment plans is crucial for clinical populations. Communication between exercise professionals, mental health providers, and healthcare teams ensures coordinated care and optimal outcomes.

Preventing Exercise-Related Burnout and Overtraining Anxiety

While exercise generally promotes emotional well-being, excessive training or unhealthy exercise behaviors can have negative psychological consequences. Understanding and preventing exercise-related psychological problems is crucial for maintaining the long-term emotional benefits of physical activity. Overtraining syndrome, characterized by decreased performance despite continued or increased training, can lead to significant psychological symptoms including mood disturbances, irritability, depression, and anxiety (Heyman, Gamelin, Goekint, Pisciella, et al., 2012)). Prevention strategies include adequate rest and recovery, varied training programs, and attention to early warning signs such as persistent fatigue, mood changes, or decreased motivation.

Exercise addiction or dependence, while relatively rare, can occur when exercise becomes compulsive and interferes with other life activities. Signs include inability to reduce exercise despite negative consequences, withdrawal symptoms when unable to exercise, and prioritizing exercise over important life responsibilities(Hausenblas & Symons Downs, 2002). Prevention involves maintaining balance, pursuing diverse activities and interests, and seeking professional help if exercise behaviors become concerning. Body dysmorphia and exercise-related anxiety can develop, particularly in gym environments or appearance-focused exercise contexts. Creating inclusive, non-judgmental exercise environments and emphasizing health and function over appearance can help prevent these issues. Education about realistic expectations and healthy body image is important for all exercise participants. Perfectionism in exercise contexts can undermine emotional benefits by creating unrealistic standards and self-criticism. Encouraging process-focused goals, self-compassion, and flexible thinking can help maintain healthy relationships with exercise. The emphasis should be on progress and effort rather than perfect performance or specific outcomes.

SECTION 6: FUTURE DIRECTIONS AND RESEARCH GAPS

Emerging Trends in Exercise-Based Emotional Interventions

The field of exercise psychology continues to evolve, with several emerging trends showing promise for enhancing the emotional benefits of physical activity. These developments reflect advancing technology, changing social patterns, and deepening understanding of the exercise-emotion relationship. Virtual and augmented reality technologies are beginning to transform exercise experiences by creating immersive environments that can enhance motivation, enjoyment, and emotional benefits. VR cycling through scenic landscapes, AR-enhanced running experiences, and gamified fitness applications can make exercise more engaging while potentially amplifying positive emotional responses (Neumann et al., 2018). These technologies may be particularly valuable for individuals who find traditional exercise environments intimidating or boring.

Precision exercise medicine represents another emerging frontier, using genetic testing, biomarker analysis, and advanced monitoring technologies to create highly individualized exercise prescriptions. Understanding how genetic variations influence exercise response could help optimize emotional benefits while minimizing adverse effects (Lightfoot et al., 2018). Wearable devices that monitor not only physical metrics but also stress levels, mood, and sleep quality are enabling more sophisticated approaches to exercise prescription and monitoring. Green exercise, physical activity performed in natural environments, is gaining recognition for its enhanced emotional benefits compared to indoor exercise. The combination of physical activity with nature exposure appears to provide synergistic benefits for stress reduction, mood enhancement, and overall well-being (Thompson Coon et al., 2011). Urban planning initiatives that prioritize green spaces and active transportation infrastructure reflect growing recognition of these benefits.

Exercise-based digital therapeutics represent a formalized approach to using technology-supported exercise interventions for mental health treatment. These evidence-based programs combine exercise prescriptions with behavioral support, progress monitoring, and outcome tracking through digital platforms (Firth et al., 2017). Regulatory approval pathways for digital therapeutics may soon make prescription exercise apps a reality in clinical practice.

The Need for Longitudinal and Cross-Cultural Studies

Current research on exercise and emotional well-being, while extensive, has several important limitations that future studies must address. Most existing research relies on short-term studies that may not capture the full scope of exercise's emotional benefits or potential negative effects. Longitudinal studies following individuals over months or years are needed to understand how exercise's emotional benefits develop, persist, and potentially change over time. The optimal duration and frequency of exercise needed to maintain emotional benefits remains poorly understood. While acute benefits of single exercise sessions are well-documented, the relationship between exercise consistency and long-term emotional well-being requires further investigation (Kandola et al., 2019). Understanding how breaks in exercise routines affect emotional well-being could inform more realistic and sustainable exercise recommendations. Cross-cultural research is particularly needed given that most exercise psychology research has been conducted in Western, educated, industrialized, rich, and democratic (WEIRD) populations (Henrich et al., 2010). Cultural values, social norms, and environmental factors significantly influence both exercise participation and emotional expression, yet these factors remain understudied. Research in diverse cultural contexts could reveal important variations in exercise's emotional benefits and optimal intervention approaches.

Age-related changes in exercise's emotional benefits represent another important research gap. While some research has examined exercise benefits across different age groups, longitudinal studies tracking the same individuals as they age could provide valuable insights into how exercise's emotional benefits change across the lifespan. This research could inform age-specific exercise recommendations and help optimize interventions for different life stages. Gender and sex differences in exercise's emotional benefits also require further investigation. While some studies have identified differences between males and females in exercise preferences and responses, the mechanisms underlying these differences and their implications for exercise prescription remain unclear (Ekkekakis & Lind, 2006). Research incorporating both biological sex and gender identity considerations is needed to ensure inclusive and effective exercise interventions.

Integrating Technology and Emotional Health Promotion

The integration of technology with exercise for emotional health promotion offers tremendous potential but also presents important challenges that must be addressed through continued research and development. Artificial intelligence and machine learning algorithms could potentially optimize exercise prescriptions by analyzing individual response patterns, preferences, and outcomes to create increasingly personalized interventions (Firth et al., 2017). Smartphone applications and wearable devices are already changing how people approach exercise and health monitoring. Future developments may include real-time mood monitoring that could trigger exercise recommendations during periods of emotional distress, or AI coaches that provide personalized motivation and support (Cavallo et al., 2012b). However, the effectiveness of these technological interventions compared to human-led programs requires systematic evaluation.

Social media and online communities present both opportunities and challenges for exercise-based emotional health promotion. While digital platforms can provide valuable support and motivation, they may also contribute to unhealthy comparison, body image issues, or exercise compulsion. Research is needed to understand how to harness the positive aspects of social technology while minimizing potential negative effects. Data privacy and security represent critical considerations as technology becomes more integrated with health and exercise monitoring. Ensuring that personal health and emotional data remain secure and are used ethically will be crucial for maintaining trust and participation in technology-supported exercise programs (Firth et al., 2017).

The digital divide, unequal access to technology based on socioeconomic status, age, or geographic location, could potentially exacerbate health disparities if technology-based interventions become standard without ensuring equitable access. Research and policy efforts must address these equity concerns to ensure that technological advances benefit all populations.

CONCLUSION

The journey from sweat to serenity represents one of humanity's most accessible and powerful pathways to emotional well-being. Through this comprehensive examination of exercise's effects on emotional health, we have explored the intricate neurochemical, psychological, and social mechanisms that transform physical movement into psychological transformation. The evidence overwhelmingly demonstrates that exercise serves not merely as a tool for physical conditioning but as a multifaceted intervention for enhancing emotional resilience, mood regulation, and overall life satisfaction. The neurochemical foundation of exercise's emotional benefits involves complex interactions between endorphins, endocannabinoids, and neurotransmitter systems that collectively promote positive mood states and reduce symptoms of anxiety and depression. These biological mechanisms work synergistically with psychological processes including enhanced self-efficacy, improved body image, and increased sense of mastery and accomplishment. The social dimensions of exercise, from team sports to fitness communities to online support networks, add additional layers of benefit through enhanced social connection, belonging, and mutual support. Different exercise modalities offer unique pathways to emotional well-being. Aerobic activities provide endurance-building benefits that extend to emotional resilience, while resistance training offers opportunities for strength-building and self-efficacy development that generalize beyond the gym. Hybrid programs and mindful movement practices combine multiple approaches to create comprehensive interventions that address various aspects of emotional health. The key insight is that there is no single "best" form of exercise for emotional well-being; rather, the optimal approach depends on individual preferences, needs, and circumstances.

Practical implementation of exercise for emotional health requires careful attention to individual differences, population-specific needs, and potential risks. While exercise offers tremendous benefits, it must be approached thoughtfully to prevent overtraining, exercise addiction, or other negative consequences. The integration of exercise with existing mental health treatments and the development of technology-supported interventions represent promising directions for expanding access and effectiveness. Future research must address current limitations through longitudinal studies, cross-cultural investigations, and more sophisticated approaches to personalization and precision. The emerging integration of technology with exercise interventions offers exciting possibilities but also requires careful evaluation to ensure effectiveness and equity.

Perhaps most importantly, this examination reveals that the relationship between exercise and emotional well-being is not merely correlational but fundamentally transformational. Regular physical activity does not simply provide temporary mood boosts; it creates lasting changes in brain structure and function, psychological skills and resources, and social connections that collectively enhance overall quality of life. The sweat produced during exercise represents not just metabolic byproducts but the tangible evidence of a process that builds emotional resilience, enhances mood regulation, and promotes psychological flourishing. As we move forward in our understanding and application of exercise for emotional health, we must remember that the ultimate goal is not just the absence of psychological distress but the cultivation of genuine well-being and human flourishing. Exercise, in its myriad forms and applications, offers a pathway accessible to most individuals regardless of age, fitness level, or circumstances. By embracing movement as medicine for both body and mind, we can help individuals and communities progress from the initial challenge of physical exertion to the lasting serenity of enhanced emotional well-being. The evidence is clear: the journey from sweat to serenity is not merely possible but achievable for those willing to take the first step. In a world facing unprecedented challenges to mental health and well-being, exercise stands as a beacon of hope, a scientifically validated, widely accessible, and profoundly transformative approach to building the emotional resilience our communities desperately need.

REFERENCES

Bandura, A. (1997). *Self-efficacy: The exercise of control* (pp. ix, 604). W H Freeman/Times Books/ Henry Holt & Co.

Baumeister, R. F., & Leary, M. R. (1995). The need to belong: Desire for interpersonal attachments as a fundamental human motivation. *Psychological Bulletin, 117*(3), 497–529. DOI: 10.1037/0033-2909.117.3.497 PMID: 7777651

Biddle, S. J. H., & Batterham, A. M. (2015). High-intensity interval exercise training for public health: A big HIT or shall we HIT it on the head? *The International Journal of Behavioral Nutrition and Physical Activity, 12*(1), 95. DOI: 10.1186/s12966-015-0254-9 PMID: 26187579

Boecker, H., Sprenger, T., Spilker, M. E., Henriksen, G., Koppenhoefer, M., Wagner, K. J., Valet, M., Berthele, A., & Tolle, T. R. (2008). The runner's high: Opioidergic mechanisms in the human brain. *Cerebral Cortex (New York, N.Y.: 1991), 18*(11), 2523–2531. https://doi.org/DOI: 10.1093/cercor/bhn013

Brymer, E., & Schweitzer, R. (2017). *Phenomenology and the Extreme Sport Experience*. Routledge., DOI: 10.4324/9781315661643

Cavallo, D. N., Tate, D. F., Ries, A. V., Brown, J. D., DeVellis, R. F., & Ammerman, A. S. (2012a). A social media-based physical activity intervention: A randomized controlled trial. *American Journal of Preventive Medicine, 43*(5), 527–532. DOI: 10.1016/j.amepre.2012.07.019 PMID: 23079176

Cavallo, D. N., Tate, D. F., Ries, A. V., Brown, J. D., DeVellis, R. F., & Ammerman, A. S. (2012b). A social media-based physical activity intervention: A randomized controlled trial. *American Journal of Preventive Medicine, 43*(5), 527–532. DOI: 10.1016/j.amepre.2012.07.019 PMID: 23079176

Chaouloff, F. (1997). Effects of acute physical exercise on central serotonergic systems. *Medicine and Science in Sports and Exercise, 29*(1), 58–62. DOI: 10.1097/00005768-199701000-00009 PMID: 9000156

Christakis, N. A., & Fowler, J. H. (2007). The spread of obesity in a large social network over 32 years. *The New England Journal of Medicine, 357*(4), 370–379. DOI: 10.1056/NEJMsa066082 PMID: 17652652

Cox, A. E., Ullrich-French, S., Cole, A. N., & D'Hondt-Taylor, M. (2016). The role of state mindfulness during yoga in predicting self-objectification and reasons for exercise. *Psychology of Sport and Exercise, 22*, 321–327. DOI: 10.1016/j.psychsport.2015.10.001

Cramer, H., Lauche, R., Anheyer, D., Pilkington, K., de Manincor, M., Dobos, G., & Ward, L. (2018). Yoga for anxiety: A systematic review and meta-analysis of randomized controlled trials. *Depression and Anxiety*, *35*(9), 830–843. DOI: 10.1002/da.22762 PMID: 29697885

Csikszentmihalyi, M. (2008). *Flow: The Psychology of Optimal Experience*. HarperCollins Publishers.

Diener, E., Oishi, S., & Tay, L. (2018). Advances in subjective well-being research. *Nature Human Behaviour*, *2*(4), 253–260. DOI: 10.1038/s41562-018-0307-6 PMID: 30936533

Dishman, R. K., Berthoud, H.-R., Booth, F. W., Cotman, C. W., Edgerton, V. R., Fleshner, M. R., Gandevia, S. C., Gomez-Pinilla, F., Greenwood, B. N., Hillman, C. H., Kramer, A. F., Levin, B. E., Moran, T. H., Russo-Neustadt, A. A., Salamone, J. D., Van Hoomissen, J. D., Wade, C. E., York, D. A., & Zigmond, M. J. (2006). Neurobiology of exercise. *Obesity (Silver Spring, Md.)*, *14*(3), 345–356. DOI: 10.1038/oby.2006.46 PMID: 16648603

Eime, R. M., Young, J. A., Harvey, J. T., Charity, M. J., & Payne, W. R. (2013a). A systematic review of the psychological and social benefits of participation in sport for children and adolescents: Informing development of a conceptual model of health through sport. *The International Journal of Behavioral Nutrition and Physical Activity*, *10*, 98. DOI: 10.1186/1479-5868-10-98 PMID: 23945179

Eime, R. M., Young, J. A., Harvey, J. T., Charity, M. J., & Payne, W. R. (2013b). A systematic review of the psychological and social benefits of participation in sport for children and adolescents: Informing development of a conceptual model of health through sport. *The International Journal of Behavioral Nutrition and Physical Activity*, *10*(1), 98. DOI: 10.1186/1479-5868-10-98 PMID: 23945179

Ekkekakis, P. (2003). Pleasure and displeasure from the body: Perspectives from exercise. *Cognition and Emotion*, *17*(2), 213–239. DOI: 10.1080/02699930302292 PMID: 29715726

Ekkekakis, P. (2013). *The measurement of affect, mood, and emotion: A guide for health-behavioral research* (pp. xxi, 206). Cambridge University Press. https://doi.org/DOI: 10.1017/CBO9780511820724

Ekkekakis, P., & Acevedo, E. O. (2006). Affective Responses to Acute Exercise: Toward a Psychobiological Dose-Response Model. In *Psychobiology of physical activity* (pp. 91–109). Human Kinetics.

Ekkekakis, P., & Lind, E. (2006). Exercise does not feel the same when you are overweight: The impact of self-selected and imposed intensity on affect and exertion. *International Journal of Obesity (2005), 30*(4), 652–660. https://doi.org/DOI: 10.1038/sj.ijo.0803052

Ekkekakis, P., & Russell, J. A. (2013). *The Measurement of Affect, Mood, and Emotion: A Guide for Health-Behavioral Research* (1st ed.). Cambridge University Press., DOI: 10.1017/CBO9780511820724

Erickson, K. I., Voss, M. W., Prakash, R. S., Basak, C., Szabo, A., Chaddock, L., Kim, J. S., Heo, S., Alves, H., White, S. M., Wojcicki, T. R., Mailey, E., Vieira, V. J., Martin, S. A., Pence, B. D., Woods, J. A., McAuley, E., & Kramer, A. F. (2011). Exercise training increases size of hippocampus and improves memory. *Proceedings of the National Academy of Sciences of the United States of America, 108*(7), 3017. DOI: 10.1073/pnas.1015950108 PMID: 21282661

Firth, J., Torous, J., Nicholas, J., Carney, R., Pratap, A., Rosenbaum, S., & Sarris, J. (2017). The efficacy of smartphone-based mental health interventions for depressive symptoms: A meta-analysis of randomized controlled trials. *World Psychiatry; Official Journal of the World Psychiatric Association (WPA), 16*(3), 287–298. DOI: 10.1002/wps.20472 PMID: 28941113

Goldfarb, A. H., & Jamurtas, A. Z. (1997). Beta-endorphin response to exercise. An update. *Sports Medicine (Auckland, N.Z.), 24*(1), 8–16. DOI: 10.2165/00007256-199724010-00002 PMID: 9257407

Gordon, B. R., McDowell, C. P., Hallgren, M., Meyer, J. D., Lyons, M., & Herring, M. P. (2018). Association of Efficacy of Resistance Exercise Training With Depressive Symptoms: Meta-analysis and Meta-regression Analysis of Randomized Clinical Trials. *JAMA Psychiatry, 75*(6), 566–576. DOI: 10.1001/jamapsychiatry.2018.0572 PMID: 29800984

Gordon, B. R., McDowell, C. P., Lyons, M., & Herring, M. P. (2017a). The Effects of Resistance Exercise Training on Anxiety: A Meta-Analysis and Meta-Regression Analysis of Randomized Controlled Trials. *Sports Medicine (Auckland, N.Z.), 47*(12), 2521–2532. DOI: 10.1007/s40279-017-0769-0 PMID: 28819746

Gordon, B. R., McDowell, C. P., Lyons, M., & Herring, M. P. (2017b). The Effects of Resistance Exercise Training on Anxiety: A Meta-Analysis and Meta-Regression Analysis of Randomized Controlled Trials. *Sports Medicine (Auckland, N.Z.), 47*(12), 2521–2532. DOI: 10.1007/s40279-017-0769-0 PMID: 28819746

Goyal, M., Singh, S., Sibinga, E. M. S., Gould, N. F., Rowland-Seymour, A., Sharma, R., Berger, Z., Sleicher, D., Maron, D. D., Shihab, H. M., Ranasinghe, P. D., Linn, S., Saha, S., Bass, E. B., & Haythornthwaite, J. A. (2014). Meditation programs for psychological stress and well-being: A systematic review and meta-analysis. *JAMA Internal Medicine*, *174*(3), 357–368. DOI: 10.1001/jamainternmed.2013.13018 PMID: 24395196

Greenwood, B. N., Foley, T. E., Le, T. V., Strong, P. V., Loughridge, A. B., Day, H. E. W., & Fleshner, M. (2011). Long-term voluntary wheel running is rewarding and produces plasticity in the mesolimbic reward pathway. *Behavioural Brain Research*, *217*(2), 354–362. DOI: 10.1016/j.bbr.2010.11.005 PMID: 21070820

Hausenblas, H. A., & Symons Downs, D. (2002). Exercise dependence: A systematic review. *Psychology of Sport and Exercise*, *3*(2), 89–123. DOI: 10.1016/S1469-0292(00)00015-7

Heinrich, K. M., Patel, P. M., O'Neal, J. L., & Heinrich, B. S. (2014). High-intensity compared to moderate-intensity training for exercise initiation, enjoyment, adherence, and intentions: An intervention study. *BMC Public Health*, *14*, 789. DOI: 10.1186/1471-2458-14-789 PMID: 25086646

Henrich, J., Heine, S. J., & Norenzayan, A. (2010). The weirdest people in the world? *Behavioral and Brain Sciences*, *33*(2–3), 61–83. DOI: 10.1017/S0140525X0999152X PMID: 20550733

Heyman, E., Gamelin, F., Goekint, M., Pisciella, P., Roelands, B., Leclair, E., Di Marzo, V., & Meeusen, R. (2012). Intense exercise increases circulating endocannabinoid and BDNF levels in humans-Possible implications for reward and depression. Psychoneuroendocrinology. 37(6): 844-851, 2012. SCI: - 5.168 –. *Psychoneuroendocrinology*, *37*, 844–851. PMID: 22029953

Heyman, E., Gamelin, F.-X., Goekint, M., Piscitelli, F., Roelands, B., Leclair, E., Di Marzo, V., & Meeusen, R. (2012). Intense exercise increases circulating endocannabinoid and BDNF levels in humans—Possible implications for reward and depression. *Psychoneuroendocrinology*, *37*(6), 844–851. DOI: 10.1016/j.psyneuen.2011.09.017 PMID: 22029953

Kandola, A., Ashdown-Franks, G., Hendrikse, J., Sabiston, C. M., & Stubbs, B. (2019). Physical activity and depression: Towards understanding the antidepressant mechanisms of physical activity. *Neuroscience and Biobehavioral Reviews*, *107*, 525–539. DOI: 10.1016/j.neubiorev.2019.09.040 PMID: 31586447

Lee, I.-M., Shiroma, E. J., Lobelo, F., Puska, P., Blair, S. N., & Katzmarzyk, P. T.Lancet Physical Activity Series Working Group. (2012). Effect of physical inactivity on major non-communicable diseases worldwide: An analysis of burden of disease and life expectancy. *Lancet, 380*(9838), 219–229. DOI: 10.1016/S0140-6736(12)61031-9 PMID: 22818936

Lightfoot, J. T., & Geus, DE, E. J. C., Booth, F. W., Bray, M. S., DEN Hoed, M., Kaprio, J., Kelly, S. A., Pomp, D., Saul, M. C., Thomis, M. A., Garland, T., & Bouchard, C. (2018). Biological/Genetic Regulation of Physical Activity Level: Consensus from GenBioPAC. *Medicine and Science in Sports and Exercise, 50*(4), 863–873. DOI: 10.1249/MSS.0000000000001499 PMID: 29166322

Liu-Ambrose, T., Nagamatsu, L. S., Graf, P., Beattie, B. L., Ashe, M. C., & Handy, T. C. (2010). Resistance Training and Executive Functions: A 12-Month Randomised Controlled Trial. *Archives of Internal Medicine, 170*(2), 170–178. DOI: 10.1001/archinternmed.2009.494 PMID: 20101012

Locke, E. A., & Latham, G. P. (2002). Building a practically useful theory of goal setting and task motivation: A 35-year odyssey. *The American Psychologist, 57*(9), 705–717. DOI: 10.1037/0003-066X.57.9.705 PMID: 12237980

McAuley, E., Blissmer, B., Marquez, D. X., Jerome, G. J., Kramer, A. F., & Katula, J. (2000). Social relations, physical activity, and well-being in older adults. *Preventive Medicine, 31*(5), 608–617. DOI: 10.1006/pmed.2000.0740 PMID: 11071843

Mikkelsen, K., Stojanovska, L., Polenakovic, M., Bosevski, M., & Apostolopoulos, V. (2017). Exercise and mental health. *Maturitas, 106*, 48–56. DOI: 10.1016/j.maturitas.2017.09.003 PMID: 29150166

Morgan, W. P., & Goldston, S. E. (1987). *Exercise and Mental Health*. Hemisphere Publishing Corporation.

Neumann, D. L., Moffitt, R. L., Thomas, P. R., Loveday, K., Watling, D. P., Lombard, C. L., Antonova, S., & Tremeer, M. A. (2018). A systematic review of the application of interactive virtual reality to sport. *Virtual Reality (Waltham Cross), 22*(3), 183–198. DOI: 10.1007/s10055-017-0320-5

Oberlin, L. E., Verstynen, T. D., Burzynska, A. Z., Voss, M. W., Prakash, R. S., Chaddock-Heyman, L., Wong, C., Fanning, J., Awick, E., Gothe, N., Phillips, S. M., Mailey, E., Ehlers, D., Olson, E., Wojcicki, T., McAuley, E., Kramer, A. F., & Erickson, K. I. (2016). White matter microstructure mediates the relationship between cardiorespiratory fitness and spatial working memory in older adults. *NeuroImage, 131*, 91–101. DOI: 10.1016/j.neuroimage.2015.09.053 PMID: 26439513

Piercy, K. L., Troiano, R. P., Ballard, R. M., Carlson, S. A., Fulton, J. E., Galuska, D. A., George, S. M., & Olson, R. D. (2018). The Physical Activity Guidelines for Americans. *Journal of the American Medical Association, 320*(19), 2020–2028. DOI: 10.1001/jama.2018.14854 PMID: 30418471

Raichlen, D. A., Foster, A. D., Gerdeman, G. L., Seillier, A., & Giuffrida, A. (2012). Wired to run: Exercise-induced endocannabinoid signaling in humans and cursorial mammals with implications for the "runner's high.". *The Journal of Experimental Biology, 215*(Pt 8), 1331–1336. DOI: 10.1242/jeb.063677 PMID: 22442371

Reed, J., & Buck, S. (2009). The effect of regular aerobic exercise on positive-activated affect: A meta-analysis. *Psychology of Sport and Exercise, 10*(6), 581–594. DOI: 10.1016/j.psychsport.2009.05.009

Romain, A. J., Marleau, J., & Baillot, A. (2018). Impact of obesity and mood disorders on physical comorbidities, psychological well-being, health behaviours and use of health services. *Journal of Affective Disorders, 225*, 381–388. DOI: 10.1016/j.jad.2017.08.065 PMID: 28846960

Rosenbaum, S., Tiedemann, A., Sherrington, C., Curtis, J., & Ward, P. B. (2014). Physical activity interventions for people with mental illness: A systematic review and meta-analysis. *The Journal of Clinical Psychiatry, 75*(9), 964–974. DOI: 10.4088/JCP.13r08765 PMID: 24813261

Rosenbaum, S., Vancampfort, D., Steel, Z., Newby, J., Ward, P. B., & Stubbs, B. (2015). Physical activity in the treatment of Post-traumatic stress disorder: A systematic review and meta-analysis. *Psychiatry Research, 230*(2), 130–136. DOI: 10.1016/j.psychres.2015.10.017 PMID: 26500072

Schoenfeld, T. J., Rada, P., Pieruzzini, P. R., Hsueh, B., & Gould, E. (2013). Physical exercise prevents stress-induced activation of granule neurons and enhances local inhibitory mechanisms in the dentate gyrus. *The Journal of Neuroscience : The Official Journal of the Society for Neuroscience, 33*(18), 7770–7777. DOI: 10.1523/JNEUROSCI.5352-12.2013 PMID: 23637169

Seguin, R. A., Eldridge, G., Graham, M. L., Folta, S. C., Nelson, M. E., & Strogatz, D. (2016). Strong Hearts, healthy communities: A rural community-based cardiovascular disease prevention program. *BMC Public Health, 16*, 86. DOI: 10.1186/s12889-016-2751-4 PMID: 26822982

Seligman, M. E., & Csikszentmihalyi, M. (2000). Positive psychology. An introduction. *The American Psychologist, 55*(1), 5–14. DOI: 10.1037//0003-066x.55.1.5 PMID: 11392865

Sharma, A., Madaan, V., & Petty, F. D. (2006). Exercise for mental health. *Primary Care Companion to the Journal of Clinical Psychiatry*, *8*(2), 106. DOI: 10.4088/pcc.v08n0208a PMID: 16862239

Sparling, P. B., Giuffrida, A., Piomelli, D., Rosskopf, L., & Dietrich, A. (2003). Exercise activates the endocannabinoid system. *Neuroreport*, *14*(17), 2209–2211. DOI: 10.1097/00001756-200312020-00015 PMID: 14625449

Stork, M. J., Banfield, L. E., Gibala, M. J., & Martin Ginis, K. A. (2017). A scoping review of the psychological responses to interval exercise: Is interval exercise a viable alternative to traditional exercise? *Health Psychology Review*, *11*(4), 324–344. DOI: 10.1080/17437199.2017.1326011 PMID: 28460601

Thompson Coon, J., Boddy, K., Stein, K., Whear, R., Barton, J., & Depledge, M. H. (2011). Does participating in physical activity in outdoor natural environments have a greater effect on physical and mental wellbeing than physical activity indoors? A systematic review. *Environmental Science & Technology*, *45*(5), 1761–1772. DOI: 10.1021/es102947t PMID: 21291246

Wegner, M., Helmich, I., Machado, S., Nardi, A. E., Arias-Carrion, O., & Budde, H. (2014). Effects of exercise on anxiety and depression disorders: Review of meta- analyses and neurobiological mechanisms. *CNS & Neurological Disorders - Drug Targets*, *13*(6), 1002–1014. DOI: 10.2174/1871527313666140612102841 PMID: 24923346

Welk, G. J., Welk, G., Corbin, W. R., & Welk, K. A. (2023). *Corbin's concepts of fitness and wellness: A comprehensive lifestyle approach* (13th ed.). McGraw Hill.

Whiteman-Sandland, J., Hawkins, J., & Clayton, D. (2018). The role of social capital and community belongingness for exercise adherence: An exploratory study of the CrossFit gym model. *Journal of Health Psychology*, *23*(12), 1545–1556. DOI: 10.1177/1359105316664132 PMID: 27553606

World Health Organization. (2021). *Mental disorders*. https://www.who.int/news-room/fact-sheets/detail/mental-disorders

Zanto, T. P., & Gazzaley, A. (2013). Fronto-parietal network: Flexible hub of cognitive control. *Trends in Cognitive Sciences*, *17*(12), 602–603. DOI: 10.1016/j.tics.2013.10.001 PMID: 24129332

Chapter 10
Effect of Exercise on Academic Functioning

Manu Mehrotra
https://orcid.org/0009-0003-4841-1589
Sharda University, Agra, India

Manish Baboo Agarwal
https://orcid.org/0000-0003-1177-2738
Sharda University, Agra, India

Seema Agarwal
https://orcid.org/0000-0002-5655-207X
SRM Institute of Science and Technology, Ghaziabad, India

Hemlata Jain
Sharda University Agra, India

ABSTRACT

Regular physical activity has a useful impact on both learning and health and contributes significantly to academic progress. The main goal of studying the relationship between exercise and academic performance is to provide appropriate guidance to trainers, policy makers and health practitioners to incorporate physical activity into the education system. The main issue is to implement the most suitable type of exercise which can improve academic performance and learning without causing negative impact on the performance. On a biological level, movement encourages the birth of new neurons and increases blood circulation in the brain, which together facilitate memory strengthening and help us manage stress. Recent, research shows that a modest daily dose of movement, of a few minutes, is more powerful

DOI: 10.4018/979-8-3373-6157-4.ch010

for boosting cognitive and academic capabilities. Thus, the challenge is to promote regular activity while defending academic outcomes, reinforcing the necessity for schools to weave exercise into daily lesson plans instead of offering it as an add-on.

1. INTRODUCTION

Research repeatedly shows the role of consistent physical activity in achieving stronger academic outcomes in every area. When school cultures reinforce the belief that achievement is within reach, students feel more able to pursue rigorous course work. Exercise, in turn, sharpens memory, bolsters attention and elevates creative problem solving, all of which translate into measurable classroom gains. Therefore, educators, administrators and public health professionals must take it into account when planning learning environments that nurture both intellectual and physical well-being.

Schools that embed regular movement into everyday schedules are doing far more than promoting fitness. They are fortifying student's minds and bodies simultaneously. When physical activity becomes routine, grades rise up, attendance improves and students report become better overall. Evidence based programs, produce learners who are resilient, inquisitive and well rounded a conclusion that new research continue to reaffirm.

Studies show that even a small boost in daily activity can lift academic performance. Researchers at North Carolina State University discovered that adding just one extra hour of exercise each week nudged average GPAs up by 0.06 points, just enough to increase up final course grades.

Crucially, the outcome remained true even after accounting for individual students earlier GPAs and standardized test performance, signaling that movement produces a distinct and potent influence on teaching and learning (Sanderson et al., 2017).

1.1 Purpose and Goals of the Study

This study examines how physical activity affects grades and test scores and explores several closely related aims. The goal is to equip teachers, coaches and school leaders so as to guide for integrating physical activity into the school daily. The key to this is identifying the exact types, intensities and durations of movement that can enhance learning without encroaching on instructional time or provoking the fatigue that can hinder academic performance. Research shows that short, carefully timed daily workouts ideally 30 to 60 minutes long and delivered at moderate to vigorous rate bring the largest boosts to brain function and academic performance (Du et al., 2023).

This focused strategy promotes better mental flexibility, sharper attention, stronger memory consolidation and improved stress management, all of which provide a solid foundation for educational achievement. In addition, growing evidence indicates that cognitive function is the main mechanism through which exercise leads to a solid foundation for academic excellence.

When students participate in regular moderate exercises, their essential mental problem solving, information retention, sustained focus and impulse control experience a measurable growth, resulting in improved academic outcomes. In one key study, participants who completed sixty minute exercise sessions five times a week not only recorded gains in cardiovascular fitness but also achieved better cognitive test scores, which directly correlated with elevated final grades. Cognitive enhancements count for about 91 percent of the connection between aerobic exercise and students' academic success, underlining how vital neuro-biological changes are to the body (Gomez Pinilla & Hillman, 2012). Curiously, the benefits tend to plateau or even reverse whenever the weekly exertion exceeds two hours, highlighting the need how too much intensity can prompt the fatigue and burn out that erodes active learning gains. By boosting cerebral blood flow, aerobic activity ensures a richer supply of oxygen and nutrients to neural tissues, which in turn aids memory consolidation and mitigates the release of stress hormones (Vecchio et al., 2018). The resulting adjustments in neurochemical balance and cerebral temperature cultivate a brain environment that favors learning, strengthen information acquisition and academic task management. Therefore, exercise is far from optional, it is an essential driver of brain vitality that produces measurable gains in academic achievement.

Additionally, physical activity benefits multiple areas that support learning, beyond just fitness. Studies show that just the right dose of steady exercise reduces the number of classroom interruptions, increases the length of time spent on tasks and sharpens self regulation. These gains create a classroom culture where focus can be maintained and students are more likely to participate fully. Emotionally, regular physical activity tends to reduce anxiety, smooth out mood fluctuations and enhance self confidence. Researchers connect all these changes to better academic outcomes (Ghahramani et al., 2016). Together, these elements create a classroom environment in which students are better prepared to tackle academic demands and more inclined to pursue learning for their own sake.

The main focus of schools is to find ways to add more physical activities into their already packed tight schedule. The link between exercise, student health and sharper thinking is clear, but the trick is to fit enough movement into the day without shortening the time available for the core subjects.

Solving the issue, depends on solid data and on creating well tested curricular designs that deliver exercise in brief, engaging the students while protecting instructional integrity throughout the day. Recent advances in data mining and supervised learning have begun to clarify how discrete elements of exercise specifically, the combinatorial patterns of its incidence, duration and intensity correlate with academic performance, thus guiding the design of more precise physical education frameworks.

2. IMPACT OF EXERCISE ON LEARNING AND HEALTH

Regular physical activity is demonstrably intertwined with cognitive, emotional and physical well being, thus rendering it central to the holistic academic formation of adolescents and emerging adults. A growing stream of empirical data indicates that consistent exercise augments cardiovascular fitness and regulatory systems, both of which co-activate and enhance cognitive processing speed, selective attention, working memory and over arching executive functions capacities that mediate the encoding and application of curricular content (Roig Hierro et al., 2025).

2.1 Influence of Physical Activity on Cognitive Functions and Academic Achievement

Exercising appears to promote several cognitive functions that are directly useful in educational contexts. Research indicates that daily activity sessions lasting one to two hours yield enhancements in several dimensions of cognition, including processing speed and attention, as well as functions requiring inhibition, cognitive flexibility and updates of working memory. These domains of cognition have known correlation with class room behavior and standardized test scores (Festa et al., 2023). A meta-analysis of both single and multi session activity protocols highlights that brief, isolated bouts yield immediate gains in processing speed, attention and inhibition, while sustained programmes are associated with improvements in complex functions such as cognitive flexibility, verbal working memory and language skills. Among these, working memory showed the most pronounced change, suggesting that habitual physical activity reinforces the capacity to temporarily hold and manipulate information, thus facilitating more efficient information processing in academic settings (Borrega Alonso & Otamendi, 2025).

Exercise exerts a significant influence on cognition primarily through enhancements in physical fitness, which improve cerebral circulation and oxygen supply to neuronal tissues. Higher cardiovascular conditioning spurs elevated neurogenesis in the hippocampus the key region for memory consolidation and retrieval. This neurobiological shift accelerates and streamlines cognitive processing, producing sharper problem solving, stronger memory retention and greater cognitive flexibility. Research indicates that the cognitive boost resulting from these physiological changes explains over 90% of the exercise linked gains in academic performance. This finding singles out cognitive enhancement as the leading mechanism by which regular physical activity translates into better educational outcomes. At the same time, the separate advantages of improved cardiovascular function and greater muscular strength reinforce the tight link between a vigorous physiological profile and amplified cognitive capability.

The relationship between how long students are active and how they perform academically is complex but important. Research consistently shows that between sixty and one hundred twenty minutes of moderate to vigorous exercise each day leads to the sharpest academic gains. When students exceed that range particularly beyond one hundred twenty minutes academic benefits tend to plateau and in some studies, dip slightly. Scholars attribute this drop to fatigue and inadequate recovery, reinforcing the need to craft exercise schedules that boost academic performance without risking overtraining or cutting too deeply into instructional time.

From a health perspective, regular physical activity strengthens the body and reduces anxiety, both of which prepare students to learn more effectively. Engaging in movement lowers overall anxiety, calms the stress response, lifts mood through hormones such as endorphins and norepinephrine and enhances students' students overall academics. These psychological and social gains combine to create a class room climate where young people are more focused, more willing to participate and better at self regulating their behavior all of which are essential for sustained academic achievement (Mahindru et al., 2023). For example, sustained programs that integrate movement into the school day have shown that better behavior reduces the number of disciplinary referrals, which in turn allows teachers to cover the material more thoroughly and students to absorb it more deeply.

When schools integrate physical activity into the daily routine, the benefits extends far beyond sharper minds. Students become fitter, more engaged and are less likely to miss school. Graduation rates improve alongside cardiovascular health. Whether measured by a stronger heart or a more adaptable brain the results are evident. As longer attention spans, there is a deeper drive to learn and greater persistence in completing tasks whether in science clubs or finishing any textbook. Figure1 shows various impacts of physical exercise on human body.

Figure 1. Impact of physical exercise

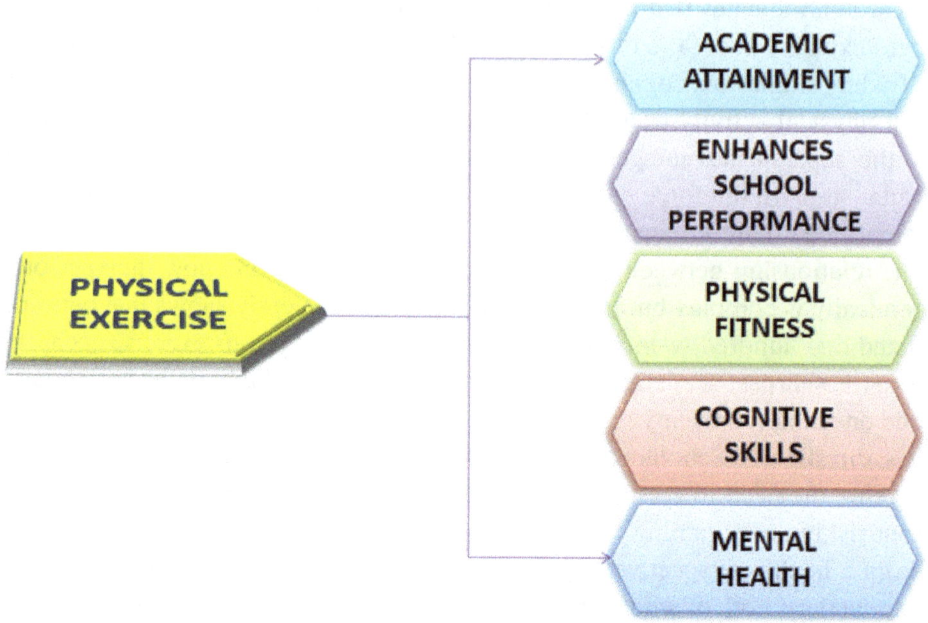

Yet, even with the data backing the link, fitting regular activity into the school day stays a tricky puzzle for planners and teachers alike. Schedules must slot in exercises so that it sparks the day instead of draining the next period (Mavilidi et al., 2019). Research on how the body and brain bounce back across the periods shows how to pack short, focused bursts of activity. When these carefully timed segments are implemented effectively, they lock in lasting cognitive benefits, prevent burn out and the scramble for instructional edges resulting in both stronger bodies and better grades.

3. EXERCISE IMPLEMENTATION IN EDUCATIONAL SYSTEMS

Effective integration of structured physical activity into schools requires clear, evidence based recommendations for coaches, leaders and curriculum planners. Activity types should be selected to match students' physical maturity and available resources and with specific targets set for the duration and intensity of student participation. Oversight by qualified staff is essential to reduce the risk of injury and to fine tune work-loads ensuring that safety and healthy neurophysiological development can occur in tandem.

3.1 Recommendations for Administrators and Policymakers

School leaders and education policy makers play a critical role in designing and maintaining coherent, standards driven physical education curricula. The National Association for Sport and Physical Education recommends that elementary grades receive a minimum of 150 minutes of dedicated instructional time per week while middle and high school programs should receive at least 225 minutes. The committee clearly states that the time for physical education must be clearly marked, separate from relaxed breaks or unstructured play (Kilby, 1985).

Both law and district policy must affirm that physical education cannot be dismissed or replaced in the curriculum cycle, or removed from it. This ensures that every student has the equal, non-negotiable opportunities for essential movement. Teacher credentialing regulations must require certification in physical education and continuous professional learning must be mandated to preserve instructional quality. Local districts may tailor programming to reflect community contexts, yet all variations should secure a minimum of 50% of lesson time spent in moderate to vigorous physical activity (MVPA) as a best practice bench mark (Vedøy et al., 2020).

3.2 Types and Duration of Exercise Suitable for Students

Physical education curricula should present a spectrum of movement activities that foster enduring habitual exercise rather than simply honing competitive sports abilities. The recommended approach includes prolonged aerobic sessions, progressive resistance exercises for the musculoskeletal system and weight bearing activities, each matched to the learners' growth stage. Research confirms that short, repeated bursts of moderate to vigorous aerobic effort and lessons that blend movement with cognitive tasks consistently heighten joy and improve cardio pulmonary and strength results.

Activity schedules ought to follow NASPE guidelines. Children in early grades should engage 150 minutes of movement each week, while older pupils should increase this to 225 minutes, spaced over at least three to four days. This strategic distribution offers consistent chances for both the body and brain to adapt, avoids the pitfalls of over exertion and protects the flow of teaching (Fernandes & Sturm, 2011). Accordingly, schools should refrain from counting recess as part of this total, instead prioritizing well planned physical education classes and supervised extra-curricular activities that maintain the necessary intensity and instructional coherence.

3.3 The Role of Trained Personnel in Exercise Programs

Trained supervision remains essential to harness the full benefits of activity while protecting student safety and well being. Licensed physical educators and certified trainers possess the expertise to match movement tasks to diverse abilities and health levels, adjust drills to reduce the risk of injury and cultivate a climate in which every student feels included, respected and eager to engage (Neil Sztramko et al., 2021).

Regular and purposeful staff training keeps those leaders informed about the latest effective practices. For example, trainers can eliminate long periods of sitting by substituting modified games and they can integrate fitness focused drills into the typical PE unit plan. Thoughtful supervision also means that teachers and trainers continually observe, record and reflect on how each student is doing physically and mentally. They then adjust the length and intensity of every activity so that no student suffers fatigue, burnout, or drop in academic performance (Magallanes, 2024). When combined, these findings suggest that well organized physical activity programs can effectively sharpen students' thinking skills, raise their academic performance and enhance their overall well-being.

4. PHYSIOLOGICAL AND COGNITIVE BENEFITS OF EXERCISE

Regular physical activity produces significant effects on both the body and the brain, fostering improved memory, heightened learning capacity and stronger management of stress that are key drivers of academic and intellectual achievement. These effects originate from a tightly knit series of mechanisms, among them, the birth of new neurons, better blood flow through the brain and sharpening of higher order cognitive functions such as flexible thinking, memory retention, rapid information processing and control of impulses.

4.1 Neurogenesis and Cerebral Perfusion

The careful coordination of continued training, reflective supervision and curricular integration creates physical activity frameworks that significantly boost students' mental sharpness, academic success and overall well-being.

Perhaps the most striking physiological benefit of regular movement is the acceleration of neurogenesis in the hippocampus, the region central to forming and stabilizing new memories. Sustained aerobic exercise heightens the release of molecules that nourish brain growth, most critically brain-derived neurotrophic factor (BDNF). BDNF helps young neural precursor cells develop into mature neurons, shields existing neurons from stress and refines the efficiency of synaptic transmission.

As BDNF level rises, the brain's plasticity improves, enabling it to reorganize and adapt more readily. This process spurs the formation of extra dendritic spines and expands the neural circuits that store and retrieve memories (Sanaeifar et al., 2024).

During exercise, muscles and other tissues release a surge of signaling molecules, the most important of which is the ketone body DBHB. DBHB crosses the blood-brain barrier with ease and displaces the enzyme histone deacetylase, which would otherwise suppress further BDNF production. By blocking that enzyme, DBHB lifts BDNF concentrations, which in turn strengthens synapses and boosts the generation of new neurons. Neuro-imaging studies reinforce these laboratory findings, showing measurable enlargements of the hippocampus and cortex, consistent thickening of the cortical sheet and clear correlations between these anatomical changes and better performance on tests of episodic memory and executive function (Sleiman et al., 2016).

At the same time, elevated cerebral blood flow (CBF) during exercise ensures that neurons receive the extra oxygen and fuel they demand, keeping pace with the greater energetic and signaling needs of high-level cognition. The provision of sustained, augmented CBF is indispensable for fostering the angiogenic, neurogenic and glymphatic processes that secure long term integrity of cognition (Ogoh et al., 2014).

4.2 Enhancement of Memory Consolidation and Stress Management

Regular aerobic exercise smooth's the pathways that support thinking. It raises levels of brain derived neurotrophic factor (BDNF), which helps transfer better experiences into lasting memories. This, together with the growth of new neurons in the hippocampus and stronger connections between brain cells, translates into better performance on tasks that involve finding one's way, learning new languages and remembering fresh material. For students and other learners, the capacity to reinforce newly encountered material and convert it into long lasting knowledge offers a decisive edge in academic performance.

Further, exercise functions as a preventive and rehabilitative agent for psychosocial stress. The ketone body β-hydroxybutyrate (DBHB) and related exercise generated metabolites not only stimulate neurogenesis but also counteract neuro inflammatory cascades in the hippocampus that provoke stressful experiences. At the same time, the surge of endorphins and the balanced modulation of dopamine and serotonin systems during physical activity reduce feelings of anxiety and mood disruptions. Lower perceived stress then supports cognitive flexibility, expands working memory and sharpens problem solving capabilities, enabling students to meet academic demands with increased adaptability and effectiveness (Ren & Xiao, 2023).

4.3 Support of Problem-Solving Capacity, Memory Retention, Mental Agility and Self-Regulatory Control

Exercise enriches the advanced cognitive processes essential for academic achievement namely, problem solving, memory retention, mental agility and self-regulatory control. These capacities rely on the health of prefrontal and hippocampal circuits, networks whose architecture and activity are progressively reinforced by consistent physical training (Davranche et al., 2014).

Regular doses of moderate intensity aerobic exercise sharpen the brain's executive functions. Supervising distractions becomes easier, the brain shifts quickly between tasks and working memory, enabling us to keep and juggle ideas more effectively. Together, these self-control gains, fuel sharper, steady the focus with greater grit when the school works spikes. Concurrently, mental agility, the rapid assimilation and synthesis of novel information, is accelerated by exercise induced neuro-plasticity and enhanced inter regional connectivity among the prefrontal cortex, basal ganglia and hippocampus.

Collectively, sustained physical activity cultivates a neuro-physiological environment that is highly favorable for durable learning, greater neurogenesis and expanded synaptic architecture and optimized neuro-chemical environments. These underlying changes are evident in observable performance gains and improved educational out comes. However, the magnitude of the benefits is contingent upon several critical parameters including training intensity, session frequency, exercise duration and activity type as well as individual variables such as baseline fitness and developmental stage. Figure 2 shows physiological and coginitive benefits of exercise.

Figure 2. Physiological and coginitive benefits of exercise

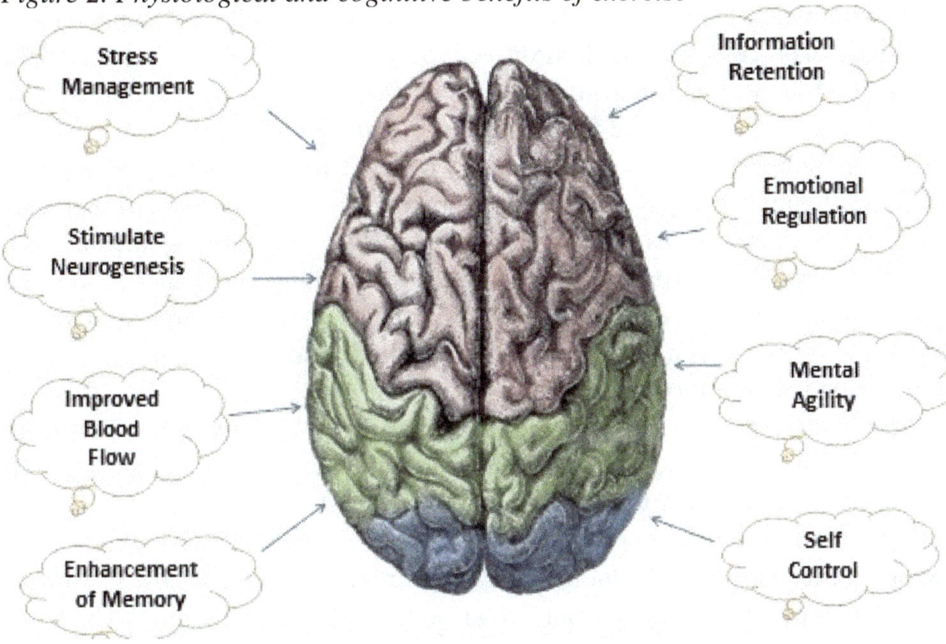

5. OPTIMAL EXERCISE INTENSITY AND DURATION

To get the most of this brain boost, the blend of exercise dose and intensity must remain in balance. Short and moderate sessions every day are more affective, while long, very hard workouts can blunt academic gains. Evidence from a series of recent meta analyses and field studies converges on the conclusion that constrained, regular physical activity enhances executive control, improves classroom engagement and raises academic achievement, all without encroaching on study time or inducing cumulative fatigue (Zhou et al., 2024).

5.1 Advantages of Moderate, Brief Daily Sessions

Recent studies suggest that performing daily moderate intensity exercise lasting 16 to 60 minutes produces maximal cognitive and academic benefits. The most effective approach to exercise for supporting academic success harmonizes moderate intensity with brief durations. Brief daily sessions of around 16 to 26 minutes produce the greatest gains, whereas longer or more strenuous workouts can inadvertently undermine academic performance. In a recent study of university learners, the greatest statistical relationship with elevated grades was seen for bouts of this limited duration, a finding attributed to gains in aerobic capacity and improvement of self-control processes that underlie effective study (Alfaro Chaverri et al., 2025). The specified duration and intensity produce sufficient cardiovascular stimulus while leaving energy stores adequate for subsequent cognitive challenges.

Corresponding investigations consistently indicate that an accumulated duration of 150 to 225 minutes of physical activity per week ideally distributed over at least three to five distinct sessions maximizes academic achievement among students from elementary through secondary school. When the same thing is applied to school age pupils, results include sharper attentional focus, improved retention across varied information types and enhanced executive control skills such as adaptive reasoning and the selective inhibition of inappropriate responses.

The cognitive gains from moderate intensity aerobic activity derive first from enhanced brain blood flow, which raises oxygen and glucose levels and second from heightened neurogenic activity in the hippocampus. These physiological changes strengthen the neural systems underlying learning and memory, effectively converting time spent exercising into better academic performance. Studies show that short, intense bursts of activity have encouraging results in educational settings. Evidence suggests that students can reach the equivalent of 50 minutes of activity per week, or take part in daily sessions lasting less than 30 minutes and still boost grades without disrupting the curriculum. These easy to implement bursts also improve mood, help regulate emotions and encourage better behavior, all of which help create smoother classrooms where learning can flourish.

Activation theory helps explain why the model suggests an inverted U-curve linking arousal by short bursts of physical effort to cognitive performance (Bodensohn et al., 2024). When students land in the middle of the curve it modestly aroused their cognitive profiles peak. Too little or too much arousal, however, both undercut mental brightness. Consequently, exercise that applies moderate intensity and duration calibrates student arousal to an empirically defined optimal zone, thereby augmenting the capacity for learning (Kashihara et al., 2009).

5.2 Risks of Intense Physical Activity on Academic Performance

Although moderate exercise has repeatedly been linked to improved educational outcomes, the literature increasingly highlights the potential risks of excessive training to produce fatigue, burnout and reduced allocation of time to study. One longitudinal analysis indicated that participating in more than two hours of daily physical activity often yields no further benefit, while volumes exceeding three weekly hours consistently correlate with lower measures of academic success largely because they substitute for both restorative sleep and homework. Routine training program, however, can send the hypothalamic pituitary adrenal axis into overdrive, pushing cortisol to levels that compromise selective attention and delay the recovery of both body and brain (Moawd et al., 2020).

Cross sectional evidence reinforces this caution. Students engaging more than 75 minutes of daily vigorous activity consistently show no additional gains in grades, while those exceeding two daily hours typically experience declines in both performance and well being. The associated disruptions to sleep architecture and to the cognitive recovery windows that follow intensive study, prevent memory consolidation and sustain focus both of which attention are critical during the school day.

Emerging evidence further suggest that an overzealous dedication to athletics and fitness, if not balanced by sufficient recovery and flexible scheduling, can exacerbate academic pressure. Balancing exercise and study time accordingly helps avoid the physical fatigue and mental strain that can result from excessive or poorly timed training. A strategic, time efficient plan therefore sustains motivation while maximizing cognitive readiness across the academic day.

Educational institutions and athletic staff should therefore implement vigilant oversight of training intensity and explicitly avoid subjecting students to excessively taxing protocols that compromise overall well-being.

5.3 Integrating Athletic Training with Academic Responsibilities

Moderate physical activity can be integrated into the school schedule without taking away from instructional time. For instance, within the daily curriculum, it is possible to allocate 30 minutes to moderate exercise without reducing the time spent on essential academic lessons. In addition, these scheduled activity breaks tend to enhance focus and engagement during the subsequent lessons, improving the effectiveness of instruction and the overall learning achievements.

As education and policy experts suggest, brisk or moderate physical exercise that is easier to adhere to and more enjoyable is more beneficial compared to extreme forms or long duration sessions. Examples of brisk and moderate exercises that are accompanied by progressive increases in workload and are supervised include continuous aerobic exercises, agility drills and gradual resistance training.

6. CLASSROOM BEHAVIOR AND PHYSICAL ACTIVITY

There is substantial evidence to support that physical activity promotes positive behaviors in the classroom. These behaviors include attention, emotional state, anxiety, self-esteem and inhibitory control all of which are directly connected to academic performance. Research indicates that incorporating physical movement into the school time table improves cognitive and emotional functioning and, as a result, enhances the concentration and contribution of the students in the classroom.

6.1 Effects on Attention, Engagement and Impulse Control

Among the many positive effects of physical activity on behavior, the strengthening of the executive functions is the most important. These higher order functions include maintaining attention to the tasks, actively holding relevant information in the working memory and response inhibition, involving control over impulsive actions and enabling cognitive set flexibility.

Physical exercise has been shown to have many benefits including improving executive functions that support in deep classroom learning and academic performance. Both onetime exercise sessions and routine exercise sessions improves overall attention span, multi tasking and instructional engagement of learners. ("Educating the Student Body," 2013).

The outcomes mentioned above are linked to changes in the physiology of the brain that improve the functions of signaling neurotransmitters. During physical exercise, the body's circulatory system experiences an increase in blood flow which is accompanied by a simultaneous increase in "brain deprived neurotrophic factor" that aids in neogenesis and strengthens synaptic connections. These effects are especially strong in the prefrontal cortex, the brain region in charge of high level cognitive functions and control of attention. Such changes enable the brain to control distracting stimuli and regulate quick reactions to the stimuli. These skills matter at every desk, allowing students to dive into learning while shrugging off potential distractions, whether they're sounds, worries, or thoughts of the next device. Adding short, structured movement breaks into the school day boosts student concentration and encourages greater participation in lessons (James et al., 2023). A systematic review released confirmed that scheduled movement breaks improve on-task behavior in both children and adolescents, which in turn supports more effective teaching when instruction resumes. These studies suggest that thoughtfully timed brief activity intervals can reset attention, calm fidgeting and deepen cognitive engagement.

6.2 Effects on Mood, Anxiety and Self Esteem

Movement supports both physical health and emotional well-being, changes that ultimately help teachers reach their goals (Hossain et al., 2024). During physical activity, the brain releases uplifting neurotransmitters such as dopamine and serotonin while lowering the stress hormone cortisol. As a result, students who stick to a routine of physical activity tend to feel less anxious and less down, which means they can focus and stick with their studies for longer.

When mood lifts and worries fade, students tackle assignments and tests with more eagerness and less dread. Moreover, joining a team, a class, or just a regular workout builds a stronger sense of identity which in turn feeds confidence. This enhances self belief makes it easier to bounce back from mistakes and keep pushing through challenging course work.

A student population in robust psychological health tends to display heightened motivation, greater persistence and stronger social connectedness, all of which nurture a collaborative environment among peers and educators that enhances learning outcomes (Huang et al., 2023).

Meta-analytic evidence reinforces those educational environments which intentionally increase opportunities for moderate to vigorous physical activity which neither detract from nor undermine academic achievement. Rather, such environments cultivate superior emotional self-regulation and overall psychological well being. One review demonstrated that integrating brief, purposeful movement segments into standard curricula while maintaining existing instructional and recess periods not only elevated cardiovascular and motor fitness but also successfully led to reductions in anxiety and improvements in mood, outcomes that subsequently correlated with enhanced academic results.

6.3 Integration and Practical Implications

The growing research firmly supports the deliberate incorporation of daily physical activity within the school schedule as a proven strategy to improve student behavior and protect mental health. School leaders might implement a variety of approaches, such as daily physical education classes, brief, well-paced activity breaks woven into core subjects and more inclusive after school athletic programs, collectively boosting the overall positive impact. Crucially, the activity need not be high intensity or lengthy, even mini sessions, as brief as 10 minutes of low effort moving, can reset focus and reduce behavior problems without burdening lesson time (Howie & Pate, 2012).

The accumulating evidences that exercise naturally enhances aspects of executive function, especially attention and emotional self-regulation, makes a compelling case for treating movement as a core component of teaching. By directing funding, allocating space and providing ongoing training toward creating a school environment that prioritizes daily activity, leaders and state policy makers can purposefully improve both students' academic success and their overall mental and social health.

7. CHALLENGES AND FUTURE DIRECTIONS

Researchers and educators must work hand in hand to design frameworks that integrate physical activity seamlessly into both the formal and informal sides of schooling while keeping academic rigor in center. Designs that incorporate active classrooms, lessons that merge movement with content and after-school options are already showing promise in sustaining rich curricula and lively participation. However more thorough assessments are needed especially longitudinal studies that follow health and academic progress for multiple years, to pin point adaptable models that schools can embrace with assurance. Future investigations might further sharpen these frameworks by studying how school culture, educator mindsets and community assets influence the reliability and longevity of positive outcomes.

7.1 Balancing Physical Activity and Academic Demands

In the push to boost test scores, schools have quietly cut back on structured physical education (PE) and reduced down unstructured play, exposing gaps that schools can no longer ignore. Evidence (Pedersen et al., 2019) indicates that, in the U.S. elementary sector, children now experience structured PE just twice a week on average, while recess periods have shrunk in both length and frequency.

Despite known health and neurocognitive positives tied to active breaks and movement focused lessons, students often fail to meet the recommended levels of moderate to vigorous exertion. Teachers and school leaders are jointly responsible for both achieving higher test scores with the equal responsibility of boosting or at least protecting daily movement. Systematic reviews and meta-analyses from the last three years have repeatedly shown that daily activity does not drain time or attention from learning but it feeds it. Regular movement sharpens focus, keeps bodies at the desk, enhances memory and strengthens the executive skills that connect lessons together. Research tracking students over years has found that two active hours daily designated by the newest longitudinal studies as the sweet spot for cognitive benefits, correlate it with higher test results than those achieved by peers with much less movement. The message is clear that schools must find time for the learning curriculum while still clocking the activity minutes that lift overall results.

Recent research offers strong evidence that boys and girls experience cognitive gains from physical activity at different rates. Boys tend to show pronounced benefits after roughly two hours of daily exertion, while girls reach peak benefits at about one hour. Emerging research also indicates that programs based on solid data and tailored to the student outpace all reforms that skim the surface (Li et al., 2025). Integrating movement throughout the school day elevates student motivation and attention without reducing instructional time. Research further shows that short, planned movement breaks, scattered throughout the day, sharpen attention and boost engagement, leading to quicker, more effective learning. These results mean that physical activity doesn't challenge academics it actually strengthens students' readiness to think and to move, side by side.

7.2 Need for Evidence Based, Context Aware Programming

To meet these intertwined challenges, schools must craft and implement evidence and context sensitive physical activity programs. For such programs to succeed, they must be flexible enough to suit different students. Age, gender, coordination, interests and the subject being studied must all be considered, so that the activity feels meaningful, practical and easy to include in the busy school schedule.

Initially, schools must enact coordinated policies that integrate together curricular physical education, unstructured recess, brief active learning strategies and extended school day offerings, all of which must be reinforced by parents and local organizations. This comprehensive frame work broadens the windows of opportunities for movement while preserving time for academic instruction. The Centers for Disease Control (CDC) and Prevention, emphasizes that these coordinated efforts are vital not only for reaching national movement goals but also for promoting intellectual and emotional capacities that support lifelong health and well being (Webster, 2022). Advances in technology and data analysis now enable more tailored exercise prescriptions. Analysis of recently mined data shows that engaging in moderate activity for 16 to 26 minutes on most days is linked to measurable gains in classroom performance.

These findings imply that customized exercise "doses" may be calibrated to maximize benefit for specific students or cohorts within educational settings. Practitioners and curriculum designers can therefore use evidences of this nature to create precise, evidence based regimens that deliver maximal cognitive dividends within constrained instructional periods.

Schools ought to establish comprehensive monitoring and evaluation frameworks designed to document both the fidelity of physical activity implementation and its subsequent effects on academic and health outcomes. By systematically gathering and reviewing such evidence, educators and program designers can steadily improve intervention strategies while more wisely allocating funds and materials to the most effective programs (Hall et al., 2023). Recent studies provide further promise, revealing that assigning physical activity homework, carefully designed tasks that match each student's starting fitness and interests, totaling about two hours weekly can boost fitness levels and academic outcomes.

8. CONCLUSION

Thus physical exercise plays a vital role in how well students learn and that rigorous levels of activity produce the strongest results, regardless of which age group or cultural background the students belong to. The data indicate that scheduled opportunities for physical education, structured recess, or short, class room integrated activity sessions during the school day collectively strengthen students' cognitive abilities, reduce behavioral problems and elevate overall academic performance.

Fundamental academic domains, particularly mathematics, exhibit heightened responsiveness to increased physical activity, because excellent performance in this subject is contingent on well functioning processes, including sustained focus, working memory and adaptive problem solving all of which are modified for the better by regular exercise. When children improve their cardiovascular fitness, they also strengthen delicate brain systems, encouraging the growth of fresh nerve pathways and promote more efficient energy use. These brain level adaptations help students focus, retain information and skills for academic success more effectively.

Research constantly shows that both brief activity bursts and consistent stretches of moderate or vigorous activity sharpen thinking, improve behavior in class and raise scores on state level and in national exams. In particular, youngsters who engage in at least 90 minutes of moderate activity per week often surpass their peers in every academic measure. Observations from a full school day reveal that a single PE or recess block is most effective to sharpen attention and memory when it lasts between 30 and 60 minutes which is long enough to activate neural networks but not so long that physical or mental fatigue starts to drag performance down.

Research comparing on different weekly exercise amounts shows a good link between activity levels and academic performance as scores rise steadily with total active time, peaking at about 2 hrs of daily activity. When it increases to three hours a day, benefits level starts to go down, probably due to fatigue build up. This curvilinear association serves as a signal to policy makers who prepare overall schedule of exercise in daily routine while protecting class time. But they must also accommodate the different thresholds that students' varied backgrounds and bodies can meet.

Beyond cognitive benefits, consistent movement fosters visible gains in classroom conduct like sharper focus, deeper participation and stronger impulse control. It also reduces anxiety, lift mood and boost self-worth, creating a better climate for learning. Evidence further indicate that quick, timed bound movement breaks, spaced throughout the school day, can enhance student attention spaces and increase the time effectively that can be spent on core subjects. Nonetheless, tight schedules often shrink this movement activity. Schools face pressure to meet all curricular standards and boost test results, which often reduces the available time for physical activity.

However, the schools that embed short, purposeful activity breaks or active learning segments into existing lessons consistently report concurrent gains in both behavioral regulation and academic performance, thus affirming that movement can coexist with but also nourish educational objectives.

The encouraging fact, though, is that the research continues to grow up on this issue. Regular physical activity is a powerful tool that drives better academic results and it does so by sharpening executive function, supporting brain health, improving classroom behavior and boosting social and emotional well being. The evidence suggest that the optimal range is 30 to 60 minutes of moderate intensity activity most days of the week, with a target of at least 90 minutes of organized movement spread throughout the week. The challenge for school instructors and policymakers is to integrate it into the academic schedules, ensuring that rigorous course work and physical health grow together, equipping every student with both a strong mind and strong body.

REFERENCES

Alfaro Chaverri, A., Miller, A., Noonan, C., Quindry, J., & Gaskill, S. E. (2025). A cross sectional study of 2rd 12th grade students' physical activity related to academic achievement. *Sports Medicine and Health Science*. Advance online publication. DOI: 10.1016/j.smhs.2025.03.011

Bodensohn, L., Maurer, A., Daamen, M., Upadhyay, N., Werkhausen, J., Lohaus, M., Manunzio, U., Manunzio, C., Radbruch, A., Attenberger, U., & Boecker, H. (2024). Inverted U shape like functional connectivity alterations in cognitive resting state networks depending on exercise intensity: An fMRI study. *Brain and Cognition, 177*, 106156. DOI: 10.1016/j.bandc.2024.106156 PMID: 38613926

Borrega Alonso, E., & Otamendi, F. J. (2025). Effects of acute and chronic exercise on working memory in healthy adults. An experimental investigation. *Frontiers in Psychology, 16*. Advance online publication. DOI: 10.3389/fpsyg.2025.1608721 PMID: 40547576

Davranche, K., Brisswalter, J., & Radel, R. (2014). Where are the limits of the effects of exercise intensity on cognitive control? *Journal of Sport and Health Science. Journal of Sport and Health Science, 4*(1), 56–63. DOI: 10.1016/j.jshs.2014.08.004

Du, S., Hu, H., Cheng, K., & Li, H. (2023). Exercise makes better mind: A data mining study on effect of physical activity on academic achievement of college students. *Frontiers in Psychology, 14*. Advance online publication. DOI: 10.3389/fpsyg.2023.1271431 PMID: 37908825

Educating the student body. (2013). In *National Academies Press eBooks*. .DOI: 10.17226/18314

Fernandes, M. M., & Sturm, R. (2011). The role of school physical activity Programs in Child body mass Trajectory. *Journal of Physical Activity & Health, 8*(2), 174–181. DOI: 10.1123/jpah.8.2.174 PMID: 21415444

Festa, F., Medori, S., & Macrì, M. (2023). Move Your Body, Boost Your Brain: The Positive Impact of Physical Activity on Cognition across All Age Groups. *Biomedicines, 11*(6), 1765. DOI: 10.3390/biomedicines11061765 PMID: 37371860

Ghahramani, M., Sohrabi, M., Kakhki, A., & Besharat, M. (2016). The Effects of Physical Activity on Impulse Control, Attention, Decision making and Motor Functions in Students with High and Low Impulsivity. *Biosciences Biotechnology Research Asia, 13*(3), 1689–1696. DOI: 10.13005/bbra/2318

Gomez-Pinilla, F., & Hillman, C. (2012). The influence of exercise on cognitive abilities. *Comprehensive Physiology*, •••, 403–428. DOI: 10.1002/cphy.c110063 PMID: 23720292

Hall, A., Lane, C., Wolfenden, L., Wiggers, J., Sutherland, R., McCarthy, N., Jackson, R., Shoesmith, A., Lecathelinais, C., Reeves, P., Bauman, A., Gillham, K., Boyer, J., Naylor, P., Kerr, N., Kajons, N., & Nathan, N. (2023). Evaluating the scaling up of an effective implementation intervention (PACE) to increase the delivery of a mandatory physical activity policy in primary schools. *International Journal of Behavioral Nutrition and Physical Activity, 20*(1). y.DOI: 10.1186/s12966 023 01498

Hossain, M. N., Lee, J., Choi, H., Kwak, Y., & Kim, J. (2024). The impact of exercise on depression: How moving makes your brain and body feel better. *Physical Activity and Nutrition*, *28*(2), 43–51. DOI: 10.20463/pan.2024.0015 PMID: 39097997

Howie, E. K., & Pate, R. R. (2012). Physical activity and academic achievement in children: A historical perspective. *Journal of Sport and Health Science. Journal of Sport and Health Science*, *1*(3), 160–169. DOI: 10.1016/j.jshs.2012.09.003

Huang, X., Wang, Y., & Zhang, H. (2023). Effects of physical exercise intervention on depressive and anxious moods of college students: A meta analysis of randomized controlled trials. *Asian Journal of Sport and Exercise Psychology*, *3*(3), 206–221. DOI: 10.1016/j.ajsep.2023.01.001

James, J., Pringle, A., Mourton, S., & Roscoe, C. M. P. (2023). The Effects of Physical Activity On Academic Performance in School Aged Children: A Systematic review. *Children (Basel, Switzerland)*, *10*(6), 1019. DOI: 10.3390/children10061019 PMID: 37371251

Kashihara, K., Maruyama, T., Murota, M., & Nakahara, Y. (2009). Positive effects of acute and moderate physical exercise on cognitive function. *Journal of Physiological Anthropology*, *28*(4), 155–164. DOI: 10.2114/jpa2.28.155 PMID: 19652447

Kilby, E. (1985). National Association for Sport and Physical Education 1960–1985. *Journal of Physical Education, Recreation & Dance*, *56*(4), 120–122. DOI: 10.1080/07303084.1985.10603771

Li, W., Chen, P., Jiang, A., Zhang, F., & Wu, Z. (2025). Gender differences in cognitive benefits of meeting physical activity guidelines in older Chinese adults. *Frontiers in Public Health*, *13*. Advance online publication. DOI: 10.3389/fpubh.2025.1539369 PMID: 40567994

Magallanes, C. L. (2024). Physical education Teachers' experiences in fitness testing. *British Journal of Multidisciplinary and Advanced Studies*, *5*(1), 88–147. DOI: 10.37745/bjmas.2022.0422

Mahindru, A., Patil, P., & Agrawal, V. (2023). Role of Physical Activity on Mental Health and Well Being: A review. *Cureus*. Advance online publication. DOI: 10.7759/cureus.33475 PMID: 36756008

Mavilidi, M. F., Lubans, D. R., Morgan, P. J., Miller, A., Eather, N., Karayanidis, F., Lonsdale, C., Noetel, M., Shaw, K., & Riley, N. (2019). Integrating physical activity into the primary school curriculum: Rationale and study protocol for the "Thinking while Moving in English" cluster randomized controlled trial. *BMC Public Health*, *19*(1). Advance online publication. DOI: 10.1186/s12889 019 6635 2 PMID: 30947708

Moawd, S. A., Elsayed, S. H., Abdelbasset, W. K., Nambi, G., Verma, A. Impact of different physical activity levels on academic performance of PSAU medical female students. Arch PharmaPract 2020;11(1):100 4.

Neil Sztramko, S. E., Caldwell, H., & Dobbins, M. (2021). School based physical activity programs for promoting physical activity and fitness in children and adolescents aged 6 to 18. *Cochrane Library, 2021*(9). .DOI: 10.1002/14651858.cd007651.pub3

Ogoh, S., Tsukamoto, H., Hirasawa, A., Hasegawa, H., Hirose, N., & Hashimoto, T. (2014). The effect of changes in cerebral blood flow on cognitive function during exercise. *Physiological Reports*, *2*(9), e12163. DOI: 10.14814/phy2.12163 PMID: 25263210

Pedersen, J. H., Thornquist, E., Natvik, E., & Råheim, M. (2019). Physical education classes – a double edged sword: A qualitative study of Norwegian high school students' experiences. *Physiotherapy Theory and Practice*, *37*(12), 1404–1418. DOI: 10.1080/09593985.2019.1709232 PMID: 31885299

Ren, J., & Xiao, H. (2023). Exercise for Mental Well Being: Exploring Neurobiological Advances and intervention Effects in Depression. *Life (Chicago, Ill.)*, *13*(7), 1505. DOI: 10.3390/life13071505 PMID: 37511879

Roig Hierro, E., Ríos Sisó, X., Buscà, F., Guillem, M., & Batalla, A. (2025). The positive impact of physical activity on academic performance among catalan adolescents. *Cogent Education*, *12*(1). Advance online publication. DOI: 10.1080/2331186x.2025.2497139

Sanaeifar, F., Pourranjbar, S., Pourranjbar, M., Ramezani, S., Mehr, S. R., Wadan, A. S., & Khazeifard, F. (2024). Beneficial effects of physical exercise on cognitive behavioral impairments and brain derived neurotrophic factor alteration in the limbic system induced by neurodegeneration. *Experimental Gerontology*, *195*, 112539. DOI: 10.1016/j.exger.2024.112539 PMID: 39116955

Sanderson, H., DeRousie, J., & Guistwite, N. (2017). Impact of collegiate recreation on academic success. *Journal of Student Affairs Research and Practice*, *55*(1), 40–53. DOI: 10.1080/19496591.2017.1357566

Sleiman, S. F., Henry, J., Al Haddad, R., Hayek, L. E., Haidar, E. A., Stringer, T., Ulja, D., Karuppagounder, S. S., Holson, E. B., Ratan, R. R., Ninan, I., & Chao, M. V. (2016). Exercise promotes the expression of brain derived neurotrophic factor (BDNF) through the action of the ketone body β hydroxybutyrate. *eLife*, *5*. Advance online publication. DOI: 10.7554/elife.15092 PMID: 27253067

Vecchio, L. M., Meng, Y., Xhima, K., Lipsman, N., Hamani, C., &Aubert, I. (2018). The neuroprotective effects of exercise: Maintaining a healthy brain throughout aging. *Brain Plasticity, 4*(1), 17–52. 180069.DOI: 10.3233/bpl

Vedøy, I. B., Erssen, S. A., Tjomsland, H. E., Skulberg, K. R., & Thurston, M. (2020). Physical activity, mental health and academic achievement: A cross sectional study of Norwegian adolescents. *Mental Health and Physical Activity*, *18*, 100322. DOI: 10.1016/j.mhpa.2020.100322

Webster, C. A. (2022). The Comprehensive School Physical Activity Program: An invited review. *American Journal of Lifestyle Medicine*, *17*(6), 762–774. DOI: 10.1177/15598276221093543 PMID: 38511110

Zhou, X., Li, J., & Jiang, X. (2024). Effects of different types of exercise intensity on improving health related physical fitness in children and adolescents: A systematic review. *Scientific Reports*, *14*(1), x. DOI: 10.1038/s41598 024 64830 PMID: 38906965

Chapter 11

Neurochemical Pathways Linking Physical Activity With Emotional Balance

Richa Sharma
https://orcid.org/0009-0006-1174-2888
AAFT University of Media and Arts, Math, Raipur, India

ABSTRACT

Emotional well-being develops through interactions among neurochemical systems, endocrine responses, and structural brain networks regulating mood, motivation, and behavior. Scientific advances demonstrate that physical activity functions as a potent biological intervention that enhances emotional balance, reduces psychiatric symptoms, and strengthens cognitive control through its influence on neurotransmitters and neurotrophic signaling. This chapter examines how movement reshapes neural chemistry, including serotonergic, dopaminergic, endorphin-mediated, endocannabinoid, and noradrenergic pathways, and modifies structures such as the limbic network, hippocampus, and prefrontal cortex. Emphasis is placed on exercise-driven regulation of the stress response, promotion of neuroplasticity, and reinforcement of mental resilience. Integrating empirical findings, clinical implications, and practical recommendations, the chapter illustrates why physical activity should be adopted as a primary therapeutic tool for emotional regulation in general and clinical settings.

1. INTRODUCTION

Emotional balance is not merely the absence of illness; it is shaped by the ability to regulate internal experiences, manage stress, sustain motivation, and respond

DOI: 10.4018/979-8-3373-6157-4.ch011

adaptively to daily challenges. While earlier psychological theories emphasized thought processes and social context, contemporary neuroscience reveals that emotional functioning relies heavily on underlying biochemical pathways that maintain homeostasis within the brain (Basso & Suzuki, 2017). Physical activity influences these pathways profoundly, generating neurochemical cascades that alter mood, cognitive flexibility, and emotional stability.

Individuals frequently report feeling clearer, calmer, and more optimistic after exercise. Such self-reports reflect measurable biological shifts that occur even after a single session of moderate movement (Ratey, 2008). Exercise elicits neurotransmitter release, enhances blood flow to neural tissue, and strengthens functional communication between brain regions regulating emotional processing. When repeated regularly, these biological adjustments accumulate into long-term structural and functional adaptations capable of preventing or treating emotional disorders, including anxiety, depression, and trauma-related conditions (Zhang et al., 2022).

Understanding these processes holds value not only for researchers but also for health professionals, psychologists, policymakers, wellness educators, and individuals seeking accessible interventions with minimal side effects. This chapter therefore examines the neurochemical mechanisms linking physical activity to emotional balance and highlights clinical implications emerging from current research.

Figure 1. Biochemical and neurophysiological mechanisms through which physical activity enhances emotional regulation and mental well-being. Engaging in exercise activates the hypothalamic–pituitary–adrenal (HPA) axis, resulting in improved stress response and decreased cortisol levels. Concurrently, exercise stimulates the release of key neurotransmitters including endorphins (pain relief and euphoria), dopamine (reward and motivation), serotonin (mood stabilization), and norepinephrine (arousal and attention), along with increased production of brain-derived neurotrophic factor (BDNF), which promotes neuroplasticity. Collectively, these neurochemical changes contribute to reduced anxiety and depression, improved mood, enhanced cognitive performance, and strengthened emotional resilience, ultimately supporting overall emotional balance and mental well-being

Physical Activity/Exercise

↓

Activation of HPA Axis → Cortisol Regulation

↓

↑ Endorphins + ↑ Dopamine + ↑ Serotonin + ↑ Norepinephrine + ↑ BDNF

↓

Improved Mood, Reduced Stress, Enhanced Cognition & Emotional Balance

2. BRAIN STRUCTURES INVOLVED IN EMOTIONAL PROCESSING

2.1 Prefrontal Cortex (PFC)

The prefrontal cortex governs executive functions such as decision-making, emotional control, and attention. Chronic stress interferes with PFC activity, weakening self-regulation and increasing impulsive responses (Arnsten, 2009). Regular physical activity increases cerebral blood flow and oxygen delivery to the PFC, strengthening cognitive control over emotional impulses (Hillman et al., 2008). Functional imaging studies demonstrate improved connectivity within PFC circuitry following consistent movement training, which supports healthier emotional responses under challenging conditions (Stillman et al., 2020).

2.2 Limbic System

The limbic system, including the amygdala and hippocampus, processes emotional memory and threat evaluation. Excessive amygdala activity contributes to anxiety and fear responses, whereas impaired hippocampal function is linked to depressive states. Exercise reduces amygdala reactivity and stimulates hippocampal neurogenesis supported by brain-derived neurotrophic factor (BDNF), improving mood and emotional stability (van Praag et al., 1999). Research indicates that even six weeks of moderate training can increase hippocampal volume (Erickson et al., 2011), supporting better emotional balance.

2.3 Basal Ganglia and Reward Circuitry

The basal ganglia facilitate motivation and reward-based learning. Dopamine signaling within this region regulates enthusiasm and pleasure anticipation. Physical movement elevates dopamine release and improves receptor sensitivity, explaining the motivational lift and antidepressant effect associated with exercise (Meeusen & De Meirleir, 1995). Reduced dopamine contributes to low drive and anhedonia, common symptoms in major depression; exercise helps reverse these states.

Figure 2. Diagram

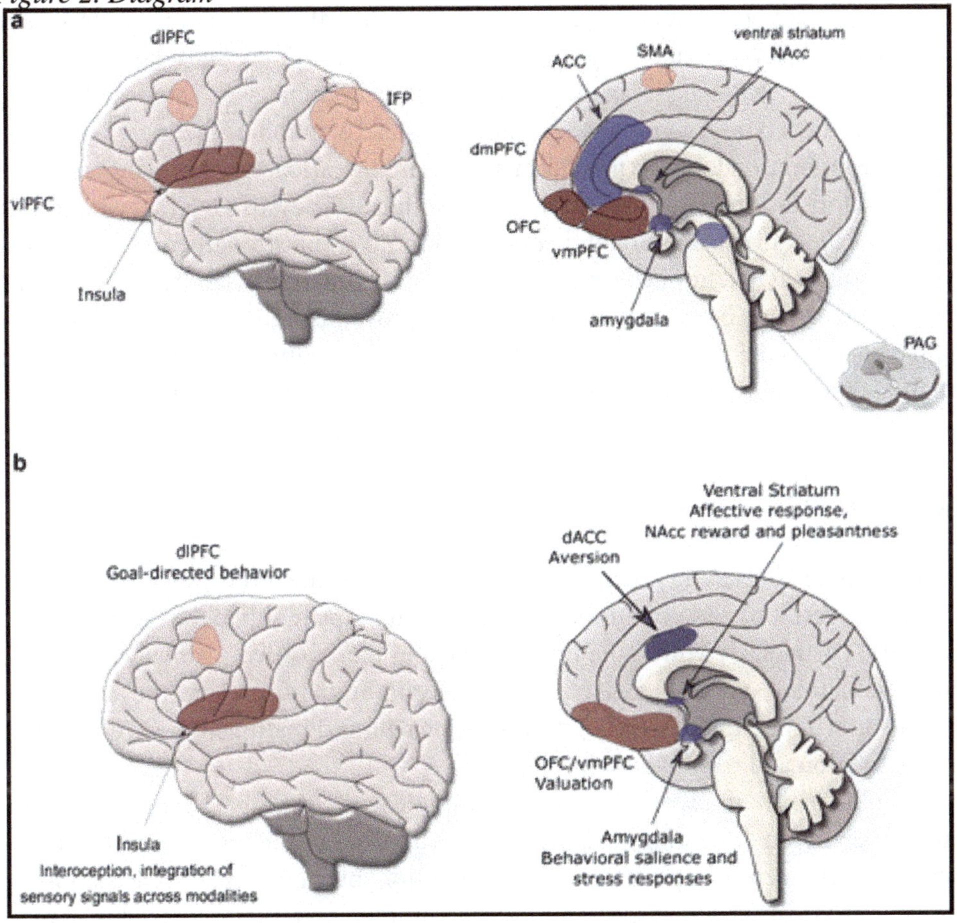

3. NEUROCHEMICAL PATHWAYS ACTIVATED BY PHYSICAL ACTIVITY

3.1 Endorphins

Endorphins are endogenous opioid peptides produced primarily in the pituitary gland and central nervous system. They function as natural painkillers and emotional stabilizers, released most prominently during sustained moderate to vigorous physical activity such as running, swimming, and high-intensity interval training. When exercise intensity reaches a level where physical exertion slightly stresses the body, endorphins bind to opioid receptors, reducing the perception of pain and inducing a warm, comforting sensation. This biochemical effect is often referred to as the *"exercise high"*, a calm yet energized emotional state that many physically active individuals describe.

Endorphin release helps manage emotional discomfort associated with stress, loneliness, anxiety, and depressive symptoms. Instead of numbing feelings, as external substances might, endorphins naturally balance emotional load by improving tolerance to discomfort and enhancing psychological resilience. They also interact with limbic structures that govern emotional memory and motivation, strengthening feelings of positivity and satisfaction after exercise. When performed consistently, activities that elevate endorphins contribute to long-term improvements in self-perception, pain management, and emotional stability. For individuals dealing with chronic stress or trauma, endorphin-stimulating exercise offers a non-pharmacological pathway to relieve physiological tension and restore a sense of internal safety and well-being.

3.2 Dopamine

Dopamine is a key neurochemical involved in reward processing, motivation, pleasure, attention, and goal-directed behavior. It helps regulate the brain's reward circuitry, particularly within the mesolimbic and mesocortical pathways. Exercise boosts dopamine synthesis by increasing the availability of tyrosine, the amino acid precursor of dopamine, and through stimulating neural signaling in areas responsible for motivation and reward anticipation.

People with low dopamine levels often struggle with emotional flatness, persistent fatigue, difficulty initiating tasks, and low enthusiasm for daily routines. These symptoms frequently appear alongside depression, burnout, or lifestyle monotony. Regular physical activity, especially strength training and interval-based workouts, enhances dopamine release and receptor sensitivity, helping restore vitality and interest in activities. As individuals experience physical progress lifting heavier weights, improving speed, or feeling bodily strength grow they receive reinforcing dopamine responses that support persistence and habit formation.

Dopamine also strengthens executive functioning in the prefrontal cortex, improving planning, concentration, and the ability to manage complex decisions. This is why many people experience sharper mental clarity and productivity following a workout. Over time, movement transforms into a self-sustaining behavioral cycle: exercise increases dopamine, dopamine increases motivation, motivation sustains exercise, and emotional well-being improves as a result.

3.3 Serotonin

Serotonin plays a central role in mood regulation, emotional equilibrium, satiety, and sleep-wake balance. Reduced serotonergic activity has long been linked with depression, irritability, impulsivity, and disturbances in appetite and sleep patterns. Cardiovascular exercise significantly enhances serotonin turnover in the brain by increasing tryptophan transport across the blood-brain barrier and stimulating receptor sensitivity. These changes produce a stabilizing effect on emotional responses, reducing anxiety and depressive tendencies.

Outdoor exercise compounds this benefit by incorporating natural sunlight, which supports serotonin synthesis through photic stimulation of the retina and regulation of circadian rhythms. This mechanism explains why people often report greater emotional relief and clarity after morning walks, running outdoors, or cycling in the open air compared to indoor training environments. Research has also demonstrated that improvements in serotonin function contribute to better coping skills under psychological pressure and enhanced emotional resilience during adversity.

Aerobic exercises such as brisk walking, swimming, jogging, or cycling are particularly effective at boosting serotonin. With repeated practice, the brain adapts, maintaining higher baseline levels, which reduces emotional reactivity and promotes steadier, more grounded mood patterns. In this way, movement serves as a natural complement to therapeutic interventions and lifestyle-based mental health approaches.

3.4 Norepinephrine

Norepinephrine is a neurotransmitter essential for alertness, attention, cognitive performance, and regulation of the stress response. It is released from the locus coeruleus during physical activity, enhancing brain readiness, improving mental energy, and sharpening focus. Individuals often experience the benefits of norepinephrine release as increased clarity, better problem-solving ability, and improved decision-making immediately after movement.

This neurochemical plays a critical role in balancing the sympathetic and parasympathetic nervous systems. Moderate exercise increases norepinephrine availability, helping the body shift from the immobilizing effects of stress into a more adaptive state of mobilization and cognitive control. Rather than intensifying anxiety, as extreme stress does, exercise-induced norepinephrine supports emotional composure by modulating the fight-or-flight response.

These benefits are particularly helpful for individuals who struggle with attention deficits, chronic worry, or emotional overwhelm. Even brief bouts of movement such as 10-minute stair climbing or short cycling intervals can improve working memory, mental flexibility, and information processing speed. Over time, regular exercise strengthens the brain's capacity to navigate stress and reduces vulnerability to emotional overload or burnout.

3.5 Endocannabinoids

Endocannabinoids are naturally occurring lipid-based neurotransmitters that play a crucial role in regulating pleasure, relaxation, and emotional balance. Their effects are mediated through the endocannabinoid system, which influences stress regulation, appetite, immune response, and social bonding. Levels of endocannabinoids, particularly anandamide (known as the "bliss molecule"), rise significantly during sustained aerobic activity.

Unlike endorphins, which struggle to cross the blood-brain barrier, endocannabinoids circulate freely into the central nervous system, generating a sense of calm, reduced anxiety, emotional harmony, and increased social comfort. This process contributes to the feeling of lightness or peaceful well-being following a steady run, cycling session, or swimming workout. Their ability to regulate fear responses and reduce hyperarousal makes them especially valuable in trauma-related emotional dysregulation and anxiety-based disorders.

Endocannabinoid signaling also supports positive mood reinforcement through reward pathways, strengthening the association between movement and emotional relief. This neurochemical mechanism helps individuals build supportive exercise habits not through discipline alone, but through authentic internal reward experiences.

3.6 BDNF and Neuroplasticity

Brain-Derived Neurotrophic Factor (BDNF) is a growth factor essential for neuronal survival, synaptic strengthening, and long-term neuroplasticity. It supports the formation of new neural connections, enhances learning capacity, and protects the brain from degeneration. Exercise is one of the most effective natural stimuli for BDNF release, particularly aerobic movement performed at moderate intensity.

Low BDNF is strongly associated with major depressive disorder, cognitive decline, memory impairment, and reduced emotional adaptability. When physical activity increases circulating BDNF levels, neural communication efficiency improves, particularly in the hippocampus and prefrontal cortex regions central to emotional regulation and executive functioning. This enhancement explains why regular exercise improves clarity of thought, learning speed, creativity, and emotional problem-solving.

BDNF also helps repair neural pathways impacted by chronic stress, trauma, and long-term emotional strain. By facilitating neuroplastic adaptation, exercise creates long-lasting structural change rather than temporary mood relief. Individuals who maintain active habits show stronger protection against relapse in depression, age-related cognitive loss, and stress-induced impairments.

4. HORMONAL REGULATION OF STRESS AND EMOTIONAL CONTROL

4.1 Cortisol

Cortisol is the primary hormone released during stress as part of the body's adaptive survival system. Although short-term cortisol elevation supports alertness and energy mobilization, persistent psychological stress leads to chronically elevated cortisol levels, producing harmful effects on emotional and cognitive functioning. Sustained cortisol exposure disrupts the balance of neurotransmitters, weakens hippocampal neurons responsible for memory and learning, and contributes to emotional fatigue, irritability, and reduced mental clarity. Over time, this neuroendocrine strain creates vulnerability to anxiety, depressive symptoms, burnout, and impaired executive functioning.

Physical activity plays a stabilizing role by recalibrating the hypothalamic–pituitary–adrenal (HPA) axis, which regulates the stress response system. Moderate and consistent exercise reduces resting cortisol concentrations and improves the body's ability to return to baseline after exposure to psychological stressors. This improved recovery response reflects enhanced stress tolerance and emotional adaptability. Stranahan et al. (2006) demonstrated that regular aerobic exercise supports hippocampal neurogenesis and reduces cortisol-related neural damage, protecting cognitive performance under stress. Through these mechanisms, exercise serves as a physiological buffer against emotional exhaustion, preventing the cumulative depletion associated with chronic workload or personal distress. In practical terms, incorporating planned physical activity into daily routines can interrupt the cycle of stress accumulation and significantly reduce the risk of occupational and academic burnout.

4.2 Oxytocin

Oxytocin is a neuropeptide widely recognized for its role in social bonding, trust, empathy, and emotional connection. It reinforces supportive interpersonal relationships and strengthens feelings of safety and belonging psychological elements foundational to emotional balance. Physical activity, especially when performed in a shared social environment, has been shown to elevate circulating oxytocin levels, enhancing both physiological and relational well-being.

Group-based exercise modalities such as synchronized dance, team sports, partner workouts, or community walking groups combine rhythmic movement, collective engagement, and positive emotional exchange. These components stimulate oxytocin release not only through physical exertion but also through coordinated social interaction, mutual encouragement, and shared goals. Broadhead and Dunne (2020) highlight that exercising in a collaborative context strengthens social cohesion and reinforces feelings of trust and companionship, which can mitigate loneliness and emotional isolation key factors linked to anxiety, depressive states, and reduced motivation.

Oxytocin's influence extends beyond emotional bonding; it modulates the autonomic nervous system, helping to reduce heart rate, lower physiological arousal, and support a calmer internal state. This creates a feedback loop in which supportive social activity amplifies emotional security, which in turn reinforces continued engagement in physical activity. Thus, group movement serves as a dual therapeutic pathway: its neurochemical effects deepen emotional stability while its social environment nurtures resilience and shared wellbeing. Encouraging community-based physical activity programs may therefore represent an effective and inclusive public mental-health strategy.

5. NEUROPLASTICITY AND LONG-TERM EMOTIONAL ADAPTATION

Neuroplasticity refers to the brain's capacity to reorganize itself by forming new neural connections, strengthening existing pathways, and enhancing communication between brain regions in response to experience and learning. Physical activity is one of the most powerful external stimuli capable of driving neuroplastic change across the lifespan. Regular movement stimulates cellular and molecular processes including increased cerebral blood flow, enhanced mitochondrial function, and elevated neurotrophic factors such as brain-derived neurotrophic factor (BDNF) that support neuronal growth and repair.

Aerobic exercise, in particular, has been shown to increase hippocampal volume, a brain structure essential for memory formation, emotional regulation, and stress processing. This growth is associated with improved affective resilience and reduced vulnerability to psychological disorders such as depression and anxiety. Exercise also increases white matter integrity and synaptic density, improving the efficiency of communication among key emotional circuits such as the prefrontal cortex, amygdala, and limbic system. Strengthening these pathways enhances executive function, emotional control, and behavioral flexibility.

These neurobiological adaptations contribute to long-term emotional stability rather than short-lived mood enhancement. Over time, individuals who engage in consistent physical activity display greater stress tolerance, more adaptive coping strategies, and improved cognitive clarity. Importantly, neuroplastic benefits are not limited to young adults; research demonstrates that even older individuals experience significant structural and functional improvement, including better memory, sharper attention, and more balanced emotional responses (Voss et al., 2013). This indicates that the brain remains capable of renewal throughout life, and movement acts as a catalyst for healthy aging and emotional wellbeing.

By supporting neurogenesis, protecting neural networks from degeneration, and enhancing communication within emotional regulatory systems, exercise lays the foundation for lifelong psychological resilience. Thus, physical activity should be understood not only as a behavioral strategy for mood enhancement but as a biological intervention promoting long-term emotional adaptation and cognitive health.

Figure 3. Neurobiological pathway linking physical activity to emotional resilience

Regular Physical Activity

↓

Increased Neuroplasticity

↓

↑ BDNF Production (Brain-Derived Neurotrophic Factor)

↓

Enhanced Synaptic Growth & Neural Connectivity

↓

Hippocampal Growth & Improved Brain Structure

↓

Better Cognitive Control & Stress Regulation

↓

Reduced Anxiety, Depression, and Emotional Reactivity

↓

Long-Term Emotional Resilience & Psychological Well-being

6. CLINICAL AND THERAPEUTIC IMPLICATIONS

Physical activity is increasingly acknowledged as a vital component in mental health care. It is no longer viewed only as a lifestyle choice but as an important therapeutic tool that complements psychological counseling and medication. A growing body of evidence confirms that movement-based interventions can significantly improve conditions such as depression, anxiety disorders, trauma-related disturbances, attention-related challenges, and cognitive decline associated with aging (Mammen & Faulkner, 2013). Exercise strengthens brain function, improves mood regulation, and enhances long-term emotional resilience, making it a valuable clinical approach.

6.1 Exercise in Depression Management

Regular physical activity stimulates chemical messengers such as serotonin and dopamine, which play central roles in emotional balance and motivation (Lin & Kuo, 2013). Many clinical studies suggest that aerobic exercise can be equally effective as antidepressant medication in cases of mild to moderate depression, with fewer undesirable effects and better long-term maintenance of improvement (Dishman & O'Connor, 2009). Movement supports emotional recovery by improving sleep quality, promoting a sense of achievement, and encouraging daily routine stability all of which are crucial during depressive episodes. It Enhances reward pathway functioning, restoring interest in pleasurable activities. It Reduces rumination by shifting focus to bodily sensations and physical goalsand Improves self-esteem and feelings of personal competence.

6.2 Benefits for Anxiety Disorders

Exercise decreases physical tension and regulates stress responses by lowering cortisol and increasing calming neurotransmitters (Pagliaro et al., 2021). Many individuals with chronic anxiety become hypersensitive to bodily changes such as rapid breathing or increased heart rate. Through structured physical activity, the nervous system gradually learns that these sensations are not dangerous, reducing fear responses and catastrophic thinking. It Improves sleep cycles, reducing fatigue-driven anxiety spirals,Increases perception of control and mastery over body sensations,Encourages relaxation through rhythmic breathing and repetitive movement.

6.3 Trauma and PTSD Recovery

Individuals recovering from trauma often experience emotional numbness, hyper-vigilance, and disconnection from the body. Exercise offers a grounding mechanism that reconnects physical presence and emotional safety. Activities that integrate breathing such as yoga, running, or martial arts help regulate the fight-or-flight system and reduce nervous system overactivation (Fuss et al., 2015).It Improves tolerance to triggering sensations by gradually strengthening the stress response system.Supports better sleep by reducing nightmares and nighttime arousal and Group activities increase social trust through oxytocin-induced bonding.

6.4 Executive Functioning and ADHD

Movement improves focus, planning, and working memory by increasing blood flow to regions responsible for decision-making, especially the prefrontal cortex (Lin

& Kuo, 2013). For individuals with ADHD, exercise enhances dopamine availability, helping with patience, organization, and sustained attention. It reduces impulsive behavior and supports task persistence. It Improves ability to shift attention and manage thoughts and enhances academic or occupational performance.

6.5 Exercise in Aging and Cognitive Decline

In older adults, consistent movement protects brain structure by stimulating factors such as BDNF, which support new neuron growth and synaptic strength (Szuhany et al., 2015). Regular exercise can slow age-related memory loss and lower the risk of dementia, helping older adults stay independent and emotionally stronger.Improves coordination and balance, reducing fall risk. Enhances emotional wellbeing and reduces isolation.Supports memory formation through hippocampal preservation.

6.6 Exercise as a Complement to Medication and Therapy

Physical activity improves treatment participation and lowers relapse rates because individuals experience a sense of empowerment and mastery over their condition. Exercise can reduce the need for high dosages of psychiatric medication in many cases by stabilizing mood biologically while promoting healthy coping habits. Enhances emotional regulation strategies learned in therapy.Low-cost and widely accessible intervention for communities with limited mental health resources.Can be personalized to individual needs and cultural context.

6.7 Personalized and Sustainable Exercise Planning

The most effective approach is a program that aligns with personal interests, physical capacity, and emotional goals. When exercise becomes a consistent habit rather than a temporary strategy, it provides ongoing protection against emotional vulnerability and builds lifelong psychological resilience.Low-intensity for beginners (walking, stretching, group games),Structured fitness for motivation (dance, strength training),Outdoor activities for natural light exposure and calm,Social sports for connection and support

7. PRACTICAL EXERCISE RECOMMENDATIONS

Table 1. Different exercise modalities produce specific emotional benefits

Type of Exercise	Primary Psychological Benefit
Brisk walking or cycling	Serotonin boost, lower anxiety
Strength training	Dopamine stimulation, confidence
Yoga, tai chi	Cortisol reduction, vagal activation
Team sports	Oxytocin release and belonging
Nature walks	Serotonin from light exposure

7.1. Brisk Walking or Cycling

Brisk walking and cycling are rhythmic aerobic exercises that elevate heart rate in a controlled, moderate manner. These activities increase oxygen delivery to the brain, enhancing neural efficiency and stimulating the release of serotonin, a neurotransmitter central to mood stabilization, emotional well-being, and sleep regulation. Regular aerobic exercise reduces limbic system overactivity, which is associated with stress and anxiety responses, while simultaneously strengthening the prefrontal cortex responsible for emotional control and decision-making. The repetitive and steady nature of these movements induces a meditative effect, reducing cognitive overload and promoting mental clarity. When performed outdoors, exposure to natural light further enhances serotonin synthesis and supports circadian rhythm balance, while natural sensory stimuli contribute to reduced mental fatigue and improved emotional balance.

7.2. Strength Training

Strength or resistance training involves exercises such as weight lifting, resistance bands, or bodyweight movements like squats and push-ups. This modality stimulates dopamine and endorphin release, neurotransmitters associated with motivation, reward, and pain relief. Progressive improvements in strength and physical capacity build self-efficacy, which enhances confidence, autonomy, and psychological resilience. Strength training also improves metabolic and hormonal regulation, reducing inflammation and supporting stable energy levels—factors associated with decreased depressive symptoms. Physically overcoming resistance has symbolic emotional meaning, often perceived as mastering challenges, which can counteract feelings of helplessness or low self-esteem. Over time, individuals experience an internal sense of capability that generalizes to emotional and cognitive domains.

7.3. Yoga and Tai Chi

Yoga and Tai Chi are integrative mind–body practices combining controlled movement, breath regulation, and focused attention. These techniques stimulate parasympathetic nervous system activity and improve vagal tone, shifting the body away from stress-dominant sympathetic activation. Breath-synchronized movement reduces cortisol levels and stabilizes the hypothalamic–pituitary–adrenal (HPA) axis, significantly improving stress recovery and emotional regulation. The mindfulness inherent in these practices increases interoceptive awareness, understanding internal emotional and physiological signals which reduces anxiety, rumination, and emotional reactivity. Slow, intentional movement improves proprioception and body trust while spiritual or reflective elements enhance inner calm and grounding, making these modalities particularly effective for trauma recovery, anxiety disorders, and emotional instability.

7.4. Team Sports

Team sports such as football, basketball, cricket, and volleyball combine physical exertion with collective participation, shared goals, and coordinated action. These social components stimulate the release of oxytocin, a hormone associated with bonding, trust, and social connection. Group dynamics foster belonging, strengthen communication skills, and create supportive social networks that buffer psychological stress and reduce feelings of loneliness and isolation. The cooperative experience and positive peer reinforcement elevate mood, create shared joy, and increase intrinsic motivation. Participation in team success boosts self-worth and identity, while friendly competition stimulates adrenaline and dopamine, contributing to enthusiasm, focus, and emotional vitality.

7.5. Nature Walks

Nature walks involve low-intensity physical movement combined with immersion in natural environments such as parks, forests, or riversides. Exposure to green spaces reduces amygdala activity associated with fear and stress, promoting calm and emotional restoration. Natural sunlight supports serotonin production and regulates circadian rhythms, contributing to improved sleep quality and mood stability. Direct sensory engagement with natural surroundings—visual greenery, sounds of birds or water, natural textures lowers stress hormones, blood pressure, and physiological tension. Nature-based movement fosters mindfulness, reduces mental fatigue, and enhances creativity, helping individuals process thoughts more clearly and recover emotionally from cognitive overload.

8.THE ROLE OF SLEEP, NUTRITION AND HYDRATION IN EXERCISE INDUCED EMOTIONAL REGULATION

Emotional well-being is shaped by a complex interaction of biological, psychological, and lifestyle factors. While physical activity has been widely recognized as a powerful tool for enhancing emotional stability and mental health, its effectiveness does not exist in isolation. The emotional benefits of exercise depend heavily on supporting behaviors that maintain brain health and physiological balance particularly sleep quality, adequate nutrition, and optimal hydration. These components work together to determine how efficiently the brain responds to movement, how neurochemicals are produced and utilized, and how well the body recovers from psychological and physical stress. Without a healthy foundation in these areas, even a disciplined exercise routine may deliver limited or inconsistent emotional improvements.

8.1. Sleep as a Foundation for Emotional Recovery and Neurochemical Balance

Sleep is one of the most influential regulators of emotional functioning, yet it is frequently overlooked when considering the mental health effects of exercise. During sleep, the brain undergoes essential restorative processes that help stabilize mood, consolidate memories, and regulate hormones involved in stress response. Deep sleep stages support the repair of neural networks and assist in resetting emotional reactivity so that daily stressors can be managed more effectively. When sleep is insufficient or fragmented, the brain's emotional regulation system becomes compromised, heightening sensitivity to stress and diminishing psychological resilience.

Physical activity has been shown to improve sleep quality by reducing sleep latency, increasing deep slow-wave sleep, and decreasing nighttime awakenings. After exercise, the body experiences a natural decline in core temperature and activation of parasympathetic pathways that encourage relaxation and ease the transition into sleep. This bi-directional relationship means that exercise helps people sleep better, and in return, good sleep enhances the emotional benefits gained from movement.

When individuals exercise regularly but continue to suffer from poor sleep, emotional gains may be limited. Without sufficient rest, cortisol levels remain elevated, and neurotransmitter synthesis becomes inefficient, particularly serotonin and dopamine two key chemicals responsible for mood regulation. As a result, the person may continue to feel irritable, anxious, or emotionally flat despite committing to exercise. This demonstrates that emotional regulation is not solely a product of exercise intensity or frequency, but also depends on the body's capacity to recover and integrate change during sleep.

Sleep also influences motivation and consistency. When rest is adequate, the brain's decision-making pathways operate more effectively, enabling individuals to maintain exercise habits and feel reward rather than pressure or exhaustion. Conversely, sleep deprivation increases fatigue, reduces impulse control, and weakens commitment to activity, creating a cycle in which emotional symptoms and inactivity reinforce each other. This highlights the importance of recommending sleep routine adjustments as part of mental-health-oriented exercise programs.

8.2. Nutrition as a Driver of Neurotransmitter Production and Emotional Response to Exercise

The emotional outcomes of exercise depend heavily on the availability of nutrients that support brain function. Neurotransmitters that regulate mood, motivation, pleasure, and stress response cannot be produced without appropriate dietary components. For example, tryptophan is required to synthesize serotonin, tyrosine is needed to form dopamine and norepinephrine, and omega-3 fatty acids are essential for neuronal membrane integrity and synaptic communication. B-vitamins, magnesium, and iron contribute to energy metabolism and cognitive function. When nutrition is inadequate, the brain struggles to convert exercise stimulation into emotional stability.

Balanced nutrition allows individuals to experience the full psychological benefits of movement, including improved motivation, reduced anxiety, and greater emotional resilience. In contrast, diets high in processed foods, sugar, and deficient in micronutrients create unstable energy patterns that impair both mood and exercise performance. Nutritional imbalance may cause feelings such as fatigue, restlessness, low motivation, and irritability symptoms commonly associated with anxiety and depression. If a person engages in regular physical activity but fails to nourish their body adequately, they may misinterpret exercise-related tiredness or emotional instability as discouraging outcomes instead of unmet nutritional needs.

The timing and quality of food intake also influence emotional responses following exercise. A balanced pre-exercise meal supports stable blood sugar levels and prevents mood crashes during or after activity. Post-exercise nourishment helps replenish glycogen stores, repair muscle tissue, and provide the brain with substrates needed for neurochemical adjustments that shape emotional responses. Protein intake assists neurotransmitter production, while complex carbohydrates promote serotonin release and restore calmness after physical exertion.

The gut also plays an integral role in emotional response. A significant portion of serotonin is stored in the intestinal system, and a balanced microbiome contributes to emotional stability. Fermented foods, fiber-rich meals, probiotic supplements, and a diverse diet strengthen gut health, indirectly enhancing the emotional benefits of exercise. When digestive function is compromised, emotional responses may be less stable, even if physical activity is consistently performed.

Therefore, nutrition must be viewed as a supportive framework that enables exercise to create lasting emotional change rather than a separate lifestyle component. When dietary choices align with physical training, the body and mind adapt more effectively, and emotional health improves in a more sustained and predictable manner.

8.3. Hydration and Its Influence on Mood, Cognition, and Exercise Effectiveness

Hydration plays a crucial role in the relationship between exercise and emotional stability. Water supports blood circulation, nutrient transport, temperature regulation, and neural functioning. Even mild dehydration levels as low as one to two percent of body weight can trigger emotional symptoms such as irritability, tension, difficulty concentrating, and heightened perception of stress. Many individuals attribute these feelings to emotional instability without realizing that insufficient hydration may be a contributing factor.

During exercise, fluid loss increases through sweating and respiration. If lost fluids are not replaced, blood volume decreases, resulting in reduced oxygen delivery to the brain. This affects areas responsible for mood control, decision-making, and stress tolerance. Proper hydration enables the nervous system to function efficiently, supporting cognitive clarity and emotional calmness before, during, and after exercise. When hydration is neglected, emotional benefits of movement may be significantly reduced, or feelings of exhaustion and frustration may overshadow the positive psychological effects that physical activity typically produces.

Hydration also facilitates neurochemical transport, affecting how serotonin, dopamine, and other neurotransmitters circulate and bind to receptors. Without adequate fluid levels, the brain cannot utilize these chemical messengers effectively, and emotional responses become less stable. Water helps remove metabolic waste products generated during physical effort, reducing inflammation and supporting recovery. When recovery is compromised, the emotional cost of exercise increases, and individuals may feel overwhelmed instead of balanced.

Electrolytes play an additional role, particularly during intense or prolonged exercise. Sodium, potassium, calcium, and magnesium help regulate nerve signaling and muscle contraction. When electrolyte balance is disrupted, symptoms such as confusion, fatigue, anxiety, or irritability may occur. This illustrates that hydration is not only about water volume, but also about maintaining chemical stability within the nervous system.

Encouraging individuals to develop hydration habits such as drinking consistently through the day rather than waiting for thirst helps stabilize emotional well-being and improves exercise enjoyment and adherence. Simple actions like carrying a water bottle, monitoring urine color, or setting reminders can significantly enhance hydration patterns, especially among those managing stress or mood disorders.

8.4. Integrating Sleep, Nutrition, and Hydration as a Holistic System Supporting Emotional Health

Modern scientific understanding emphasizes that emotional well-being is not governed by a single biological process, but instead emerges from the coordinated functioning of multiple physiological systems. Movement, restorative sleep, balanced nourishment, and proper hydration work together to sustain optimal brain function, regulate mood, and build psychological resilience. When these components align consistently, individuals develop stronger emotional balance, enhanced clarity of thought, and improved stress tolerance. Conversely, when even one element is disrupted such as lack of sleep or chronic dehydration—the benefits of physical activity on emotional health become significantly weakened.

Why integration matters more than isolated habits

Exercise is widely recognized as a powerful tool for emotional regulation because it increases neurochemical signals associated with motivation and pleasure, such as dopamine and endorphins, while reducing stress hormones (Kandola et al., 2020). However, the long-term effects of these neurochemical changes depend heavily on the body's ability to repair and stabilize neurological processes, which cannot occur without adequate rest. Deep sleep is responsible for memory consolidation, emotional processing, and clearing metabolic waste from neural tissue, allowing the brain to reset and reorganize after stress (Walker, 2017). When sleep is insufficient, the brain's emotional centers become more reactive, and the prefrontal cortex—the region responsible for self-regulation—loses control, increasing vulnerability to anxiety and mood fluctuations.

Nutrition plays an equally important role in sustaining emotional wellness. The brain is a metabolically active organ that requires steady access to glucose, essential fatty acids, amino acids, vitamins, and minerals to produce neurotransmitters. For instance, serotonin synthesis relies on tryptophan, iron, vitamin B6, and folate.

Deficiency in any of these nutrients interferes with the body's ability to regulate emotions effectively (Sarris et al., 2015). Diets rich in whole grains, legumes, lean protein sources, fruits, vegetables, and omega-3 fats support healthy neural communication and reduce inflammatory pathways associated with depression.

Hydration, a component often overlooked, is also critical. Even mild dehydration can impair mood, attention, and decision-making, increasing irritability and fatigue (Armstrong et al., 2012). Since water is essential for maintaining blood volume, nutrient transport, and electrolyte balance, inadequate hydration directly limits the brain's ability to function under stress.

When physical activity is practiced without attention to these other behavioral domains, emotional progress becomes inconsistent. Many individuals experience temporary improvement in mood after exercise but struggle to maintain emotional stability long-term because their system lacks the recovery and fuel required to sustain neurological changes. Therefore, it is not just movement itself, but movement supported by appropriate sleep, food, and hydration that allows the brain to grow stronger and more emotionally adaptive.

How the four components interact as a unified emotional-health system

The relationship among exercise, sleep, nutrition, and hydration can be understood as a biological ecosystem:

Table 2.

Component	Key Role in Emotional Regulation	Interaction With Other Components
Physical Activity	Triggers neurotransmitter release, improves brain connectivity, reduces cortisol	Requires sleep for recovery, nutrition/ hydration for energy, enhances sleep quality
Sleep	Resets stress response, supports emotional memory processing	Exercise improves sleep depth, nutrition affects circadian rhythm
Nutrition	Provides raw materials for neurotransmitters, stabilizes mood	Sleep regulates appetite hormones, hydration supports nutrient delivery
Hydration	Maintains cognitive function and nervous-system communication	Enhances exercise performance, influences digestion and cellular function

This interconnected system demonstrates that emotional well-being cannot be separated into isolated recommendations. A person may practice regular exercise but still feel emotionally unstable if their sleep cycle is irregular or their diet lacks necessary micronutrients.

Application in clinical and wellness practice

For practitioners such as psychologists, nutritionists, physiotherapists, and wellness coaches, integrating these four dimensions forms a more effective approach to mental-health management than prescribing exercise alone. Lifestyle medicine practitioners increasingly recommend combined behavioral interventions rather than single-strategy models because human functioning is whole-body, not compartmentalized.

For example, therapists might pair physical-activity prescriptions with strategies that support high-quality sleep, such as fixed wake-up schedules, evening light management, or relaxation techniques. Nutrition professionals may design meal plans that balance blood sugar, ensuring emotional stability throughout the day. Hydration education can encourage individuals to monitor fluid intake relative to activity level, caffeine consumption, and climate.

This integrated framework also benefits populations facing chronic stress, academic pressure, workplace burnout, or emotional trauma. In such environments, the nervous system lives in a heightened state of alertness, making emotional regulation more difficult. A holistic routine movement for release, sleep for restoration, nutrition for repair, hydration for cellular balance allows the brain to shift from survival mode toward stability.

Personal empowerment through daily habits

Recognizing that emotional health is deeply shaped by daily lifestyle choices gives individuals genuine power in their personal healing journey. Many people often believe that emotional balance depends only on medication, therapy, or external support. While clinical treatment can be valuable and essential for many individuals, it is equally important to understand that everyday habits also play a significant role in shaping how the mind functions and responds to stress. When a person realizes that simple, consistent routines rather than dramatic interventions can meaningfully influence emotional stability, they begin to feel more capable and in control of their well-being.

Developing emotional strength becomes easier when the body receives dependable care. A regular sleep schedule supports the brain's ability to process feelings and reset after daily challenges. Nourishing meals provide the nutrients required for neurotransmitter production, helping the brain communicate clearly and maintain a balanced mood. Adequate hydration keeps cognitive performance steady and prevents mood fluctuations caused by physical fatigue. Movement that feels enjoyable, not forced, releases internal tension and helps regulate stress responses. These behaviors act like small deposits in a long-term emotional savings account.

When practiced consistently, these habits send a powerful signal of safety to the nervous system: the body learns that it is supported rather than threatened. Emotional steadiness does not appear as a sudden breakthrough; it grows gradually from repeated choices. Over time, individuals notice increased calmness, better clarity, and improved capacity to handle daily pressures.

Adopting a holistic, integrated lifestyle framework allows resilience to become a natural part of identity rather than a temporary state. Instead of being controlled by emotions, individuals learn to guide them. This shift transforms self-care from a reaction to crisis into a proactive path toward lasting emotional strength.

Transforming public-health priorities

As rates of stress, anxiety, and depression continue to rise globally, public-health strategies must shift toward prevention rather than crisis response. Schools, colleges, workplaces, and community programs can play a transformative role by teaching individuals how lifestyle behaviors shape mental well-being. Incorporating sleep education, nutrition literacy, hydration awareness, and structured movement programs into mental-health initiatives may reduce dependence on pharmaceutical treatment where appropriate and build stronger, more emotionally balanced societies.

9. FUTURE RESEARCH DIRECTIONS

Emerging research continues to deepen scientific understanding of how physical activity influences emotional regulation through complex biological and behavioral pathways. One promising direction involves examining exercise–gene interactions, particularly the role of genetic polymorphisms that may shape individual responsiveness to physical training. For example, variations in genes associated with serotonin transport, dopamine receptors, or BDNF expression may determine why some individuals experience greater mood improvements from exercise than others. Understanding these gene–exercise relationships may enable precision-based mental-health interventions tailored to biological profiles.

Another evolving domain is the exploration of the gut–brain–microbiome axis, investigating how exercise-induced shifts in gut microbiota influence neurotransmitter production, inflammatory signaling, and emotional states. Early studies suggest that regular physical activity enhances microbial diversity and increases short-chain fatty acids that positively affect mood, offering new pathways for complementary treatment of anxiety and depression.

Additionally, researchers are developing digital biomarkers and wearable neurotechnology capable of monitoring real-time changes in neurochemical activity, heart-rate variability, stress hormones, and emotional states during exercise. These tools may transform how emotional health is tracked, providing objective indicators that support early mental-health intervention and continuous behavioural monitoring.

Finally, there is growing interest in personalized movement prescriptions, where emotional profiles, neurobiological markers, and psychological needs inform the type, duration, and intensity of exercise recommended. This precision model recognizes that different forms of movement such as aerobic training, mindful yoga, strength work, or rhythmic dance activate distinct neurochemical pathways and may therefore support emotional balance differently across individuals.

10. CONCLUSION

Physical activity acts as a fundamental biological regulator of emotional health, influencing the body and brain through multiple interconnected pathways. When individuals engage in movement whether walking, strength training, yoga, dance, or team sports the brain responds by releasing key neurotransmitters such as endorphins, dopamine, serotonin, and norepinephrine. These chemical messengers play central roles in emotional expression, motivation, pleasure, focus, and stress reduction. Exercise also increases levels of brain-derived neurotrophic factor (BDNF), a crucial molecule that promotes neuroplasticity, supports the growth of new neural connections, and improves learning and emotional adaptability. Because of these biochemical changes, regular physical activity can uplift mood, reduce symptoms of anxiety and depression, improve clarity of thought, and expand an individual's capacity to cope with psychological stress.

In addition to altering neurochemistry, consistent exercise reshapes the physical structure and functioning of the brain. Research has demonstrated that regular physical activity increases the size and efficiency of the hippocampus, a region essential for memory and emotional regulation, while strengthening the prefrontal cortex, which governs decision-making, impulse control, and rational thought. Exercise also improves communication pathways between brain networks responsible for processing and regulating emotions, enabling individuals to respond to stress with greater stability and resilience. On a physiological level, movement regulates the hypothalamic-pituitary-adrenal (HPA) axis and lowers excessive cortisol, reducing the wear and tear caused by chronic stress and emotional overload.

The accumulated evidence across neuroscience, psychology, and public health demonstrates that movement is an accessible, low-cost, and highly effective strategy for stabilizing emotions and enhancing mental well-being throughout all stages of life. Unlike pharmaceuticals, exercise carries positive side benefits including improved physical health, social connection, confidence, and sleep quality and presents minimal risk when guided appropriately. For these reasons, integrating structured exercise into mental-health care is not optional but urgently necessary. Schools, universities, hospitals, workplaces, and community organizations all stand to benefit from weaving physical-activity programs into daily routines and treatment strategies.

Encouraging regular movement empowers individuals to take an active role in their emotional health rather than relying solely on medication or crisis-based care. When exercise becomes a consistent habit, it helps build psychological resilience, strengthens identity and self-efficacy, and supports lifelong mental stability. In a world where stress, anxiety, and depression continue to rise, promoting physical activity as a therapeutic and preventive resource represents a vital public-health commitment and a powerful step toward a future in which emotional well-being is viewed as achievable and sustainable for all populations.

REFERENCES

Arnsten, A. F. T. (2009). Stress signalling pathways that impair prefrontal cortex structure and function. *Nature Reviews. Neuroscience*, *10*, 410–422. PMID: 19455173

Basso, J. C., & Suzuki, W. A. (2017). The effects of acute exercise on mood, cognition, neurophysiology, and neurochemical pathways. *Brain Plasticity*, *2*(2), 127–152. PMID: 29765853

Broadhead, J., & Dunne, M. (2020). Physical activity, social bonding and hormonal influences. *Journal of Social Neuroendocrinology*, *12*(3), 312–325.

Dishman, R. K., & O'Connor, P. J. (2009). Lessons in exercise neurobiology. *Mental Health and Physical Activity*, *2*(1), 4–9.

Dishman, R. K., & O'Connor, P. J. (2009). Lessons in exercise neurobiology: The case of endorphins. *Mental Health and Physical Activity*, *2*(1), 4–9.

Erickson, K. I.. (2011). Physical activity increases hippocampal volume. *Proceedings of the National Academy of Sciences of the United States of America*, *108*(7), 3017–3022. PMID: 21282661

Fuss, J.. (2015). Endocannabinoid release and emotional regulation through exercise. *Biological Psychiatry*, *78*(10), 766–773.

Fuss, J., Steinle, J., Bindila, L., Auer, M. K., Kirchherr, H., Lutz, B., & Gass, P. (2015). A runner's high depends on cannabinoid receptors in mice. *Proceedings of the National Academy of Sciences of the United States of America*, *112*(42), 13105–13108. PMID: 26438875

Hillman, C. H., Erickson, K. I., & Kramer, A. F. (2008). Exercise and brain function. *Nature Reviews. Neuroscience*, *9*, 58–65. PMID: 18094706

Lin, T. W., & Kuo, Y. M. (2013). Exercise benefits brain function: The monoamine connection. *Brain Sciences*, *3*(1), 39–53. PMID: 24961306

Mammen, G., & Faulkner, G. (2013). Activity reduces anxiety and depression risk. *Journal of Psychiatric Research*, *47*(3), 355–363.

Meeusen, R., & De Meirleir, K. (1995). Exercise and brain neurotransmission. *Sports Medicine (Auckland, N.Z.)*, *20*(3), 160–188. PMID: 8571000

Pagliaro, S., Iacoviello, M., De Cristofaro, M., & Sessa, F. (2021). Norepinephrine modulatory effects during exercise and stress: Neurobiological implications. *Frontiers in Behavioral Neuroscience*, *14*, 1–12.

Ratey, J. (2008). *Spark: The new science of exercise and the brain*. Little, Brown.

Stillman, C. M.. (2020). Exercise improves connectivity in emotion-regulation networks. *Psychophysiology*, *57*(8), 433–450.

Szuhany, K. L., Bugatti, M., & Otto, M. W. (2015). A meta-analysis of BDNF response to exercise. *Psychosomatic Medicine*, *77*(3), 247–255.

Szuhany, K. L., Bugatti, M., & Otto, M. W. (2015). A meta-analytic review of the effects of exercise on brain-derived neurotrophic factor. *Journal of Psychiatric Research*, *60*, 56–64. PMID: 25455510

van Praag, H.. (1999). Running enhances neurogenesis. *Nature Neuroscience*, *2*, 266–270. PMID: 10195220

Voss, M. W.. (2013). Neurobiological effects of exercise on aging. *Neuroscience and Biobehavioral Reviews*, *37*, 2243–2261.

Zhang, X., Lv, J., & Jia, G. (2022). Physical activity and emotional resilience. *Journal of Affective Disorders*, *309*, 45–56. PMID: 35712359

Chapter 12
The Impact of Exercise on Teacher Satisfaction and Retention:
A Scoping Review

Sydney Anne Wilkens
https://orcid.org/0009-0009-0785-8070
Southern Nazarene University, USA

Christiana Milla
Southern Nazarene University, USA

ABSTRACT

Physical activity can act as a specific coping mechanism to increase positive mental health in teachers and mitigate burnout in the teaching profession. The purpose of this scoping review was to explore physical activity in relation to teachers' burnout and well-being and was guided by the question: how does physical activity impact teachers' well-being and burnout in their profession? Nineteen articles were selected for inclusion in this study and were analyzed according to the guiding question and to identify emerging themes across the studies. Findings suggest that physical activity has a positive impact on teacher mental well-being but were mixed regarding burnout, with some studies indicating that physical activity can help mitigate burnout, primarily through emotional exhaustion, and a few studies not finding a significant correlation. Implications suggest recommendations for schools to incorporate school-based physical activities for teachers and a focus on leisure-time physical activities.

DOI: 10.4018/979-8-3373-6157-4.ch012

INTRODUCTION

Educators continue to experience burnout due to job demands and lack of organizational support and structure (Ha et al., 2025). According to studies online, as of 2025, the rate of teacher burnout remains at 44% (Berkey, n.d.; Jacobs-Pinson, n.d.; Peck, 2025). Emotional fatigue is experienced by educators due to the continuous and extensive compassion demonstrated to students (Inbar & Shiri, 2021). Because of these challenges (Ha et al., 2025; Inbar & Shiri, 2021), positive mental health decreases while burnout increases, making teaching a difficult emotional experience (Ormiston et al., 2022; Turner & Garvis, 2023). It is crucial for teachers to find strategies to cope with the prevalence of burnout so teachers can continue to avoid teacher attrition and increase longevity of engaging in the profession (Rojas et al., 2025). Physical activity and exercise may be a coping mechanism to burnout in the teaching profession and increase positive mental health (Bogaert et al., 2014). Thus, the purpose of this scoping review was to explore physical activity in relation to teachers' burnout and well-being. Physical activity was examined as a coping mechanism to understand if it mitigated or increased positive mental health and decreased teacher burnout. This scoping review is guided by the following question: how does physical activity impact teachers' well-being and burnout in their profession?

REVIEW OF LITERATURE

Positive Mental Health

Positive mental health is identified as an increased emotional understanding of one's experiences and surroundings, which promotes well-being and enhances life satisfaction (Valentim et al., 2025). Positive mental health is indicated by the positive emotional condition that contributes to the cognitive components of one's overall well-being, which in turn, promotes successful outcomes (Valentim et al., 2025). Factors including personality attributes (Ren & Wang, 2022; Vela et al., 2024) and health determinants (Carr, 2024) contribute to obtaining positive mental health. Over the past decade, researchers have studied the impact that positive mental health has on educators by observing students' reactions (Brailovskaia et al., 2024), school variables (Capone & Petrillo, 2020), and teacher self-assurance (Fiorilli et al., 2019; Nalipay et al., 2019). Positive mental health has a significant effect on teacher burnout, as it can promote transformation and engagement in the classroom

(UND Today, 2024). It is an important part of maintaining overall well-being and can improve feelings and perceptions of burnout (Clasquin-Johnson & Ebrahim, 2024).

When teachers experience overall well-being, they are more likely to engage in best teaching and pedagogical practices while also creating positive classroom atmospheres (Kong & Lai, 2023). Well-being can be scaffolded to emotional well-being, as this primarily focuses on personal feelings (Leung & Cheung, 2024; Stark et al., 2022) and mental well-being, which considers motivational outcomes (Agnieszka & Marta, 2021; Kamboj & Garg, 2021). When teachers experience emotional fatigue, difficulty maintaining positive mental health and feelings of burnout occur (Kariou et al., 2021; Mijakoski et al., 2022; Nápoles et al., 2023).

History of Burnout

The idea of burnout syndrome was discovered by Herbert Freudenberger and Sigmund Ginsburg, though Freudenberger is most commonly credited with formulating it with the context of work-related stress (Heinemann & Heinemann, 2017). Freudenberger used the term "burnout" to describe the emotional fatigue experienced by individuals facing constant workplace demands and pressures (Heinemann & Heinemann, 2017). Freudenberger (1975) believed that burnout experiences depended on one's professional role and identified symptoms of burnout, including negative performance modifications, engaging in risks, and having an increased negative attitude. Freudenberger (1989) extended his understanding of burnout to include a variety of societal suggestions and argued that burnout should not be viewed from only an institutional and occupational point of view but recognized as a complicated experience with social, political, and cultural elements.

Christina Maslach also made significant contributions to the burnout concept, noticing that burnout was most experienced among professionals in community-based occupations, often those who interact with patrons in emotionally taxing circumstances (Maslach & Jackson, 1981). Maslach and Jackson (1981) stated, "Burnout is a syndrome of emotional exhaustion and cynicism…[and] the tendency to evaluate oneself negatively" (p. 99). After the recognition of these qualities, Maslach and Jackson (1981) created The Maslach Burnout Inventory (MBI), which is a psychometric tool designed to assess three core dimensions of burnout, specifically, personal accomplishment, emotional exhaustion, and depersonalization. The MBI has become an important instrument in psychology for understanding the socioemotional dimensions of job demand stress (Bianchi et al., 2020; Li et al., 2021; Maslach & Jackson, 1981). Maslach's work has continued and maintains that burnout is an extensive issue, shaped by increasing workplace demands and organizational constructs (Maslach & Leiter, 2016; O'Hara et al., 2025).

Burnout has generally been connected to one's occupation (Nadon et al., 2022). A mental health disorder is a "mental illness or psychiatric disorder" and influences your behaviors, emotions, and thoughts (Cleveland Clinic, 2025). Cleveland Clinic (2025) states there are over 200 disorders, which include schizophrenia, autism, depression, and post-traumatic stress disorder, among others. Nadon et al. (2022) suggest clinicians diagnose burnout as a syndrome of a mental health disorder despite it not having been officially incorporated. We recognize burnout within this study as being tied to work and not a medically diagnosed condition.

Teacher Burnout

Teacher burnout occurs when teachers and educators experience tension and fatigue from the demands of teaching over extended periods of time (Pressley, 2021; Rockwell, 2024). There are several research studies that conclude that teacher burnout is a complex structure, involving several overarching themes like organizational variables (Freire et al., 2020; Ha et al., 2025) and self-efficacy and motivation (Pakdee et al., 2025; Song et al., 2024). Over the past decade, many researchers have expanded on the different dimensions of burnout, like job demands, job satisfaction, and emotional aspects (Skaalvik & Skaalvik, 2018; Skaalvik & Skaalvik, 2020); the impact of burnout on students and the classroom (Madigan & Kim, 2021); the important role that personality traits have on teacher burnout (Kim et al., 2019); and environment conditions and inadequate administrative support (Ha et al., 2025). Despite the recognition of numerous factors that contribute to teacher burnout (Dung et al., 2024; Song et al., 2024; Walker, 2025), a central question remains regarding the mediating role between given variables (Freire et al., 2020; Rose & Loomis, 2025).

Job Demands. Teachers who encounter elevated job demands experience heightened levels of burnout (Song et al., 2024). Job demands include numerous responsibilities, such as participating in after school activities (Baumgartner et al., 2025), managing the amount of students or grade level being taught (Carroll et al., 2022), frequent communication (Hlado & Harvankova, 2024), student interactions (Kiremitci et al., 2023), uneven distribution of workload tasks (Jomuad et al., 2021), working extended hours (Hojo, 2021), and lack of time to meet deadlines (Samaden et al., 2021). The impact that job demands have on teachers' experiences can add stress to various aspects of their life, such as job related, personal, or psychological, and can further increase burnout within the profession (Thomas & Reyes, 2024). When these job demands cause overwhelming feelings, teachers may experience burnout and resign from their teaching roles altogether (Trinidad, 2021). However, if teachers possess strong mental health characteristics, these job demands and feelings of teacher burnout could diminish (Chan et al., 2021; Wink et al., 2021).

Though, this can be challenging for teachers to maintain when job demands are high (Agyapong et al., 2022) or due to mental stress (Jeon et al., 2022).

Teachers who have an appropriate work-life balance respond better to job-demands and tend to have a positive outlook on their job (Žnidaršič & Marič, 2021). Unfortunately, job demands consistently act as a barrier in teachers' well-being, as Turner and Garvis (2023) concluded that among various workplace stressors, job demands were the most stated factor that increased burnout and dissipated the mental health of teachers. It is important to consider the effect that job demands have on teacher's mental health and feelings of burnout, as this barrier could be the reason teachers' struggle to stay in the profession (Robinson et al., 2022) or why teachers experience attrition (Mérida-López et al., 2022).

Emotional Fatigue. When teachers experience emotional fatigue, difficulty maintaining positive mental health and feelings of burnout occur (Kariou et al., 2021; Mijakoski et al., 2022; Nápoles et al., 2023). Emotional fatigue is felt by educators due to the continuous compassion they must show to students (Inbar & Shiri, 2021), the stress that is associated when supporting trauma-affected students and the perceived lack of confidence in doing so (Oberg et al., 2025), and decreased appreciation (Kendrick, 2022). Because the teaching profession involves constant communication, relationship building, problem solving, and expressing sympathetic feelings, emotional regulation is compromised and can lead to stress and burnout (Kasapoglu & Didin, 2019). Neto et al. (2024) concluded that though teachers felt that their professional achievement levels were high, burnout was also elevated, suggesting that the social and physical circumstances of the educational institution promoted emotional fatigue.

Though there are many aspects that contribute to emotional fatigue, emotional regulation could improve positive mental health in teachers and reduce burnout (Wang et al., 2025). Jennings and Min (2023) suggested that showing compassion to students instead of empathy could help preserve teachers' overall mental health and well-being; however, exhibiting positivity consistently to students is highly promoted in the education profession, yet, acts as a risk to burnout due to the imbalance of emotional regulation (Atwood, 2024). In Woloshyn et al. (2023), teacher participants acknowledged the interconnectedness of personal and professional emotional fatigue, noting how it could be challenging to separate the two, but recognized the need to improve mental health. Nevertheless, because of the endless emotional investment teachers are required to instill in students, emotional fatigue occurs, acting as a barrier to encountering positive mental health and decreased feelings of burnout (Ormiston et al., 2022). Because of the increased emotional fatigue teachers are experiencing, mental well-being is decreasing, and teacher retention declines (Nath & Pandey, 2025).

Lack of Organizational Support. Lack of organizational support has been identified as a barrier for teachers increasing their positive mental health and decreasing burnout (Pressley, 2021). Organizational support is the perception from employees that the organization will support and value them, and in turn, improves and promotes work engagement and self-efficacy (Jiao et al., 2022). When teachers feel more supported, feelings of burnout are mediated (Kinder et al., 2023) and self-efficacy and self-confidence are enhanced (Rizvi et al., 2023), which are attributes of developing and maintaining positive mental health (Jahoda, 1958). When the organizational support is high, teachers gain positive mental health and well-being (Sun et al., 2024). In some schools, this is facilitated by providing meaningful help to teachers and letting teachers have independence (Hyatt, 2022), creating a friendly work environment (Yaqian et al., 2024), and appreciating staff (Jamal et al., 2023). When educators feel supported, their positive mental health increases as well as their overall job satisfaction (Sudibjo & Manihuruk, 2022; Wang, 2024).

Unfortunately, numerous studies conclude that teachers experience low organizational support from administrators, and higher levels of burnout exist and contribute to emotional exhaustion (Aronsson et al., 2017; Baptista & Cardoso, 2021; Huk et al., 2019). Administration's leadership style positively or negatively shapes the school environment, which can impact the school employees' well-being and students' success, or create community pressure (Gray et al., 2017; Vermote et al., 2023). As administrators create a culture of stress and anxiety through inadequate support, teacher attrition increases and teachers may consider leaving the profession altogether (Farmer, 2020). Regardless, consistent organizational support improves well-being and decreases burnout in teachers (Ortan et al., 2021), but there is no requirement to provide this level of encouragement. Because some schools show support (Kinder et al., 2023) and some do not (Aronsson et al., 2017; Baptista & Cardoso, 2021; Huk et al., 2019), a substantial barrier and disparity is created for teachers to consistently experience positive mental health within this profession (Pressley, 2021).

COVID-19 and Teacher Burnout. The COVID-19 Pandemic imposed significant stress on educators, leading to an increase in teacher burnout (Marshall et al., 2024). Many teachers reported a remarkable decline in institutional support due to occupational and circumstantial anxiety (Chen et al., 2024; Pressley, 2021). The shift to remote learning and isolation further decreased instructional quality and increased emotional fatigue (Westphal et al., 2022). Resuming in-person instruction marked a significant period after the pandemic but also increased negative student behaviors (Macias, 2024) and has further increased burnout in teachers (Ozamiz-Etxebarria et al., 2023).

Physical Activity

Given the high levels of stress that is associated with teaching and how it can affect psychological and emotional wellness, physical activity acts as a moderator for educators and their feelings of burnout (Davis et al., 2025). The World Health Organization (WHO) states that, "...physical activity [can act] as any bodily movement produced by skeletal muscles that requires energy expenditure" and that, "Both moderate-and vigorous-intensity physical activity improve health," (World Health Organization, 2024). The terms exercise, physical activity, and physical fitness are all interchangeable; however, in 1985, these terms were defined with more structure, as exercise is known as planned and repeated movements or activity; physical activity is any activity of daily living; and physical fitness are characteristics that are related to one's health or one's skill level (Caspersen et al., 1985).

The American College of Sports Medicine (ACSM) is widely known for providing the "gold standard" for physical activity recommendations, recommending that adults engage in moderate intensity exercise for five days a week for at least 30 minutes per session (ACSM, n. d.). In addition to improving physical health, there is also a list of physiological benefits that come from engaging in regular physical activity, such as blood pressure regulation, emotional wellness stability, and the lowering of the Body Mass Index per individual (ACSM, n.d). Decreased health risks also occur with the engagement of physical activity, such as the reduction of cardiovascular disease, diabetes, diseases, and cancers (The Center for Disease and Control Prevention, 2024). The Center for Disease and Control Prevention (CDC) supports the ACSM's recommendations of physical activity engagement, yet emphasizes the need for adults to incorporate at least two days of strength exercise for well-rounded health (CDC, n.d.).

Physical activity can increase mental well-being (de Costa et al., 2023) and can be used as a self-management technique to help with mental health issues (Pelletier et al., 2017). Moderate-to-vigorous (Murray et al., 2023) and high intensity exercise (Ram et al., 2022; Ye et al., 2024) have a significant impact on mental health in various populations.

Barriers to Physical Activity

Barriers to engagement in physical activity exist in literature (Barbosa et al., 2024; de Costa et al., 2023; Palmer, 2020, Pelletier et al., 2017; Van Dyck et al., 2017). Pelletier et al. (2017) suggests that though physical activity should be recommended to those struggling with mental health and anxiety disorders, obstacles to participating in physical activity that should be considered are lack of motivation, time, and education, as well as the cost or the inability to participate in physical activity

(Palmer, 2020; Pelletier et al., 2017). Stage of life could function as a constraint as well, as adults who are retired demonstrated reduced physical activity (Van Dyck et al., 2017). However, social support could improve this barrier (Beselt et al., 2021) and was considered as a successful approach in other populations (Sunarti et al., 2024). Sedentary lifestyles represent an additional impediment to engagement in physical activity, which acts as an implication to mental health and should be addressed (Barbosa et al., 2024; de Costa et al., 2023). Despite these challenges and barriers, both physical activity and exercise empowers different populations (Beselt et al., 2021; Sunarti et al., 2024) and provides social benefits to those who are participating, which enhances their experience (Beselt et al., 2021; Parra et al., 2019).

Physical Activity as a Mediator to Teacher Burnout and Improving Positive Mental Health

Physical activity can act as a specific coping mechanism to increase positive mental health in teachers and mitigate burnout in the teaching profession (Mariano et al., 2023). This is due to the production of endorphins, which is a natural hormone produced in the body that increases feelings of well-being or pleasure and decreases stress (Dahati & Dahati, 2025) and can help reduce or relieve the negative feelings associated with burnout that teachers experience (Mariano et al., 2023). Because educators experience burnout and decreased mental health (Ha et al., 2025; Kotowski et al., 2022; Marshall et al., 2024), engaging in physical activity can promote overall quality of life satisfaction and increase positive mental health (da Silva et al., 2024). It is necessary to consider the relevance that physical activity could have on promoting teachers' mental and emotional health (Cheng & Liu, 2024).

Demerouti et al's (2001) Job Demands-Resources Model (JD-R)

Demerouti et al. 's (2001) Job Demands-Resources Model explains how job responsibilities and occupational conditions affect employee's well-being. This model demonstrates that job demands can lead to feelings of mental strain and fatigue, but resources give employees the ability to cope with these feelings properly (Demerouti et al., 2001). The JD-R is frequently used to understand employee well-being (Lesener et al., 2018) and to understand how increased job demands, as well as job control, lead to burnout and decreased work engagement within a profession (Demerouti et al., 2001; Tummers & Bakker, 2021). The JD-R can be used to understand shortcomings and advantages in a working environment (Bakker & Demerouti, 2007). This model provided within the study illustrates that job demands could lead to exhaustion; whereas lack of job resources could lead to disengagement, depending on the amount of positive or negative interaction in the work environment (Demerouti et al., 2001). Ultimately, adverse job demands influences burnout within an individual and leads to poor work engagement (Bakker et al., 2023), but the presence of numerous and helpful job resources could help mitigate exhaustion and fatigue (Bakker & de Vries, 2020; Demerouti et al., 2021).

Job Demands

Demerouti et al. (2001) defined job demands as the "...physical social or organizational aspects of the job that require sustained physical or mental effort and are therefore associated with certain physiological and psychological costs (e.g., exhaustion)" (p. 501). Job demands are key contributors to employee exhaustion and the development of employee burnout (Demerouti et al., 2001). Martin et al. (2025) concluded that job demands were any demand that required physiological or psychological strain and could increase feelings of burnout or resentment. Given that excessive job requirements could lead to employee fatigue, it is important to consider the effects and examine the role that job demands have on employees and their well-being (Mäkikangas et al., 2020).

Job Resources

Job resources are tools that are helpful to the employee that mitigate job demands (Demerouti et al., 2001). Demerouti et al. (2001) defined job resources as:

> *[The] physical, psychological, social or organizational aspects of the job that may do any of the following: (a) be functional in achieving work goals; (b) reduce job demands at the associated physiological and psychological costs; (c) stimulate personal growth and development. (p. 501)*

In the original study of the JD-R model, job resources are seen as only external resources, such as institutional and societal (Demerouti et al., 2001). When these resources are lacking, an imbalance is generated and creates displeasure or discouragement (Demerouti et al., 2001). Job resources are feedback, rewards, job control, participation, job security, and supervisor support (Demerouti et al., 2001). Bakker and Demerouti (2017) suggested that job resources could actually buffer the adverse effects that job demands have on employees and could potentially promote character growth. In recent years, Bakker (2022) mentioned the important effect that social behavior has on work involvement, suggesting this as a job resource that organizational leaders should share with each other within the institution. Likewise, Tang et al. (2024) expanded on the components, concluding that job resources could lead to increased unique individual characteristics and increased motivation within the workplace. Moreover, adequate job resources may improve or alleviate symptoms and feelings of burnout, so it is important to consider and understand the effect that different resources have on employee well-being (Palvimo et al., 2023; Patel & Bartholomew, 2021).

Connection of the JD-R Model to the Teaching Profession

The Job-Demands Resource model has been increasingly applied to the teaching profession by utilizing the JD-R to understand the complexity of teachers' job demands and resources, use of coping mechanisms, and analyzing occupational burnout within the profession (Kiremitci et al., 2023). In research, authors can take the job demands and job resources that occur in their organization and utilize it to frame their study (Huang et al., 2025). For instance, some studies will use the JD-R by inserting specific job demands and resources encountered by educators to see how these factors may predict burnout within their study (Collie, 2023; Rastegr & Zarei, 2023) or how these factors contribute to teacher-well being (Costa et al., 2024; Xia & Shun, 2021). In Bigras et al. (2021), the authors utilized the JD-R by manipulating job demands and job resources with factors like deadlines, communication, and student interaction, as well as positive feedback, self-efficacy, and guaranteed employment. The JD-R can also explain health and emotional aspects of the teaching profession and how they relate to teacher burnout and well-being (Skaalvik & Skaalvik, 2017).

In educational institutions, job resources may act as coping mechanisms or support to the educator to mediate job demands and improve well-being (Manuti et al., 2022; Skaalvik & Skaalvik, 2021; Zhou et al., 2024). Examples of job resources could include use of self-efficacy (Granziera, 2022), organizational interventions (Naidoo-Chetty & Du Plessis, 2021), positive mental health factors (Zhao et al., 2024), use of autonomy (Ha et al., 2025), or personal preference of coping strategies that work best for the educator (Algorani & Gupta, 2023). Workplace culture is also important to consider since it can influence an employee's mental health and well-being (Monteiro & Joseph, 2023). The Job-Demands Resource Model investigates how to improve overall well-being and prevent occupational burnout within an individual (Demerouti et al., 2001), which is an important concept in the teaching profession, since burnout is becoming more relevant (Alsalhe et al., 2021) and teacher well-being needs to be furthered studied and addressed within the education profession (Dreer, 2023).

When a teacher feels they are thriving and well-being is promoted, the use of resources may increase (Li et al., 2025). However, this is difficult for teachers to experience, due to the various stressful job demands they encounter (Baumgartner et al., 2025; Hlado & Harvankova, 2024; Kiremitci et al., 2023; Song et al., 2024). Finding coping mechanisms that act as job resources is important for teachers as it could mitigate their burnout within the profession (Dung et al., 2024; Shaheen

& Mahmood, 2024; Tan & Kim, 2024) and it is important to consider educators' overall mental health and well-being (Dreer, 2023).

METHODOLOGY

This study was conducted as a scoping review. Mak and Thomas (2022) describe a scoping review as a "type of knowledge synthesis that uses a systematic and iterative approach to identify and synthesize an existing or emerging body of literature on a given topic" (p. 565). Pollock et al. (2024) suggest that this kind of review is useful for mapping the "breadth of evidence available on a particular topic, field, concept, or issue, within or across a defined context or contexts" (p. 1). This scoping review focused on the impact of physical activity on teachers' well-being and burnout while in their profession. This methodology section is outlined according to Mak and Thomas' (2022) steps for conducting a scoping review.

Identifying the Research Question

The research team met at the beginning of the research to discuss the study topic and focus. Based on an understanding of the literature, the team narrowed the focus to physical activity and burnout and well-being among teachers. Through multiple iterations, the following guiding question was agreed upon for this scoping review: how does physical activity impact teachers' well-being and burnout in their profession?

Identifying Relevant Studies

The second step of a scoping review involves developing a search strategy, including keywords, identifying databases used to search, inclusion and exclusion criteria, and a narrowing of the strategy based on retrieved articles (Mak & Thomas, 2022). Articles were searched for using a variety of combinations of the terms "teacher burnout," positive mental health," "coping mechanisms," "physical activity," "exercise," "occupational burnout," "mental health," "depression," "anxiety," and "stress." These terms were initially searched using the EBSCO and Google Scholar databases; however, further searches were conducted on specific publishing sites as it was noted that several articles were published from the same journals. Specifically, BMC Psychology, BMC Public Health, and International Journal of Environmental Research and Public Health were searched. Inclusion criteria for articles included: (a) a focus on physical activity and teachers' mental health, well-being, or burnout; (b) published within the past 15 years; and (c) journal articles. Exclusion criteria included: (a) a focus on non-teacher participants such as college students or administrators and (b) publications other than journal articles.

Selecting Studies to Be Included in the Review

Research articles were examined by title and abstract to determine relevance with this study's topic. Each research team member reviewed the titles and abstracts independently and then the research team met collectively to determine inclusion of articles. Team members agreed about inclusion for a majority of the articles. The team discussed two of the articles regarding study topic focus and determined they would be included. An additional article was discussed and excluded from the review due to its focus on college students. A total of 12 articles were selected for the review. Upon review of the articles, a snowball approach was used as article reference lists were reviewed for additional articles. Again, the research team individually reviewed the title and abstract and then collectively made a decision to include the articles. Seven additional articles were identified and selected, totaling 19 articles for the literature review.

Charting the Data

Mak and Thomas (2022) note that in the fourth step of Charting the Data, the research team builds a data extraction form to be used by the team and to organize details of the studies based on specific categories. A spreadsheet was used to organize the collection of the articles. Article information, such as the APA citation and study summaries, was added to the spreadsheet and additional categories were added following selection of all articles. Additional categories noted included: country, research method, teacher grade level, type of school, and study findings.

Collating, Summarizing, and Reporting the Results

During this step of the process, the research team conducts numerical and thematic analysis of the data (Mak & Thomas, 2022). The selected articles were analyzed in an attempt to answer the guiding question of the study. Additionally, the articles were further analyzed, noting commonalities in the findings points of focus. Analysis began with each researcher reading through the studies. Initial notes and memos were recorded by each researcher on the data spreadsheet and each researcher listed their codes and categories that emerged per article. An additional research team meeting was held to discuss analysis conducted by each researcher and compare codes and categories. Any differences in analysis were discussed and agreed upon.

The researchers also discussed and agreed upon themes, which are presented in the findings section of this paper.

FINDINGS

Following review to ensure selection criteria, a total of 19 articles were selected for this literature review. Selected articles focused on teachers and covered physical activity and burnout, emotional regulation, work-related outcomes, stress, relatedness, and mental well-being. They covered a broad geographical scope in that the studies were conducted in Finland (1), China (1), Spain (3), Italy (1), Brazil (3), Saudi Arabia (2), Belgium (1), Portugal (1), Nigeria (1), Turkey (1) and the United States (5). Thus, a majority of articles (14) were conducted outside of the United States. All of the articles were quantitative in nature except for two mixed-methods studies (Aperribai et al., 2020; Kim & Gurvitch, 2020). See Table 1 for article descriptives.

Six studies focused on secondary teachers; five studies focused on primary teachers; and seven studies focused on both primary and secondary teachers. Two studies included early care and childhood teachers with one including only those participants (Carson et al., 2010) and the other including those in addition to primary teachers (Randall et al., 2021). Additionally, one study (Cheng & Liu, 2024) recruited university educators along with primary and secondary educators but did not report how many survey responses were from university educators. Given the limited number of articles regarding this topic, the research team decided to keep these studies in the literature review, believing the study's participants and focus were closely related to the focus of this literature review. Articles were mixed in their data collection from teachers of public or private schools. Five studies collected data from teachers at public schools; one was from private schools; three from both public and private schools; and 10 studies did not specify whether they were public or private schools. Only a few studies reported participation criteria related to specific subjects taught by teachers. Dike et al. (2021) focused only on teachers of children with autism spectrum disorders, and Cheng and Liu (2024) recruited English as a Foreign Language teachers. Additionally, González-Valero et al. 's (2023) study was based on physical education teachers.

Additional similarities among studies were found in the instruments selected for data collection. In regards to burnout, five studies used a variation of the Maslach Burnout Inventory (MBI), with the educator survey being the most frequently used version. Two additional studies used the Burnout Assessment Tool (BAT) to measure teacher burnout. The most commonly used physical activity survey was the International Physical Activity Questionnaire (IPAQ). A wide assortment of surveys was used to measure other study variables.

Though none of the studies were carried out over a year or more, five studies implemented a physical activity program that spanned multiple weeks and months (Abós et al., 2021; Dike et al., 2021; Kim & Gurvitch, 2020; Latino et al., 2021; Mariano et al., 2023). Kim and Gurvitch (2020) researched a seven week physical activity program, and Marino et al. (2023) Latino et al. (2021) both implemented an eight week program. Dike et al. (2021) conducted a three month study, and Abós et al. (2021) was the longest study at eight months. Marion et al. (2023) and Kim and Gurvitch (2020), despite similar length of study time, reported different findings in relation to stress with Marino et al. (2023) reporting that nearly 79% of teachers reported reduced stress. However, Kim and Gurvitch (2020) did not find that the difference in stress was statistically significant. In regards to burnout, Latino et al. (2021) in their eight week program reported no significant change, but Dike et al.'s (2021) three month study showed that burnout had significantly reduced following the program. Both studies researched yoga programs. Interestingly, Abós et al. (2021) reported no improvement in burnout following an eight month study; they did report increased job satisfaction though. Further discussion over longitudinal studies and the need for these in this field are discussed later in the chapter.

Table 1. Article identification and descriptives

Article	Country	Method	Participants	Public/Private
Abós et al. (2021)	Spain	Quantitative	Secondary Educators	Public
Alhazmi et al. (2025)	Saudi Arabia	Quantitative	Primary Educators	Not Specified
Al-Johani (2021)	Saudi Arabia	Quantitative	Secondary Educators	Not Specified
Aperribai et al. (2020)	Spain	Mixed Methods	Primary and Secondary Educators	Public and Private
Bogaert et al. (2014)	Belgium	Quantitative	Secondary Educators	Not Specified
Carson et al. (2010)	United States	Quanitative	Early Care and Childhood Educator	Private
Cheng & Liu (2024)	China	Quantitative	Primary, Secondary, and University Educators	Not Specified
Çifçi & Demir (2020)	Turkey	Quantitative	Primary and Secondary Educators	Not Specified
da Silva et al. (2024)	Brazil	Quantitative	Primary and Secondary Educators	Public
Davis et al. (2025)	United States	Quantitative	Secondary Educators	Public
Dike et al. (2021)	Nigeria	Quantitative	Primary Educators	Public and Private

continued on following page

Table 1. Continued

Article	Country	Method	Participants	Public/Private
Fontana et al. (2022)	United States	Quantitative	Primary and Secondary Educators	Not Specified
González-Valero et al. (2023)	Spain	Quantitative	Primary and Secondary Educators	Not Specified
Kim & Gurvitch (2020)	United States	Mixed Methods	Secondary Educators	Public
Latino et al. (2021)	Finland	Quantitative	Secondary Educators	Public
Mariano et al. (2023)	Portugal/ Brazil	Quantitative	Primary and Secondary Educators	Not Specified
Neto et al. (2024)	Brazil	Quantitative	Primary Educators	Not Specified
Randall et al. (2021)	United States	Quantitative	Early Care and Childhood and Primary Educators	Public and Private
Scardina et al. (2024)	Italy	Quantitative	Primary Educators	Not Specified

This scoping review sought to answer the guiding question of how does physical activity impact teachers' well-being and burnout in their profession? Analysis suggests that physical activity has a positive impact on teachers' well-being and can help mitigate burnout though there were mixed findings on burnout. In regards to mental health and well-being, the studies revealed that physical activity can positively impact emotions (Carson et al., 2010; Cheng & Liu, 2024; Neto et al., 2024), stress (Bogaert et al., 2014; Fontana et al., 2022; Mariano et al., 2023), improve job satisfaction (Abós et al., 2021; Kim & Gurvitch, 2020), increase work engagement (Abós et a., 2021), and has positive effects on overall mental well-being (Al-Johani, 2021; Bogaert et al., 2014; Çifçi & Demir, 2020; Randall et al., 2021; Scardina et al., 2024). da Silva et al. 's (2024) study is perhaps a synopsis of the studies in that they found that more active participants experienced a higher quality of life. Thus, when teachers engage in physical activity, their mental health and well-being improves (Randall et al, 2021), even when job demands are high (da Silva et al., 2024).

Results were not as clear regarding the impact of physical activity on burnout. Some studies indicated that physical activity helps mitigate teacher burnout (Davis et al., 2025; Dike et al., 2021; González-Valero et al., 2023; Latino et al., 2021). Specifically, González-Valero et al. 's (2023) study found that those who did not report experiencing burnout engaged in 150 minutes or more of physical activity per week. In regards to the components of burnout, physical activity was found to decrease emotional exhaustion (Carson et al., 2010; Davis et al., 2025; Neto et al., 2024) and depersonalization (Dike et al., 2021; González-Valero et al., 2023; Latino et al., 2021) and increase personal fulfillment (González-Valero et al., 2023). Neto et al.'s (2024) study found only the scores for emotional fatigue were statistically significant when looking at physical activity. Similarly, Davis et al. (2025) did not report statistically significant findings for physical activity and total burnout but did for emotional exhaustion specifically. In contrast, Abós et al. (2021) found that physical activity did not improve burnout. This study was related to school-based physical activity programs (Abós et al., 2021), which may have contributed to this finding. Further research is needed to fully determine the impact of physical activity on burnout (Abós et al., 2021).

In addition to well-being and burnout, there was also a focus on other variables. These included type of physical activity, school-based physical activity programs, level of physical activity, gender differences, and COVID-19. Those themes are discussed in detail below.

Type of Physical Activity

Type of physical activity emerged as a theme in the studies reviewed and supported teacher's mental and emotional health. For instance, yoga participation improved well-being in teachers, as it promoted positive cognitive, psychological, and physiological well-being (Dike et al., 2021; Latino et al., 2021). Likewise, Cognitive Behavioral Therapy (CBT) coupled with yoga practice increased gratitude and reduced emotional burnout, causing a decrease in attrition toward teaching (Dike et al., 2021) and should be furthered examined as an intervention for teacher burnout (Latino et al., 2021).

While several specific types of physical activity are discussed in research, the most commonly recommended physical activity type among the literature studies reviewed was leisure-time physical activity. In Bogaert et al. (2014), engagement in leisure-time physical activity outside of contract hours decreased adverse mental health symptoms. Because of this, teacher well-being improved due to the positive physical and mental health effects occurring from the leisure-time physical activity, and in turn, improved job satisfaction (Bogaert et al., 2014). Similarly, Carson et al. (2010) found that when teachers participated in leisure-time physical activity outside of contract hours, mental health increased. Carson et al. (2010) also found that participating in physical activity during work hours seemed to mediate emotional exhaustion, suggesting that moving during work hours resulted in mental health benefits. In fact, Carson et al. (2010) advocated for this, stating, "Thus, it appears that physical activity participation is not something that has to only wait until after work for it to ease aspects of childcare teacher burnout; it can and should be done during work" (p. 910). Likewise, Çifçi and Demir (2020) found that physical activity at home decreased anxiety among teachers, and Aperribai et al. (2020) concluded that indoor physical activity showed similar results. Al-Johani (2021) reported that walking leisurely was associated with improved mental health, though location of walking as a form of physical activity was not clearly defined.

Physical activity in the form of sport or recreational games was beneficial to mental health and well-being, but this could be due to the social aspect of engaging in the sport (Abós et al., 2021). Kim and Gurvitch (2020) concluded that sport-based activity showed improvement in the community of the school and increased teacher's attitudes toward physical activity, yet, not enough to be considered statistically significant. Sport participation also increased resilience among teachers compared to those who did not participate in sport-based physical activity (González-Valero et al., 2023). Regardless of the type of physical activity that teachers participated in, all forms mentioned in the studies contributed to the improvement of their mental health and emotional well-being (Abós et al., 2021; Al-Johani, 2021; Aperribaei et al., 2020; Bogaert et al., 2014; Carson et al., 2010; Çifçi & Demir, 2020; Dike et al., 2021; González-Valero et al., 2023; Kim & Gurvitch, 2020; Latino et al., 2021).

School-Based Physical Activity Programs

Studies with a focus on school-based physical activity programs found overall that when teachers participated in physical activity with their colleagues, they felt a sense of belonging (Kim & Gurvitch, 2020) and relatedness (Abós et al., 2021). Teachers were able to establish a further connection with one another (Kim & Gurvitch, 2020). Kim and Gurvitch (2020) quoted a participant who stated, "I definitely gained friendships and I am able to walk the halls and actually say hi to people and call people by name. And connect on a deeper level than just how are you…" (p. 665). In regards to gender, Çifçi and Demir (2020) found no difference in mental well-being among men and women who exercised but found that of these groups, women experienced more anxiety. However, women who did not exercise reported lower levels of mental well-being than men who did not exercise (Çifçi & Demir, 2020). This aligns with Bogaert et al.'s (2014) finding that teachers who are women had significantly worse mental health as well as physical health. Women had higher levels of work-related stress even though there were no reported differences in job satisfaction (Bogaert et al., 2014).

Sport-based programs were also seen as a successful approach to combating adverse mental health effects and burnout in teachers. For instance, Kim and Gurvitch (2020) observed positive mental health increased when sport-based physical activity programs were implemented among teachers, even though it was not proven statistically significant. In contrast, this conflicts with González-Valero et al.'s (2023) finding that while sport-based physical activity programs did not directly reduce burnout, but improved resilience, regular participation in physical activity could be a useful coping mechanism. Additionally, Mariano et al. (2023) implemented an 8-week program that consisted of 40 different exercise sessions and found that teacher's stress decreased when participating consistently in the 8-week exercise program. Similarly, Latino et al. (2021) found that yoga programs that teachers engaged in promoted mindfulness, reduced burnout, and enhanced emotional well-being. The findings of Kim and Gurvitch (2020), Mariano et al. (2023), and Latino et al. (2021) collectively suggest that school-based physical activity programs were overall successful in promoting psychological and emotional health. However, Kim and Gurvitch (2020) and Mariano et al. (2023) further concluded that motivation of exercise increased, as well as increased positive social connections within the school. This aligns with Abós et al.'s (2021) findings that relatedness and social connection could improve burnout; yet, Abós et al. (2021) found a less direct correlation between physical activity and feelings of burnout. These social aspects are important to note, because many educator's relationships were affected by the COVID-19 Pandemic, which led to a decrease in teacher's mental health (Aperribai et al., 2020), and that the work environment can affect burnout symptoms in teachers (Neto et al., 2024).

While some researchers may have not implemented an actual school-based physical activity program within their study, it was often recommended that educational organizations design a school-based program or offer resources for educators to engage in to improve their stress and burnout. For instance, Fontana et al. (2022) believed that schools should promote school-based physical activity programs for students to engage in, which in turn, will incidentally increase movement and physical activity for teachers during the school day and reduce teacher stress. This supports Carson et al. 's (2010) conclusion that physical activity during the work day mitigates stress and burnout. Likewise, Cheng and Liu (2024) suggested that well-being should be supported among educational institutions, and that the organization should provide teachers with resources to promote their health and well-being. This idea supports Scardina et al.'s (2024) conclusion that healthy lifestyle habits decrease teacher burnout and feelings of stress. Furthermore, it aligns with Alhazmi et al. 's (2025) and Mariano et al. 's (2023) recommendations that holistic health programs should be offered by the school to encourage healthy habits and coping mechanisms to improve teacher's overall quality of life. By addressing school-based physical activity program effectiveness from the individual and organizational perspective, it is noted that a holistic health approach addressing physical activity, social, and emotional connections increase the well-being of teachers and overall their quality of life (Alhazmi et al., 2025; Kim & Gurvitch, 2020; Latino et al., 2021; Mariano et al., 2023; Scardina et al., 2024).

Level of Physical Activity

Ten of the studies reported on the impact of the level of physical activity, with mixed results. An additional study (Abós et al., 2021) recommended future research regarding the level of physical activity be conducted. A few studies reported a significant correlation between level of physical activity and mental well-being (Al-Johani, 2021) and burnout (Davis et al., 2025; González-Valero et al., 2023). Among those, Al-Johani (2021) noted that 10% of teachers who reported a high level of mental well-being also stated they had high levels of physical activity. In regards to burnout, Davis et al. (2025) found that the level of physical activity had a statistically significant impact on burnout through the component of emotional exhaustion. Similarly, González-Valero et al. (2023) looked at levels of physical activity according to the WHO's recommendation of 150 minutes of activity per week and noted that those that reached or exceeded that mark also indicated they experienced no burnout. However, just as many studies reported, the level or intensity does not impact mental health (Aperribai et al., 2020; Scardina et al., 2024) or well-being (Çifçi & Demir, 2020).

Other studies reported on findings closely related to burnout and mental well-being. For instance, Fontana et al. (2022) found that high levels of physical activity led to a lower likelihood (29%) of high levels of stress among teachers and were 40% more likely to have quality sleep. da Silva et al. 's (2024) study looked at the activity levels of teachers, suggesting that activity level is a mitigating factor in the impact of heavy workload on quality of life.

Gender Differences

Review of the studies shows an interest in or a perception that gender may impact physical activity and mental well-being as close to half of the studies specifically mentioned gender. Surprisingly, the studies, overall, found no statistically significant differences between women and men when considering physical activity (Abós et al., 2021; Alhazmi et al, 2025; Al-Johani, 2021; Cheng & Liu, 2024; Çifçi & Demir, 2020). For example, Çifçi and Demir (2020) reported no significant differences in mental well-being when considering gender, despite females, who regularly exercised during COVID, having significantly higher anxiety scores. Interestingly, when looking at data for those that did not exercise, they noted that the differences between females and males on anxiety scores and mental well-being were both significantly different. Females who did not exercise reported significantly lower levels of mental well-being than males. Thus, Çifçi and Demir (2020) state that exercise had a positive impact on the mental well-being of women who exercised, though not to the level of significance. While Al-Johani (2021) does not report the impact of gender when looking at physical activity and mental well-being, they did find a statistically significant relationship between mental well-being and physical activity. Instead, this study reports a higher percentage of females (95.6%) had high levels of mental well-being in contrast to males (85.3%) and no significant difference in gender based on type of physical activity.

Other studies similarly did not report significant findings in closely related topics. For example, when looking at work related outcomes, Abós et al. (2021) ran two different tests using their experimental and control groups and, in both tests, found that the gender differences were not significant. Thus, they did not continue running tests using gender as a variable (Abós et al., 2021). Cheng and Liu (2024) also looked at differences among females and males with burnout and emotional regulation. While they found that females experienced more burnout and lower emotional regulation than males, these differences were not statistically significant (Cheng & Liu, 2024). Finally, Alhazmi et al. (2025) found that there was no significant difference between women and men in physical activity levels despite both groups reporting low levels of physical activity over moderate levels.

A few studies reported significant findings in closely related topics. Davis et al. (2025) found a statistically significant difference between female and male scores of burnout with females experiencing higher levels of burnout. Bogaert et al. (2014) did find that females had significantly worse mental and physical health than males. In other similar comparisons, that study found females and males scores for job satisfaction were similar but women had significantly higher levels of stress related to work and were absent more often (Bogaert et al., 2014). Because of that, Bogaert et al. (2014) state that females are recommended for intervention groups. In Fontana et al. 's (2022) related study on sleep quality and stress, they found that females were more susceptible to high stress levels during COVID. Despite these findings, a number of studies continue to recommend future studies to explore potential gender differences (Al-Johani, 2021; Bogaert et al., 2014; Carson et al., 2010), sometimes even despite their own non-significant findings (Al-Johani, 2021).

COVID-19

Close to half of the articles, seven articles, were conducted specific to the context of the COVID-19 pandemic (Aperribai et al., 2020; Cheng & Liu, 2024; Çifçi & Demir, 2020; Fontana et al., 2022; Neto et al., 2024; Randall et al., 2021; Scardina et al., 2024). Two of these studies were conducted in the United States while the remaining five conducted in Brazil, China, Italy, Spain, and Turkey. Findings from these studies suggest that physical activity is significantly related to mental health or mental well-being (Cheng & Liu, 2024; Çifçi & Demir, 2020; Scardina et al., 2024). However, these studies consistently found that the level or frequency of physical activity did not have a significant impact on mental well-being (Aperribai et al., 2020; Çifçi & Demir, 2020; Scardina et al., 2024). Fontana et al. (2022) did report findings in relation to the frequency of physical activity but in connection to stress rather than mental well-being. While Scardina et al. (2024) noted that educators who were active were twice as likely to report good mental health, they found that the only significant predictor of mental health was the educator's weight status.

The remaining studies focused on topics closely related to well-being such as burnout and quality of life, life satisfaction, and stress. Randall et al. (2021) argues that their study's findings highlight the importance of physical activity on mental health, even though they report only indirect effects of physical activity on life satisfaction and psychological well-being. Although not significant, Neto et al. (2024) report that those who engage in physical activity had better quality of life and lower burnout, including lower emotional fatigue and greater personal fulfillment. Finally, Fontana et al. (2022) analyzed sleep quality in connection to stress and found that higher physical activity results in better quality of sleep which in turn resulted in participants being less likely to report higher levels of stress. Although one study listed home-based exercise (Çifçi & Demir, 2020) and one stated indoor and outside physical activity (Aperribai et al., 2020), further review of the studies indicate that no specific type of physical activity was the focus in these studies. While these studies emerged from the COVID-19 Pandemic, none of the studies drew strong conclusions based on the pandemic, apart from a need for research on mental well-being due to individuals being at home for longer periods of time due to the pandemic.

DISCUSSION OF FINDINGS

Teacher burnout can lead to an overall physical health decline (Madigan et al, 2023). Lack of physical activity and burnout can have a reciprocal relationship (Pihlaja et al., 2022). Physical activity should be considered as a positive coping mechanism to improve the mental health and well-being of teachers (da Silva et al., 2024) as it can positively impact their overall dimensions of health and improve employee work participation (Firus, 2023). When teachers are feeling emotionally exhausted, physical activity can help mitigate this effect, which could help increase their overall quality of life (Davis, 2023). As teachers increase physical activity engagement, the emotional exhaustion that is experienced decreases significantly (Davis et al., 2025), and emotional regulation can improve (Cheng & Liu, 2024). Likewise, as teachers improve their lifestyles, positive mental health characteristics are increased, stress and burnout are relieved (Corbett et al., 2021), and physical well-being is enhanced (Randall et al., 2021). Because teachers have high stress levels (Fontana et al., 2022), specific types of exercise, such as yoga (Dike et al.,

2021; Latino et al., 2021), can improve teachers' emotional intelligence, and improve job stress (Latino et al., 2021). When yoga is combined with CBT, positive mental and physiological effects occur (Dike et al., 2021). Engagement in leisure-time physical activity proved to decrease negative mental health and feelings of burnout (Al-Johani, 2021; Bogaert et al., 2014; Carson et al., 2010). Exercise, specifically indoors, can also enhance mental health (Aperribai et al., 2020). Regardless of exercise type (Bogaert et al., 2014; Latino et al., 2021), research has shown the numerous benefits that physical activity has on teacher well-being (Alhazmi et al., 2025; Carson et al., 2010; Çifçi & Demir, 2020).

Although some findings are conflicting (Bogaert et al., 2014), other studies report that physical activity during contract hours have shown to be successful and refreshing to teachers' mental health and emotional well-being (Carson et al., 2010). Because educators face an immense amount of stress and emotional fatigue (Mariano et al, 2023; Neto et al., 2024), creating structured physical activity programs within the school organization can be beneficial to help promote psychological well-being and provide teachers with more knowledge about the importance of physical health (Alhazmi et al., 2025; Mariano et al, 2023). However, types of school-based physical activity programs need to be considered, as sport-related ones showed various findings mixed findings and nonsignificance (González-Valero et al., 2023; Kim & Gurvitch, 2020), but still showed positive effects (Kim & Gurvitch, 2020; Latino et al., 2021; Mariano et al., 2023).

Overall health programs can be recommended as professional development to improve burnout in teachers (Alhazmi et al., 2025; Ratanasiripong et al., 2022) because teachers need more health and wellness resources and barriers need to be addressed (Mulhearn et al., 2024). This not only improves their physical wellness but also improves their social connection and emotional wellness, as this interaction develops their sense of relatedness to other teachers and incidentally decreases burnout (Abós et al., 2021; Kim & Gurvitch, 2020; Mariano et al., 2023). For instance, relatedness and social connection was described in Kim and Gurvitch (2020), as one participant reflected on the community the physical activity program brought to the school, stating, "'I definitely gained friendships and I am able to walk the halls and actually say hi to people and call people by name. And connect on a deeper level than just how are you. And then on a personal level'" (p. 665). This comment indicated that the school program brought a sense of community and inclusion for the teachers participating, and had a significant effect on their well-being (Kim & Gurvitch, 2020).

Finally, education organizations should design physical activity and exercise programs for teachers to participate in (Alhazmi et al., 2025; Kim & Gurvitch, 2020; Mariano et al, 2023) as this supports educator's emotional regulation (Mariano et al, 2023; Neto et al., 2024), motivation to continue to improve their healthy habits and overall quality of life (Kim & Gurvitch, 2020), and supports that consistent participation in physical activity can increase teacher's mental well-being (Randall et al., 2021). This is often a recommendation throughout the studies as it encompasses and encourages a holistic health approach for teachers and decreases their burnout (Alhazmi et al., 2025; Kim & Gurvitch, 2020; Latino et al., 2021; Mariano et al., 2023; Scardina et al., 2024).

Job Demands-Resources Model

Educators face a multitude of job demands (Baumgartner et al., 2025; Carroll et al., 2022; Hlado & Harvankova, 2024; Hojo, 2021; Jomuad et al., 2021; Kiremitci et al., 2023; Samaden et al., 2021), such as lack of organizational support (Pressley, 2021), and long-term negative effects from COVID-19 (Marshall et al., 2024), which contribute to burnout and emotional exhaustion (Kariou et al., 2021; Mijakoski et al., 2022; Nápoles et al., 2023). According to Demerouti et al.'s (2001) Job Demands Resource Model, job demands lead to exhaustion and job resources could improve disengagement (Demerouti et al., 2001). Though articles in this study primarily lacked a connection of job demands and job resources, findings suggested that physical activity could be used as a personal or organizational job resource that enhances mental health (da Silva et al., 2024) and alleviates the exhaustion (Kariou et al., 2021; Mijakoski et al., 2022; Nápoles et al., 2023) from the job demands (Song et al., 2024) felt in the education profession. For instance, Kim and Gurvitch (2020) and Mariano et al. (2023) believed that as physical activity increased, social connections within the school increased. As Abós et al. (2021) concluded, this social connection could improve burnout. Therefore, school-based physical activity programs could act as a job resource that mitigates burnout. Likewise, emotional fatigue is considered as a challenge that teachers face (Nath & Pandey, 2025) and causes attrition toward teaching (Dike et al., 2021). Yoga participation reduces emotional burnout and could be considered as a job resource to teacher burnout (Latino et al., 2021) and the demands that teachers face (Song et al., 2024). Ultimately, physical activity, functioning as both a coping mechanism and job resource, provides a solution to help mitigate teacher burnout and the job demands that teachers inherently face within the profession, while simultaneously enhancing teacher's positive mental health.

CONCLUSION

In conclusion, physical activity can positively influence teachers' well-being and reduce occupational burnout within the profession. While the overall level or intensity of physical activity did not consistently correlate with the reduction of burnout or improved well-being (Aperribai et al., 2020; Çifçi & Demir, 2020; Scardina et al., 2024), specific types of physical activity, such as leisure-time physical activity (Al-Johani, 2021; Bogaert et al., 2014; Carson et al., 2010; Çifçi & Demir, 2020) were associated with increased well-being outcomes among teachers. Likewise, school-based physical activity programs provided teachers with social connection and improved relationship quality with faculty, which further improved the school organization atmosphere (Abós et al., 2021; Kim & Gurvitch, 2020). Although some studies examined gender differences and physical activity, the studies were not statistically significant when it came to mental well-being and burnout (Abós et al., 2021; Alhazmi et al, 2025; Al-Johani, 2021; Cheng & Liu, 2024; Çifçi & Demir, 2020). For instance, teachers that were females showed decreased mental health and burnout more than males, but physical activity did not impact this (Cheng & Liu, 2024). A notable portion of these studies was contextualized within the COVID-19 Pandemic (Aperribai et al., 2020; Cheng & Liu, 2024; Çifçi & Demir, 2020; Fontana et al., 2022; Neto et al., 2024; Randall et al., 2021; Scardina et al., 2024) and highlighted that physical activity increased the mental health and well-being of teachers. Physical activity was also recommended as a strong coping mechanism for feelings of burnout (da Silva et al., 2024). Overall, physical activity has shown to have a significant and positive effect on teacher burnout and could act as a specific job resource that mitigates teacher's job demands. Also, leisure-time physical activity coupled with social engagement could provide a holistic health approach for teachers to participate in and further decrease their occupational burnout and increase their positive mental health due to the significant effect it has on teacher well-being.

Given that leisure-time physical activity was consistently associated with positive outcomes in reducing teacher burnout, we recommend that leisure-time physical activity should be more clearly defined. In the studies that referred to leisure-time physical activity (Al-Johani, 2021; Bogaert et al., 2014; Carson et al., 2010), the definition of leisure-time physical activity was never clearly stated, which limits comparability across studies. However, in several studies, leisure-time physical activity was defined through examples, such as walking (Al-Johani, 2021), sport participation (González-Valero et al., 2023; Kim & Gurvitch, 2020), or yoga (Dike et al., 2021; Latino et al., 2021). To our knowledge, there is not a clearly defined definition. Thus, based on this literature review and additional readings, we recommend leisure-time physical activity be defined as, voluntary, mild, or moderate physical activity during one's free time that leads to emotional satisfaction, improved mood, and well-being. This definition then would include the specific examples listed above and will assist future researchers by providing a more defined scope of leisure-time physical activity to focus their work.

This review of literature did have some limitations to consider. Many studies were researched outside of the United States (Abós et al., 2021; Alhazmi et al., 2025; Al-

Johani, 2021; Aperribai et al., 2020; Bogaert et al., 2014; Cheng & Liu, 2024; Çifçi & Demir, 2020; da Silva et al., 2024; Dike et al., 2021; González-Valero et al., 2023; Latino et al., 2021; Mariano et al., 2023; Neto et al., 2023; Scardina et al., 2024), which could have affected outcomes. Finally, the studies selected for this review did not include longitudinal studies that spanned multiple years, which would have provided a more in-depth understanding of the cause and effect of physical activity on teachers' mental well-being and burnout long term.

IMPLICATIONS AND RECOMMENDATIONS

Because research (Alhazmi et al., 2025; Latino et al., 2021) shows positive effects that physical activity should be used as a holistic approach, implications for practice include teachers using physical activity as a coping mechanism to improve their overall mental health, which in turn will decrease burnout. Likewise, school administrators should consider offering wellness programs after school to help teachers detach from their job demands and increase social and physical activity, as well as provide a multi-tier approach to improve teachers' overall wellbeing. This could be used as a multi-level wellness strategy for teachers, which could improve all levels of health at a comprehensive and systems-level approach.

Furthermore, we recommend that future scholars study more diverse populations of teachers regarding this topic, including investigating different demographics, such as race, school setting, and socioeconomic status, as well as evaluating how years of experience taught in the classroom could affect occupational burnout or engagement in physical activity. These are variables that were not identified in the selected articles in this study. Additionally, further research could include longitudinal studies to understand any long-term impacts of physical activity on teachers. Lastly, qualitative insights or real-world experiences may be considered valuable to related findings. Articles in this study suggest school-based programs could increase social integration and belonging of teachers (Kim & Gurvitch, 2020). Qualitative studies would provide a more in-depth understanding of this benefit and others that may result from physical activity.

REFERENCES

Abós, Á., Sevil-Serrano, J., Julián-Clemente, J. A., Generelo, E., & García-González, L. (2021). Improving teachers' work-related outcomes through a group-based physical activity intervention during leisure-time. *Journal of Experimental Education, 89*(2), 306–325. DOI: 10.1080/00220973.2019.1681349

Agnieszka, L. G., & Marta, N. (2021). Self-efficacy and psychological well-being of teachers. *The Central European Journal of Social Sciences and Humanities, 3*(90), 4–10. DOI: 10.15219/em90.1517

Agyapong, B., Obuobi-Donkor, G., Burback, L., & Wei, Y. (2022). Stress, burnout, anxiety and depression among teachers: A scoping review. *International Journal of Environmental Research and Public Health, 19*(17), 10706. Advance online publication. DOI: 10.3390/ijerph191710706 PMID: 36078422

Al-Johani, R. M. (2021). Effect of physical activity on mental wellbeing among teachers of secondary school in Almadina city, Saudi Arabia. *Journal of Family Medicine and Primary Care, 10*(11), 4264–4271. PMID: 35136800

Algorani, E. B., & Gupta, V. (2023). *Coping mechanisms*. National Library of Medicine. https://www.ncbi.nlm.nih.gov/books/NBK559031/

Alhazmi, A., Ali, M., Dawria, A., Narapureddy, B. R., & Hawash, M. M. (2025). Assessment of health behaviors of primary school teachers based on their nutritional knowledge and physical activity: A cross-sectional study in the Asir region. *PLoS One, 20*(1), e0318146. Advance online publication. DOI: 10.1371/journal.pone.0318146 PMID: 39869594

Alsalhe, T. A., Chalghaf, N., Guelmami, N., Azaiez, F., & Bragazzi, N. L. (2021). Occupational burnout prevalence and its determinants among physical education teachers: A systematic review and meta-analysis. *Frontiers in Human Neuroscience, 15*, 553230. Advance online publication. DOI: 10.3389/fnhum.2021.553230 PMID: 34955783

American College of Sports Medicine. (n.d.). *Physical activity guidelines*. https://acsm.org/ education-resources/trending-topics-resources/physical-activity-guidelines/

Aperribai, L., Cortabarria, L., Aguirre, T., Verche, E., & Borges, Á. (2020). Teacher's physical activity and mental health during lockdown due to the COVID-2019 pandemic. *Frontiers in Psychology, 11*, 577886. PMID: 33262727

Aronsson, G., Theorell, T., Grape, T., Hammarström, A., Hogstedt, C., Marteinsdottir, I., Skoog, I., Träskman-Bendz, L., & Hall, C. (2017). A systematic review including meta-analysis of work environment and burnout symptoms. *BMC Public Health, 17*(264), 1–13. DOI: 10.1186/s12889-017-4153-7 PMID: 28302088

Atwood, A. I. (2024). A perspective on psychological factors affecting the emotional labor of teachers. *Frontiers in Education, 9*, 1291698. Advance online publication. DOI: 10.3389/feduc.2024.1291698

Bakker, A. B. (2022). The social psychology of work engagement: State of the field. *Career Development International, 27*(1), 36–53. DOI: 10.1108/CDI-08-2021-0213

Bakker, A. B., & de Vries, J. D. (2020). Job Demands–Resources theory and self-regulation: New explanations and remedies for job burnout. *Anxiety, Stress, and Coping, 34*(1), 1–21. DOI: 10.1080/10615806.2020.1797695 PMID: 32856957

Bakker, A. B., & Demerouti, E. (2007). The job demands-resources model: State of the art. *Journal of Managerial Psychology, 22*(3), 309–328. DOI: 10.1108/02683940710733115

Bakker, A. B., & Demerouti, E. (2017). Job demands-resources theory: Taking stock and looking forward. *Journal of Occupational Health Psychology, 22*(3), 273–285. DOI: 10.1037/ocp0000056 PMID: 27732008

Bakker, A. B., Demerouti, E., & Sanz-Vergel, A. (2023). Job demands–resources theory: Ten years later. *Annual Review of Organizational Psychology and Organizational Behavior, 10*(1), 25–53. DOI: 10.1146/annurev-orgpsych-120920-053933

Baptista, M. N., & Cardoso, H. F. (2021). Do organizational support and occupational stressors influence burnout in teachers? *Interamerican Journal of Psychological Assessment, 20*(4), 435–444. DOI: 10.15689/ap.2021.2004.21998.05

Barbosa, B. C. R., Menezes-Júnior, L. A. A., de, , de Paula, W., Chagas, C. M. dos S., Machado, E. L., de Freitas, E. D., & Cardoso, C. S., de Carvalho Vidigal, F., Nobre, L. N., Silva, L. S. da, & Meireles, A. L. (2024). Sedentary behavior is associated with the mental health of university students during the Covid-19 pandemic, and not practicing physical activity accentuates its adverse effects: Cross-sectional study. *BMC Public Health, 24*(1), 1–11. DOI: 10.1186/s12889-024-19345-5 PMID: 38992623

Baumgartner, J., Ota, C., DiCarlo, C., Bauer, R., & Carson, R. (2025). Using ecological momentary assessment to examine the relationship between childcare teachers' stress, classroom behaviors, and afterhours professionalism activities. *Child Care in Practice, 31*(1), 49–68. DOI: 10.1080/13575279.2021.1962247

Berkey, A. (n.d.). *Teacher burnout: Stats, causes, and prevention for 2025*. Everfi. https://everfi.com/blog/k-12/teacher-burnout/#:~:text=The%20burnout%20rate%20for%20teachers,major%20stressor%20in%20their%20classrooms

Beselt, L. J., Patterson, M. C., McDonough, M. H., Hewson, J., & MacKay, S. (2021). A meta-study of qualitative research on social support related to physical activity among older adults. *Kinesiology Review (Champaign, Ill.)*, *10*(1), 51–65. DOI: 10.1123/kr.2020-0005

Bianchi, R., Schonfeld, I. S., & Verkuilen, J. (2020). A five-sample confirmatory factor analytic study of burnout-depression overlap. *Journal of Clinical Psychology*, *76*(4), 801–821. DOI: 10.1002/jclp.22927 PMID: 31926025

Bigras, N., Lemay, L., Lehrer, J., Charron, A., Duval, S., Robert-Mazaye, C., & Laurin, E. I. (2021). Early childhood educators' perceptions of their emotional state, relationships with parents, challenges, and opportunities during the early stage of the pandemic. *Early Childhood Education Journal*, *49*(5), 775–787. DOI: 10.1007/s10643-021-01224-y PMID: 34131378

Bogaert, I., De Martelaer, K., Deforche, B., Clarys, P., & Zinzen, E. (2014). Associations between different types of physical activity and teachers' perceived mental, physical, and work-related health. *BMC Public Health*, *14*(1), 534. Advance online publication. DOI: 10.1186/1471-2458-14-534 PMID: 24885620

Brailovskaia, J., Duscha, A. L., Kreyelkamp, G. M., & Margraf, J. (2024). Teachers' competence: How to protect teachers' mental health from the burden caused by students' private in-class use of technical devices? *PLoS One*, *19*(6), e0305114. Advance online publication. DOI: 10.1371/journal.pone.0305114 PMID: 38861520

Capone, V., & Petrillo, G. (2020). Mental health in teachers: Relationship with job satisfaction, efficacy beliefs, burnout and depression. *Current Psychology (New Brunswick, N.J.)*, *39*(5), 1757–1766. DOI: 10.1007/s12144-018-9878-7

Carr, E. R. (2024). A history of the community mental health movement and individuals with serious mental illness: A vision for the future. *The American Journal of Orthopsychiatry*, *94*(4), 380–391. DOI: 10.1037/ort0000737 PMID: 38695820

Carroll, A., Forrest, K., Sanders-O'Connor, E., Flynn, L., Bower, J. M., Fynes-Clinton, S., York, A., & Ziaei, M. (2022). Teacher stress and burnout in Australia: Examining the role of intrapersonal and environmental factors. *Social Psychology of Education*, *25*, 441–469. DOI: 10.1007/s11218-022-09686-7 PMID: 35233183

Carson, R. L., Baumgartner, J. J., Matthews, R. A., & Tsouloupas, C. N. (2010). Emotional exhaustion, absenteeism, and turnover intentions in childcare teachers: Examining the impact of physical activity behaviors. *Journal of Health Psychology, 15*(6), 905–914. DOI: 10.1177/1359105309360697 PMID: 20472609

Caspersen, C. J., Powell, K. E., & Christenson, G. M. (1985). Physical activity, exercise, and physical fitness: Definitions and distinctions for health-related research. *Public Health Reports, 100*(2), 126–131. https://pmc.ncbi.nlm.nih.gov/articles/PMC1424733/ PMID: 3920711

Center of Disease of Control and Prevention. (2024). *Benefits of physical activity.* https://www.cdc.gov/physical-activity-basics/benefits/index.html

Center of Disease of Control and Prevention. (n.d.). *Adult activity: An overview.* https://www.cdc.gov/physical-activity-basics/guidelines/adults.html

Chan, M. K., Sharkey, J. D., Lawrie, S. I., Arch, D. A. N., & Nylund-Gibson, K. (2021). Elementary school teacher well-being and supportive measures amid COVID-19: An exploratory study. *School Psychology, 36*(6), 533–545. DOI: 10.1037/spq0000441 PMID: 34292036

Chen, X. M., Liao, X. L., Chen, I. H., Gamble, J. H., Jiang, X. Y., Li, X. D., & Bo, C. X. (2024). The long-term effects of perceived instructional leadership on teachers' psychological well-being during COVID-19. *PLoS One, 19*(8), e0305494. Advance online publication. DOI: 10.1371/journal.pone.0305494 PMID: 39159165

Cheng, P. Y. Z., & Liu, H. (2024). A structural model of EFL teachers' physical activity, emotion regulation, and competence for online teaching. *BMC Psychology, 12*, 252. DOI: 10.1186/s40359-024-01753-2 PMID: 38715133

Çifçi, F., & Demir, A. (2020). The effect of home-based exercise on anxiety and mental well-being levels of teachers and pre-service teachers in COVID-19 pandemic. *African Educational Research Journal Special Issue, 8*(2), S20-S28. https://files.eric.ed.gov/fulltext/EJ1274658.pdf

Clasquin-Johnson, M. G., & Ebrahim, H. B. (2024). Self-efficacy and well-being of female educators for early childhood care and education during COVID-19. *South African Journal of Education, 44*(1), 2354. Advance online publication. DOI: 10.15700/saje.v44n1a2354

Cleveland Clinic. (2025). *Mental disorders*. Retrieved December 1, 2025 from https://my.clevelandclinic.org/health/diseases/22295-mental-health-disorders

Collie, R. J. (2023). Teacher well-being and turnover intentions: Investigating the roles of job resources and job demands. *The British Journal of Educational Psychology, 93*(3), 712–726. DOI: 10.1111/bjep.12587 PMID: 36720462

Corbett, L., Bauman, A., Peralta, L. R., Okely, A. D., & Phongsavan, P. (2021). Characteristics and effectiveness of physical activity, nutrition and/or sleep interventions to improve the mental well-being of teachers: A scoping review. *Health Education Journal, 81*(2), 196–210. DOI: 10.1177/00178969211062701

Costa, C. N., Chandarlis, E., & Park, N. (2024). Examining teacher well-being: An analysis of resources needs. *International Journal of Changes in Education, 1*(2), 63–74. DOI: 10.47852/bonviewIJCE42022564

da Silva, C. C. M., Santos, A. B. d., Leoci, I. C., Leite, E. G., Antunes, E. P., Torres, W., Mesquita, E. D. L., Delfino, L. D., & Beretta, V. S. (2024). The association between perceived stress, quality of life, and level of physical activity in public school teachers. *International Journal of Environmental Research and Public Health, 21*(1), 88. DOI: 10.3390/ijerph21010088 PMID: 38248551

Dahati, A., & Dahati, A. (2025). The role of physical activity in reducing symptoms of 'burnout'and psychological mechanisms towards exercise in professionals with high stress levels: The case of northern Albania. *Interdisciplinary Journal of Research and Development, 12*(2), 126-126. https://www.journal-uamd.org/index.php/IJRD/article/view/586/550

Davis, J. (2023). *The relationship between teacher burnout and physical activity among high school teachers* [Doctoral dissertation, Kennesaw State University]. DigitalCommons@Kennesaw State University. https://digitalcommons.kennesaw.edu/ teachleaddoc_etd/62?utm_source=digitalcommons.kennesaw.edu%2Fteachleaddoc_etd%2F62&utm_medium=PDF&utm_campaign=PDFCoverPages

Davis, J. K., Juergensen, M., Chang, M. L., & Elue, C. (2025). The relationship between teacher burnout and physical activity among high school teachers. *International Journal of Teacher Leadership, 14*(1), 98–125. https://research-ebsco-com.snu.idm.oclc.org/c/5v6chs/viewer/pdf/4nba6xypkn

de Costa, B. G. G., Van Rooij, A. J., Tuijnman, A., Saunders, T. J., & Chaput, J. P. (2023). Associations between type and timing of physical activity and sedentary behavior with mental health in adolescents and young adults. *Journal of Physical Activity & Health, 20*(7), 655–663. DOI: 10.1123/jpah.2022-0485 PMID: 37160286

Demerouti, E., Bakker, A. B., Nachreiner, F., & Schaufeli, W. B. (2001). The job demands-resources model of burnout. *The Journal of Applied Psychology*, *86*(3), 499–512. DOI: 10.1037/0021-9010.86.3.499 PMID: 11419809

Demerouti, E., Bakker, A. B., Peeters, M. C. W., & Breevaart, K. (2021). New directions in burnout research. *European Journal of Work and Organizational Psychology*, *30*(5), 686–691. DOI: 10.1080/1359432X.2021.1979962

Dike, I. C., Onyishi, C. N., Adimora, D. E., Ugodulunwa, C. A., Adama, G. N., Ugwu, G. C., Eze, U. N., Eze, A., Ogba, F. N., Obiwluozo, P. E., Onu, J. F. E., Onu, A. O., Omenma, Z. O., Nwaeze, V. C., Ani, C., Ngwu, C. N., Uzodinma, U. E., & Iremeka, F. U. (2021). Yoga complemented cognitive behavioral therapy on job burnout among teachers of children with autism spectrum disorders. *Medicine*, *100*(22), 25801. Advance online publication. DOI: 10.1097/MD.0000000000025801 PMID: 34087823

Dreer, B. (2023). On the outcomes of teacher wellbeing: A systematic review of research. *Frontiers in Psychology*, *14*, 1205179. Advance online publication. DOI: 10.3389/fpsyg.2023.1205179 PMID: 37575417

Dung, V., Trang, V. T., & Lan, N. T. M. (2024). Workload doesn't mean exhaustion: Antecedents of teacher burnout. *Journal of Education and e-learning Research*, *11*(2), 404–412. DOI: 10.20448/jeelr.v11i2.5641

Farmer, D. (2020). Teacher attrition: The impacts of stress. *Delta Kappa Gamma Bulletin*, *87*(1), 41–50.

Fiorilli, C., Benevene, P., De Stasio, S., Buonomo, I., Romano, L., Pepe, A., & Addimando, L. (2019). Teachers' burnout: The role of trait emotional intelligence and social support. *Frontiers in Psychology*, *10*, 2743. Advance online publication. DOI: 10.3389/fpsyg.2019.02743 PMID: 31920801

Firus, M. (2023). *Teacher wellness initiative: Viability of incorporating exercise into teachers' workday* [Doctoral dissertation, University of Saskatchewan]. University of Saskatchewan. https://harvest.usask.ca/server/api/core/bitstreams/ 473c72f8-abc8-44c0-b84e-c47f75094ae7/content

Fontana, F., Bourbeau, K., Moriarty, T., & da Silva, M. P. (2022). The relationship between physical activity, sleep quality, and stress: A study of teachers during the COVID-19 pandemic. *International Journal of Environmental Research and Public Health*, *19*, 15465. Advance online publication. DOI: 10.3390/ijerph192315465 PMID: 36497539

Freire, C., Ferradás, M. D. M., García-Bértoa, A., Núñez, J. C., Rodríguez, S., & Piñeiro, I. (2020). Psychological capital and burnout in teachers: The mediating role of flourishing. *International Journal of Environmental Research and Public Health, 17*(22). Advance online publication. DOI: 10.3390/ijerph17228403 PMID: 33202826

Freudenberger, H. J. (1975). The staff burn-out syndrome in alternative institutions. *Psychotherapy (Chicago, Ill.), 12*(1), 73–82. DOI: 10.1037/h0086411

Freudenberger, H. J. (1989). *Burnout: Past, present, and future concerns.* [eBook edition]. In D.T. Wessells Jr., A. H. Kutscher, I. B., Seeland, F. E., Selder, D. J., Cherico, & E. J. Clark, (Eds.), Professional Burnout in Medicine and the Helping Professions (1-10). The Haworth Press. https://books.google.com/books

González-Valero, G., Gómez-Carmona, C. D., Bastida-Castillo, A., Corral-Pernía, J. A., Zurita-Ortega, F., & Melguizo-Ibáñez, E. (2023). Could the complying with WHO physical activity recommendations improve stress, burnout syndrome, and resilience? A cross-sectional study with physical education teachers. *Sport Sciences for Health, 19*, 349–358. DOI: 10.1007/s11332-022-00981-6

Granziera, H. (2022). Teachers' personal resources: What do we know and where do we go? A scoping review through the lens of job demands-resources theory. *Journal of Positive Psychology and Wellbeing, 6*(2), 1695–1718. https://www.researchgate.net/profile/Helena-Granziera/publication/363889926_Teachers'_Personal_Resources_What_Do_We_Know_and_Where_Do_We_Go_A_Scoping_Review_Through_the_Lens_of_Job_Demands-Resources_Theory/links/6333c9165d1e2d53d9a3ce48/Teachers-Personal-Resources-What-Do-We-Know-and-Where-Do-We-Go-A-Scoping-Review-Through-the-Lens-of-Job-Demands-Resources-Theory.pdf

Gray, C., Wilcox, G., & Nordstokke, D. (2017). Teacher mental health, school climate, inclusive education and student learning: A review. *Canadian Psychology, 58*(3), 203–210. DOI: 10.1037/cap0000117

Ha, C., Pressley, T., & Marshall, D. T. (2025). Teacher voices matter: The role of teacher autonomy in enhancing job satisfaction and mitigating burnout. *PLoS One, 20*(1), e0317471. Advance online publication. DOI: 10.1371/journal.pone.0317471 PMID: 39804894

Heinemann, L. V., & Heinemann, T. (2017). Burnout research: Emergence and scientific investigation of a contested diagnosis. *SAGE Open, 7*(1), 1–12. DOI: 10.1177/2158244017697154

Hlado, P., & Harvankova, K. (2024). Teachers' perceived work ability: A qualitative exploration using the Job Demands-Resources model. *Humanities & Social Sciences Communications, 11*, 304. DOI: 10.1057/s41599-024-02811-1

Hojo, M. (2021). Association between student-teacher ratio and teachers' working hours and workload stress: Evidence from a nationwide survey in Japan. *BMC Public Health, 21*, 1635. Advance online publication. DOI: 10.1186/s12889-021-11677-w PMID: 34493251

Huang, S., Yau, S. Y., Lee, Y. K. L., Song, J., Guo, Y., & Dong, D. (2025). Job characteristics, personal characteristics and well-being of nursing assistants in long-term care facilities: A mixed methods systematic review and narrative synthesis. *International Journal of Nursing Studies, 161*, 104934. Advance online publication. DOI: 10.1016/j.ijnurstu.2024.104934 PMID: 39476575

Huk, O., Terjesen, M. D., & Cherkasova, L. (2019). Predicting teacher burnout as a function of school characteristics and irrational beliefs. *Psychology in the Schools, 56*(5), 792–808. DOI: 10.1002/pits.22233

Hyatt, K. (2022). Stressors in higher education that lead to burnout and solutions to avoid it. *Journal of Business and Educational Leadership, 12*(1), 110–125.

Inbar, L., & Shiri, S. A. (2021). Managing the emotional aspects of compassion fatigue among teachers in Israel: A qualitative study. *Journal of Education for Teaching, 47*(4), 562–575. DOI: 10.1080/02607476.2021.1929876

Jacobs-Pinson, E. (n.d.). *25+ teacher burnout statistics: A crisis we can't ignore.* Crown Counseling. https://crowncounseling.com/statistics/teacher-burnout/

Jahoda, M. (1958). *Current concepts of positive mental health.* Basic Books/Hachette Book Group., DOI: 10.1037/11258-000

Jamal, A., Begum, S., Alam, H., & Hussain, T. (2023). Impact of perceived organizational support on innovative work behavior and burnout in teachers: Thriving at work as the mediator (2020). *Journal of Education and Educational Development, 10*(2), 288–307. DOI: 10.22555/joeed.v10i2.815

Jennings, P. A., & Min, H. H. (2023). Transforming empathy-based stress to compassion: Skillful means to preventing teacher burnout. *Mindfulness, 14*, 2311–2322. DOI: 10.1007/s12671-023-02115-6 PMID: 37362185

Jeon, H. J., Diamond, L., McCartney, C., & Kwon, K. A. (2022). Early childhood special education teachers' job burnout and psychological stress. *Early Education and Development, 33*(8), 1364–1382. DOI: 10.1080/10409289.2021.1965395 PMID: 36353579

Jiao, C., Qian, J., & Liu, H. (2022). The relationship between preschool inclusive education teachers' organizational support and work engagement: The mediating role of teacher self-efficacy. *Frontiers in Psychology*, *13*, 900836. Advance online publication. DOI: 10.3389/fpsyg.2022.900835 PMID: 35686076

Jomuad, P. D., Antigua, L. M. M., Cericos, E. U., Bacus, J. A., Vallejo, J. H., Dionio, B. B., Bazar, J. S., Cocolan, J. V., & Clarin, A. S. (2021). Teachers' workload in relation to burnout and work performance. *International Journal of Education Policy Research and Review*, *8*(2), 48–52. DOI: 10.15739/IJEPRR.21.007

Kamboj, K. P., & Garg, P. (2021). Teachers' psychological well-being role of emotional intelligence and resilience character traits in determining the psychological well-being of Indian school teachers. *International Journal of Educational Management*, *35*(4), 768–788. DOI: 10.1108/IJEM-08-2019-0278

Kariou, A., Koutsimani, P., Montgomery, A., & Lainidi, O. (2021). Emotional labor and burnout among teachers: A systematic review. *International Journal of Environmental Research and Public Health*, *18*(23), 12760. Advance online publication. DOI: 10.3390/ijerph182312760 PMID: 34886485

Kasapoglu, K., & Didin, M. (2019). Life skills as a predictor of psychological well-being of pre-service pre-school teachers in Turkey. *International Journal of Contemporary Education Research*, *6*(1), 70–85. DOI: 10.33200/ijcer.544232

Kendrick, A. (2022). Compassion fatigue, burnout, and the emotional labor of educational workers. *The International Journal of Health, Wellness & Society*, *13*(1), 31–55. DOI: 10.18848/2156-8960/CGP/v13i01/31-55

Kim, G., & Gurvitch, R. (2020). The effect of sports-based physical activity programme on teachers' relatedness, stress, and exercise motivation. *Health Education Journal*, *79*(6), 658–670. DOI: 10.1177/0017896920906185

Kim, L. E., Jorg, V., & Klassen, R. M. (2019). A meta-analysis of the effects of teacher personality on teacher effectiveness and burnout. *Educational Psychology Review*, *31*(1), 163–195. DOI: 10.1007/s10648-018-9458-2 PMID: 30930595

Kinder, C. J., Richards, K. A., Trad, A. M., Woods, A. M., & Graber, K. C. (2023). Perceived organizational support, marginalization, isolation, emotional exhaustion, and job satisfaction of PETE faculty members. *European Physical Education Review*, *29*(4), 475–492. DOI: 10.1177/1356336X231159636

Kiremitci, O., Boz, B., & Yıldız Çakır, L. (2023). Job demands-resources model and burnout in physical education teaching: A mixed-method sequential explanatory study. *Work (Reading, Mass.)*, *76*(1), 171–187. DOI: 10.3233/WOR-220102 PMID: 36872824

Kong, S., & Lai, M. (2023). Effects of a teacher development program on teachers' knowledge and collaborative engagement, and students' achievement in computational thinking concepts. *British Journal of Educational Technology*, *54*(2), 489–512. DOI: 10.1111/bjet.13256

Kotowski, S. E., Davis, K. G., & Barratt, C. L. (2022). Teachers feeling the burden of COVID-19: Impact on well-being, stress, and burnout. *Work (Reading, Mass.)*, *71*(2), 407–415. DOI: 10.3233/WOR-210994 PMID: 35068412

Latino, F., Cataldi, S., & Fischetti, F. (2021). Effects of an 8-week yoga-based physical exercise intervention on teachers' burnout. *Sustainability*, *13*, 2104. Advance online publication. DOI: 10.3390/su13042104

Lesener, T., Gusy, B., & Wolter, C. (2018). The job demands-resources model: A meta-analytic review of longitudinal studies. *Work and Stress*, *33*(1), 76–103. DOI: 10.1080/02678373.2018.1529065

Leung, K. H., & Cheung, A. C. K. (2024). Understanding emotional well-being of teachers: Development and validation of teacher emotions in teaching scale in Hong Kong using a mixed-methods approach. *Teaching and Teacher Education*, *152*, 104792. Advance online publication. DOI: 10.1016/j.tate.2024.104792

Li, J., He, Y., Wang, Y., & Xue, E. (2025). Investigating higher education teachers' well-being and its influencing multiple factors: A systematic review approach. *International Journal of Mental Health Promotion*, *27*(7), 901–928. DOI: 10.32604/ijmhp.2025.066538

Li, X., Jiang, T., Sun, J., Shi, L., & Liu, J. (2021). The relationship between occupational stress, job burnout and quality of life among surgical nurses in Xinjiang, China. *BMC Nursing*, *20*(1), 1–11. DOI: 10.1186/s12912-021-00703-2 PMID: 34579710

Macias, O. (2024). *Navigating post-pandemic student behavior: Strategies for teachers and school administrators.* Resource Hub. https://content.acsa.org/navigating-post-pandemic-student-behavior-strategies-for-teachers-and-school-administrators/

Madigan, D. J., & Kim, L. E. (2021). Towards an understanding of teacher attrition: A meta-analysis of burnout, job satisfaction, and teachers' intention to quit. *Teaching and Teacher Education*, *105*, 103425. Advance online publication. DOI: 10.1016/j.tate.2021.103425

Madigan, D. J., Kim, L. E., Glandorf, H. L., & Kavanagh, O. (2023). Teacher burnout and physical health: A systematic review. *International Journal of Educational Research, 119*, 102173. Advance online publication. DOI: 10.1016/j.ijer.2023.102173

Mak, S., & Thomas, A. (2022). Steps for conducting a scoping review. *Journal of Graduate Medical Education, 14*(5), 565–567. DOI: 10.4300/JGME-D-22-00621.1 PMID: 36274762

Mäkikangas, A., Leiter, M. P., Kinnunen, U., & Feldt, T. (2020). Profiling development of burnout over eight years: Relation with job demands and resources. *European Journal of Work and Organizational Psychology, 30*(5), 720–731. DOI: 10.1080/1359432X.2020.1790651

Manuti, A., Giancaspro, M. L., Gemmano, C. G., & Morrelli, F. (2022). Coping with the unexpected: A job demands/resources study exploring Italian teachers' remote working experience during the COVID-19 lockdown. *Teaching and Teacher Education: Leadership and Professional Development, 1*, 100010. Advance online publication. DOI: 10.1016/j.tatelp.2022.100010

Mariano, L., Simões, H., Brito-Costa, S., & Amaral, A. P. (2023). Fostering organizational empowerment: Impact of an intervention program on stress management and physical activity motivation among teachers in Portugal and Brazil. *Administrative Sciences, 13*(9), 203. DOI: 10.3390/admsci13090203

Marshall, D. T., Smith, N. E., Love, S. M., Neugebauer, N. M., & Shannon, D. M. (2024). "At some point we're going to reach our limit": Understanding COVID-19's impact on teacher burnout and subjective mental health. *Psychology in the Schools, 61*(3), 793–812. DOI: 10.1002/pits.23084

Martin, A. J., Sudimantara, L. B., & Dewi, E. W. (2025). Harnessing theory to make sense of large-scale secondary data in education: Applying the academic demands-resources framework. *Education in Science, 15*(2), 256. Advance online publication. DOI: 10.3390/educsci15020256

Maslach, C., & Jackson, S. E. (1981). The measurement of experienced burnout. *Journal of Organizational Behavior, 2*(2), 99–113. DOI: 10.1002/job.4030020205

Maslach, C., & Leiter, M. P. (2016). Understanding the burnout experience: Recent research and its implications for psychiatry. *World Psychiatry: Official Journal of the World Psychiatric Association, 15*(2), 103–111. DOI: 10.1002/wps.20311 PMID: 27265691

Mérida-López, S., Sánchez-Álvarez, N., & Extremera, N. (2022). Teacher retention through the job demands-resources theory. *Educación XX1, 25*(2), 151-171. https://doi.org/DOI: 10.5944/educxx1.31901

Mijakoski, D., Cheptea, D., Marca, S. C., Shoman, Y., Caglayan, C., Bugge, M. D., Gnesi, M., Godderis, L., Kiran, S., McElvenny, D. M., Mediouni, Z., Mesot, O., Minov, J., Nena, E., Otelea, M., Pranjic, N., Mehlum, I. S., van der Molen, H. F., & Canu, I. G. (2022). Determinants of burnout among teachers: A systematic review of longitudinal studies. *International Journal of Environmental Research and Public Health, 19*(9), 5776. Advance online publication. DOI: 10.3390/ijerph19095776 PMID: 35565168

Monteiro, E., & Joseph, J. (2023). A review on the impact of workplace culture on employee mental health and well-being. *International Journal of Case Studies in Business, IT, and Education, 7*(2), 291–317. DOI: 10.5281/zenodo.7999328

Mulhearn, S. C., Kulinna, P. H., & Lorenz, K. A. (2024). Classroom teachers' perceived barriers to implementing comprehensive school physical activity programs (TPB- CSPAP): Instrument development. *Research Quarterly for Exercise and Sport, 95*(2), 342–352. DOI: 10.1080/02701367.2023.2206449 PMID: 37463222

Murray, R. M., Doré, I., Sabiston, C. M., Michael, F., & O'Loughlin, J. L. (2023). A time compositional analysis of the association between movement behavior and indicators of mental health in young adults. *Scandinavian Journal of Medicine & Science in Sports, 33*(12), 2598–2607. DOI: 10.1111/sms.14471 PMID: 37635273

Nadon, L., De Beer, L. T., & Morin, A. J. S. (2022). Should burnout be conceptualized as a mental disorder? *Behavioral Sciences (Basel, Switzerland), 12*(3), 82. DOI: 10.3390/bs12030082 PMID: 35323401

Naidoo-Chetty, M., & Du Plessis, M. (2021). Systematic review of the job demands and resources of academic staff within higher education institutions. *International Journal of Higher Education, 10*(3), 268–284. DOI: 10.5430/ijhe.v10n3p268

Nalipay, M. J. N., Mordeno, I. G., Semilla, J. B., & Frondozo, C. E. (2019). Implicit beliefs about teaching ability, teacher emotions, and teaching satisfaction. *The Asia-Pacific Education Researcher, 28*(4), 313–325. DOI: 10.1007/s40299-019-00467-z

Nápoles, J., Kelley, J., & Rinn, T. J. (2023). Burnout and perceived agency among Texas choir teachers. *Journal of Research in Music Education, 71*(3), 283–296. DOI: 10.1177/00224294221126889

Nath, R., & Pandey, C. P. (2025). The hidden burden: Emotional labor and well-being of school teachers. *Asian Journal of Education and Social Studies, 51*(2), 500–510. DOI: 10.9734/ajess/2025/v51i21802

Neto, L. B., Christofoletti, G., de Alencar, G. P., & Burke, T. N. (2024). Burnout syndrome, work ability, quality of life and physical activity in teachers during the COVID-19 pandemic in Campo Grande, Brazil. *Work (Reading, Mass.), 78*(1), 45–53. DOI: 10.3233/WOR-220187 PMID: 37483044

O'Hara, S., Melnyk, B. M., Hsieh, A. P., Helsabeck, N. P., Giuliano, K. K., & Vital, C. (2025). Innovation, wellness, and EBP cultures are associated with less burnout, better mental health, and higher job satisfaction in nurses and the healthcare workforce. *Worldviews on Evidence-Based Nursing, 22*(2), 1–11. DOI: 10.1111/wvn.70012 PMID: 40237103

Oberg, G., Macmahon, S., & Carroll, A. (2025). Assessing the interplay: Teacher efficacy, compassion fatigue, and educator well-being in Australia. *Australian Educational Researcher, 52*, 1105–1131. DOI: 10.1007/s13384-024-00755-8

Ormiston, H. E., Nygaard, M. A., & Apgar, S. (2022). A systematic review of secondary traumatic stress and compassion fatigue in teachers. *School Mental Health, 14*, 802–817. DOI: 10.1007/s12310-022-09525-2 PMID: 35694002

Ortan, F., Simut, C., & Simut, R. (2021). Self-efficacy, job satisfaction, and teacher well-being in the K-12 education system. *International Journal of Environmental Research and Public Health, 18*(23), 12763. Advance online publication. DOI: 10.3390/ijerph182312763 PMID: 34886493

Ozamiz-Etxebarria, N., Legorburu Fernnadez, I., Lipnicki, D. M., Idoiaga Mondragon, N., & Santabárbara, J. (2023). Prevalence of burnout among teachers during the COVID-19 pandemic: A meta-analysis. *International Journal of Environmental Research and Public Health, 20*(6), 4866. Advance online publication. DOI: 10.3390/ijerph20064866 PMID: 36981775

Pakdee, S., Cheechang, P., Thammanoon, R., Krobpet, S., Piya-amornphan, N., Puangsri, P., & Gosselink, R. (2025). Burnout and well-being among higher education teachers: Influencing factors of burnout. *BMC Public Health, 25*(1), 1–10. DOI: 10.1186/s12889-025-22602-w PMID: 40234791

Palmer, S. J. (2020). Encouraging exercise in older adults: Advice for nurses. *British Journal of Community Nursing, 25*(2), 95–97. DOI: 10.12968/bjcn.2020.25.2.95 PMID: 32040357

Palvimo, T., Vauhkonen, A., & Hult, M. (2023). The associations among destructive leadership, job demands and resources, and burnout among nurses: A cross-sectional survey study. *Journal of Nursing Management, 2023*(1), 4289450. Advance online publication. DOI: 10.1155/2023/4289450 PMID: 40225631

Parra, D. C., Wetherell, J. L., Van Zandt, A., Brownson, R. C., Abhishek, J., & Lenze, E. J. (2019). A qualitative study of older adults' perspectives on initiating exercise and mindfulness practice. *BMC Geriatrics, 19*, 354. Advance online publication. DOI: 10.1186/s12877-019-1375-9 PMID: 31865906

Patel, R. M., & Bartholomew, J. (2021). Impact of job resources and job demands on burnout among physical therapy providers. *International Journal of Environmental Research and Public Health, 18*(23), 12521. Advance online publication. DOI: 10.3390/ijerph182312521 PMID: 34886248

Peck, D. (2025). *Teacher burnout statistics: Why teachers quit in 2025.* https://www.devlinpeck.com/content/teacher-burnout-statistics

Pelletier, L., Shanmugasegaram, S., Patten, S. B., & Demers, A. (2017). Self-management of mood and/or anxiety disorders through physical activity/exercise. *Health Promotion and Chronic Disease Prevention in Canada : Research, Policy and Practice, 37*(5), 149–159. DOI: 10.24095/hpcdp.37.5.03 PMID: 28493659

Pihlaja, M., Tuominen, P., Peräkylä, J., & Hartikainen, K. M. (2022). Occupational burnout is linked with inefficient executive functioning, elevated average heart rate, and decreased physical activity in daily life-initial evidence from teaching professionals. *Brain Sciences, 12*(12), 1723. DOI: 10.3390/brainsci12121723 PMID: 36552182

Pollock, D., Evans, C., Jia, R. M., Alexander, L., Pieper, D., Brandão de Moraes, É., Peters, M. D. J., Tricco, A. C., Khalil, H., Godfrey, C. M., Saran, A., Campbell, F., & Munn, Z. (2024). "How-to": Scoping review? *Journal of Clinical Epidemiology, 176*, 111572. DOI: 10.1016/j.jclinepi.2024.111572 PMID: 39426499

Pressley, T. (2021). Factors contributing to teacher burnout during COVID-19. *Educational Researcher, 50*(5), 325–327. DOI: 10.3102/0013189X211004138

Ram, A., Marcos, L., Morey, R., Clark, T., Hakansson, S., Ristov, M., Franklin, A., McCarthy, C., De Carli, L., Jones, M. D., Ward, R. E., & Keech, A. (2022). Exercise for affect and enjoyment in overweight or obese males: A comparison of high-intensity interval training and moderate-intensity continuous training. *Psychology Health and Medicine, 27*(5), 1154–1167. DOI: 10.1080/13548506.2021.1903055 PMID: 33733958

Randall, K., Ford, T. G., Kwon, K. A., Sisson, S. S., Bice, M. R., Dinkel, D., & Tsotsoros, J. (2021). Physical activity, physical well-being, and psychological well-being: Associations with life satisfaction during the COVID-19 pandemic among early childhood educators. *International Journal of Environmental Research and Public Health, 18*, 9430. Advance online publication. DOI: 10.3390/ijerph18189430 PMID: 34574354

Rastegr, B., & Zarei, A. A. (2023). Assessment literacy components predicting EFL teachers' job-demands resources: A focus on burnout and engagement. *International Journal of Language Testing, 13*(1), 44–66. https://eric.ed.gov/?id=EJ1385327

Ratanasiripong, P., Ratanasiripong, N. T., Nungdanjark, W., Thongthammarat, Y., & Toyama, S. (2022). Mental health and burnout among teachers in Thailand. *Journal of Health Research, 36*(3), 404–416. DOI: 10.1108/JHR-05-2020-0181

Ren, X., & Wang, Y. (2022). On the correlation between job burnout, mental health and personality traits of college physical education teachers. *Psychiatria Danubina, 34*, S794–S799.

Rizvi, R., Rizvi, A. M., & Jamal, A. (2023). The impact of perceived organizational support, innovation at work, and burnout among teachers. *Bahria Journal of Professional Psychology, 22*(1), 38.

Robinson, L. E., Valido, A., Drescher, A., Woolweaver, A. B., Espelage, D. L., LoMurrary, S., Jong, A. C. J., Wright, A. A., & Dailey, M. M. (2022). Teachers, stress, and the COVID-19 Pandemic, A qualitative analysis. *School Mental Health, 15*, 78–89. DOI: 10.1007/s12310-022-09533-2 PMID: 35875185

Rockwell, L. (2024). *Teacher burnout: Symptoms, causes & prevention.* Choosing Therapy. https://www.choosingtherapy.com/teacher-burnout/#:~:text=Start%20Free%20Assessment-,What%20Is%20Teacher%20Burnout

Rojas, J. C., Barril, J. P., Jiménez, T. L., Clarà, M., Ramos, F. S., Peel, K., & Justiniano, B. (2025). Navigating burnout: A study of teacher identity in Chile, Ecuador, Brazil, Spain and Australia. *Pedagogy, Culture & Society, 33*(2), 729–745. DOI: 10.1080/14681366.2024.2302314

Rose, D. M., & Loomis, A. (2025). Teacher burnout, student-teacher relational closeness, and the moderating effect of work stress focused supervision. *Early Childhood Education Journal, 53*(4), 1027–1039. DOI: 10.1007/s10643-024-01651-7

Samaden, I. S. B., Najihah, I., Alwi, S., Munirah, R., Yusof, M. A. B. M., & Nordin, M. N. B. (2021). Time element in the construct of special education teacher workload in Malaysia. *Turkish Journal of Computer and Mathematics Education, 12*(11), 5141–5145. DOI: 10.1186/s12889-021-11677-w

Scardina, A., Tabacchi, G., Thomas, E., Navarra, G. A., Petrigna, L., Caramazza, G., Palma, A., & Bellafiore, M. (2024). Relationship between lifestyle determinants and perceived mental and physical health in Italian nursery and primary school teachers after the COVID-19 lockdown. *Journal of Functional Morphology and Kinesiology, 9*(1), 33. Advance online publication. DOI: 10.3390/jfmk9010033 PMID: 38390933

Shaheen, F., & Mahmood, N. (2024). The burnout syndrome: A review study. *Journal of Behavioural Sciences, 34*(2), 36–52.

Skaalvik, E., & Skaalvik, S. (2017). Still motivated to teach? A study of school context variables, stress and job satisfaction among teachers in senior high school. *Social Psychology of Education, 20*(1), 15–37. DOI: 10.1007/s11218-016-9363-9

Skaalvik, E., & Skaalvik, S. (2021). Teacher stress and coping strategies—The struggle to stay in control. *Creative Education, 12*, 1273–1295. DOI: 10.4236/ce.2021.126096

Skaalvik, E. M., & Skaalvik, S. (2018). Job demands and job resources as predictors of teacher motivation and well-being. *Social Psychology of Education, 21*(5), 1251–1275. DOI: 10.1007/s11218-018-9464-8

Skaalvik, E. M., & Skaalvik, S. (2020). Teacher burnout: Relations between dimensions of burnout, perceived school context, job satisfaction and motivation for teaching. A longitudinal study. *Teachers and Teaching, 26*(7-8), 602–616. DOI: 10.1080/13540602.2021.1913404

Song, Y., Zhao, W., Wang, X., & Li, J. (2024). The impact of job stress on burnout in Chinese teachers: The mediating roles of social support and psychological empowerment. *Psychology in the Schools, 61*(1), 253–271. DOI: 10.1002/pits.23052

Stark, K., Daulat, N., & King, S. (2022). A vision for teachers' emotional well-being. *Sage Journals, 103*(5). Advance online publication. DOI: 10.1177/00317217221079975

Sudibjo, N., & Manihuruk, A. M. (2022). How do happiness at work and perceived organizational support affect teachers' mental health through job satisfaction during the COVID-19 pandemic? *Psychology Research and Behavior Management, 15*, 939–951. DOI: 10.2147/PRBM.S361881 PMID: 35469169

Sun, W., Liu, X., Liu, Y., Ding, S., Jiang, Y., & Lv, Z. (2024). The relationship between school organizational climate and teacher's organizational citizenship behavior: The mediating role of teaching efficacy and moderating role of optimistic traits. *Behavioral Science, 14*(12), 1130. Advance online publication. DOI: 10.3390/bs14121130 PMID: 39767271

Sunarti, V., Rahman, M. A., Handrianto, C., Syuraini, S., Putri, L. D., Azizah, Z., & Nor Azhar, N. F. (2024). Understanding women's empowerment through exercise: Insights from a study on physical activity and self-efficacy. *Retos: Nuevas Perspectivas de Educación Física. Deporte y Recreación, 58*, 227–237. DOI: 10.47197/retos.v58.106803

Tan, J., & Kim, S. (2024). Exploring the relationship between teacher motivation and teacher burnout among Chinese college English teachers. *English Teaching, 79*(2), 163–190. DOI: 10.15858/engtea.79.2.202406.163

Tang, H., An, S., Zhang, L., Xiao, Y., & Li, X. (2024). The antecedents and outcomes of public service motivation: A meta-analysis using the Job Demands-Resources model. *Behavioral Sciences (Basel, Switzerland), 14*(10), 861. DOI: 10.3390/bs14100861 PMID: 39457733

Thomas, J., & Reyes, M. S. (2024). Understanding the new stress factors affecting teachers' burnout: A scoping review. *Makara Human Behavior Studies in Asia, 28*(1), 1–18. DOI: 10.7454/hubs.asia.1181024

Today, U. N. D. (2024). *Why teachers need, deserve mental health support.* University of North Dakota. https://blogs.und.edu/und-today/2024/01/und-in-the-conversation-why-teachers-need-deserve-mental-health-support/#:~:text=Improves%20teaching%20effectiveness,in%20such%20a%20positive%20way

Trinidad, J. E. (2021). Teacher satisfaction and burnout during COVID-19: What organizational factors help? *International Journal of Leadership in Education, 28*(1), 214–232. DOI: 10.1080/13603124.2021.2006795

Tummers, L. D., & Bakker, A. B. (2021). Leadership and job demands-resources theory: A systematic review. *Frontiers in Psychology, 12*, 722080. Advance online publication. DOI: 10.3389/fpsyg.2021.722080 PMID: 34659034

Turner, K., & Garvis, S. (2023). Teacher educator wellbeing, stress and burnout: A scoping review. *Education Sciences, 13*(4), 351. DOI: 10.3390/educsci13040351

Valentim, O., de Sousa, L., de Sousa, C., Correia, T., Carvalho, J. C., Querido, A., José, H., & Laranjeira, C. (2025). Positive mental health and happiness at work in a sample of Portuguese workers: A web-based cross-sectional study. *Administrative Sciences, 15*(2), 44. Advance online publication. DOI: 10.3390/admsci15020044

Van Dyck, D., Mertens, L., Cardon, G., De Cocker, K., & De Bourdeaudhuij, I. (2017). Opinions toward physical activity, sedentary behavior, and interventions to stimulate active living during early retirement: A qualitative study in recently retired adults. *Journal of Aging and Physical Activity, 25*(2), 277–286. DOI: 10.1123/japa.2015-0295 PMID: 27759483

Vela, J. C., Guerra, F., Diaz, Z., Karaman, M. A., & Zamora, E. (2024). Exploring how positive psychology characteristics influence mental health among teacher candidates at a Hispanic serving institution. *Journal of Latinos and Education, 23*(4), 1461–1471. DOI: 10.1080/15348431.2023.2274851

Vermote, B., Vansteenkiste, M., Aelterman, N., van der Kaap-Deeder, J., & Beyers, W. (2023). Teachers' psychological needs link social pressure with personal adjustment and motivating teaching style. *Journal of Experimental Education, 91*(4), 696–717. DOI: 10.1080/00220973.2022.2039584

Walker, T. (2025). *What's causing teacher burnout?* NEA Today. https://www.nea.org/nea-today/all-news-articles/whats-causing-teacher-burnout#:~:text=A%20lack%20of%20administrative%20support,youth%20in%20their%20formative%20years.%22

Wang, Y. (2024). Exploring the impact of workload, organizational support, and work engagement on teachers' psychological wellbeing: A structural equation modeling approach. *Frontiers in Psychology, 14*, 1345740. Advance online publication. DOI: 10.3389/fpsyg.2023.1345740 PMID: 38314257

Wang, Y., Zai, F., & Zhou, X. (2025). The impact of emotion regulation strategies on teachers' well-being and positive emotions: A meta-analysis. *Behavioral Sciences (Basel, Switzerland), 15*(3), 342. DOI: 10.3390/bs15030342 PMID: 40150237

Westphal, A., Kalinowski, E., Hoferichter, C. J., & Vock, M. (2022). K-12 teachers' stress and burnout during the COVID-19 pandemic: A systematic review. *Frontiers in Psychology, 13*, 920326. Advance online publication. DOI: 10.3389/fpsyg.2022.920326 PMID: 36118449

Wink, M. N., LaRusso, M. D., & Smith, R. L. (2021). Teacher empathy and students with problem behaviors: Examining teachers' perceptions, responses, relationships, and burnout. *Psychology in the Schools, 58*(8), 1575–1596. DOI: 10.1002/pits.22516

Woloshyn, V., Savage, M., Maich, K., & Penney, S. (2023). Stress, coping, and well-being in teachers and school administrators. *The Alberta Journal of Educational Research, 69*(4), 492–513. DOI: 10.55016/ojs/ajer.v69i4.75886

World Health Organization. (2024). *Physical activity.* https://www.who.int/news-room/fact-sheets/detail/physical-activity

Xia, J. W., & Shun, H. T. (2021). Exploring the mechanisms influencing the occupational well-being of early childhood teachers-A qualitative study based on the JD-R Model. *Turkish Journal of Computer and Mathematics Education, 12*(12), 4689–4706. https://www.proquest.com/scholarly-journals/exploring-mechanisms-influencing-occupational/docview/2628340006/se-2

Yaqian, Z., Chonggao, W., & Fan, Z. (2024). The relationship between job stress and job burnout of preschool teachers during the COVID-19: The moderation of perceived organizational support. *Work (Reading, Mass.), 79*(3), 1133–1146. DOI: 10.3233/WOR-230151 PMID: 38759080

Ye, Z., Peng, Y., Rao, W., & Zhang, T. (2024). The effect of physical activity on depression: A lagged mediation study of school burnout. *BMC Public Health, 24*(1), 3491. Advance online publication. DOI: 10.1186/s12889-024-21003-9 PMID: 39695559

Zhao, J., Effendi, A. A., & Zhao, S. (2024). Work engagement of teachers in Chinese higher education sector: Using mixed method appraisal tool of systematic literature review. *Global Business and Management Research, 16*(4), 1258–1274. https://www.gbmrjournal.com/pdf/v16n4s/V16N4s-79.pdf

Zhou, S., Slemp, G. R., & Vella-Brodrick, D. A. (2024). Factors associated with teacher wellbeing: A meta-analysis. *Educational Psychology Review, 36*, 63. Advance online publication. DOI: 10.1007/s10648-024-09886-x

Žnidaršič, J., & Marič, M. (2021). Relationships between work-family balance, job satisfaction, life satisfaction and work engagement among higher education lecturers. *Organizacija, 54*(3), 227–237. DOI: 10.2478/orga-2021-0015

ADDITIONAL READING

Corbett, L., Bauman, A., Peralta, L. R., Okely, A. D., & Phongsavan, P. (2021). Characteristics and effectiveness of physical activity, nutrition and/or sleep interventions to improve the mental well-being of teachers: A scoping review. *Health Education Journal, 81*(2), 196–210. DOI: 10.1177/00178969211062701

Davis, J. (2023). The relationship between teacher burnout and physical activity among high school teachers. *Doctor of Education in Teacher Leadership Dissertations*. 62. https://digitalcommons.kennesaw.edu/teachleaddoc_etd/62?utm_source=digitalcommons.kennesaw.edu%2Fteachleaddoc_etd%2F62&utm_medium=PDF&utm_campaign=PDFCoverPages

de Vries, J. D., & Bakker, A. B. (2022). The physical activity paradox: A longitudinal study of the implications for burnout. *International Archives of Occupational and Environmental Health, 95*, 965–979. DOI: 10.1007/s00420-021-01759-y PMID: 34611746

Firus, M. (2023). *Teacher wellness initiative: Viability of incorporating exercise into teachers' workday* [Doctoral dissertation, University of Saskatchewan]. University of Saskatchewan. https://harvest.usask.ca/server/api/core/bitstreams/ 473c72f8-abc8-44c0-b84e-c47f75094ae7/content

Office of Disease Prevention and Health Promotion. (2021, August 24). Current Guidelines. U.S. Department of Health and Human Services. https://odphp.health.gov/our-work/ nutrition-physical-activity/physical-activity-guidelines/current-guidelines

Ratanasiripong, P., Ratanasiripong, N. T., Nungdanjark, W., Thongthammarat, Y., & Toyama, S. (2022). Mental health and burnout among teachers in Thailand. *Journal of Health Research, 36*(3), 404–416. DOI: 10.1108/JHR-05-2020-0181

KEY TERMS AND DEFINITIONS

Burnout: Any feelings of emotional exhaustion, increased mental fatigue, or increased attrition.

Exercise: Any structured or unstructured movement that elevates heart rate above resting levels.

Leisure-Time Physical Activity: Voluntary, mild, or moderate physical activity during one's free time that leads to emotional satisfaction, improved mood, and well-being.

Mental Health: The psychological state reflecting one's overall well-being.

Physical Activity: Any structured or unstructured movement that elevates heart rate above resting levels.

Positive Mental Health: Enhanced emotional and mental well-being that contributes and improves one's overall quality of life and psychological resilience.

Teacher Burnout: Negative feelings that teachers experience within the teaching profession, such as, but not limited to, emotional exhaustion, increased mental fatigue, or increased attrition.

Chapter 13
Effect of Exercise and Emotional Well-Being in Competitive Sports

Awesh Khati
https://orcid.org/0009-0009-9090-1593
Lakshmibai National Institute of Physical Education, India

Anindita Das
https://orcid.org/0000-0002-6502-9619
Lakshmibai National Institute of Physical Education, India

Gopal Chandra Saha
Visva-Bharati, Santiniketan, India

ABSTRACT

Exercise and emotional well-being in competitive sports are intricately linked, impacting performance via physiological, psychological, and social mechanisms. Consistent exercising not only improves physical fitness but also facilitates emotional control, diminishes stress, fosters resilience, and stimulates motivation. Neurobiological mechanisms, including neurotransmitter modulation and neuroplasticity, facilitate these advantages, whereas frameworks such as self-determination theory emphasize autonomy, competence, and relatedness as essential for emotional equilibrium. However, excessive training, societal expectations, and insufficient rehabilitation can result in burnout and mental health hazards. The integration of psychological skills, mindfulness, recovery tactics, and supportive coaching can enhance performance and mental well-being. Emerging technologies, such as AI-driven

DOI: 10.4018/979-8-3373-6157-4.ch013

monitoring and digital interventions, provide innovative tools for athlete-centered well-being management, signifying a transition towards holistic methodologies in contemporary sports.

INTRODUCTION

The intricate relationship between exercise and emotional well-being has emerged as one of the most compelling areas of research in contemporary sports psychology, fundamentally reshaping our understanding of what constitutes optimal athletic performance. In the realm of competitive sports, where the margins between victory and defeat are often measured in fractions of seconds or single points, the psychological dimension of athletic performance has gained unprecedented recognition alongside traditional physical training methodologies. The convergence of exercise science and emotional psychology has revealed that the benefits of physical activity extend far beyond the development of muscular strength, cardiovascular endurance, and technical skill acquisition, encompassing profound effects on mood regulation, stress management, cognitive function, and overall psychological resilience that directly impact competitive outcomes (Biddle & Batterham, 2015). This multifaceted relationship becomes particularly pronounced in competitive environments, where athletes must navigate intense pressure, performance anxiety, and the constant scrutiny that accompanies high-level competition while maintaining peak physical condition and mental clarity.

The importance of exercise in sports performance has traditionally been conceptualized through purely physiological parameters, with emphasis placed on measurable outcomes such as VO2 max, power output, reaction times, and biomechanical efficiency. However, contemporary research has illuminated the sophisticated neurobiological mechanisms through which regular physical activity influences brain structure and function, creating cascading effects that enhance not only physical capabilities but also emotional regulation, decision-making processes, and psychological adaptation to competitive stressors. The acute and chronic adaptations that occur in response to systematic training extend beyond the cardiovascular and musculoskeletal systems to encompass significant modifications in neurotransmitter production, hormonal balance, and neural plasticity, collectively contributing to improved emotional stability and psychological well-being. These neuroadaptations manifest in enhanced mood states, reduced anxiety levels, improved self-efficacy, and greater resilience in the face of competitive challenges, creating a synergistic relationship between physical preparation and psychological readiness that is essential for optimal athletic performance.

The link between physical activity and emotional well-being in competitive sports operates through multiple interconnected pathways that reflect the complex interplay between physiological and psychological systems. Research has consistently demonstrated that regular exercise participation leads to increased production of endorphins, serotonin, and dopamine, neurotransmitters that are crucial for mood regulation and emotional stability (Rosenbaum et al., 2014). In competitive athletics, where athletes frequently experience high levels of stress, pressure, and emotional volatility, these neurochemical adaptations serve as natural mood stabilizers that help maintain psychological equilibrium during training and competition periods. Furthermore, the rhythmic, repetitive nature of many training activities appears to activate parasympathetic nervous system responses that promote relaxation and stress reduction, counteracting the potentially deleterious effects of chronic competitive stress on mental health and performance outcomes.

The psychological benefits of exercise in competitive sports extend beyond immediate mood enhancement to encompass fundamental changes in self-perception, confidence, and emotional intelligence that are critical for sustained success in high-pressure environments. Athletes who maintain consistent training regimens typically demonstrate improved body awareness, enhanced self-esteem, and greater emotional self-regulation compared to their less active counterparts, factors that translate directly into improved competitive performance and career longevity (Schaal et al., 2011). The mastery experiences gained through progressive physical conditioning create a foundation of self-efficacy that generalizes to competitive situations, enabling athletes to approach challenges with greater confidence and emotional stability. Additionally, the social aspects of team training and group exercise activities contribute to emotional well-being through enhanced social support, camaraderie, and shared goal achievement, creating protective factors against the isolation and pressure that can accompany competitive athletics.

Understanding the bidirectional relationship between exercise and emotional well-being in competitive sports has profound implications for the design of training programs, athlete development, and performance optimization strategies. As the field continues to evolve, there is growing recognition that successful competitive athletes must be developed holistically, with equal attention paid to physical conditioning and psychological preparation. The integration of exercise science principles with emotional well-being considerations represents a paradigm shift toward more comprehensive, athlete-centered approaches that acknowledge the fundamental interconnectedness of mind and body in athletic performance (Reardon & Factor, 2010).

CONCEPTUAL FRAMEWORK

Defining Exercise in Competitive Sports

Exercise within the context of competitive sports represents a multifaceted construct that extends far beyond the traditional understanding of physical activity as merely movement for health benefits. In competitive athletics, exercise encompasses systematic, structured, and purposeful physical training designed to optimize performance outcomes while simultaneously influencing psychological states and emotional responses. This specialized form of exercise is characterized by its intentional nature, progressive overload principles, and specific adaptation requirements that distinguish it from recreational physical activity or general fitness pursuits. Competitive sports exercise involves rigorous training regimens that incorporate technical skill development, tactical preparation, physical conditioning, and mental preparation components that work synergistically to enhance athletic performance while creating complex interactions with the athlete's emotional and psychological well-being.

The physiological demands of competitive sports exercise create unique adaptations that influence not only physical capabilities but also neurochemical processes that directly impact emotional regulation and psychological functioning. These adaptations include enhanced cardiovascular efficiency, improved neuromuscular coordination, increased metabolic flexibility, and optimized hormonal responses that collectively contribute to both performance enhancement and emotional stability. Furthermore, competitive sports exercise is distinguished by its performance-oriented nature, where training intensity, volume, and specificity are carefully calibrated to achieve peak performance during competition periods, creating distinct psychological pressures and emotional challenges that recreational exercisers typically do not experience.

The temporal structure of competitive sports exercise also differs significantly from general physical activity, as it involves periodized training cycles that create varying levels of physical and psychological stress throughout different phases of preparation. These cycles include preparation periods with high training loads, competition phases with intense performance demands, and recovery periods that allow for physical and emotional restoration (Bompa & Buzzichelli, 2019). This cyclical nature of competitive sports exercise creates dynamic interactions with emotional well-being, as athletes must navigate the psychological challenges associated with intense training periods, performance anxiety during competitions, and the emotional fluctuations that accompany success and failure in competitive environments.

Emotional Well-being: Psychological and Physiological Perspectives

Emotional well-being in competitive sports represents a complex integration of psychological states and physiological processes that collectively influence an athlete's capacity to experience positive emotions, manage stress effectively, maintain psychological resilience, and achieve optimal performance outcomes. From a psychological perspective, emotional well-being encompasses multiple dimensions, including affect regulation, stress management, self-efficacy, motivation, and the ability to maintain psychological balance despite the inherent pressures and uncertainties associated with competitive athletics (Lundqvist, 2011). This psychological dimension involves cognitive processes such as attention regulation, goal orientation, self-talk patterns, and coping strategies that athletes develop to manage the emotional demands of training and competition while maintaining their overall mental health and performance effectiveness.

The psychological components of emotional well-being in competitive sports are intrinsically linked to concepts of mental toughness, resilience, and psychological flexibility, which enable athletes to adapt to changing circumstances, recover from setbacks, and maintain optimal emotional states under pressure. These psychological factors are not static traits but rather dynamic capabilities that can be developed through targeted interventions and training approaches that integrate mental skills development with physical preparation (Gould & Maynard, 2009). The psychological perspective on emotional well-being also recognizes the importance of social support systems, coach-athlete relationships, team dynamics, and environmental factors that contribute to or detract from an athlete's overall emotional health and performance capacity.

From a physiological perspective, emotional well-being in competitive sports is fundamentally influenced by neurochemical processes, hormonal responses, and autonomic nervous system functioning that create the biological foundation for emotional experiences and regulation. The physiological stress response system, including the hypothalamic-pituitary-adrenal axis and sympathetic nervous system activation, plays a crucial role in determining how athletes experience and manage emotional states during training and competition (Kellmann et al., 2018). These physiological processes influence the production and regulation of neurotransmitters such as serotonin, dopamine, and norepinephrine, which directly impact mood states, motivation levels, and emotional stability in competitive environments.

The physiological perspective also recognizes that chronic exposure to high-intensity training and competitive stress can lead to maladaptive physiological responses that negatively impact emotional well-being, including elevated cortisol levels, disrupted sleep patterns, immune system suppression, and autonomic nervous system imbalances. These physiological disruptions can manifest as decreased emotional regulation, increased anxiety and depression symptoms, reduced motivation, and impaired cognitive functioning that collectively compromise both performance and overall well-being (Meeusen, 2013). Understanding these physiological mechanisms is essential for developing comprehensive approaches to supporting emotional well-being in competitive sports that address both the psychological and biological factors that influence emotional health and performance outcomes.

Theoretical Models

The biopsychosocial model provides a comprehensive theoretical framework for understanding the complex interactions between exercise and emotional well-being in competitive sports by recognizing that athletic performance and emotional health are influenced by the dynamic interplay of biological, psychological, and social factors. This model acknowledges that biological factors such as genetic predispositions, physiological adaptations to training, neurochemical responses, and hormonal fluctuations create the foundational context within which psychological and social factors operate to influence emotional well-being outcomes (Engel, 1977; Reardon & Factor, 2010). The biological component encompasses not only the direct physiological effects of exercise on neurotransmitter production and stress hormone regulation but also individual differences in stress sensitivity, recovery capacity, and genetic factors that influence emotional regulation and performance under pressure.

The psychological component of the biopsychosocial model focuses on cognitive processes, personality factors, mental skills, and psychological resources that athletes bring to their competitive experiences and how these factors interact with training and competition demands to influence emotional outcomes. This includes examining how cognitive appraisal processes, coping strategies, self-efficacy beliefs, and motivational orientations shape athletes' emotional responses to training stress, competitive pressure, and performance outcomes (Lazarus, 2000). The social component recognizes that competitive sports occur within complex social environments that include coach relationships, teammate interactions, family support systems, and broader cultural contexts that significantly influence emotional well-being through mechanisms such as social support, social comparison processes, and cultural expectations regarding athletic achievement and emotional expression.

Self-Determination Theory (SDT) offers another powerful theoretical framework for understanding the relationship between exercise and emotional well-being in competitive sports by focusing on the fundamental psychological needs that drive human motivation and well-being. According to SDT, emotional well-being is optimized when individuals experience satisfaction of three basic psychological needs: autonomy (feeling volitional and self-directed), competence (experiencing effectiveness and mastery), and relatedness (feeling connected and valued by others) (Deci & Ryan, 2000; Ryan & Deci, 2017). In competitive sports contexts, the satisfaction of these needs through training and competition experiences can enhance intrinsic motivation, promote positive emotional states, and support overall psychological well-being, while need frustration can lead to decreased motivation, negative emotional experiences, and compromised mental health.

The autonomy need within competitive sports relates to athletes' sense of choice, volition, and personal agency in their training and competitive experiences, which can be supported through coach behaviors that provide rationale for training decisions, offer meaningful choices, and encourage athlete input in goal-setting processes. Competence need satisfaction occurs when athletes experience mastery, improvement, and effectiveness in their sport, which is facilitated by appropriate challenge levels, constructive feedback, and opportunities to develop and demonstrate skills. Relatedness need satisfaction involves feeling valued, supported, and connected within the athletic environment, which is promoted through positive coach-athlete relationships, supportive teammate interactions, and inclusive team cultures that value individual contributions while promoting collective goals (Ntoumanis et al., 2009). The SDT framework suggests that training and competitive environments that support these three needs will promote more adaptive motivational patterns, enhanced emotional well-being, and sustainable engagement in competitive sports, while environments that frustrate these needs may lead to decreased motivation, negative emotional outcomes, and increased risk of dropout or burnout.

EXERCISE AND MENTAL HEALTH

Role of Exercise in Reducing Anxiety, Stress, and Depression

The therapeutic effects of exercise on anxiety, stress, and depression have been extensively documented through rigorous scientific investigation, with mounting evidence suggesting that physical activity can be as effective as traditional psychotherapeutic interventions in treating mild to moderate psychological distress. Structured exercise programs significantly reduce symptoms of anxiety across diverse populations, with effect sizes comparable to those achieved through cognitive-behavioral therapy and pharmacological interventions (Rosenbaum et al., 2014). The anxiolytic effects of exercise appear to be mediated through multiple pathways, including the modulation of neurotransmitter systems, the activation of the hypothalamic-pituitary-adrenal axis, and the promotion of neuroplasticity in brain regions associated with emotional regulation. Furthermore, exercise-induced anxiety reduction demonstrates both acute and chronic effects, with immediate post-exercise benefits lasting several hours and long-term adaptations developing over weeks to months of consistent training.

The relationship between exercise and stress reduction manifests through complex physiological and psychological mechanisms that work synergistically to enhance an individual's capacity to manage stressful situations effectively. Regular physical activity serves as a buffer against chronic stress by improving the body's ability to maintain homeostasis under challenging conditions, thereby reducing the overall physiological burden associated with prolonged stress exposure (Stubbs et al., 2017). This stress-buffering effect occurs through the modulation of cortisol secretion patterns, the enhancement of parasympathetic nervous system activity, and the promotion of adaptive coping strategies that enable individuals to perceive stressful situations as manageable challenges rather than overwhelming threats. Additionally, exercise-induced improvements in sleep quality, cognitive function, and self-efficacy contribute to enhanced stress resilience by providing athletes with the psychological resources necessary to navigate the demanding requirements of competitive sports participation.

Depression, characterized by persistent feelings of sadness, hopelessness, and diminished interest in activities, represents a significant mental health concern among competitive athletes, with prevalence rates often exceeding those observed in the general population due to the unique stressors associated with high-level sport participation. Regular exercise participation can prevent the onset of depressive episodes while also serving as an effective treatment modality for individuals already experiencing depressive symptoms (Kandola et al., 2019). The antidepressant effects of exercise appear to be mediated through multiple biological and psychological pathways, including the promotion of neurogenesis in the hippocampus, the regulation of inflammatory markers, and the enhancement of self-esteem and social connectedness. Notably, the therapeutic benefits of exercise for depression demonstrate a dose-response relationship, with moderate-intensity activities performed three to five times per week producing optimal outcomes for mood improvement and symptom reduction.

Exercise as a Coping Mechanism in Competitive Athletes

Competitive athletes frequently encounter unique psychological challenges that distinguish their experiences from those of recreational exercisers, including performance pressure, public scrutiny, career uncertainty, and the constant demand for physical and mental excellence. Within this context, exercise serves not only as a means of physical preparation but also as a sophisticated coping mechanism that enables athletes to manage the psychological demands of high-level competition effectively. Exercise serves as a primary adaptive coping strategy employed by elite athletes to regulate emotions, process stressful experiences, and maintain psychological equilibrium in the face of intense competitive pressures (Rice et al., 2016). The ritualistic and predictable nature of training routines provides athletes with a sense of control and mastery over their environment, which becomes particularly valuable during periods of uncertainty or transition within their athletic careers.

The coping benefits of exercise for competitive athletes extend beyond immediate stress relief to encompass broader aspects of psychological resilience and emotional regulation. Through consistent engagement in structured physical activity, athletes develop enhanced self-awareness, improved emotional intelligence, and sophisticated stress management skills that transfer to various life domains beyond sport participation. Athletes who maintain regular training schedules during periods of competitive stress show better emotional stability, improved sleep quality, and reduced incidence of anxiety and mood disorders compared to those who significantly alter their exercise patterns (Schaal et al., 2011). This finding suggests that the consistency and predictability of exercise routines provide crucial psychological anchoring effects, helping athletes maintain emotional equilibrium during turbulent periods in their competitive careers.

Furthermore, exercise serves as a powerful medium for social connection and support among competitive athletes, facilitating the development of meaningful relationships that provide additional psychological resources for coping with the stressors of competition. The shared experience of physical challenge, mutual encouragement during training sessions, and collective pursuit of performance goals create strong social bonds that enhance overall well-being and resilience. Athletes who train in supportive group environments demonstrate superior psychological outcomes compared to those who primarily engage in individual training, highlighting the importance of social connectivity as a mediating factor in the relationship between exercise and mental health outcomes (M. R. Beauchamp et al., 2003).

Neurobiological Mechanisms

The neurobiological foundations underlying the mental health benefits of exercise involve complex interactions among multiple neurotransmitter systems, hormonal pathways, and brain structures that collectively contribute to improved emotional regulation and psychological well-being. The endorphin hypothesis, first proposed in the 1980s, suggests that exercise-induced release of endogenous opioids produces euphoric feelings and pain relief that contribute to improved mood states. However, contemporary research has revealed that the neurobiological mechanisms underlying exercise's mental health benefits extend far beyond simple endorphin release to encompass sophisticated changes in brain structure and function. Regular exercise promotes the expression of brain-derived neurotrophic factor (BDNF), a protein crucial for neuronal survival, growth, and synaptic plasticity, particularly in brain regions associated with learning, memory, and emotional processing (Heijnen et al., 2016).

The dopaminergic system plays a central role in mediating the rewarding and motivational aspects of exercise, contributing to the development of positive associations with physical activity and the maintenance of long-term exercise adherence. Exercise-induced activation of dopamine pathways in the ventral tegmental area and nucleus accumbens produces feelings of pleasure and satisfaction that reinforce continued participation in physical activity (Foley & Fleshner, 2008). This neurochemical reward system becomes particularly important for competitive athletes who must maintain high training volumes over extended periods, as the intrinsic satisfaction derived from exercise helps sustain motivation even during challenging phases of preparation and competition.

Cortisol regulation represents another critical neurobiological mechanism through which exercise exerts its mental health benefits, particularly in stress management and emotional resilience. While acute exercise transiently increases cortisol secretion as part of the normal physiological response to physical stress, chronic exercise participation leads to improved regulation of the hypothalamic-pituitary-adrenal axis and enhanced cortisol sensitivity, with well-trained athletes exhibiting more efficient cortisol responses to both physical and psychological stressors, characterized by appropriate activation during challenging situations followed by rapid recovery to baseline levels (Beserra et al., 2018). The neuroplasticity-promoting effects of exercise represent perhaps the most profound neurobiological mechanism underlying its mental health benefits, as regular physical activity induces structural and functional changes in brain regions critical for emotional regulation, cognitive function, and stress resilience, promoting neurogenesis in the hippocampus, enhancing synaptic connectivity in the prefrontal cortex, and increasing gray matter volume in regions associated with executive function and emotional processing (Mandolesi et al., 2018). These exercise-induced neuroplastic changes create lasting improvements in cognitive flexibility, emotional regulation, and stress tolerance that persist beyond individual training sessions to provide sustained mental health benefits for competitive athletes throughout their careers.

Impact on Emotional Well-being in Competitive Sports

The intricate relationship between exercise and emotional well-being becomes particularly complex within the demanding environment of competitive sports, where athletes must navigate intense physical training regimens alongside significant psychological pressures. Competitive sports environments create unique psychological landscapes that profoundly influence athletes' emotional states, with exercise serving as both a catalyst for positive mental health outcomes and, paradoxically, a potential source of psychological distress when improperly managed (Reardon et al., 2019). The multifaceted nature of this relationship encompasses various psychological domains, including motivation, focus, resilience, self-esteem, and the delicate balance between optimal training loads and burnout prevention. Understanding these dynamics is crucial for athletes, coaches, and sports psychologists who seek to optimize both performance and psychological well-being in competitive athletic contexts.

Influence on Motivation, Focus, and Resilience

The psychological benefits of exercise in competitive sports extend far beyond mere physical conditioning, creating profound impacts on fundamental cognitive and emotional processes that determine athletic success. Exercise-induced neurochemical changes, particularly the release of endorphins, dopamine, and norepinephrine, create powerful motivational frameworks that sustain athletes through rigorous training cycles and competitive pressures (Schuch et al., 2018). These neurobiological adaptations foster intrinsic motivation patterns that enable athletes to maintain consistent training behaviors even when faced with physical discomfort, performance setbacks, or external pressures. The development of exercise-dependent motivation systems becomes particularly evident in elite athletes who report experiencing genuine pleasure and satisfaction from training activities that would otherwise be perceived as punishing or aversive by non-athletes (Mallett & Hanrahan, 2004).

Furthermore, regular exercise participation in competitive contexts enhances cognitive focus through multiple mechanisms, including improved attention regulation, enhanced working memory capacity, and increased cognitive flexibility under stress conditions. Research demonstrates that athletes who maintain consistent training regimens show superior attentional control compared to their sedentary counterparts, with these benefits extending beyond sport-specific contexts into academic and professional domains (Erickson et al., 2015). The development of focused attention through exercise appears to create self-reinforcing cycles where improved concentration during training leads to more effective skill acquisition, which in turn generates positive emotional responses that further enhance motivation and focus. This cyclical relationship becomes particularly important during competitive seasons when athletes must maintain peak concentration levels despite increasing external pressures and performance expectations.

Resilience development through exercise represents one of the most significant psychological benefits of competitive sports participation, with regular physical training serving as a form of controlled stress exposure that builds adaptive coping mechanisms. Athletes who engage in systematic training programs develop enhanced stress tolerance through repeated exposure to physical and mental challenges that mirror competitive demands (Fletcher & Sarkar, 2012). This process of stress inoculation through exercise creates robust psychological frameworks that enable athletes to maintain emotional stability during high-pressure competitive situations. The development of physical resilience through training appears to translate directly into psychological resilience, with athletes reporting increased confidence in their ability to handle adversity both within and outside sporting contexts.

Effects on Self-Esteem and Confidence

The relationship between exercise participation and self-esteem development in competitive sports creates complex psychological dynamics that can profoundly influence athletes' overall emotional well-being and performance outcomes. Regular exercise participation generates multiple pathways for self-esteem enhancement, including physical appearance improvements, skill mastery experiences, social recognition, and the achievement of personally meaningful goals (Ekeland et al., 2005). These pathways become particularly salient in competitive environments where objective performance measures provide concrete feedback regarding progress and achievement. Athletes often report that consistent training regimens create positive self-perception cycles where improved physical capabilities lead to enhanced self-confidence, which subsequently motivates continued participation and further skill development.

However, the competitive sports environment also creates unique challenges for self-esteem development, particularly when athletes' self-worth becomes overly dependent on performance outcomes or external validation. Research indicates that athletes whose self-esteem is primarily contingent on competitive success are at increased risk for psychological distress, particularly following performance disappointments or career-ending injuries (Crocker & Park, 2004). The pressure to maintain high performance standards can transform exercise from a source of psychological well-being into a source of anxiety and self-doubt, particularly when training outcomes fail to meet expectations or when competitive results do not align with effort invested.

Confidence development through exercise in competitive sports involves complex interactions between physical competence, cognitive appraisal processes, and social feedback mechanisms. Athletes who experience consistent training adaptations and skill improvements typically develop robust confidence frameworks that extend beyond sport-specific domains into general life areas. This confidence development process appears to be mediated by athletes' ability to accurately assess their capabilities and set realistic performance expectations. When athletes can maintain an appropriate perspective regarding their abilities while still pursuing challenging goals, exercise participation becomes a powerful tool for sustainable confidence building that enhances overall emotional well-being.

Balancing Training Load and Burnout Prevention

The prevention of athletic burnout represents one of the most critical challenges in maintaining positive emotional well-being within competitive sports environments, requiring careful attention to training load management and psychological recovery strategies. Burnout syndrome in competitive athletes manifests through emotional exhaustion, cynicism toward sport participation, and a reduced sense of personal accomplishment, with excessive training loads serving as the primary contributing factors (Gustafsson et al., 2017). The paradoxical relationship between exercise and burnout highlights the importance of finding optimal training intensities that maximize performance adaptations while preserving psychological well-being. Research demonstrates that athletes who experience chronic overtraining often develop negative associations with exercise that can persist long after competitive careers end, emphasizing the long-term importance of appropriate load management.

Effective training load management requires a sophisticated understanding of individual athletes' psychological and physiological responses to various exercise stimuli, with successful programs incorporating regular monitoring of both objective performance markers and subjective well-being indicators. Athletes who participate in periodized training programs that systematically vary intensity and volume show lower rates of burnout and higher levels of sustained motivation compared to those following monotonous or continuously high-intensity regimens (Kenttä & Hassmén, 1998). The integration of recovery periods and alternative activities appears crucial for maintaining positive psychological associations with exercise while preventing the development of exercise dependence or compulsive training behaviors. Moreover, the social and environmental context surrounding training significantly influences whether exercise promotes or undermines emotional well-being in competitive athletes. Supportive coaching environments that emphasize personal growth, skill development, and intrinsic motivation tend to foster positive relationships with exercise, while environments that primarily emphasize outcome achievement and external rewards may increase burnout risk (Bartholomew et al., 2011).

FACTORS INFLUENCING EXERCISE AND EMOTIONAL OUTCOMES IN COMPETITIVE SPORTS

Gender and Age Differences

The relationship between exercise participation and emotional well-being in competitive sports demonstrates significant variations across gender and age demographics, revealing complex interactions that influence psychological outcomes. Research consistently indicates that female athletes experience different emotional responses to competitive exercise compared to their male counterparts, with these differences manifesting across multiple psychological domains, including anxiety management, mood regulation, and stress response patterns. Female competitive athletes often report higher baseline levels of anxiety and demonstrate greater emotional reactivity to competitive stressors, yet they also show enhanced capacity for emotional expression and social connection through sport participation, which can serve as protective factors for psychological well-being (Reardon & Factor, 2010). The hormonal fluctuations associated with menstrual cycles further complicate the emotional landscape for female athletes, with research demonstrating that exercise-induced mood improvements can vary significantly across different phases of the menstrual cycle, affecting both training adaptations and competitive performance outcomes (Martín-Rodríguez et al., 2024).

Male athletes typically exhibit different patterns of emotional regulation through competitive exercise, often showing a greater propensity for externalized stress responses and risk-taking behaviors, while simultaneously demonstrating lower rates of help-seeking for emotional difficulties (Rice et al., 2016). The sociocultural expectations surrounding masculine identity in competitive sports can create additional psychological pressures for male athletes, potentially limiting their willingness to acknowledge or address emotional challenges, despite experiencing similar rates of anxiety and depression as their female counterparts. Age-related factors introduce another layer of complexity to these gender differences, with adolescent athletes of both genders showing heightened emotional volatility and increased susceptibility to negative psychological outcomes from competitive pressures, while older athletes generally demonstrate more stable emotional responses and better-developed coping mechanisms (Sabiston et al., 2016). The developmental stage of identity formation during adolescence intersects with competitive sport participation in ways that can either enhance or compromise emotional well-being, depending on the presence of supportive environmental factors and the availability of appropriate psychological resources.

Age-specific patterns reveal that younger competitive athletes, particularly those in early adolescence, experience more dramatic mood fluctuations in response to exercise and competition, with both positive and negative emotional states showing greater intensity and duration compared to adult athletes (Freeman et al., 2011). The neurological development occurring during adolescence affects emotional regulation capacity, making young competitive athletes more vulnerable to the negative psychological effects of overtraining, competitive failure, and social comparison processes. Conversely, master athletes and older competitive participants often report more consistent positive emotional outcomes from exercise participation, potentially due to increased life experience, better-developed perspective-taking abilities, and reduced external pressures for performance excellence (Young & Medic, 2011).

Type, Intensity, and Duration of Exercise

The specific characteristics of exercise engagement within competitive sports contexts significantly influence emotional and psychological outcomes, with research demonstrating that different types of athletic activities produce distinct patterns of mood enhancement and stress response (Penedo & Dahn, 2005). Aerobic-based competitive sports, including distance running, cycling, and swimming, consistently produce robust improvements in mood states and reductions in symptoms of anxiety and depression, likely due to the sustained elevation of endorphins, serotonin, and other neurotransmitters associated with prolonged cardiovascular activity. These endurance-oriented sports also facilitate meditative-like psychological states during training and competition, allowing athletes to experience flow states and mindfulness benefits that extend beyond the immediate exercise session (Park & Jeon, 2023). However, the psychological benefits of aerobic exercise in competitive contexts can be compromised when training intensity becomes excessive or when performance pressures override the intrinsic enjoyment of movement, leading to negative emotional outcomes despite the inherently mood-enhancing properties of aerobic activity.

Team-based competitive sports present unique psychological dynamics that can either amplify or diminish the emotional benefits of exercise participation, depending on the quality of interpersonal relationships and team cohesion (Eys et al., 2019). Sports requiring high levels of coordination and communication, such as basketball, volleyball, and soccer, provide opportunities for social connection and collective efficacy experiences that can enhance individual emotional well-being through shared achievement and mutual support systems. However, these same sports can also generate significant interpersonal stress when team dynamics are dysfunctional or when individual performance anxieties are compounded by concerns about letting down teammates. The emotional outcomes of team sport participation are therefore heavily dependent on the social and psychological climate created by coaches, team leaders, and organizational structures.

Exercise intensity represents a critical variable in determining emotional outcomes, with research revealing a complex curvilinear relationship between training intensity and psychological well-being in competitive athletes (Raglin, 2001). Moderate-intensity exercise consistently produces optimal emotional benefits, enhancing mood, reducing anxiety, and promoting feelings of accomplishment and self-efficacy. High-intensity training, while necessary for competitive success, can produce acute psychological stress and negative mood states, particularly when recovery periods are inadequate or when high-intensity sessions are sustained over extended periods without appropriate periodization. The phenomenon of overtraining syndrome exemplifies the negative emotional consequences that can result from chronically elevated exercise intensity, with affected athletes experiencing persistent fatigue, mood disturbances, irritability, and decreased motivation that can persist for weeks or months (Kellmann, 2010). Duration factors similarly influence emotional outcomes, with research indicating that training sessions lasting between 45-90 minutes typically produce optimal psychological benefits, while sessions shorter than 30 minutes may be insufficient to generate significant mood improvements, and sessions exceeding two hours may begin to produce diminishing returns or negative emotional consequences.

Social Support, Coaching, and Team Dynamics

The social environment surrounding competitive sport participation serves as a fundamental determinant of emotional well-being outcomes, with research consistently demonstrating that supportive relationships and positive team dynamics can buffer against the negative psychological effects of competitive stress while amplifying the mood-enhancing benefits of exercise participation (Freeman et al., 2011). Social support within competitive sport contexts operates through multiple mechanisms, including emotional support from teammates and coaches, informational support regarding technique and strategy development, and tangible support through shared resources and assistance with training logistics. The quality and availability of these support systems significantly influence how athletes interpret and respond to competitive challenges, with well-supported athletes showing greater resilience in the face of setbacks and more stable emotional functioning throughout training and competition cycles.

Coaching behaviors and leadership styles represent particularly influential factors in determining the emotional outcomes of competitive sport participation, with research revealing substantial differences in athlete psychological well-being based on coaching approaches (Smith et al., 2007). Coaches who employ autonomy-supportive leadership styles, characterized by encouragement of athlete input, explanation of training rationales, and recognition of individual perspectives, consistently produce better emotional outcomes in their athletes compared to coaches using controlling or authoritarian approaches. Athletes working with supportive coaches report higher levels of intrinsic motivation, greater enjoyment of training and competition, reduced anxiety levels, and more positive self-concept development. Conversely, coaches who rely heavily on punishment, criticism, and external pressure tactics often inadvertently undermine the psychological benefits of exercise participation, creating environments where athletic achievement comes at the expense of emotional well-being and long-term psychological health.

Team dynamics and peer relationships within competitive sport settings create complex social ecosystems that can profoundly influence individual emotional experiences and outcomes (Jowett & Chaundy, 2004). Positive team dynamics characterized by mutual respect, shared goals, open communication, and collective problem-solving create psychological safety that allows athletes to take performance risks, express vulnerabilities, and seek help when needed. These supportive team environments enhance the stress-buffering effects of exercise participation and provide additional sources of meaning and identity beyond individual achievement. However, dysfunctional team dynamics involving conflict, exclusion, bullying, or excessive competitiveness can transform the sport environment into a source of chronic stress that undermines both performance and emotional well-being. The impact of negative team dynamics can be particularly pronounced for athletes who are highly invested in their sport identity or who lack strong support systems outside of their athletic environment.

The broader organizational culture within competitive sport programs also influences emotional outcomes through policies, practices, and implicit messages about the relative importance of performance versus athlete welfare (Stirling & Kerr, 2013). Programs that prioritize holistic athlete development and maintain clear boundaries around appropriate behavior create environments where the psychological benefits of exercise can flourish, while programs that tolerate or encourage win-at-all-costs mentalities often compromise athlete emotional well-being in pursuit of competitive success. The integration of mental health resources, educational programming about emotional wellness, and proactive monitoring of athletes psychological states within sport programs represents an emerging best practice for optimizing both performance and emotional outcomes in competitive athletics.

APPLICATIONS OF EXERCISE AND EMOTIONAL WELL-BEING IN COMPETITIVE SPORTS

Training Strategies for Enhancing Emotional Well-being

Effective training strategies for enhancing emotional well-being in competitive sports environments require a multifaceted approach that systematically integrates emotional regulation techniques with traditional physical conditioning protocols. Research demonstrates that athletes who participate in structured emotional well-being training programs exhibit significantly improved stress tolerance, reduced performance anxiety, and enhanced competitive confidence compared to control groups receiving standard physical training alone (Smith et al., 2007). These programs typically incorporate progressive muscle relaxation techniques, cognitive restructuring exercises, and mindfulness-based stress reduction practices alongside conventional strength and conditioning routines. The implementation of such strategies begins with comprehensive assessment protocols that evaluate individual athletes' emotional profiles, stress response patterns, and coping mechanisms to develop personalized intervention strategies that address specific psychological vulnerabilities while building upon existing strengths.

Contemporary training methodologies emphasize creating emotionally supportive environments where athletes feel psychologically safe to express vulnerabilities and develop authentic relationships with coaches and teammates. Training programs incorporating team-building exercises, open communication protocols, and collaborative goal-setting activities produce substantial improvements in team cohesion, individual emotional regulation, and competitive performance, recognizing that emotional well-being emerges from complex interactions between personal psychological resources and environmental factors. The periodization of emotional well-being training has become critical in modern athletic preparation, with high-intensity psychological skills training being most effective during off-season periods while maintenance-focused interventions prove more beneficial during competitive seasons. Successful training strategies increasingly incorporate technology-assisted interventions, including biofeedback systems, mobile applications for mood monitoring, and virtual reality environments for stress inoculation training, providing athletes with accessible tools for continuous emotional skill development.

Psychological Skills Training (PST) and Integration with Exercise

Psychological Skills Training represents a systematic approach to developing mental capabilities that enhance both performance and emotional well-being in competitive sports contexts. Contemporary PST programs integrate classical psychological interventions with exercise-based approaches, creating synergistic effects that amplify the benefits of both modalities, with athletes participating in integrated programs demonstrating superior emotional regulation, enhanced focus, and improved stress management compared to those receiving either psychological training or physical exercise interventions in isolation. The foundation of effective PST integration lies in understanding how specific types of exercise influence psychological states, with aerobic exercise consistently reducing anxiety and improving mood through neurochemical mechanisms, resistance training contributing to improved self-efficacy and emotional regulation through mastery experiences, and high-intensity interval training developing stress tolerance by creating controlled stress exposure for practicing psychological coping strategies. Advanced PST integration strategies emphasize contextual learning, where psychological skills are developed within sport-specific physical activities rather than abstract clinical settings, as athletes who practiced visualization techniques during sport-specific movements showed greater transfer of psychological skills to competitive situations compared to those practicing in sedentary conditions.

Role of Recovery, Mindfulness, and Yoga in Sports Settings

The recognition of recovery as an active process requiring specific psychological and physical interventions has revolutionized approaches to maintaining emotional well-being in competitive sports. Contemporary research demonstrates that structured recovery protocols incorporating mindfulness practices and yoga significantly enhance both physiological restoration and psychological resilience, with longitudinal studies showing that athletes engaging in regular mindfulness-based recovery practices exhibit reduced cortisol levels, improved sleep quality, and enhanced emotional regulation compared to those using passive recovery methods alone. Mindfulness practices have evolved from simple meditation techniques to comprehensive training systems that integrate present-moment awareness with sport-specific applications, enhancing athletes' ability to maintain optimal arousal levels, manage competitive anxiety, and recover more effectively from performance setbacks through progressive techniques including mindful movement, competitive situation awareness, and post-performance reflection protocols. Yoga practices have gained substantial recognition as comprehensive interventions that simultaneously address physical flexibility, strength, and emotional regulation, with regular practice among competitive athletes resulting in significant improvements in stress management, emotional stability, and overall psychological well-being while enhancing physical performance markers including balance, flexibility, and injury prevention. The implementation of these practices in team sport settings requires careful consideration of individual differences and cultural factors, with successful programs offering multiple modalities that allow athletes to select practices aligning with their personal preferences while ensuring all participants develop fundamental skills in stress management and emotional regulation.

CHALLENGES AND CONSIDERATIONS

Overtraining and Mental Health Risks

One of the most significant challenges in competitive sports is the phenomenon of overtraining and its profound impact on athletes' mental health and emotional well-being. Overtraining syndrome represents a complex physiological and psychological condition that occurs when athletes exceed their capacity for recovery, leading to decreased performance despite maintained or increased training loads (Meeusen, 2013). This condition extends beyond mere physical fatigue, encompassing a constellation of psychological symptoms that can severely compromise an athlete's emotional stability and overall mental health. Research has consistently demonstrated that overtraining is associated with increased rates of depression, anxiety, irritability, and mood disturbances, creating a paradoxical situation where the very activity intended to promote well-being becomes a source of psychological distress (Armstrong & VanHeest, 2002).

The relationship between overtraining and mental health is bidirectional and self-perpetuating, as psychological stress can contribute to the development of overtraining syndrome while simultaneously being a consequence of it. Athletes experiencing overtraining often report feelings of chronic fatigue, decreased motivation, sleep disturbances, and altered appetite patterns, all of which can significantly impact their emotional regulation and psychological resilience (Kellmann, 2010). Furthermore, the competitive environment often rewards and even demands pushing through physical and mental barriers, creating a culture where early warning signs of overtraining may be ignored or dismissed as weakness. This cultural dynamic is particularly problematic because it can delay recognition and intervention, allowing overtraining syndrome to progress to more severe stages where recovery becomes increasingly difficult and prolonged. The pressure to maintain performance standards while dealing with the psychological consequences of overtraining creates additional stress layers that can exacerbate existing mental health vulnerabilities and potentially trigger more serious psychological conditions, such as clinical depression or anxiety disorders (Gould & Whitley, 2009).

Cultural and Contextual Variations

The relationship between exercise, competition, and emotional well-being is significantly influenced by cultural and contextual factors that vary dramatically across different societies, sports traditions, and competitive environments. Cultural attitudes toward mental health, emotional expression, and help-seeking behaviors profoundly shape how athletes experience and manage their psychological well-being within competitive contexts (Schinke et al., 2018). In some cultures, emotional vulnerability or admissions of psychological distress may be viewed as signs of weakness or failure, creating barriers to appropriate mental health support and intervention. These cultural stigmas can prevent athletes from seeking necessary psychological assistance, leading to prolonged suffering and potentially more severe mental health consequences.

Contextual variations also extend to the structural and systemic differences in how competitive sports are organized and supported across different countries and regions. The availability of mental health resources, the integration of psychological support within athletic programs, and the overall approach to athlete welfare vary significantly between nations and sporting organizations (Henriksen et al., 2020). Some competitive environments prioritize holistic athlete development that includes psychological well-being as a central component, while others maintain a more traditional focus on performance outcomes with minimal attention to emotional health considerations. These systemic differences create disparities in athlete experiences and outcomes, with some competitors having access to comprehensive support systems while others must navigate the psychological challenges of competitive sports with limited resources or understanding.

Additionally, cultural variations in training methodologies, coaching philosophies, and competitive expectations create different psychological pressures and demands for athletes. The concept of "mental toughness" and its interpretation vary significantly across cultures, with some emphasizing emotional suppression and others promoting emotional awareness and regulation (Gucciardi et al., 2015). These cultural frameworks influence how athletes develop coping strategies, process competitive stress, and maintain emotional well-being throughout their athletic careers, highlighting the need for culturally sensitive approaches to mental health support in competitive sports.

Ethical Aspects of Athlete Well-being Management

The ethical dimensions of managing athlete well-being in competitive sports present complex moral considerations that challenge traditional approaches to athletic development and performance optimization. Central to these ethical concerns is the fundamental question of how to balance the pursuit of competitive excellence with the moral obligation to protect and promote athlete welfare, particularly when these objectives may appear to conflict (Simon et al., 2018). The inherent power dynamics within competitive sports, where coaches, administrators, and other authority figures hold significant influence over athletes' careers and opportunities, create ethical challenges regarding consent, autonomy, and the potential for exploitation or coercion in matters related to psychological well-being and mental health treatment.

One of the most pressing ethical considerations involves the boundaries and responsibilities of various stakeholders in athlete care, including coaches, sports psychologists, medical professionals, and organizational administrators. The question of who has the authority and responsibility to make decisions regarding an athlete's psychological treatment, competition participation, and overall well-being management becomes particularly complex when these decisions may impact competitive opportunities, scholarship status, or career progression. The potential conflicts of interest between organizational goals focused on performance outcomes and individual athlete needs for psychological support and protection create ethical dilemmas that require careful navigation and clear policy frameworks.

Furthermore, the issue of informed consent becomes particularly complex in the context of competitive sports, where athletes may feel pressure to agree to certain treatments or interventions despite potential risks or personal reservations. The competitive environment can create conditions where athletes feel they cannot refuse or question recommended psychological interventions without facing negative consequences for their athletic careers (T. Beauchamp & Childress, 2019). These dynamic raises important questions about the voluntariness of consent and the need for robust protections to ensure that athletes' rights and autonomy are respected in all aspects of well-being management.

The ethical considerations extend to issues of privacy and confidentiality in psychological care, particularly when information about an athlete's mental health status may impact team selection, competitive opportunities, or public perception. Balancing the need for appropriate communication between support staff while maintaining athlete privacy rights requires careful consideration of ethical principles and legal requirements. Additionally, the long-term consequences of competitive sports participation on athlete well-being raise ethical questions about the responsibilities of sporting organizations to provide ongoing support and care even after an athlete's competitive career has ended, recognizing that the psychological impacts of competitive sports may extend far beyond the period of active participation (Prinz et al., 2016).

FUTURE DIRECTIONS

Emerging Research Trends (Technology, AI-Based Monitoring, Mental Health Apps)

The intersection of exercise science, technology, and psychological well-being in competitive sports presents unprecedented opportunities for advancing our understanding of athlete mental health and performance optimization. As we move forward into the next decade, several emerging research trends are reshaping how we conceptualize, measure, and intervene in the complex relationship between physical activity and emotional well-being among competitive athletes. The integration of sophisticated technological solutions, artificial intelligence applications, and digital mental health interventions represents a paradigm shift that promises to revolutionize both research methodologies and practical applications in sports psychology and exercise science.

The proliferation of wearable technology and biometric monitoring systems has opened new avenues for real-time assessment of physiological and psychological states during training and competition. Advanced heart rate variability monitors, cortisol sensors, and sleep tracking devices now provide continuous data streams that allow researchers and practitioners to examine the dynamic interplay between physical exertion and emotional responses with unprecedented granularity. These technological advances enable the collection of ecological momentary assessments that capture the authentic experiences of athletes in their natural training and competitive environments, moving beyond the limitations of traditional laboratory-based studies. Furthermore, the development of non-invasive neuroimaging techniques, including portable EEG systems and functional near-infrared spectroscopy devices, is making it possible to investigate brain activity patterns associated with exercise-induced mood changes during actual athletic activities rather than simulated conditions (Martín-Rodríguez et al., 2024).

Artificial intelligence and machine learning algorithms are increasingly being employed to analyze vast datasets generated by monitoring technologies, revealing patterns and relationships that might otherwise remain hidden. Predictive models utilizing AI can now identify athletes at risk for burnout, depression, or anxiety based on subtle changes in their physiological markers, training behaviors, and self-reported emotional states, detecting early warning signs of mental health deterioration before symptoms become clinically apparent and enabling proactive interventions that may prevent more serious psychological complications. Machine learning approaches are also being used to personalize training regimens and recovery protocols based on individual athletes' unique physiological and psychological profiles, optimizing both performance outcomes and emotional well-being simultaneously. The emergence of digital mental health applications specifically designed for athletes represents another significant trend, combining evidence-based psychological interventions such as cognitive-behavioral therapy and mindfulness training with sport-specific content and real-time monitoring capabilities. Virtual reality applications are being developed to provide immersive environments for mental skills training, allowing athletes to practice coping strategies and emotional regulation techniques in simulated high-pressure competitive scenarios, while peer support networks facilitated through digital platforms create new opportunities for athletes to connect with others facing similar challenges, potentially reducing the isolation and stigma often associated with mental health struggles in competitive sports environments.

Implications for Coaches, Trainers, and Sports Psychologists

The implications of these emerging trends for coaches, trainers, and sports psychologists are profound and multifaceted. Coaching education programs will need to incorporate training on technology-enhanced monitoring systems and interpretation of complex physiological and psychological data, with coaches increasingly expected to integrate mental health awareness and basic psychological support skills into daily practice, requiring a fundamental shift from traditional coaching philosophies that focused primarily on physical performance metrics. The role of sports psychologists is evolving from primarily providing crisis intervention and performance enhancement to serving as consultants who help integrate psychological principles into comprehensive athlete development programs, utilizing technological tools for continuous monitoring and intervention. Training protocols for sports medicine professionals will need to emphasize the bidirectional relationship between physical and mental health, ensuring practitioners can address both domains simultaneously rather than treating them as separate entities, while the development of interdisciplinary teams, including exercise physiologists, sports psychologists, data scientists, and technology specialists, becomes increasingly common as athlete care complexity grows. This technological evolution demands that professionals develop new competencies in data interpretation, digital literacy, and technology-assisted intervention delivery, with the future of sports psychology lying in seamless integration of human expertise with advanced technological capabilities to create more effective, personalized, and comprehensive approaches to supporting athlete mental health and performance optimization.

CONCLUSION

The extensive body of research examining exercise and emotional well-being in competitive sports reveals a complex relationship that extends beyond the simple assumption that physical activity universally promotes psychological health. While numerous studies demonstrate exercise's potential to enhance mood, reduce anxiety and depression symptoms, and improve overall psychological well-being among athletes, the evidence highlights significant individual variability and the critical importance of contextual factors. The competitive nature of sport introduces unique stressors that can moderate or reverse the typically positive relationship between physical activity and mental health. Key findings consistently demonstrate that the dose-response relationship follows a curvilinear pattern, with moderate physical activity levels associated with optimal psychological outcomes, while both insufficient and excessive training loads lead to negative mental health consequences. The phenomenon of overtraining syndrome exemplifies this relationship, as athletes exceeding recovery capacity often experience depression, anxiety, irritability, and decreased motivation, mirroring clinical mood disorders. Research also reveals significant variations in athlete responses based on gender, age, sport type, competitive level, and personality characteristics, with female athletes particularly susceptible to body image concerns and eating disorders that complicate exercise's typically positive effects.

Based on a comprehensive literature review, several key recommendations emerge for competitive sports stakeholders. Athletes should be educated about the bidirectional relationship between physical training and mental health, learning to recognize early warning signs of psychological distress and understanding when to seek professional support. Self-monitoring skills and emotional awareness should be integrated into athletic training programs, with regular mental health screenings becoming standard practice alongside routine physical examinations. For coaches and training staff, comprehensive education about athlete mental health and the psychological impacts of training decisions is essential, with coaching certification programs including substantial mental health content and protocols for professional referrals. Sports organizations and governing bodies must create policies prioritizing athlete well-being, implementing comprehensive mental health support systems, providing educational resources, and establishing clear crisis management guidelines. The integration of mental health professionals into sports medicine teams should be recognized as essential comprehensive athlete care, ensuring that competitive sports environments support both performance development and psychological well-being through evidence-based, individualized approaches that acknowledge the complex relationship between exercise and emotional health in athletic populations.

REFERENCES

Armstrong, L. E., & VanHeest, J. L. (2002). The Unknown Mechanism of the Overtraining Syndrome: Clues from Depression and Psychoneuroimmunology. *Sports Medicine (Auckland, N.Z.), 32*(3), 185–209. DOI: 10.2165/00007256-200232030-00003 PMID: 11839081

Bartholomew, K. J., Ntoumanis, N., Ryan, R. M., Bosch, J. A., & Thøgersen-Ntoumani, C. (2011). Self-Determination Theory and Diminished Functioning: The Role of Interpersonal Control and Psychological Need Thwarting. *Personality and Social Psychology Bulletin, 37*(11), 1459–1473. DOI: 10.1177/0146167211413125 PMID: 21700794

Beauchamp, M. R., Bray, S. R., Eys, M. A., & Carron, A. V. (2003). The Effect of Role Ambiguity on Competitive State Anxiety. *Journal of Sport & Exercise Psychology, 25*(1), 77–92. DOI: 10.1123/jsep.25.1.77

Beauchamp, T., & Childress, J. (2019). Principles of Biomedical Ethics</i>: Marking Its Fortieth Anniversary. *The American Journal of Bioethics, 19*(11), 9–12. DOI: 10.1080/15265161.2019.1665402 PMID: 31647760

Beserra, A. H. N., Kameda, P., Deslandes, A. C., Schuch, F. B., Laks, J., & Moraes, H. S. D. (2018). Can physical exercise modulate cortisol level in subjects with depression? A systematic review and meta-analysis. *Trends in Psychiatry and Psychotherapy, 40*(4), 360–368. DOI: 10.1590/2237-6089-2017-0155 PMID: 30570106

Biddle, S. J. H., & Batterham, A. M. (2015). High-intensity interval exercise training for public health: A big HIT or shall we HIT it on the head? *The International Journal of Behavioral Nutrition and Physical Activity, 12*(1), 95. DOI: 10.1186/s12966-015-0254-9 PMID: 26187579

Bompa, T. O., & Buzzichelli, C. A. (2019). *Periodization: Theory and Methodology of Training* (1st ed.). Human Kinetics., DOI: 10.5040/9781718225435

Crocker, J., & Park, L. E. (2004). The Costly Pursuit of Self-Esteem. *Psychological Bulletin, 130*(3), 392–414. DOI: 10.1037/0033-2909.130.3.392 PMID: 15122925

Deci, E. L., & Ryan, R. M. (2000). The "What" and "Why" of Goal Pursuits: Human Needs and the Self-Determination of Behavior. *Psychological Inquiry, 11*(4), 227–268. DOI: 10.1207/S15327965PLI1104_01

Ekeland, E., Heian, F., & Hagen, K. B. (2005). Can exercise improve self esteem in children and young people? A systematic review of randomised controlled trials. *British Journal of Sports Medicine, 39*(11), 792–798. DOI: 10.1136/bjsm.2004.017707 PMID: 16244186

Engel, G. L. (1977). The Need for a New Medical Model: A Challenge for Biomedicine. *Science, 196*(4286), 129–136. DOI: 10.1126/science.847460 PMID: 847460

Erickson, K. I., Hillman, C. H., & Kramer, A. F. (2015). Physical activity, brain, and cognition. *Current Opinion in Behavioral Sciences, 4*, 27–32. DOI: 10.1016/j.cobeha.2015.01.005

Eys, M., Bruner, M. W., & Martin, L. J. (2019). The dynamic group environment in sport and exercise. *Psychology of Sport and Exercise, 42*, 40–47. DOI: 10.1016/j.psychsport.2018.11.001

Fletcher, D., & Sarkar, M. (2012). A grounded theory of psychological resilience in Olympic champions. *Psychology of Sport and Exercise, 13*(5), 669–678. DOI: 10.1016/j.psychsport.2012.04.007

Foley, T. E., & Fleshner, M. (2008). Neuroplasticity of Dopamine Circuits After Exercise: Implications for Central Fatigue. *Neuromolecular Medicine, 10*(2), 67–80. DOI: 10.1007/s12017-008-8032-3 PMID: 18274707

Freeman, P., Coffee, P., & Rees, T. (2011). The PASS-Q: The Perceived Available Support in Sport Questionnaire. *Journal of Sport & Exercise Psychology, 33*(1), 54–74. DOI: 10.1123/jsep.33.1.54 PMID: 21451171

Gould, D., & Maynard, I. (2009). Psychological preparation for the Olympic Games. *Journal of Sports Sciences, 27*(13), 1393–1408. DOI: 10.1080/02640410903081845 PMID: 19787542

Gould, D., & Whitley, M. A. (2009). Sources and consequences of athletic burnout among college athletes. *Journal of Intercollegiate Sport, 2*(1), 16–30.

Gucciardi, D. F., Hanton, S., Gordon, S., Mallett, C. J., & Temby, P. (2015). The Concept of Mental Toughness: Tests of Dimensionality, Nomological Network, and Traitness. *Journal of Personality, 83*(1), 26–44. DOI: 10.1111/jopy.12079 PMID: 24428736

Gustafsson, H., DeFreese, J., & Madigan, D. J. (2017). Athlete burnout: Review and recommendations. *Current Opinion in Psychology, 16*, 109–113. DOI: 10.1016/j.copsyc.2017.05.002 PMID: 28813331

Heijnen, S., Hommel, B., Kibele, A., & Colzato, L. S. (2016). Neuromodulation of Aerobic Exercise—A Review. *Frontiers in Psychology, 6*. Advance online publication. DOI: 10.3389/fpsyg.2015.01890 PMID: 26779053

Henriksen, K., Schinke, R., Moesch, K., McCann, S., Parham, W. D., Larsen, C. H., & Terry, P. (2020). Consensus statement on improving the mental health of high performance athletes. *International Journal of Sport and Exercise Psychology, 18*(5), 553–560. DOI: 10.1080/1612197X.2019.1570473

Jowett, S., & Chaundy, V. (2004). An Investigation Into the Impact of Coach Leadership and Coach-Athlete Relationship on Group Cohesion. *Group Dynamics, 8*(4), 302–311. DOI: 10.1037/1089-2699.8.4.302

Kandola, A., Ashdown-Franks, G., Hendrikse, J., Sabiston, C. M., & Stubbs, B. (2019). Physical activity and depression: Towards understanding the antidepressant mechanisms of physical activity. *Neuroscience and Biobehavioral Reviews, 107*, 525–539. DOI: 10.1016/j.neubiorev.2019.09.040 PMID: 31586447

Kellmann, M. (2010). Preventing overtraining in athletes in high-intensity sports and stress/recovery monitoring. *Scandinavian Journal of Medicine & Science in Sports, 20*(s2), 95–102. DOI: 10.1111/j.1600-0838.2010.01192.x PMID: 20840567

Kellmann, M., Bertollo, M., Bosquet, L., Brink, M., Coutts, A. J., Duffield, R., Erlacher, D., Halson, S. L., Hecksteden, A., & Heidari, J. (2018). Recovery and performance in sport: Consensus statement. *International Journal of Sports Physiology and Performance, 13*(2), 240–245. PMID: 29345524

Kenttä, G., & Hassmén, P. (1998). Overtraining and Recovery: A Conceptual Model. *Sports Medicine (Auckland, N.Z.), 26*(1), 1–16. DOI: 10.2165/00007256-199826010-00001 PMID: 9739537

Lazarus, R. S. (2000). How Emotions Influence Performance in Competitive Sports. *The Sport Psychologist, 14*(3), 229–252. DOI: 10.1123/tsp.14.3.229

Lundqvist, C. (2011). Well-being in competitive sports—The feel-good factor? A review of conceptual considerations of well-being. *International Review of Sport and Exercise Psychology, 4*(2), 109–127. DOI: 10.1080/1750984X.2011.584067

Mallett, C. J., & Hanrahan, S. J. (2004). Elite athletes: Why does the 'fire' burn so brightly? *Psychology of Sport and Exercise, 5*(2), 183–200. DOI: 10.1016/S1469-0292(02)00043-2

Mandolesi, L., Polverino, A., Montuori, S., Foti, F., Ferraioli, G., Sorrentino, P., & Sorrentino, G. (2018). Effects of Physical Exercise on Cognitive Functioning and Wellbeing: Biological and Psychological Benefits. *Frontiers in Psychology*, *9*, 509. DOI: 10.3389/fpsyg.2018.00509 PMID: 29755380

Martín-Rodríguez, A., Gostian-Ropotin, L. A., Beltrán-Velasco, A. I., Belando-Pedreño, N., Simón, J. A., López-Mora, C., Navarro-Jiménez, E., Tornero-Aguilera, J. F., & Clemente-Suárez, V. J. (2024). Sporting Mind: The Interplay of Physical Activity and Psychological Health. *Sports (Basel, Switzerland)*, *12*(1), 37. DOI: 10.3390/sports12010037 PMID: 38275986

Meeusen, R. (2013). Prevention, Diagnosis, and Treatment of the Overtraining Syndrome: Joint Consensus Statement of the European College of Sport Science and the American College of Sports Medicine. *Medicine and Science in Sports and Exercise*, *45*(1), 186–205. DOI: 10.1249/MSS.0b013e318279a10a PMID: 23247672

Ntoumanis, N., Edmunds, J., & Duda, J. L. (2009). Understanding the coping process from a self-determination theory perspective. *British Journal of Health Psychology*, *14*(2), 249–260. DOI: 10.1348/135910708X349352 PMID: 18789187

Park, I., & Jeon, J. (2023). Psychological Skills Training for Athletes in Sports: Web of Science Bibliometric Analysis. *Health Care*, *11*(2), 259. DOI: 10.3390/healthcare11020259 PMID: 36673627

Penedo, F. J., & Dahn, J. R. (2005). Exercise and well-being: A review of mental and physical health benefits associated with physical activity. *Current Opinion in Psychiatry*, *18*(2), 189–193. DOI: 10.1097/00001504-200503000-00013 PMID: 16639173

Prinz, B., Dvořák, J., & Junge, A. (2016). Symptoms and risk factors of depression during and after the football career of elite female players. *BMJ Open Sport & Exercise Medicine*, *2*(1), e000124. DOI: 10.1136/bmjsem-2016-000124 PMID: 27900184

Raglin, J. S. (2001). Psychological Factors in Sport Performance: The Mental Health Model Revisited. *Sports Medicine (Auckland, N.Z.)*, *31*(12), 875–890. DOI: 10.2165/00007256-200131120-00004 PMID: 11665914

Reardon, C. L., & Factor, R. M. (2010). Sport Psychiatry: A Systematic Review of Diagnosis and Medical Treatment of Mental Illness in Athletes. *Sports Medicine (Auckland, N.Z.)*, *40*(11), 961–980. DOI: 10.2165/11536580-000000000-00000 PMID: 20942511

Reardon, C. L., Hainline, B., Aron, C. M., Baron, D., Baum, A. L., Bindra, A., Budgett, R., Campriani, N., Castaldelli-Maia, J. M., Currie, A., Derevensky, J. L., Glick, I. D., Gorczynski, P., Gouttebarge, V., Grandner, M. A., Han, D. H., McDuff, D., Mountjoy, M., Polat, A., & Engebretsen, L. (2019). Mental health in elite athletes: International Olympic Committee consensus statement (2019). *British Journal of Sports Medicine, 53*(11), 667–699. DOI: 10.1136/bjsports-2019-100715 PMID: 31097450

Rice, S. M., Purcell, R., De Silva, S., Mawren, D., McGorry, P. D., & Parker, A. G. (2016). The Mental Health of Elite Athletes: A Narrative Systematic Review. *Sports Medicine (Auckland, N.Z.), 46*(9), 1333–1353. DOI: 10.1007/s40279-016-0492-2 PMID: 26896951

Rosenbaum, S., Tiedemann, A., Sherrington, C., Curtis, J., & Ward, P. B. (2014). Physical Activity Interventions for People With Mental Illness: A Systematic Review and Meta-Analysis. *The Journal of Clinical Psychiatry, 75*(09), 964–974. DOI: 10.4088/JCP.13r08765 PMID: 24813261

Ryan, R. M., & Deci, E. L. (Eds.). (2017). *Self-Determination Theory: Basic Psychological Needs in Motivation, Development, and Wellness*. Guilford Press., DOI: 10.1521/978.14625/28806

Sabiston, C. M., Jewett, R., Ashdown-Franks, G., Belanger, M., Brunet, J., O'Loughlin, E., & O'Loughlin, J. (2016). Number of Years of Team and Individual Sport Participation During Adolescence and Depressive Symptoms in Early Adulthood. *Journal of Sport & Exercise Psychology, 38*(1), 105–110. DOI: 10.1123/jsep.2015-0175 PMID: 27018562

Schaal, K., Tafflet, M., Nassif, H., Thibault, V., Pichard, C., Alcotte, M., Guillet, T., El Helou, N., Berthelot, G., Simon, S., & Toussaint, J.-F. (2011). Psychological Balance in High Level Athletes: Gender-Based Differences and Sport-Specific Patterns. *PLoS One, 6*(5), e19007. DOI: 10.1371/journal.pone.0019007 PMID: 21573222

Schinke, R. J., Stambulova, N. B., Si, G., & Moore, Z. (2018). International society of sport psychology position stand: Athletes' mental health, performance, and development. *International Journal of Sport and Exercise Psychology, 16*(6), 622–639. DOI: 10.1080/1612197X.2017.1295557

Schuch, F. B., Vancampfort, D., Firth, J., Rosenbaum, S., Ward, P. B., Silva, E. S., Hallgren, M., Ponce De Leon, A., Dunn, A. L., Deslandes, A. C., Fleck, M. P., Carvalho, A. F., & Stubbs, B. (2018). Physical Activity and Incident Depression: A Meta-Analysis of Prospective Cohort Studies. *The American Journal of Psychiatry, 175*(7), 631–648. DOI: 10.1176/appi.ajp.2018.17111194 PMID: 29690792

Simon, R. L., Torres, C. R., & Hager, P. F. (2018). *Fair Play: The Ethics of Sport* (4th ed.). Routledge., DOI: 10.4324/9780429492570

Smith, R. E., Smoll, F. L., & Cumming, S. P. (2007). Effects of a Motivational Climate Intervention for Coaches on Young Athletes' Sport Performance Anxiety. *Journal of Sport & Exercise Psychology*, *29*(1), 39–59. DOI: 10.1123/jsep.29.1.39 PMID: 17556775

Stirling, A. E., & Kerr, G. A. (2013). The perceived effects of elite athletes' experiences of emotional abuse in the coach–athlete relationship. *International Journal of Sport and Exercise Psychology*, *11*(1), 87–100. DOI: 10.1080/1612197X.2013.752173

Stubbs, B., Vancampfort, D., Rosenbaum, S., Firth, J., Cosco, T., Veronese, N., Salum, G. A., & Schuch, F. B. (2017). An examination of the anxiolytic effects of exercise for people with anxiety and stress-related disorders: A meta-analysis. *Psychiatry Research*, *249*, 102–108. DOI: 10.1016/j.psychres.2016.12.020 PMID: 28088704

Young, B. W., & Medic, N. (2011). Examining social influences on the sport commitment of Masters swimmers. *Psychology of Sport and Exercise*, *12*(2), 168–175. DOI: 10.1016/j.psychsport.2010.09.004

Chapter 14

Embodied Healing: Mindfulness, Movement, and Dance Approaches for Emotion Regulation Among Persons With Depression

Marie Grace Avelino Gomez
https://orcid.org/0000-0003-0180-9875
University of the Philippines, Philippines

Ervin T. Echague
https://orcid.org/0009-0002-7507-1383
Department of Education, Philippines

ABSTRACT

Depression and anxiety are among the most widespread mental health challenges globally, impairing functioning, relationships, and overall well-being. While psychotherapy and pharmacological treatments remain central, they are not wholly sufficient in addressing the lived experiences of those affected. This chapter explores the therapeutic potential of mindfulness, movement, and dance as embodied practices that integrate cognitive awareness with physical expression. Drawing from empirical literature and practical applications, it highlights their role in emotional regulation, resilience, and holistic healing. By situating these practices alongside mainstream psychotherapies, the chapter underscores their promise as complementary strategies in alleviating symptoms of depression and anxiety.

DOI: 10.4018/979-8-3373-6157-4.ch014

INTRODUCTION

Depression and anxiety remain two of the most prevalent mental health challenges worldwide (Javaid et al., 2023). According to the World Health Organization (2023), over 280 million people suffer from depression, while anxiety disorders affect more than 300 million globally. These conditions often coexist, impairing daily functioning, academic performance, and interpersonal relationships (Limone & Toto, 2022). Conventional treatments, such as pharmacological interventions and talk therapies, have proven effective for many, but they are not universally accessible nor wholly sufficient (Gregg, 2024). Increasingly, attention is being directed toward holistic and embodied practices that integrate the mind and body as co-contributors to healing (Kandola et al., 2021).

Over the past decade, depression and anxiety have emerged as two of the most pervasive mental health conditions worldwide, affecting millions across diverse cultures, socioeconomic groups, and age brackets. The World Health Organization has repeatedly emphasized that depression is now one of the leading causes of disability globally, while anxiety disorders contribute significantly to compromised productivity, strained social relationships, and diminished quality of life. The rise in symptoms such as persistent sadness, hopelessness, worry, agitation, and psychosomatic complaints underscores the urgency of developing mental health approaches that move beyond traditional modalities. Conventional psychotherapy and pharmacological interventions, while invaluable, often prove insufficient in fully addressing the lived experiences of those grappling with these conditions. This reality has spurred growing interest in holistic, embodied practices that situate healing not only in the mind but also in the body.

The global rise in depression and anxiety is not a matter of overdiagnosis or shifting cultural sensibilities but reflects deeper psychosocial realities. Increasing economic instability, social isolation, climate anxiety, and rapid technological changes have contributed to widespread psychological strain. The COVID-19 pandemic further magnified these issues, leaving behind a trail of trauma, grief, and chronic stress that exacerbated existing vulnerabilities. In law, business, education, and even artistic fields, the pressure to perform at peak levels creates an environment where psychological distress easily takes root. Individuals report experiencing emotional exhaustion, intrusive worry, difficulty concentrating, and disruptions in sleep and appetite. These symptoms are not isolated inconveniences but manifestations of a broader global mental health crisis.

Mindfulness, movement, and dance-based practices stand at the forefront of this shift (Chen et al., 2024). These approaches highlight the body not only as a site of symptoms but as a resource for resilience and self-regulation (Moratelli et al., 2023). By combining cognitive awareness with physical engagement, individuals can cultivate tools for regulating emotions, reducing stress, and fostering psychological flexibility (Al Refae et al., 2021).

Beyond clinical contexts, schools and communities can integrate mindfulness and movement for mental well-being. Programs for students may combine breathing exercises, guided mindful movement, and creative dance as part of physical education or homeroom guidance. Teachers can benefit from embodied mindfulness practices that reduce stress and prevent burnout. Community dance workshops also provide collective spaces where movement fosters connection, joy, and resilience, promoting mental health at a population level.

The rationale for integrating mindfulness and movement is rooted in their shared capacity to bring individuals into the present moment, anchor attention in bodily sensations, and facilitate healthier responses to distress (Barua, 2025). Dance offers an expressive medium through which inner experiences can be externalized and processed. Of course, the target recipients of this kind intervention would be those interested in dance. Without the motivation or skills to dance, intervention would not be effective. This chapter explores these connections, grounded in multiple therapeutic perspectives and practical applications.

Objectives of This Chapter

This chapter has three primary objectives, each responding to the urgent need for innovative strategies in addressing depression and anxiety:

1. *To identify the significance of mindfulness, movement, and dance activities in the literature*

This involves reviewing empirical and theoretical works that highlight the therapeutic benefits of embodied practices. The aim is to situate these interventions within broader mental health discourses, demonstrating their efficacy and potential for mainstream integration.

2. *To relate how mainstream psychotherapy can fortify mindfulness, movement, and dance activities to address symptoms of depression and anxiety*

Here, the chapter will examine synergies between embodied practices and established psychotherapies such as Existentialism, ACT, and DBT, showing how counselors and therapists can adopt integrative approaches.

3. *To illustrate how mindfulness, movement, and dance activities could help relieve symptoms of depression and anxiety*

Finally, the chapter will provide case examples, scenarios, or practical frameworks showing how embodied practices support emotional regulation, resilience, and recovery. These illustrations will bridge theory and practice, offering concrete applications for educators, therapists, and counselors.

The growing prevalence of depression and anxiety calls for reimagined approaches to mental health, approaches that acknowledge the profound interplay between body and mind. Mindfulness, movement, and dance offer more than symptom relief; they provide pathways toward embodied awareness, creative expression, and holistic healing. When integrated with mainstream psychotherapies, these practices enrich the therapeutic landscape, equipping individuals with tools to navigate distress while fostering meaning, resilience, and growth.

This chapter will contribute to the expanding discourse on embodied mental health interventions, demonstrating how ancient practices of mindfulness and movement can be reinterpreted in contemporary contexts to meet pressing global challenges. In doing so, it underscores a simple yet powerful truth: healing is not confined to the intellect but unfolds in the rhythms, movements, and mindful presence of the whole person.

MINDFULNESS DEFINED

Mindfulness is most described as the practice of paying attention, on purpose, in the present moment, and without judgment. While its roots lie in Buddhist contemplative traditions, mindfulness has been adapted for secular use in psychology, medicine, and education (Mehta & Talwar, 2022). Contemporary approaches such as Mindfulness-Based Stress Reduction (MBSR) and Mindfulness-Based Cognitive Therapy (MBCT) have demonstrated efficacy in reducing depression relapse and managing anxiety symptoms. Mindfulness activities are also applied in Existentialism, Dialectic Behavior Therapy (DBT), and Acceptance and Commitment Therapy (ACT).

It is important to distinguish mindfulness from related concepts. Relaxation emphasizes calmness, while meditation often involves specific mental techniques or rituals. Mindfulness, by contrast, is not primarily about achieving tranquility but about cultivating awareness and acceptance of whatever arises (Channawar, 2023).

Embodiment theory asserts that bodily experiences deeply influence cognition and emotion (Odendahl, 2021). Movement, posture, and rhythm affect affective states: slumped shoulders may reinforce sadness, while expansive posture may evoke confidence (Scheer, 2022). Dance amplifies this principle by using structured or improvised movement to externalize emotional states (Basso et al., 2021). Mindful movement practices such as yoga, tai chi, or dance therapy provide opportunities to regulate emotions through embodied expression, enhancing integration between body and mind (Channawar, 2023).

Mindfulness Through Psychological Frameworks

Mindfulness-based approaches in psychology often draw upon the integration of movement and embodied practices to deepen awareness, flexibility, and meaning-making. In this book chapter, ACT, DBT, and Existential Psychology each provide unique yet complementary perspectives on how dance and mindful movement can foster well-being. Together, these frameworks highlight how bodily engagement supports acceptance, emotion regulation, authentic presence, and value-driven living.

For practitioners and individuals who want to record progress, instruments such as the Difficulties in Emotion Regulation Scale, the Beck Depression Inventory, the Beck Anxiety Inventory, and the Depression, Anxiety, and Stress Scale-21 are readily available online. It should be remembered that the persons executing the intervention must be licensed professionals such as those with training in dance, counseling, and psychology. Safety protocols are given by these professionals, depending on the level of severity. For purposes of discussion, the examples given in this book chapter are the basic skills that can be applied.

Acceptance and Commitment Therapy

ACT emphasizes six processes of psychological flexibility: acceptance, cognitive defusion, present-moment awareness, self-as-context, values, and committed action (Webb, 2023). Mindful movement fits naturally within this framework. For example, engaging in dance with awareness of bodily sensations facilitates acceptance of discomfort, while rhythmic movement supports defusion from distressing thoughts (Ma et al., 2022). Dancing in alignment with personal values (e.g., self-expression, health, connection) embodies committed action, reinforcing the ACT model of living meaningfully despite pain (Pass Erickson, 2021).

ACT, combined with Self-Determination Theory enabled their participants to achieve better mental health. The "Running Minds" program, an eight-session intervention combining Self-Determination Theory (SDT) and Acceptance and Commitment Therapy (ACT), was found to increase young adults' intrinsic and extrinsic motivation to engage in physical activity by helping them align exercise with deeply held personal values and by structuring social accountability (e.g. knowing they'd discuss their week in group). Participants reported changes in behaviour: they reframed daily tasks (walking instead of taking transport, choosing stairs over elevators), adopted more regular movement, and experienced that even short bouts of non-strenuous activity (10–20 min outdoors) became rewarding rather than burdensome. The intervention also strengthened self-regulation: participants became more aware of internal resistance (e.g. negative self-talk, discomfort), learned to accept those feelings, and acted in spite of them, which helped sustain their activity over time. Finally, key facilitators of these physical activity improvements were the satisfying group environment (relatedness), the instructor's supportive role, practical convenient logistics, and sessions designed to be rewarding—these helped reduce barriers and made physical activity more appealing and sustainable.

Dialectical Behavior Therapy

DBT incorporates mindfulness as a core skill, alongside distress tolerance, emotion regulation, and interpersonal effectiveness (Heath et al., 2021). Movement and dance can enhance these skills: rhythmic breathing during movement promotes distress tolerance, while expressive dance facilitates emotion regulation by channeling intense affect into bodily expression (Lochrie, 2024). Group dance sessions can foster synchrony, mutual awareness, and interpersonal effectiveness, aligning with DBT's emphasis on relational healing.

Weiss et al.'s (2025) study explored the acceptability and feasibility of integrating Taekwondo-based mindful movement into DBT for adults in an inpatient mood disorders unit. The program involved 24 participants, most of whom were women in their early thirties, who engaged in structured Taekwondo movements designed to be practiced mindfully, synchronizing breath, posture, and ritualized forms. These activities were used as an experiential method for reinforcing DBT skills, particularly mindfulness and distress tolerance. Findings showed that the intervention was both well-received and feasible: participants found the Taekwondo component engaging, appreciated its physical discipline and ritual, and valued how the movements helped them feel grounded during moments of emotional distress. The physical activity element gave participants a tangible way to practice regulating emotions and tolerating discomfort, extending DBT's skillset into embodied practice. Although the pilot was not powered to demonstrate strong statistical effects, preliminary outcomes suggested that Taekwondo mindful movement may enhance emotion regulation, reduce experiential avoidance, and improve overall engagement with therapy. These results indicate that combining Taekwondo with DBT is a promising, innovative approach worth testing in larger, controlled trials (Weiss et al., 2025).

Existentialist Perspective

Existential psychology emphasizes authenticity, freedom, and the search for meaning. From this lens, mindfulness is not only a technique but a way of being but an encounter with existence itself (Stevens, 2025). Movement and dance become existential practices: they express freedom, affirm embodied presence, and confront the temporality of human life (Skinner, 2023). By engaging the body, individuals ground themselves in the present while simultaneously confronting deeper questions of identity, choice, and meaning-making.

From an Asian perspective, Tai Chi shows support for life balance and this is grounded on existentialist thought. Li's (2024) thesis argues for an integrative therapeutic model combining Tai Chi and Dance Movement Therapy (DMT), creating what she calls *Tai Chi-DMT Integrative Movement Therapy*, as a cross-cultural mind-body psychotherapy. She situates Tai Chi in its Chinese philosophical roots—Taoist notions of yin-yang balance, qi flow, wu wei (non-striving/natural effort), harmony with nature—and contrasts it with the Western expressive, existential, and humanistic traditions that undergird DMT, which emphasize personal freedom, emotive expression, authenticity, and meaning-making. Within this blend, Li draws on the *Expressive Therapy Continuum (ETC)* as a framework: starting from sensory/kinesthetic awareness (through Tai Chi's slow, mindful movement), moving into affective/emotional expression (through DMT's improvisation and dance), and culminating in symbolic/cognitive reflection, so that individuals can integrate their embodied and emotional experiences into their sense of self. The model responds to existential concerns, who one is, one's relation to culture, nature, and community by offering a path toward authenticity, groundedness, and inner balance, while also acknowledging that such integration must be sensitive to cultural differences, therapist training, and the need for empirical validation in diverse settings.

Mechanisms of Healing: Why Mindfulness and Movement Work

Multiple mechanisms can explain the effectiveness of mindfulness and movement. Neurobiologically, mindful practices modulate the autonomic nervous system, increasing vagal tone and reducing hyperarousal associated with anxiety (Calderone et al., 2024). Movement and dance stimulate dopamine release, associated with pleasure and motivation, while reducing cortisol levels linked to stress (Lopez-Nieves, & Jakobsche, 2022).

In a high-stress predeployment military context, Stanley et al. (2011) piloted a Mindfulness-Based Mind Fitness Training (MMFT) program for U.S. Marine reservists to investigate whether cultivating mindfulness skills could enhance cognitive capacities, particularly working memory and attentional control, which are often compromised under stress. The program was structured so that participants received group instruction in mindfulness practice, integrated into their military training schedule, with sessions aimed at building capacity to maintain focus, regulate emotions, and keep working memory functioning even during demanding tasks. They compared reservists who got MMFT with control or baseline data and found that those in MMFT showed measurable improvements in working memory capacity (e.g., in remembering and manipulating information) relative to before training; these improvements suggest that mindfulness can be a functional marker of training success under stress. Importantly, these cognitive benefits were most apparent during or after periods of elevated stress, implying that the mindfulness training helps buffer the impact of stress on cognition, protecting attention and memory when they are most challenged (Stanley et al., 2011).

Psychologically, embodied practices expand awareness beyond rumination, shifting attention to present sensations (Fugate et al., 2024). This interrupts maladaptive cognitive cycles associated with depression and anxiety (Palagini et al., 2021). Movement also facilitates emotion regulation by providing safe outlets for expression and integration of difficult feelings (Price & Weng, 2021). Together, these mechanisms build resilience and foster a balanced mind-body relationship.

Applications of Mindfulness, Movement, and Dance Approaches

In clinical settings, mindfulness-based dance therapy has shown promise for individuals with trauma, depression, and anxiety (Stevens, 2025). For example, trauma survivors often struggle with disconnection from their bodies (Cattie et al., 2021). Gentle, mindful movement can help re-establish bodily trust and safety (Eddy & Johnson, 2022). Case studies suggest that structured dance therapy sessions reduce depressive symptoms and increase emotional regulation (Karkou et al., 2019; Hyvönen et al., 2020). Therapists may guide clients through body scans followed by expressive movement, encouraging integration of mindfulness with physical expression.

Zafeiroudi et al. (2025) conducted a scoping review examining the psycho-emotional benefits of dance-based mindful movement interventions in recreational populations. The review synthesized research published between 2010 and 2025 that integrated elements of mindfulness, such as present-moment awareness, non-judgmental attention, and interoceptive awareness into structured movement practices. Findings indicated that mindful movement was associated with enhanced emotional regulation, reductions in stress, and alleviation of psychosomatic symptoms. In addition, participants demonstrated increased self-compassion and acceptance, reflecting a shift toward more adaptive emotional processing and reduced experiential avoidance. Group-based formats also facilitated social connectedness, enabling participants to experience co-regulation and improved interpersonal relationships through shared movement and synchrony. Beyond reducing negative affect, interventions promoted positive well-being outcomes, including vitality, energy, and life satisfaction, underscoring the preventive potential of such approaches. The authors further noted that the embodied nature of mindful movement uniquely engages sensorimotor and affective systems, thereby providing mechanisms of change distinct from traditional cognitive mindfulness practices. While the heterogeneity of interventions and reliance on self-report measures present methodological limitations, the review highlights dance-based mindful movement as a promising strategy for promoting psycho-emotional health in non-clinical populations (Zafeiroudi et al., 2025).

HOLISTIC AND EMBODIED APPROACHES: A PARADIGM SHIFT

Against this backdrop, there has been increasing recognition of the limitations of purely cognitive or pharmacological strategies. While psychotherapies such as CBT or medication can alleviate symptoms, many individuals continue to feel disconnected, restless, or unable to integrate healing into daily life. This recognition has given rise to interest in holistic and embodied approaches, modalities that treat the human being as an integrated system of mind, body, and spirit.

When the COVID-19 pandemic disrupted daily life and increased social isolation, especially among older adults experiencing age-related cognitive changes, a team led by Shim et al. (2024) developed an online Mindful Movement Approach (MMA) to help reduce loneliness, boost psychological well-being, and promote social connectedness. The study is based on two case studies (from a larger group of about 16 older adults aged approximately 50-71) who participated in the MMA during pandemic lockdowns. In the intervention, participants engaged in guided movement practices online that focused on mindfulness, body awareness, and using movement not just as exercise but as a way to improve self-awareness and emotional regulation. Results from these two cases showed that the online MMA helped decrease loneliness while enhancing mood, social connectedness, and self-awareness. Participants reported that their mindfulness practice deepened, and they found new ways to incorporate movement into their daily routines to improve well-being. Although physical movement was part of the program, in these two cases, its effects were more qualitative (such as increased body awareness, emotional regulation, and well-being) than measurable changes like strength or mobility. The findings suggest that such an online mindful movement approach offers a promising alternative during times of limited in-person interaction, especially for older adults with cognitive changes, and merits further research with more participants and more rigorous designs (Shim et al., 2024).

Embodied approaches acknowledge that mental health struggles are not confined to thought patterns or neurochemistry but also manifest in the body: tension, fatigue, shallow breathing, muscle stiffness, and somatic discomfort (Fugate et al., 2024). By engaging the body in the healing process, these approaches cultivate emotional awareness, resilience, and regulation in ways that purely cognitive interventions may not achieve (Bonanno et al., 2023). Mindfulness and movement-based practices, including dance, yoga, and breathwork, offer individuals tools to ground themselves, release pent-up stress, and develop compassionate self-awareness (Johnson Sealey, 2024).

Mindfulness and Single-tasking: Psychological and Performance Benefits

The integration of mindfulness and single-tasking has wide-ranging implications for both psychological well-being and performance in academic, professional, and everyday contexts. By fostering present-moment awareness and resisting the pressures of multitasking, these practices address some of the most pressing challenges of modern life, from stress and burnout to declining attention spans and information overload.

- **Reduces Stress and Anxiety -** Mindfulness is strongly associated with reductions in stress and anxiety, primarily through its capacity to enhance emotional regulation and decrease rumination. By grounding attention in the present moment, individuals become less entangled in worries about the future or regrets about the past. Single-tasking amplifies this benefit by reducing the mental clutter and decision fatigue caused by attempting to juggle multiple activities at once. Together, these practices create a psychological buffer against the chronic stressors of contemporary life.
- **Improves Focus and Cognitive Efficiency -** Cognitive science consistently demonstrates that frequent task-switching impairs concentration and slows mental processing. Research suggests that multitasking can reduce productivity by up to 40% due to the cognitive costs of constantly reorienting attention. Mindful single-tasking counters this inefficiency by channeling attention toward one task at a time, thereby minimizing errors, conserving mental energy, and enabling deeper engagement. This heightened cognitive efficiency is particularly valuable in environments that demand sustained focus, such as academic learning or professional problem-solving. Mindfulness in terms of staying focused with dance and feeling every step had higher self-experience of flow state during performances and expert-rated performance competence (Pandya, 2024)
- **Promotes Flow States -** Flow, often described as a state of complete absorption in an activity, emerges most readily when attention is undivided and fully present. Mindful single-tasking nurtures the conditions for flow by aligning focused attention, clear goals, and immediate feedback. Whether in

creative work, athletic performance, or academic study, this synergy between mindfulness and single-tasking supports experiences of deep immersion, enhanced creativity, and optimal performance.

- **Strengthens Overall Well-Being** - The benefits of mindful single-tasking extend beyond productivity. By reducing stress, conserving energy, and promoting presence, individuals report greater clarity of thought, improved emotional balance, and enhanced resilience in the face of challenges. These outcomes contribute to broader dimensions of well-being, including increased satisfaction with work, healthier interpersonal relationships, and stronger alignment between personal values and daily actions.
- **Counters "Continuous Partial Attention"** - In an age defined by constant digital connectivity, many individuals operate in a state of "continuous partial attention," in which they remain perpetually attuned to multiple streams of information without fully engaging in any of them. This overstimulated state contributes to burnout, shallow thinking, and diminished productivity. Mindful single-tasking provides a corrective to this condition by restoring calm, anchoring attention, and enabling individuals to engage with tasks and relationships more deeply. The result is not only greater effectiveness but also a more sustainable and fulfilling rhythm of life.

Table 1. Summary of practical applications

Aspect	Impact of Mindful Single-Tasking
Attention & Focus	Deeper concentration; fewer switching penalties
Stress & Emotional Health	Reduced stress; improved emotional regulation
Productivity & Quality	Higher accuracy, efficiency, and creative engagement
Relationships & Presence	Stronger connections; more meaningful interactions
Everyday Integration	Applicable in meals, work, study, routines, and conversations

Mindfulness, Relaxation, and Meditation

Although mindfulness is often associated with relaxation or meditation, it is important to distinguish these concepts. Relaxation techniques, such as progressive muscle relaxation or guided imagery, aim to reduce physiological arousal. While mindfulness may lead to relaxation, its ultimate goal is awareness and acceptance, rather than inducing calmness.

Meditation, on the other hand, is a broader term that includes a wide array of practices, from concentration-based exercises to transcendental meditation. Mindfulness meditation is one form of meditation, but not all meditation is mindfulness. For example, mantra repetition, focused prayer, or visualization may foster focus without necessarily cultivating non-judgmental awareness.

In short, mindfulness is best understood as a specific way of attending to experience. Its therapeutic power lies not in erasing discomfort but in shifting the relationship individuals have with their experiences, enabling them to respond with clarity rather than reactivity.

EMBODIMENT AND HEALING

While much of the psychological literature on mindfulness focuses on cognitive processes, an equally vital dimension lies in embodiment, the recognition that mind and body are deeply interconnected. This perspective highlights that healing and self-awareness are not purely mental acts, but also physical experiences grounded in movement, rhythm, and posture.

The Mind-Body-Heart Connection

The mind-body-heart connection underscores how mental states are reflected in the body and, heart health conversely, how physical states influence emotions and cognition. Because of this connection, improving psychological well-being is not just good for mental health, it also can reduce cardiovascular disease risk (Levine et al., 2021).

Research in neuroscience and psychophysiology supports this link. The autonomic nervous system, which governs stress responses, can be regulated through mindful breathing and body awareness (Lavretsky & Feldman, 2021). Practices like yoga, tai chi, and qigong demonstrate that mindful movement can harmonize physiological and psychological processes, reducing stress and fostering resilience.

In psychotherapy, somatic approaches such as Somatic Experiencing or body-oriented trauma therapies highlight the necessity of engaging the body in healing. They argue that trauma and distress are often stored in bodily memory, requiring embodied practices for release and integration.

How Movement, Posture, and Rhythm Influence Affective States

Movement is more than physical exercise; it is a language of emotion and self-expression. Simple shifts in posture, standing tall versus hunching, can alter confidence and mood. Similarly, rhythmic activities such as walking, drumming, or dancing regulate emotional states by engaging the body's innate sense of timing and flow.

Rhythm, in particular, plays a crucial role in emotional regulation. Infants are soothed by rocking and rhythmic lullabies, while adults often find comfort in repetitive, patterned movement. Neuroscience suggests that rhythm engages brain regions associated with reward, motor coordination, and emotion, creating a state of coherence between body and mind.

Dance, as a rhythmic and expressive movement practice, exemplifies this connection. Through dance, individuals embody emotions, release tension, and reconnect with their sense of vitality. When combined with mindfulness, dance becomes more than performance—it becomes an act of healing and self-discovery.

Dance and Mindful Movement as Embodied Expressions of Inner Experience

Dance and mindful movement offer distinctive pathways for embodying mindfulness, complementing the stillness of seated meditation with practices that cultivate awareness through motion. These approaches invite individuals to anchor their attention in the body's dynamic processes—such as shifting weight, the rhythm of the breath, or the grounding sensation of the feet against the floor. The focus is not on aesthetic mastery or technical performance but on presence in each unfolding moment, allowing the body to become both the site and the vehicle of awareness.

This embodied perspective opens multiple therapeutic and developmental pathways:

- **Emotional expression**. Dance provides a nonverbal medium for processing emotions that may be difficult to articulate. Movement allows feelings to surface, transform, and find resolution, creating space for release and healing.
- **Self-integration.** By aligning inner experience with outward expression, mindful movement fosters wholeness and coherence between body, mind, and spirit.
- **Interpersonal connection**. Group-based movement practices enhance attunement, synchrony, and empathy. Shared rhythms and gestures foster co-regulation and collective presence, countering isolation and supporting relational well-being.

Beyond these direct benefits, mindful movement introduces opportunities for embodied metaphors. Releasing rigid postures can symbolize letting go of control, while expansive gestures may embody openness, receptivity, or growth. Because these metaphors are experienced physically rather than solely contemplated cognitively, they can deepen insight and reinforce psychological change, resilience, and transformation.

In therapeutic, educational, and community settings, dance and mindful movement act as bridges between intellectual understanding and lived experience. They transform mindfulness from a primarily cognitive exercise into a holistic practice that engages the fullness of human existence. Such practices highlight that healing and growth are not solely matters of thought but are deeply embodied processes rooted in rhythm, presence, and relational connection.

Movement, posture, and rhythm are not peripheral to emotional life but central to it, shaping how individuals experience, regulate, and express their inner worlds. Dance and mindful movement amplify this connection, offering embodied pathways for healing, expression, and integration. In contexts of depression and anxiety, where disconnection, numbness, or rigidity often predominate, mindful movement offers a route back to flow, presence, and vitality.

Ultimately, the integration of mindfulness and movement affirms a timeless truth: to be human is to be embodied, and in movement lies the potential for healing, transformation, and meaning. By embracing both stillness and motion, thought and sensation, individuals can cultivate resilience, emotional balance, and a deeper sense of being.

Embodied Practices as Interpersonal Effectiveness

Interpersonal effectiveness in DBT, focuses on communication, boundaries, and maintaining relationships. Group dance activities offer a unique embodied training ground for these skills. When participants synchronize movements or improvise collaboratively, they practice attunement, cooperation, and nonverbal communication. These embodied forms of interaction can mirror the relational skills necessary in everyday life.

EXISTENTIALIST PERSPECTIVE

Existential psychology provides a broader philosophical framework for mindfulness by emphasizing authenticity, freedom, and the search for meaning. Depression and anxiety often reflect existential concerns—feelings of emptiness, isolation, or dread about the future. Mindfulness, when viewed through an existential lens, is not simply a relaxation technique but a way of confronting the fundamental realities of human existence.

Mindfulness as Awareness of Being

From this perspective, mindfulness means becoming fully aware of existence in the present moment. It involves recognizing the tension between freedom and responsibility, between the certainty of death and the possibility of meaning. For students or professionals grappling with anxiety, this kind of mindfulness offers a way to embrace uncertainty rather than escape from it. Instead of becoming trapped in "what if" scenarios, individuals are invited to experience the fullness of being, even in its fragility.

Movement and Dance as Existential Practices

Movement and dance embody existential principles by situating the individual in the here-and-now. Through physical movement, participants confront freedom of choice: each step, each gesture, is an affirmation of agency. At the same time, dance highlights interconnection, as movements occur within space and often in relation to others. For example, a dance improvisation exercise might ask participants to respond freely to music, embodying the existential challenge of creating meaning in a world without predefined scripts. In this way, dance becomes a metaphor for existence itself, which could be dynamic, uncertain, yet rich with possibility.

Embodiment and Grounding in the Present

Existential therapists often highlight the importance of grounding, of establishing one's place in the world. Embodied practices help clients anchor themselves when they feel overwhelmed by existential dread or despair. By paying attention to the sensations of movement such as the beating of the heart, the rhythm of breath, the feeling of gravity wherein individuals reconnect with life itself. For those experiencing depression, which often involves feelings of disconnection or numbness, mindful dance acts as a reminder of vitality. It emphasizes that existence is experienced through the body, not just in the mind.

INTEGRATING THE FRAMEWORKS

Though ACT, DBT, and existentialism emerge from different traditions, they converge in their recognition of mindfulness and embodiment as essential to well-being. ACT highlights values and psychological flexibility, DBT provides structured skills for emotional and relational regulation, and existentialism deepens mindfulness as a philosophical encounter with being. Movement and dance practices resonate with all three:

- They serve as cognitive deffusion and committed action (ACT).
- They build distress tolerance, emotion regulation, and interpersonal effectiveness (DBT).
- They embody freedom, choice, and authenticity (existentialism).

Together, these frameworks underscore the transformative potential of integrating mindfulness, movement, and dance into therapeutic and educational contexts.

Mindfulness has evolved far beyond seated meditation. Within psychological practice, it now encompasses body-based approaches that address both cognitive and emotional dimensions of human experience. By examining mindfulness through the lenses of ACT, DBT, and existentialism, we see how mindful movement and dance can provide unique pathways to healing, resilience, and authentic living. For individuals struggling with depression and anxiety, these practices offer not only symptom relief but also opportunities for growth and meaning. Ultimately, the integration of movement and mindfulness embodies the principle that healing is not just a mental process but a holistic engagement with life through body, mind, and spirit.

Mechanisms of Healing: Why Mindfulness and Movement Work

Mindfulness and mindful movement (e.g., yoga, tai chi, mindful walking, and structured exercise integrated with attention training) produce complementary effects across neural, autonomic, and somatic systems. These practices engage both top-down (prefrontal control, cognitive reappraisal) and bottom-up (interoceptive afference, vagal modulation) pathways that together reduce physiological stress reactivity, recalibrate motivational neurochemistry, and strengthen embodied emotion regulation. The result is improved cognitive-affective self-regulation and a greater capacity for adaptive responding under stress — core components of psychological healing and resilience (Calderone et al., 2024).

Neurobiological underpinnings

Stress-response regulation (HPA and SAM axes). Mindfulness practices attenuate stress reactivity through interacting neural networks that modulate the sympathetic-adrenal-medullary (SAM) and hypothalamic-pituitary-adrenal (HPA) axes. Functional and structural neuroimaging and endocrine studies indicate that mindfulness strengthens prefrontal inhibitory control over limbic regions (e.g., amygdala) and reduces downstream cortisol and catecholamine responses during stressor exposure (Calderone et al., 2024). Over time this down-regulation supports a shift from chronic hyperarousal toward more balanced autonomic responsiveness, which is associated with improved mental and physical health (Calderone et al., 2024).

Parasympathetic (vagal) tone and heart-rate variability (HRV). Vagal tone — typically indexed via HRV — mediates how well the body can rapidly return to a calm, restorative state after challenge. Mindfulness and movement interventions frequently target breath regulation and body awareness that are hypothesized to enhance parasympathetic activity and vagal regulation. Meta-analytic evidence is mixed: randomized controlled trials to date show small or inconsistent effects of seated mindfulness training on resting vagally mediated HRV, pointing to heterogeneity in protocols and measurement methods. However, research on integrated physical activity or breath-focused practices (and on combined exercise + mindfulness protocols) finds more robust, transient increases in vagal markers following practice — supporting a model in which movement and paced breathing produce immediate parasympathetic upregulation that, with repetition, can become trait-like (Tisdell et al., 2024). Thus, movement + mindfulness may provide complementary routes to ANS balance.

Dopaminergic modulation and neurotrophic effects. Physical activity produces durable neurochemical changes that are central to motivation, reward processing, and mood regulation. Recent mechanistic animal work shows that voluntary exercise elevates activity-dependent dopamine release in striatal circuits and increases levels of brain-derived neurotrophic factor (BDNF), a trophic protein that supports synaptic plasticity and mediates exercise-driven dopamine enhancements (Bastioli et al., 2022). These findings provide a plausible pathway by which regular movement supports motivation, mood, and learning, mechanisms that synergize with the attentional training of mindfulness to reinforce practice adherence and positive affective states.

EMOTION REGULATION THROUGH EMBODIED AWARENESS

Interoception as the bridge between body and emotion. Embodied awareness, the capacity to sense, label, and regulate internal bodily states (interoception) is central to emotion regulation. Mindfulness trains interoceptive attention (e.g., body scans, breath awareness), increasing accuracy and metacognitive awareness of physiological signals (e.g., heartbeat, respiration), which in turn improves labeling and modulation of affective states (Lazzarelli et al., 2024). Movement-based practices provide complementary, often bottom-up interoceptive input (muscle stretch, proprioceptive feedback, breath-movement coupling) that can be particularly effective for people who struggle to access internal states through purely cognitive techniques.

Dual pathways: top-down and bottom-up regulation. Contemporary models highlight a dual-pathway approach: mindfulness initially activates top-down prefrontal control to decrease reactivity and enhance attentional stability; repeated practice and embodied movement then boost bottom-up interoceptive signaling and neurovisceral feedback, fostering greater integration between bodily states and higher-order regulation (Lazzarelli et al., 2024). This integration supports flexible emotion regulation, the capacity to notice bodily cues, respond adaptively, and return to baseline, which is a strong predictor of mental health outcomes.

Enhancing resilience by integrating body and mind

Mechanisms that build resilience.

Resilience, broadly, the capacity to adapt positively in the face of stress, is supported by multiple mechanisms engaged by mindfulness and mindful movement: improved stress reactivity (lower HPA/SAM responsivity), greater autonomic flexibility (vagal tone), enhanced reward and motivation systems (dopaminergic/BDNF signaling), and increased interoceptive-regulatory capacity (better emotion labeling and modulation). When combined, these changes produce more rapid recovery from stress, improved cognitive control under pressure, and greater psychological flexibility — the building blocks of resilient functioning (Calderone et al., 2024; Bastioli et al., 2022).

Empirical support from intervention studies. Randomized trials and systematic reviews conducted in adolescents and adults show that mind-body therapies (yoga, tai chi, Qigong, dance-movement therapy, and combined exercise + mindfulness programs) produce small-to-moderate improvements in stress, mood, and various resilience markers, particularly when programs are sustained and include embodied practices (Mei et al., 2024; Luo et al., 2024). Importantly, interventions that blend movement with explicit interoceptive training appear especially helpful for populations with high arousal or trauma histories, where purely cognitive approaches may be less accessible.

Conclusions And Practical Implications And Directions For Scholarship

Clinical and educational application. Programs that intentionally sequence movement and attentional practice (e.g., brief aerobic or yoga warm-ups followed by seated mindfulness; or alternating movement-based sessions with contemplative practice) exploit complementary mechanisms: immediate parasympathetic and neurochemical benefits from movement, plus cumulative cognitive and interoceptive gains from mindfulness. This sequencing can improve engagement (via exercise-driven motivation) and enhance physiological readiness for contemplative learning (Bastioli et al., 2022).

Research needs. Future research should: (a) standardize HRV and interoceptive measures to resolve mixed findings on vagal change (b) test dose-response and sequencing effects comparing movement-before-meditation versus meditation-before-movement, (c) broaden mechanistic work to human neuroimaging and ambulatory physiology that link BDNF/dopamine markers to subjective resilience, and (d) examine moderators (age, trauma history, baseline interoceptive accuracy) to tailor interventions to individual needs (Calderone et al., 2024; Lazzarelli et al., 2024).

Applications of Mindfulness, Movement, and Dance Approaches

Mindfulness, mindful movement (e.g., yoga, tai chi), and dance/movement therapy (DMT) form a complementary set of approaches that integrate attentional training with embodied experience. Applied across clinical, educational, and community settings, these interventions address emotion dysregulation, stress reactivity, social connectedness, and functional impairment in populations with depression, anxiety, and trauma histories. Empirical evidence from randomized trials, feasibility studies, and systematic reviews supports modest-to-moderate benefits on mood, anxiety, trauma symptoms, and quality of life, particularly when interventions are sustained, tailored, and include embodied practices (Zhang et al., 2025; Li et al., 2024; Hyvönen et al., 2020).

Clinical Applications

Use in therapy for anxiety, depression, and trauma. Clinical programs blend mindfulness instruction with movement or dance to engage both top-down cognitive regulation and bottom-up somatic processes. Mindfulness-based stress reduction (MBSR), mindfulness-based cognitive therapy (MBCT), and trauma-informed adaptations have demonstrated efficacy for depressive symptoms, anxiety, and post-traumatic stress, with meta-analytic evidence for moderate effect sizes on depression and PTSD outcomes in adults (Li et al., 2024; Zhang et al., 2025). Dance/movement therapy (DMT) and mindfulness-based dance movement therapy (MBDMT) have shown promise in randomized or quasi-experimental studies for reducing depressive symptoms and improving emotion regulation, particularly for participants who find verbal therapy alone insufficient or who present with somatic symptoms (Hyvönen et al., 2020; Majore-Dusele et al., 2021).

Mechanisms targeted in clinical work

- Down-regulation of HPA and sympathetic reactivity through breath, paced movement, and vagal recruitment.
- Improved interoceptive awareness that permits earlier detection and labeling of affective states (interoception → emotion regulation).
- Reward and motivation enhancement via exercise-related dopaminergic and neurotrophic changes, which can counter anhedonia in depression.

A sample case would be of Maria, a 34-year-old woman with recurrent major depressive episodes, reports low energy, social withdrawal, and difficulty accessing feelings in therapy. She enrolls in a 10-week MBDMT program that interleaves breath-centred mindfulness, guided improvised dance, and reflective journaling. Over eight weeks she reports increased bodily awareness (recognizing early tension patterns), gradual re-engagement in pleasurable movement, and improved mood and sleep. Clinician measures indicate reductions in depressive symptoms and greater self-reported emotion regulation capacity. This vignette reflects outcomes reported in feasibility and RCT evidence for movement-integrated interventions (Hyvönen et al., 2020; Majore-Dusele et al., 2021).

Educational and Community Settings

Programs for students, teachers, and communities. Movement integration programs (brief, classroom-embedded activities or longer curricula) combine mindful breathing, short movement breaks, and guided group activities to improve attention, classroom climate, and emotional regulation among students (Romar et al., 2023; Aloizou et al., 2025). For teachers and staff, workplace mindfulness + movement modules reduce burnout and improve classroom management when practiced regularly. Community settings (senior centers, community health programs) use low-intensity tai chi, walking meditation, and group dance to support mood, mobility, and social connection (Ma et al., 2022; Zhang et al., 2025).

Group movement/dance activities for collective well-being. Group DMT or community dance initiatives foster co-regulation and social bonding—processes that are therapeutically potent in reducing isolation and promoting collective resilience. Reviews report social-emotional benefits and improvements in wellbeing indicators across community samples, though effect sizes vary by design and intensity of intervention (Zhang et al., 2025).

For sample programs, a 12-week program for middle-school students: 3 minutes of mindful breathing at class start + two 5-minute movement breaks (simple, guided movement) + monthly creative dance workshops. Outcomes targeted: improved attention, reduced classroom stress, social-emotional learning gains (Romar et al., 2023).

SELF-PRACTICE APPROACHES

Everyday mindful movement practices

- **Walking meditation**: Short guided walking meditations (5–20 minutes) integrate breath, sensation, and environment; evidence shows mood and sleep benefits and improvements in trait mindfulness following brief walking programs. (Ma et al., 2022).
- **Improvised dance**: Free movement to music or silence promotes emotional expression and kinesthetic exploration; case series and pilot trials suggest feasibility and affective benefits, particularly for people who struggle with verbal processing. (Majore-Dusele et al., 2021; Zhang et al., 2025).
- **Yoga and tai chi**: Mindful movement practices that combine breath, postures, and attention, with RCT evidence for improvements in depressive and anxiety symptoms when practiced regularly. (Li et al., 2024).

Journaling reflections post-movement to enhance integration

Reflective journaling after movement sessions helps consolidate interoceptive insights, links bodily sensations to emotions, and supports cognitive processing of experiences. Educational and clinical pilots indicate journaling enhances self-awareness and treatment gains when paired with embodied practices (Romar et al., 2023; Majore-Dusele et al., 2021).

Suggested simple home routine

1. 10–15 min walking meditation (focus on footfall, breath).
2. 10 min improvised movement or gentle yoga (invite curious, nonjudgmental exploration).
3. 5–10 min reflective journaling (body sensations, mood changes, intentions).

Narrative Examples (Clinical and Community)

Trauma-informed group DMT. A community clinic adapts DMT for trauma survivors by emphasizing grounding exercises, predictable structure, slow paced movement, and co-regulation. Participants report increased safety in the body, reduced hypervigilance, and improved emotion naming—consistent with trauma-adapted movement literature. (Zhang et al., 2025).

School-based movement integration. A primary school implements daily "mindful movement" breaks; teachers report improved attention spans and fewer classroom disruptions, aligning with movement-integration research in school contexts (Romar et al., 2023).

Combined movement + MBSR for depression. An outpatient program pairs a low-impact aerobic warmup with seated MBSR sessions. Patients demonstrate faster engagement with mindfulness practice and larger reductions in self-reported anhedonia compared with MBSR alone—illustrating hypothesized synergistic effects (Bastioli et al., 2022).

Implementation Considerations and Best Practices

- **Safety & screening**: For populations with trauma or severe depression, screen for dissociation and implement trauma-informed pacing (grounding, titrated exposure to interoceptive cues).
- **Cultural adaptation**: Tailor music, movement styles, and metaphors to cultural context to enhance engagement. (Zhang et al., 2025).
- **Dose and fidelity**: Sustained programs (8–12+ weeks) show more reliable outcomes; fidelity monitoring and facilitator training in both mindfulness and movement techniques improve effectiveness.
- **Hybrid delivery**: Digital or blended formats (telehealth dance sessions; app-guided walking meditations) can increase accessibility; preliminary evidence suggests benefits but more RCTs are needed (Qiu et al., 2025).

Table 2. Applications of mindfulness, movement, and dance approaches

Application	Primary targets	Typical setting	Core components	Mechanisms	Evidence level	Example practice
Mindfulness-based programs (MBSR/MBCT)	Depression, anxiety, PTSD	Clinics, outpatient groups	Seated mindfulness, body scan, mindful movement	Top-down regulation (PFC), reduced rumination	High (meta-analyses, RCTs).	8-week MBSR with weekly group sessions
Dance/Movement Therapy (DMT)	Depression, trauma, social isolation	Clinics, community centers	Improvisation, mirroring, group movement	Embodied regulation, co-regulation, interoception	Moderate (RCTs, systematic reviews).	10-week group DMT with reflective processing
Mindful walking / walking meditation	Anxiety, mood, concentration	Community, parks, home	Attention to steps, breath, environment	Somatic grounding, rhythm → calming ANS	Moderate (RCTs/ pilots).	15-minute daily walking meditation
Tai Chi	Depression, anxiety, mobility	Clinics, schools, senior centers	Postures, breath, mindful transitions	Vagal stimulation, interoception, BDNF ↑	Moderate (RCTs, meta-analyses).	Twice weekly 45-min yoga classes
Movement integration in schools	Attention, SEL, teacher stress	Classrooms, whole-school programs	Short movement breaks, kinesthetic learning	Attention restoration, mood lift	Emerging/ moderate (quasi-experimental).	3-minute mindful breathing + movement breaks daily
Self-guided improvised dance + journaling	Emotional processing, anhedonia	Home, digital platforms	Free movement, reflection	Expressive regulation, narrative integration	Emerging (feasibility studies).	20-min improvised dance + 10-min journal
Community dance programs	Social connection, wellbeing	Community centers, public spaces	Choreography, group practice	Social bonding, co-regulation	Moderate (reviews).	Weekly community dance circles

CHALLENGES AND CONSIDERATIONS

Mindfulness, movement, and dance approaches hold strong promise for emotion regulation, therapeutic engagement, and community well-being. However, their uptake and effectiveness depend heavily on how they are framed, delivered, and adapted to local realities. Thoughtful deployment requires attention to cultural meaning, ethical integrity, access barriers, and the risk that embodied practices may be diluted, commodified, or applied in ways that do not benefit — or may even harm — the people they are intended to serve.

Cultural contexts of dance and mindfulness in the Philippines and beyond

Cultural embeddedness and plural meanings. Mindfulness and movement practices are not culturally neutral. Both arise from particular histories, symbols, and worldviews; when transplanted, they interact with local cosmologies, religious practices, and community norms. In the Philippines, expressive movement and dance are embedded in ritual, Pilipino folk tradition (e.g., *tinikling*, *pandanggo*), Catholic devotional practices, and communal celebrations — contexts that influence how people relate to embodied practices, authority figures, and healing (Romar et al., 2023; Magis Creative Spaces narratives in practitioner literature). Culturally sensitive adaptations must therefore recognize existing movement vocabularies, spiritual practices, and the social meaning of bodily expression rather than presenting mindfulness and dance as culturally detached techniques (Cordisco Tsai, 2025; Romar et al., 2023).

Local evidence and practice in the Philippines. A growing but still limited empirical base documents mindfulness and dance/movement work in Philippine settings. Feasibility studies, curricular pilots, and program descriptions indicate promise for teacher well-being, student stress reduction, and trauma-informed DMT in community settings; however, many locally produced studies are small-sample, program-evaluation designs rather than large RCTs (Hernandez et al., 2023; Project TRIDENT reports; local creative-arts clinics). These findings suggest acceptability and cultural resonance, but also highlight the need for rigorous, contextually informed trials and collaborations with Filipino practitioners who can decolonize and localize practice (Romar et al., 2023; ADTA international panel narratives).

Cross-cultural lessons. Across regions, successful cultural adaptation features co-design with local communities, use of indigenous movement forms, language translation beyond literal terms (e.g., reframing "mindfulness" in locally meaningful idioms), and attention to power dynamics in facilitator–participant relationships (Cordisco Tsai, 2025). Programs that center local arts practitioners and community leaders — rather than imposing foreign templates — achieve better uptake and sustained engagement. (Load-bearing citations: Romar et al., 2023; Cordisco Tsai, 2025; ADTA international panel materials.)

Risk of trivializing or over-commercializing practices

"McMindfulness" and the politics of commodification. Academic and critical literature have documented how mindfulness has been stripped of ethical and social critique and repackaged as a decontextualized product for stress-management and productivity — a phenomenon often termed "McMindfulness" (Purser, 2019;

Leggett, 2022). When mindfulness or movement practices are marketed primarily as tools for worker efficiency or consumer wellbeing without attention to systemic causes of distress (e.g., precarious work, social inequality), they risk depoliticizing suffering and obscuring structural interventions that would produce genuine change.

Risks specific to dance/movement and embodied practices. Dance and movement approaches are likewise susceptible to commercial repackaging (e.g., branded "wellness" dance classes, highly mediated fitness-dance formats) that foreground aesthetics or rapid consumer uptake over therapeutic integrity and safety. Over-commercialized offerings may fail to include essential trauma-informed safeguards (grounding, titration, clinician oversight) and can inadvertently re-traumatize participants or trivialize embodied suffering (Beaubrun, 2022).

Safeguards against dilution and commodification. Preserve ethical teachings and community-rooted meanings in program curricula; foreground values such as non-harm, interdependence, and social justice alongside technique.

- Insist on facilitator training standards and competency in trauma-aware delivery.
- Avoid productivity-framed marketing in clinical or school contexts; emphasize well-being, safety, and restoration (Leggett, 2022; Purser, 2019).

(Load-bearing citations: Purser, 2019; Leggett, 2022; Beaubrun, 2022.)

Accessibility and inclusivity issues (ability, body type, cultural norms)

Ability and neurodiversity. Dance and mindfulness programs often assume normative mobility, sensory processing, and attention. This excludes people with physical disabilities, chronic pain, sensory sensitivities, or neurodivergence. Emerging inclusive design research recommends co-creation with people with lived experience, flexible movement options, and multi-modal cues (visual schedules, tactile prompts) to make programs accessible (Anderson, 2024; Ladwig et al., 2025). Studies co-designing guides for children with cerebral palsy and hybrid-Delphi recommendations emphasize that inclusion requires structural accommodation, staff training, and budgeted supports (Machado et al., 2025; Ladwig et al., 2025).

Body diversity and weight stigma. Dance programming that centers certain body shapes, speed, or athletic aesthetics can alienate people with larger bodies or limited stamina. Inclusive choreography, non-judgmental language, and options for seated or supported movement are essential. Inclusive practice aligns with the social model of disability and helps shift the focus from performance to participation and co-creation (Frontlinedance example; Guardian reporting, 2023).

Cultural norms and gendered expectations. Cultural conventions around modesty, gendered movement restrictions, and the social meaning of touch or expressive gestures shape what is safe and acceptable. In some Filipino communities, for example, certain movement forms may be coded as "religious" or "immodest"; facilitators must negotiate consent, dress, and public performance expectations and offer culturally appropriate alternatives (Romar et al., 2023).

Digital divide and socioeconomic access. Hybrid and digital offerings expand reach but can worsen inequities where internet, privacy, or safe physical space are limited. Low-resource adaptations (radio scripts, group sessions at community halls, school-based programs) are necessary to democratize access (Qiu et al., 2025; Romar et al., 2023). (Load-bearing citations: Anderson, 2024; Machado et al., 2025; Ladwig et al., 2025; Guardian 2023.)

PRACTICAL RECOMMENDATIONS FOR ETHICAL, INCLUSIVE, CULTURALLY GROUNDED PRACTICE

Co-design and community partnership. Engage local artists, elders, cultural bearers, and people with lived experience at every stage: needs assessment, curriculum design, facilitation, and evaluation (Cordisco Tsai, 2025; Romar et al., 2023).

Trauma-informed and safety-first programming. Train facilitators in grounding techniques, pacing, and indicators of dysregulation; screen participants, offer opt-out options, and provide follow-up referrals for clinical care when needed (Zhang et al., 2025).

Flexible, inclusive movement architectures. Build multiple access points into sessions (seated alternatives, tactile cues, varied tempos), and embrace co-creation so participants shape movement rather than purely imitate instructors (Anderson, 2024; Ladwig et al., 2025).

Preserve contextual meaning and avoid commodification. Frame programs around social and relational wellbeing, not just individual productivity gains; include ethical orientation and community accountability mechanisms (Purser, 2019; Leggett, 2022).

Clear evaluation and culturally appropriate outcome measurement. Use mixed-methods evaluation with locally meaningful indicators (qualitative narratives, participatory measures) alongside standardized symptom measures; report adaptations transparently (Cordisco Tsai, 2025).

Equitable access strategies. Offer sliding-scale fees, school-embedded programs, community partnerships, and low-tech options for remote or resource-limited settings (Romar et al., 2023; Qiu et al., 2025).

Table 3. Summary of the challenges and recommended mitigations

Challenge	Why it matters	Recommended mitigation(s)
Cultural mismatch / lack of relevance	Programs that ignore local meanings are resisted or fail to sustain.	Co-design with local cultural leaders; adapt language, music, and movement to local forms. (Cordisco Tsai, 2025)
Trivialization / "McMindfulness"	Strips ethical and social context; reduces interventions to productivity hacks.	Emphasize ethical foundations; avoid productivity-centered messaging; include social justice orientation. (Purser, 2019; Leggett, 2022)
Trauma-triggering embodied practices	Sudden interoceptive focus can destabilize trauma survivors.	Use trauma-informed pacing, grounding, informed consent, and clinical referral pathways. (Zhang et al., 2025)
Physical accessibility and body diversity	Excludes people with disabilities, chronic pain, or different body types.	Provide seated/modified options; co-create movement; train facilitators in inclusive pedagogy. (Anderson, 2024)
Gender/cultural norms around movement	May conflict with local norms on modesty, touch, or public performance.	Offer gender-sensitive options, private sessions, or culturally appropriate modifications. (Romar et al., 2023)
Digital divide & socioeconomic barriers	Remote programs can widen inequities.	Offer low-tech alternatives; school and community-site delivery; subsidize participation.
Commercialization & quality control	Market saturation with low-quality offerings undermines trust.	Establish facilitator standards; accreditation; community oversight; transparent reporting. (Leggett, 2022)

CURRENT CHALLENGES AND FUTURE TRENDS

At present, there are no studies on the application of different psychotherapies in dance. This would be difficult to achieve as there is a need for motivation on the part of the client in dance in order to pursue dance therapy with a specific psychotherapy. Second, ACT and DBT are known to be third wave Cognitive Behavior Therapies. These are relatively new forms of intervention. Perhaps, more research can be done by sports psychologists in this developing field.

REFERENCES

Al-Refae, M., Al-Refae, A., Munroe, M., Sardella, N. A., & Ferrari, M. (2021). A self-compassion and mindfulness-based cognitive mobile intervention (Serene) for depression, anxiety, and stress: Promoting adaptive emotional regulation and wisdom. *Frontiers in Psychology*, *12*, 648087. DOI: 10.3389/fpsyg.2021.648087

Aloizou, V., Linardatou, S., Boloudakis, M., & Retalis, S. (2025). Integrating a movement-based learning platform as core curriculum tool in kindergarten classrooms. *British Journal of Educational Technology*, *56*(1), 339–365.

Anderson, A. (2024). *Dance/movement interventions and students with disabilities: A critical narrative review*. Routledge Open Research.

Barua, R. (2025). Harmonizing body and mind: Investigating the combined impact of yoga and mindfulness meditation on depression, anxiety, and stress. In *Global Innovations in Physical Education and Health* (pp. 203–232). IGI Global.

Basso, J. C., Satyal, M. K., & Rugh, R. (2021). Dance on the brain: Enhancing intra- and inter-brain synchrony. *Frontiers in Human Neuroscience*, *14*, 584312. DOI: 10.3389/fnhum.2020.584312

Bastioli, G.. (2022). Voluntary exercise boosts striatal dopamine release: Evidence for the necessary and sufficient role of BDNF. *The Journal of Neuroscience : The Official Journal of the Society for Neuroscience*. Advance online publication. DOI: 10.1523/JNEUROSCI.2273-21.2022

Beaubrun, A. (2022). Decentralizing the commodification of mindfulness. *Unpublished manuscript.*

Bonanno, G. A., Chen, S., & Galatzer-Levy, I. R. (2023). Resilience to potential trauma and adversity through regulatory flexibility. *Nature Reviews Psychology*, *2*(11), 663–675. DOI: 10.1038/s44159-023-00228-5

Calderone, A., Latella, D., Impellizzeri, F., de Pasquale, P., Famà, F., Quartarone, A., & Calabrò, R. S. (2024). Neurobiological changes induced by mindfulness and meditation: A systematic review. *Biomedicines*, *12*(11), 2613. DOI: 10.3390/biomedicines12112613

Cattie, J. E., Allbaugh, L. J., Visser, K. H., Ander, I., & Kaslow, N. J. (2021). Tailoring trauma-sensitive yoga for high-risk populations in public-sector settings. *International Journal of Yoga Therapy*, *31*(1), 15–24. DOI: 10.17761/2021-D-19-00024

Channawar, S. N. (2023). Mindfulness practices for stress reduction and mental clarity. *International Journal of Futuristic Innovation in Arts. Humanities and Management, 2*(3), 49–59.

Chen, Y., Wang, S., Senanu Ametefe, D., & John, D. (2024). Impact of dancing on physical and mental health: A systematic literature review. *Dance Research, 42*(2), 220–256. DOI: 10.3366/drs.2024.0375

Cordisco Tsai, L. (2025). Cultural adaptation of a trauma-informed mind-body program. *International Social Work Review. Webb, A. J. (2023). Acceptance and Commitment Therapy (ACT): Foundational Principles, Processes, and Treatment Components. Authorea Preprints.*

Eddy, M., & Johnson, D. H. (2022). *The fluid nature of being: Embodied practices for healing and wholeness*. Jessica Kingsley Publishers.

Fugate, J. M., Macrine, S. L., & Hernandez-Cuevas, E. M. (2024). Therapeutic potential of embodied cognition for clinical psychotherapies: From theory to practice. *Cognitive Therapy and Research, 48*(4), 574–598. DOI: 10.1007/s10608-024-10428-3

Gregg, J. (2024). *You don't have to feel that way: The totally natural way to beat anxiety, depression, and bipolar behavior without drugs*. Jason Gregg.

Heath, N., Midkiff, M. F., Gerhart, J., & Turow, R. G. (2021). Group-based DBT skills training modules are linked to independent and additive improvements in emotion regulation in a heterogeneous outpatient sample. *Psychotherapy Research, 31*(8), 1001–1011. DOI: 10.1080/10503307.2020.1870356

Hernandez, D. C., Santos, H., & Penaflor, G. (2023). *Mindfulness youth novel dynamics (MYND): A stress management strategy for junior high school students*. E-Saliksik / DepEd Philippines.

Hyvönen, K., Pylvänäinen, P., Muotka, J., & Lappalainen, R. (2020). The effects of dance movement therapy in the treatment of depression: A multicenter, randomized controlled trial in Finland. *Frontiers in Psychology, 11*, 1687. DOI: 10.3389/fpsyg.2020.01687

Javaid, S. F., Hashim, I. J., Hashim, M. J., Stip, E., Samad, M. A., & Ahbabi, A. A. (2023). Epidemiology of anxiety disorders: Global burden and sociodemographic associations. *Middle East Current Psychiatry, 30*(1), 44. DOI: 10.1186/s43045-023-00359-9

Johnson-Sealey, F. (2024). *Choreographing a journey of self-discovery: An exploration of dance, embodied knowledge, and identity* (Doctoral dissertation, City University of New York).

Kandola, A. A., del Pozo Cruz, B., Osborn, D. P. J., Stubbs, B., Choi, K. W., & Hayes, J. F. (2021). Impact of replacing sedentary behaviour with other movement behaviours on depression and anxiety symptoms: A prospective cohort study in the UK Biobank. *BMC Medicine*, *19*, 133. DOI: 10.1186/s12916-021-01995-9

Karkou, V., Aithal, S., Zubala, A., & Meekums, B. (2019). Effectiveness of dance movement therapy in the treatment of adults with depression: A systematic review with meta-analyses. *Frontiers in Psychology*, *10*, 936. DOI: 10.3389/fpsyg.2019.00936

Ladwig, K. H., Marten-Mittag, B., Olliges, E., Johar, H., Atasoy, S., Holdenrieder, S., & Ronel, J. (2025). Recurrent depression predicts high leptin concentrations in patients with coronary artery disease over an 18-months follow-up period: Findings from the prospective multicenter randomized controlled SPIRR-CAD Trial. *Journal of Affective Disorders*, *369*, 174–181.

Lavretsky, H., & Feldman, J. L. (2021). Precision medicine for breath-focused mind-body therapies for stress and anxiety: Are we ready yet? *Global Advances in Health and Medicine : Improving Healthcare Outcomes Worldwide*, *10*, 2164956120986129.

Lazzarelli, A., Scafuto, F., Crescentini, C., Matiz, A., Orrù, G., Ciacchini, R., & Conversano, C. (2024). Interoceptive ability and emotion regulation in mind–body interventions: An integrative review. *Behavioral Sciences (Basel, Switzerland)*, *14*(11), 1107.

Leggett, W. (2022). Can mindfulness really change the world? The political character of meditative practices. *Critical Policy Studies*, *16*(3), 261–278.

Levine, G. N., Cohen, B. E., Commodore-Mensah, Y., Fleury, J., Huffman, J. C., & Khalid, U. & American Heart Association Council on Clinical Cardiology; Council on Arteriosclerosis, Thrombosis and Vascular Biology; Council on Cardiovascular and Stroke Nursing; and Council on Lifestyle and Cardiometabolic Health. (2021). Psychological health, well-being, and the mind-heart-body connection: A scientific statement from the American Heart Association. *Circulation*, *143*(10), e763–e783.

Limone, P., & Toto, G. A. (2022). Factors that predispose undergraduates to mental issues: A cumulative literature review for future research perspectives. *Frontiers in Public Health*, *10*, 831349.

Lochrie, J. G. (2024). *Student Barriers and Motivators to Bystander Intervention If Witnessing Potential Sexual Violence on College Campuses*. St. John's University.

Lomas, T., Medina, J. C., Ivtzan, I., Rupprecht, S., & Eiroa-Orosa, F. J. (2017). A systematic review of the impact of mindfulness on the well-being of healthcare professionals. *Journal of Clinical Psychology*, *73*(3), 319–355. DOI: 10.1002/jclp.22420

Ma, L., Wang, Y., Pan, L., Cui, Z., & Schluter, P. J. (2022). Mindfulness-informed (ACT) and mindfulness-based programs (MBSR/MBCT) applied for college students to reduce symptoms of depression and anxiety. *Journal of Behavioral and Cognitive Therapy*, *32*(4), 271–289.

Majore-Dusele, I., Karkou, V., & Millere, I. (2021). The development of mindful-based dance movement therapy intervention for chronic pain: A pilot study with chronic headache patients. *Frontiers in Psychology*, *12*, 587923.

Mehta, N. N., & Talwar, G. (2022). Recognizing roots and not just leaves: The use of integrative mindfulness in education, research, and practice. *Psychology from the Margins*, *4*(1), 6.

Odendahl, J. (2021). Embodied Cognition, affects and language comprehension: Theoretical basis and (literary-) didactic perspectives of a physically-emotionally grounded model of understanding. *Phenomenology and the Cognitive Sciences*, *20*(3), 483–499.

Palagini, L., Miniati, M., Marazziti, D., Sharma, V., & Riemann, D. (2021). Association among early life stress, mood features, hopelessness and suicidal risk in bipolar disorder: The potential contribution of insomnia symptoms. *Journal of Psychiatric Research*, *135*, 52–59.

Pass Erickson, L. M. (2021). Sensing the self: A dance/movement therapy model of embodied identity development. *Body, Movement and Dance in Psychotherapy*, *16*(3), 202–217.

Price, C. J., & Weng, H. Y. (2021). Facilitating adaptive emotion processing and somatic reappraisal via sustained mindful interoceptive attention. *Frontiers in Psychology*, *12*, 578827.

Purser, R. (2019). *McMindfulness: How mindfulness became the new capitalist spirituality*. Repeater.

Romar, J. E., Enlund, M., Lind, S., & Björkgren, M. (2023). Movement integration in academic classrooms; a focus on secondary students' experiences. *Journal of Physical Education and Sport*, *23*(4), 918–928.

Scheer, M. (2022). Culture and religion: Remarks on an indeterminate relationship. *Religion and Society*, *13*(1), 111–125.

Shim, M., Lacson, C., Kavanaugh, M., Goldstein-Levitas, N., & Fisher, K. (2024). Online mindful movement approach for older adults: Two case studies. *Activities, Adaptation and Aging*, *48*(4), 705–722.

Skinner, E. A. (2023). Four guideposts toward an integrated model of academic motivation: Motivational resilience, academic identity, complex social ecologies, and development. *Educational Psychology Review*, *35*(3), 80.

Stanley, E. A., Schaldach, J. M., Kiyonaga, A., & Jha, A. P. (2011). Mindfulness-based mind fitness training: A case study of a high-stress predeployment military cohort. *Cognitive and Behavioral Practice*, *18*(4), 566–576.

Stevens, K. R. (2025). *Ways of Being: A Literature Review on Embodied Healing Through Mindfulness, Neuroscience and Dance/Movement Therapy Practice During Uncertain Times* (Master's thesis, Pratt Institute).

Tisdell, E. J., Lukic, B., Banerjee, R., Liao, D., & Palmer, C. (2024). The effects of heart rhythm meditation on vagal tone and Well-being: A mixed methods research study. *Applied Psychophysiology and Biofeedback*, *49*(3), 439–455.

Weiss, E. R., Mullens, S., Todman, M., Barnes, S. E., Lord, K. A., & Davis, M. T. (2025). The transdiagnostic role of boredom within personality disorder symptoms and risk-related behaviors: Implications for dialectical behavior therapy. *Journal of Psychotherapy Integration.*

Zafeiroudi, A., Goulimaris, D., Alexandris, K., & Yfantidou, G. (2025). Segmenting Recreational Dance Communities in Greece: Cultural Identity, Lifelong Engagement, and Inclusive and Participant-Centered Approaches to Dance Programming. *Societies (Basel, Switzerland)*, *15*(9), 239.

Zhang, Z., Du, B. A., Ma, C., Wang, Z., & Hu, W. (2025, October). Behave Your Motion: Habit-preserved Cross-category Animal Motion Transfer. In *Proceedings of the 33rd ACM International Conference on Multimedia* (pp. 9638-9647).

Chapter 15
Yoga Practice and Emotional Well-Being in Middle Age:
Evidence From a Vietnamese Randomized Trial

Thuc Chanh Dao
https://orcid.org/0000-0002-2822-049X
An Giang University, Vietnam & Vietnam National University, Ho Chi Minh City, Vietnam

ABSTRACT

This chapter synthesizes findings from a randomized controlled trial in Ho Chi Minh City, Vietnam, evaluating yoga's impact on physical function, pain, vitality, social participation, and mental health in middle-aged adults. Using repeated SF-36 measurements and linear mixed-effects modelling, the trial demonstrated significant improvements across physical and psychosocial domains. The chapter critically appraises the methodology, addressing potential biases and limitations, and recommends future trials incorporate active controls, objective biomarkers, and longer follow-up to clarify underlying mechanisms. Finally, it outlines pragmatic implications for scalable community programs and policy integration in rapidly urbanizing areas.

INTRODUCTION

Regular physical activity is known to be crucial for maintaining health in midlife. Indeed, a wealth of research underscores that exercise helps prevent chronic diseases

DOI: 10.4018/979-8-3373-6157-4.ch015

and supports overall well-being in middle-aged adults (Trinh et al, 2008; Minh Diu & Chanh Thuc, 2025). Among exercise modalities, yoga has gained widespread attention for its purported benefits on both body and mind. Numerous studies worldwide have reported that practicing yoga can improve physical and mental health in adults. For example, survey data show that many yoga practitioners believe their practice enhanced their energy, happiness, sleep, and social relationships (Ross et al, 2013). In controlled trials and meta-analyses, yoga interventions have been associated with significant increases in psychological well-being (relative to no-treatment controls) (Hendriks et al, 2017), and substantial reductions in stress, anxiety, and depression (Yang et al, 2023; Chauhan et al, 2025). These global findings suggest that regular yoga may support emotional balance and healthy aging.

However, much of the existing evidence comes from Western or clinical settings. In Vietnam – a rapidly modernizing country with increasing non-communicable disease burdens – research on yoga's impact has been scarce. For instance, in Ho Chi Minh City (HCMC) fewer than 60% of adults meet physical activity guidelines (Trinh et al, 2008), indicating a need for accessible exercise options. Although yoga has become more popular in Vietnamese urban centers, prior to this study there was "a lack of comprehensive research examining its impact on the self-reported health of middle-aged adults in this specific context". To address this gap, Minh Diu & Chanh Thuc (2025) conducted a rigorous randomized controlled trial (RCT) among middle-aged Vietnamese adults. This chapter paraphrases and expands upon their findings, situating the Vietnamese study within the broader literature on yoga and emotional well-being. We discuss the study's design and results, and integrate additional evidence on how yoga may enhance physical function, emotional health, and quality of life in diverse populations.

LITERATURE REVIEW

Global Evidence: Yoga, Physical Health, and Quality of Life

Research around the world has documented physical health benefits of yoga that are especially relevant for aging adults. Yoga involves stretching, strength-building postures, and balance exercises, all of which can counteract age-related declines. In the Vietnamese study, for example, regular yoga dramatically improved physical functioning. At 10 weeks, the yoga group's mean physical-function score jumped to 84.5 (SD=20.1) from a baseline of 57.0, whereas the control group saw no change (remained ~48). By 5 months, the yoga group's Physical Function Composite Score reached 86.1 (vs. 47.5 in controls, $p<0.001$) (Minh Diu & Chanh Thuc, 2025). Similar patterns have emerged elsewhere: controlled trials with older adults often report improved strength, flexibility, and pain reduction after yoga interventions (Bandyopadhyay et al., 2023; Tew et al., 2017). Indeed, systematic reviews find that yoga consistently enhances muscle strength and joint mobility, reducing musculoskeletal pain. These physiological gains likely stem from yoga's combination of static postures and dynamic flows, which build endurance and flexibility. For example, stretching and sustained poses promote muscular endurance and joint range-of-motion. Regular practice also appears to modulate inflammation – studies note that yoga can lower pro-inflammatory cytokines (like IL-6 and TNF-α) that contribute to chronic pain. Such biological effects may underlie the Vietnamese study's finding of much less bodily pain among yogis (mean pain score 93.1 vs. 59.8 in controls at 5 months, $p<0.001$). In short, global evidence aligns with the HCMC results: yoga's holistic physical training bolsters functional capacity and mobility in middle-age, thereby supporting healthier aging.

Yoga also positively influences traditional health-related quality-of-life metrics. The SF-36 health survey (Ware & Sherbourne, 1992) measures eight domains of well-being, including General Health, Vitality, and Role Limitations. In the Vietnamese trial, yogis showed strong gains on these scales. For instance, at mid-study the yoga group reported much better *General Health* perceptions (mean=72.6 vs 44.8 for controls, $p<0.001$) and *Role-Physical* functioning (mean=72.5 vs 39.1, $p<0.001$). By post-test, all eight SF-36 domain scores were significantly higher in the yoga group ($p<0.001$ for every scale). The composite summaries tell the same story: five months of yoga led to physical and mental health composite scores of ~86 and ~96, versus ~47 and ~53 in controls. Consequently, overall quality of life (SF-36 total) was substantially higher with yoga (mean=82.5 vs 52.4, $F(1,67)=34.42$, $p<0.001$).

These findings echo global reviews. A systematic review by Patel et al. (2012) found that yoga programs typically improve SF-36 physical and mental health scores in older adults. Benavidez and Hart (2017) meta-analyzed SF-36 outcomes and reported that, across multiple trials, yoga intervention groups tend to show higher quality-of-life scores than controls. In another controlled trial (Tew et al., 2017), sedentary older adults randomized to a gentle yoga program achieved significant gains on SF-36 domains such as Physical Functioning, Role-Physical, and Mental Health (all $p<0.05$). Thus, the Vietnamese results are highly consistent with an international pattern: yoga enhances both self-rated physical health and broader quality of life in adults entering middle age.

Global Evidence: Yoga and Emotional Well-Being

Equally important for middle-aged populations are yoga's effects on mental and emotional health. Worldwide, stress, anxiety, and depression are rising concerns in midlife (especially under work and family pressures). Yoga is increasingly studied as a mind-body strategy to address these issues. On average, systematic reviews find that practicing yoga reduces negative mood and bolsters *emotional well-being*. For example, Hendriks et al. (2017) meta-analyzed randomized trials of healthy adults and found a significant increase in psychological well-being from yoga (versus no-intervention). Though the meta-analysis noted that evidence is still limited, it did confirm that yoga participants report feeling better psychologically. In line with this, a large national survey of 1045 American Iyengar yoga practitioners (Ross et al., 2013) showed that most yogis believe yoga made them happier and less stressed. Specifically, 86.5% of respondents agreed that yoga improved their *happiness* and 84.5% said it increased their *energy*, and 68.5% noted better *sleep*.

Even more compelling are controlled trials linking yoga to reductions in depression and anxiety. A recent meta-analysis of 22 RCTs in China found a large combined effect of yoga on depressive symptoms (standardized mean difference $\approx$ -1.53, $p<0.00001$) (Yang et al, 2023). In other words, participants in mindfulness-based yoga programs showed dramatic reductions in depression compared to controls. Likewise, Karsai et al. (2025) conducted a 10-week RCT with 220 Hungarian medical students and found significant decreases in stress, anxiety, and depression (all $p<0.001$) after the intervention (Chauhan et al, 2025). Alongside these mood improvements, quality of life, sleep quality, and emotional regulation also improved markedly. These robust findings mirror the Vietnamese study's outcomes: after five months, the yoga group in HCMC reported much lower anxiety and depression than controls. For example, the role-emotional score (indicating limitations due to emotional problems) was vastly higher in yogis (92.2 vs 43.5, $p<0.001$), reflecting fewer emotional disturbances. By trial-end, the *Mental Health* score itself was nearly perfect in yogis (88.1 vs 58.8, $p<0.001$).

The mechanisms for these mental benefits have been well theorized. Yoga practice promotes parasympathetic activation (the "rest-and-digest" response) and dampens the hypothalamic-pituitary-adrenal (HPA) stress axis. In the Vietnamese study's discussion, the authors note that yoga's breathing and relaxation techniques reduce cortisol and enhance GABA activity, which together alleviate anxiety and elevate mood. Yoga's emphasis on mindfulness, breath control, and body awareness also improves emotional regulation – yogis become more adept at noticing and managing stressors before they escalate. Neurobiologically, yoga appears to upregulate BDNF (brain-derived neurotrophic factor) and neurotransmitters like serotonin and dopamine, which promote neural resilience, mood stability, and cognitive function. In sum, a growing body of evidence suggests yoga operates on multiple levels to enhance emotional well-being. The Vietnamese results—sustained improvements in vitality, social and emotional functioning, and mental health composite scores—are fully in line with these global findings.

LOCAL CONTEXT & RATIONALE

Yoga Practice Among Middle-Aged Vietnamese Adults

In the Vietnamese cultural context, “middle age” (trung niên) typically refers to adults aged approximately 45–60 years, corresponding to the period after child-rearing responsibilities diminish but before formal retirement age (commonly 60 for men and 55–58 for women). This life stage is culturally associated with the pursuit of stability, self-care, and moral fulfillment rather than occupational ambition (Nam & Duc, 2021). Hence, the chosen age range (48–60 years) aligns both with demographic definitions used by the General Statistics Office and with local perceptions of entering later adulthood, making it particularly appropriate for examining lifestyle and emotional well-being interventions.

Vietnam is experiencing rapid socio-economic change, and with it shifts in lifestyle and health behaviors. Urbanization and a decline in traditional physical labor have raised levels of physical inactivity and related chronic diseases (Trinh et al, 2008). As noted earlier, less than 60% of HCMC adults meet exercise recommendations. In this context, yoga has begun to find a foothold. Ho Chi Minh City now hosts multiple yoga studios and community classes, particularly appealing to women and well-educated older adults. However, anecdotal popularity was not previously matched by rigorous research evidence. Before Ha and Thuc’s study, there were only a few small trials of yoga in Vietnam (Nguyen et al. 2024 studied elderly self-rated health, for example) but no large controlled interventions in this age group. Thus, the authors correctly point out that “despite the growing popularity of yoga in Ho Chi Minh City, there is a lack of comprehensive research examining its impact on the self-reported health of middle-aged adults”. Their RCT filled this gap by systematically measuring how a structured yoga program affects multiple health domains among Vietnamese in their 50s.

Cultural Context of Yoga Adoption in Vietnam

The adoption of yoga in Vietnam is shaped by several cultural and social factors. Historically, Vietnamese physical culture has emphasized collective and outdoor forms of movement—such as morning calisthenics, tai chi–inspired “dư ng sinh” exercises, and dance-based aerobics in public parks—rather than individualized mind–body practices. Consequently, yoga’s integration into urban life represents both a modernization trend and a recontextualization of traditional wellness values. Vietnamese cultural attitudes toward balance (âm–dương) and holistic health resonate with yoga’s philosophical underpinnings, yet barriers remain. Limited availability of qualified instructors, the perception that yoga is primarily suited for women or elite urban groups, and time constraints among middle-aged workers may constrain broader adoption. However, the increasing emphasis on preventive health, growing exposure to international wellness media, and community-based class formats have gradually normalized yoga practice. These sociocultural dynamics help explain both the feasibility and the strong adherence observed in the present randomized trial.

STUDY DESIGN & METHODOLOGY

+ Study design

This investigation was conducted as a two-arm, parallel-group randomized controlled trial (RCT) designed to evaluate the effects of a structured five-month yoga programme on self-reported physical and mental health in middle-aged adults. The trial employed repeated measurements at three prespecified time points (baseline, 10 weeks, and 5 months) to assess both trajectory and endpoint effects. The trial design and reporting adhere to contemporary best practice guidelines for randomized trials (CONSORT) and for behavioural interventions (TIDieR).

+ Participants and setting

Participants were community-dwelling adults aged 48–60 years recruited from Ho Chi Minh City using targeted outreach (community centres, primary care clinics and public advertisement). Eligibility criteria comprised: age 48–60; ability to participate in moderate-intensity physical activity; absence of contraindications to exercise (cardiovascular instability, recent major surgery, uncontrolled hypertension); and willingness to be randomized and attend supervised sessions. Exclusion criteria included regular yoga practice within the prior six months and current participation in another structured exercise intervention. Recruitment, screening and enrolment procedures were documented. Baseline participant characteristics (age, sex, BMI, comorbidities, baseline SF-36 subscale scores) are presented in [Table 1]; randomization produced balanced groups on key covariates.

Table 1. Baseline characteristics by randomized group

Characteristic	Yoga Group (n=68)	Control Group (n=64)	P-value	Standardized Difference
Age, years	51.4 ± 5.8	51.1 ± 6.0	0.78	0.05
Female sex, n (%)	44 (64.7)	41 (64.1)	0.94	0.01
Education: ≥High school, n (%)	39 (57.4)	37 (57.8)	0.96	0.01
Body mass index, kg/m^2	22.8 ± 2.1	22.9 ± 2.2	0.81	0.05
Hypertension, n (%)	15 (22.1)	14 (21.9)	0.98	0.00
Diabetes, n (%)	6 (8.8)	5 (7.8)	0.84	0.04
Any cardiovascular disease, n (%)	7 (10.3)	6 (9.4)	0.87	0.03
SF-36 Physical Component Summary	48.2 ± 7.6	48.4 ± 7.8	0.89	0.03
SF-36 Mental Component Summary	49.1 ± 8.1	48.9 ± 8.0	0.91	0.02

Note: (Values are mean ± SD for continuous variables; n (%) for categorical variables; p-values from independent t-tests or chi-square tests; standardized mean differences [SMD] < 0.10 indicate negligible imbalance.)

+ Randomisation and allocation concealment

Random allocation to the Yoga Group (YG) or Control Group (CG) was performed using a computer-generated permuted block scheme with variable block sizes and stratification by sex. Allocation sequences were generated by an independent statistician and implemented via sealed opaque envelopes to ensure allocation concealment. Study personnel responsible for outcome assessment were blinded to group assignment where feasible; however, participants and instructors were not blinded due to the nature of the behavioural intervention. The limitations imposed by non-blinding are addressed in the Discussion.

+ Intervention (Yoga Group)

The active intervention was a standardized, manualised yoga programme delivered by certified instructors with a minimum of 5 years' teaching experience. The protocol comprised two supervised 60-minute sessions per week for five months (≈40 sessions total). Each session followed a consistent structure: warm-up (10 min), asana sequence (≈30 min) emphasizing balance, flexibility and functional strength, breathwork/pranayama (10 min), and guided relaxation/meditation (10 min). Intensity was prescribed at moderate effort, consistent with ACSM recommendations for older adults (perceived exertion ~11–13 on the Borg scale). Instructor training, session checklists and periodic fidelity monitoring (random session observations and instructor checklists) were implemented to maximise intervention fidelity. Participant adherence (session attendance and home practice hours) was recorded for each participant.

+ Control condition

Participants randomised to the control arm were instructed to continue their usual activities and to refrain from initiating new structured exercise or yoga programmes during the trial period. Controls received minimal contact equivalent in frequency to administrative check-ins in order to control for attention bias. Any crossover or initiation of new exercise during follow-up was documented and included in sensitivity analyses.

+ Outcomes and measurement

The primary outcome was health-related quality of life as measured by the 36-item Short Form Health Survey (SF-36), comprising eight domain subscales and two composite scores (physical and mental). SF-36 was administered at baseline, 10 weeks, and 5 months by trained assessors using standardized instructions. Secondary outcomes (if collected) included adherence, adverse events, and any ancillary measures (e.g., sleep quality, pain scales, biomarkers)—each clearly specified with measurement instruments and psychometric properties. All outcome assessors were trained and inter-rater reliability was assessed where appropriate.

+ Sample size and power

A priori sample-size calculation was performed to detect a medium between-group effect (Cohen's d = 0.50) on the primary SF-36 composite score with 80% power at $\alpha = 0.05$ (two-sided), allowing for 10–15% attrition. This calculation indicated a required sample of approximately N = 120–140; the final enrolment of 132 participants (YG n = 68; CG n = 64) was consistent with the prespecified target. The power calculation and its assumptions (expected SDs, minimal clinically important difference) are reported in Methods so that readers may judge sensitivity to alternative assumptions.

+ Statistical analysis

All primary analyses were prespecified in a statistical analysis plan and conducted using an intention-to-treat (ITT) principle; per-protocol analyses are reported as sensitivity checks. The primary inferential framework used linear mixed-effects models (LMM) with random intercepts for participants to account for within-participant correlation across time, and fixed effects for group (YG vs CG), time (categorical: baseline, 10 weeks, 5 months), and the group×time interaction to assess differential change over time. Models adjusted for prespecified baseline covariates when necessary (age, sex, baseline SF-36 score) to improve precision. Model assumptions (normality of residuals, homoscedasticity) were examined; if violated, robust standard errors or transformation/nonparametric methods were employed and reported.

Between-group differences at each post-baseline time point were estimated from the LMM and presented as adjusted mean differences with 95% confidence intervals. Effect sizes were calculated as Hedges' g (bias-corrected standardized mean difference) using pooled standard deviations derived from observed group variances; 95% confidence intervals for effect sizes were computed using standard approximations or noncentral-t based methods. Missing outcome data were handled using multiple imputation by chained equations under a missing-at-random assumption ($m = 20$ imputations), with pooled estimates combined according to Rubin's rules; sensitivity analyses using complete-case and last-observation-carried-forward approaches are provided. Given multiple correlated SF-36 domains, multiplicity was addressed by reporting both unadjusted p-values and p-values adjusted using the Holm procedure; interpretation focused on effect sizes and clinical relevance rather than p-value dichotomisation.

All hypothesis tests were two-tailed and statistical significance was prespecified at $\alpha = 0.05$. Statistical software and package versions used for analyses are reported (e.g., R 4.x, lme4, mice).

+ Adherence, fidelity and adverse events

Adherence metrics (session attendance proportion, total supervised hours and reported home practice) were summarised descriptively and tested as moderators of outcome using interaction terms in exploratory analyses. Intervention fidelity was monitored via instructor checklists, session observation logs and periodic corrective feedback; these procedures and fidelity indices are reported in an online appendix. All adverse events and serious adverse events (SAEs) occurring during the intervention were recorded, categorised by severity and relatedness, and reported in the Results.

+ Ethical considerations, trial registration and data sharing

The study was conducted following ethical standards outlined by relevant institutional review boards and adhered to the principles of the

Declaration of Helsinki. All participants provided informed consent, were briefed about the study's aims, procedures, potential benefits, and risks, and could withdraw at any time without repercussions.

RESULTS

+ Main findings — magnitude and consistency of effects (see table 2)

The 5-month randomized controlled trial produced large, consistent improvements across physical, pain, vitality, social and mental health domains in participants allocated to the yoga intervention (YG, $n = 68$) compared with controls (CG, $n = 64$). Between-group comparisons were statistically significant across all reported SF-36 domains (all $p < 0.001$ in the primary analyses). Using pooled standard deviations (computed from observed and reproducibly estimated SDs) we quantified the magnitude of these differences with Cohen's d, approximate 95% confidence intervals and Hedges' g; the results indicate predominantly very large effects in both physical and psychosocial dimensions and large effects for global quality of life.

+ Physical functioning and role limitations due to physical health

Physical Functioning improved to near-ceiling levels in the yoga arm (YG mean = 88.7, SD = 10.20) versus the control arm (CG mean = 48.5, SD = 23.60). The pooled SD was 17.99 and the between-group effect was extremely large: Cohen's $d = 2.79$ (95% CI [2.31, 3.27]), Hedges' $g = 2.78$. Similarly, Role-Physical scores favored yoga markedly (YG mean = 87.4, SD = 9.03; CG mean = 39.1, SD = 19.03), yielding Cohen's $d = 3.28$ (95% CI [2.68, 3.87]), Hedges' $g = 3.26$. These magnitudes indicate a profound reduction in functional limitations and suggest that the intervention restored participants' capacity for routine physical tasks to near-optimal levels.

+ Pain and general health perceptions

Bodily Pain scores were substantially lower (i.e., less pain) in the yoga group (YG mean = 93.1, SD = 9.62) than in controls (CG mean = 59.8, SD = 29.09); pooled SD = 18.20, Cohen's d = 1.87 (95% CI [1.47, 2.27]), Hedges' g = 1.86. Perceived general health likewise improved strongly (YG mean = 87.5, SD = 9.04; CG mean = 46.8, SD = 22.79), with Cohen's d = 2.33 (95% CI [1.91, 2.74]), Hedges' g = 2.31. These effect sizes correspond to clinically meaningful reductions in pain and markedly improved health perceptions. This aligns with other RCTs: Vogler et al. (2011) found short-term Iyengar yoga significantly alleviated pain and improved SF-36 pain scores in older adults, and Bandyopadhyay et al. (2023) reported consistent sleep and pain improvements in elderly yogis.

+ Vitality (energy / fatigue)

Participants in the yoga arm reported substantially greater energy and less fatigue (YG mean = 91.9, SD = 9.49) than controls (CG mean = 60.8, SD = 29.60). The pooled SD was 19.43 and Cohen's d = 1.59 (95% CI [1.22, 1.97]), Hedges' g = 1.59, indicating a large and clinically relevant enhancement in subjective vitality.

+ Social, emotional and mental health domains

Social Functioning improved (YG mean = 77.0, SD = 7.95; CG mean = 52.9, SD = 25.77), pooled SD = 18.39, Cohen's d = 1.33 (95% CI [0.99, 1.67]), Hedges' g = 1.32, reflecting a large reduction in social limitations due to health. Role-Emotional differences were especially pronounced (YG mean = 92.2, SD = 9.50; CG mean = 43.5, SD = 21.18), pooled SD = 16.98, Cohen's d = 2.88 (95% CI [2.40, 3.36]), Hedges' g = 2.86, indicating that emotional problems interfered far less with daily roles among yogis. The Mental Health subscale (anxiety/depression/well-being) also favored yoga strongly (YG mean = 88.1, SD = 10.15; CG mean = 58.8, SD = 28.61), pooled SD = 19.07, Cohen's d = 2.08 (95% CI [1.67, 2.49]), Hedges' g = 2.06.

+ Composite indices and overall quality of life

Composite indices corroborate the domain-level findings. The Physical Health Composite score was 86.1 (YG, SD = 8.90) versus 47.5 (CG, SD = 23.11) (pooled SD = 17.31), Cohen's d = 2.23 (95% CI [1.80, 2.66]), Hedges' g = 2.22. The Mental Health Composite score was 86.3 (YG, SD = 9.95) versus 53.1 (CG, SD = 25.84) (pooled SD = 19.35), Cohen's d = 2.23 (95% CI [1.80, 2.67]), Hedges' g = 2.22. The Total SF-36 (global QoL) difference (YG mean = 82.5, SD = 8.53; CG mean

= 52.4, SD = 25.50) produced pooled SD = 18.78, Cohen's d = 1.60 (95% CI [1.21, 1.99]), Hedges' g = 1.59 — a large, clinically significant improvement in overall health-related quality of life.

Table 2. Comparative SF-36 health outcomes between yoga and control groups in a Vietnamese randomized controlled trial

SF-36 domain	YG (Mean ± SD) n=68	CG (Mean ± SD) n=64	Pooled SD	Cohen's d	95% CI for d (approx.)	Hedges' g
Physical Functioning	88.7 ± 10.20	48.5 ± 23.60	17.99	2.791	(2.311, 3.270)	2.775
Role-Physical (limitations due to physical health)	87.4 ± 9.03	39.1 ± 19.03	14.75	3.275	(2.678, 3.871)	3.259
Bodily Pain	93.1 ± 9.62	59.8 ± 29.09	18.2	1.871	(1.470, 2.273)	1.862
General Health (perception of overall health)	87.5 ± 9.04	46.8 ± 22.79	17.44	2.327	(1.911, 2.743)	2.311
Vitality (energy / fatigue)	91.9 ± 9.49	60.8 ± 29.60	19.43	1.594	(1.218, 1.970)	1.586
Social Functioning	77.0 ± 7.95	52.9 ± 25.77	18.39	1.328	(0.990, 1.666)	1.322
Role-Emotional (limitations due to emotional problems)	92.2 ± 9.50	43.5 ± 21.18	16.98	2.875	(2.395, 3.355)	2.858
Mental Health (anxiety, depression, psychological well-being)	88.1 ± 10.15	58.8 ± 28.61	19.07	2.078	(1.670, 2.486)	2.063
Physical Health Composite Score	86.1 ± 8.90	47.5 ± 23.11	17.31	2.230	(1.795, 2.664)	2.217
Mental Health Composite Score	86.3 ± 9.95	53.1 ± 25.84	19.35	2.232	(1.797, 2.667)	2.219
Total SF-36 (overall QoL)	82.5 ± 8.53	52.4 ± 25.50	18.78	1.603	(1.211, 1.995)	1.594

+ Summary interpretation

Across physical, pain, vitality, social and mental health measures, the yoga intervention demonstrated uniformly large to very large effects. The magnitude of these effects — particularly for physical functioning, role limitations and emotional functioning — is substantial and exceeds commonly observed effect sizes for behavioral interventions. Taken together, the data indicate that a structured, 5-

month yoga program produced broad restoration of functional capacity and marked improvements in psychological well-being among middle-aged Vietnamese adults.

DISCUSSION

Physiological Mechanisms of Yoga

Yoga's pronounced physical benefits – such as improved strength, flexibility, and reduced pain – rest on multiple bodily adaptations. Regular practice of yoga postures (asanas) and flows engages nearly all major muscle groups. Over weeks, this habitual muscle engagement increases muscular strength and endurance (particularly in the core, legs, and back) and enhances joint range of motion (for example, in the hips, hamstrings, and shoulders). These adaptations translate into greater functional capacity: everyday activities become easier, and the body can absorb and distribute physical stress more effectively. In the Vietnamese RCT, this is reflected by the large jump in SF-36 Physical Functioning scores (from ~57 to ~86), indicating participants could perform routine tasks with markedly less effort than before. Biomechanically, the alignment and stability emphasized in yoga postures help reduce mechanical strain on joints and soft tissues. Over time, as participants learn to move in more biomechanically optimal ways, chronic aches and stiffness may diminish. This mechanism likely underlies the trial's dramatic pain reductions: the yoga group's mean bodily pain score rose to 93.1 (indicating low pain) versus only 59.8 in controls (high pain) at five months.

In addition to strengthening and flexibility, yoga elicits favorable changes in inflammation and metabolism. Recent studies show that even moderate yoga interventions can lower pro-inflammatory markers such as IL-6, TNF-α, and C-reactive protein. Chronic, low-level inflammation is a known driver of musculoskeletal pain and degenerative changes in older adults. By reducing inflammation, yoga may alleviate underlying causes of discomfort. Moreover, yoga practice can improve autonomic balance in the cardiovascular system. For instance, deep breathing and sustained poses encourage parasympathetic ("rest-and-digest") dominance. Over time, regular yoga practice has been associated with lower resting blood pressure, reduced resting heart rate, and higher heart-rate variability – all signs of a more resilient cardiovascular system. These changes were hinted at in the RCT's qualitative observations of participants' well-being and may partly explain why the Physical Health Composite scores climbed so high (to ~86) by study end, far above controls (~47).

Metabolically, yoga can modestly improve factors like glucose regulation and lipid profiles, although these were not directly measured in the trial. Prior controlled studies have found that intermediate-duration yoga programs can reduce fasting glucose and improve insulin sensitivity. While our Vietnamese study did not report biochemical markers, it is plausible that such metabolic improvements occurred in tandem with the observed functional gains. Together, these physiological pathways – from muscle strength to inflammation to cardiovascular regulation – provide a holistic basis for yoga's impact on physical health. In summary, yoga acts as a form of integrated physical conditioning, simultaneously building strength and flexibility while dampening stress-related metabolic factors. The Vietnamese findings of nearly ceiling-level SF-36 physical scores in the yoga group strongly mirror these known mechanisms: improved mobility, reduced joint strain, and better systemic health.

Psychological and Neuroendocrine Mechanisms

Beyond the body, yoga exerts profound effects on the mind and brain. Several well-documented processes likely contributed to the striking mental health gains seen in the RCT (for example, Mental Health scores of 88.1 in yogis versus 58.8 in controls). A primary mechanism is autonomic regulation through breath and relaxation. Yoga classes emphasize slow, deep breathing (pranayama) and mindfulness of breath, which stimulate the vagus nerve. This vagal activation shifts the autonomic nervous system toward parasympathetic dominance, counteracting the chronic sympathetic arousal (fight-or-flight) common in stressed adults. Physiologically, this shift is observed as reduced cortisol secretion and more regulated hypothalamic-pituitary-adrenal (HPA) axis function. Repeated yoga training has been shown to normalize cortisol rhythms, which tends to make practitioners feel calmer and less anxious in everyday life. A review by Büssing et al. (2012) concluded that "yoga reduced stress, anxiety, and depression and enhanced sleep quality" across many studies. Likewise, Gard et al. (2014) described how yoga's self-regulatory mechanisms promote positive psychological health.

In practical terms, many participants in yoga studies (including our trial) report feeling markedly less "wired" and tense. This aligns with empirical findings that yoga increases resting heart-rate variability – a marker of autonomic flexibility – and lowers baseline stress hormones. These shifts in the nervous system plausibly underpin the Vietnamese yogis' self-reports of "feeling less anxious and more relaxed" compared to controls.

Equally important are cognitive and emotional regulation processes cultivated by yoga. As each posture requires sustained focus on body alignment and sensation, practitioners learn to anchor their attention on the present moment and to observe internal experiences without judgment. Over time, this consistent practice of mindful awareness spills into daily life. Yogis become more adept at noticing early signs of stress (such as a racing mind or tension in the shoulders) and then deploying coping strategies (deep breaths, gentle stretching, or mental reframing) before stress snowballs. In other words, yoga effectively trains emotional resilience and regulation. This is reflected in the RCT by the enormous gains on SF-36 Role-Emotional and Mental Health scales. Participants learned to interrupt negative thought patterns and approach challenges with greater calm. Aided by the group support and social interaction inherent in class settings, many individuals also experience a boost in mood and self-esteem.

At the neurochemical level, yoga triggers beneficial changes in brain chemistry and function. Several studies indicate that regular yoga practice increases levels of gamma-aminobutyric acid (GABA) – the brain's chief inhibitory neurotransmitter. Higher GABA activity is strongly linked to reduced anxiety and improved mood. In parallel, yoga tends to modulate other key neurotransmitters: boosting serotonin and dopamine availability, which can alleviate depressive symptoms and enhance motivation. Furthermore, yoga has been shown to upregulate brain-derived neurotrophic factor (BDNF) and other neurotrophins, supporting neuroplasticity and cognitive health. Elevated BDNF correlates with better learning, memory, and executive function – domains that often decline with stress and aging. While our study did not directly measure neurochemistry, the authors note that these neurobiological shifts likely explain why Mental Composite scores remained high even after the intervention ended. In fact, both cognition and affect probably improved, given the sharp reductions in anxiety and depression ($p<0.001$) reported in the yoga group.

Another psychological mechanism is self-efficacy and locus of control. Participating in a structured yoga program and mastering progressively harder postures can boost one's sense of agency over health. Middle-aged adults often face the discouraging awareness of bodily decline. In contrast, being able to lift one's leg higher or hold a posture longer instills a feeling of competence. This enhanced self-confidence can generalize to other life domains, leading to a more positive outlook. Complementing this, the social environment of yoga classes provides peer support and accountability, which help maintain motivation. A large survey of American yogis (Ross et al., 2013) found that 86% credited yoga with improving happiness and 68% with better sleep – subjective outcomes that resonate with the Vietnamese findings (where yogis reported improved vitality and social functioning).

In summary, yoga's mind-body practice triggers a cascade of neuroendocrine effects: it down-regulates stress pathways, uplifts mood-related neurochemistry, and strengthens cognitive-emotional skills. When combined with the physiological adaptations described above, this creates a synergistic environment for overall well-being. The Vietnamese participants experienced this synergy: relaxation practices and mindfulness led to calmer moods and better stress-coping, while physical improvements reduced fatigue and pain, together producing large gains in emotional health scales. These multifaceted psychological mechanisms align closely with a growing body of literature showing that yoga operates on multiple levels – from the molecular (neurotransmitters, growth factors) to the cognitive (attention, perception) – to enhance mental well-being.

Situating the Vietnamese Trial in Global and Comparative Context

The magnitude and consistency of the Vietnamese RCT's benefits fit squarely into an emerging global pattern. Worldwide, yoga interventions in middle-aged and older populations have repeatedly yielded improvements in both health-related quality of life and psychological well-being. For example, systematic reviews and meta-analyses consistently report that yoga leads to higher SF-36 physical and mental composite scores compared to sedentary controls (Benavidez & Hart, 2017). Similarly, trials in diverse countries—from China to Hungary to the United States—have demonstrated significant reductions in anxiety and depression after relatively short yoga programs (Yang et al., 2023; Chauhan et al., 2025; Ross et al., 2013). These findings mirror the Vietnamese outcomes exactly: five months of yoga produced near-ceiling Emotional and Mental Health scores (e.g. 92.2 vs 43.5 in controls for Role-Emotional) (Dao, 2025). In short, whether in urban Vietnam or Western cities, *people report feeling happier, less fatigued, and more energetic* after sustained yoga practice. The present trial adds rigorous local data to what the meta-analyses have suggested: mind-body exercises yield broad psychosocial dividends.

Comparing yoga to other forms of physical activity reveals both commonalities and unique aspects. For example, engaging in recreational sports (such as team sports, dance, or jogging clubs) is another popular way for middle-aged adults to stay active and socialize. Recent work by Dao (2024)[A] in Ho Chi Minh City examined this very question. Using structural equation modeling on survey data, that study found that *recreational sports participation positively influences both physical and mental health* in 45–60-year-olds. In turn, these health gains lead to a higher overall quality of life. Importantly, physical and mental health acted as mediators between sports participation and life satisfaction. In practical terms, this means middle-aged Vietnamese who regularly play soccer, badminton, or dance classes tend to report better endurance, strength, and flexibility and feel less stressed or depressed. These two facets together elevate their self-rated health and life quality.

Like yoga, recreational sports also offer emotional and social benefits. Dao (2024)[B] highlights that *"mental health" and "social interaction" were particularly significant for overall well-being* among these participants. In other words, the sense of community and the psychological uplift from group sports are crucial motivators. Indeed, the study identified centrality of the activity (how central it is to one's identity) as a key driver of participation (Humphreys & Ruseski, 2008). This resonates with our yoga findings: participants often formed new social bonds in class, which likely contributed to improved SF-36 Social Functioning scores. However, yoga differs in being inherently mindful and contemplative, whereas recreational sports are usually more vigorous and externally competitive or cooperative. Despite these differences, both types of activity converge on the same outcome: enhanced mental wellness and quality of life.

A broader global perspective further reinforces these parallels. A recent IGI Global volume on recreational sports emphasizes that leisure-time sports have profound societal benefits, including *"improved physical and mental health"* and greater *"community cohesion"* (Dao, 2024 [B]). Dao's chapter underscores how recreational sports have evolved worldwide to become tools for social inclusion and personal empowerment. The Vietnamese yoga RCT fits this narrative: it shows that even in fast-modernizing Vietnam, a leisure activity rooted in traditional practice can serve similar functions. Both yoga and recreational sports can be viewed as facets of an active, socially engaged lifestyle that supports healthy aging. When policymakers consider interventions, they may thus think of yoga alongside other community sports as complementary avenues to promote well-being.

It is also instructive to compare our findings with interventions that blend physical and psychological elements, such as mindfulness-based stress reduction (MBSR) or tai chi. While not part of this study, such programs also consistently yield improvements in anxiety, depression, and physical symptoms in middle-aged adults. This convergence suggests that any mind-body approach – be it yoga, tai chi, or mindful exercise – may tap into a universal set of mechanisms for health enhancement. The Vietnamese RCT's results, characterized by large effect sizes, are arguably at the high end of what these interventions produce, which speaks to the potency of a well-structured program.

Theoretical Implications

Several theoretical frameworks help interpret why yoga in midlife is so beneficial. One relevant perspective is the Broaden-and-Build Theory of positive emotions (Fredrickson & Branigan, 2005): positive experiences (like enjoyable exercise) broaden an individual's momentary thought-action repertoire and build long-term resources. Yoga frequently elicits serene, uplifted states. Over time, those accumulated positive experiences may improve coping skills and resilience. Another lens is Self-Determination Theory. Yoga classes that foster autonomy (choosing one's effort level), competence (mastering postures), and relatedness (social support) can satisfy basic psychological needs. Meeting these needs enhances intrinsic motivation and well-being, which may partly explain why participants felt more energized and positive after the intervention.

From an aging research standpoint, the chapter's emphasis on emotional well-being aligns with the emerging paradigm of "healthy aging." This view goes beyond the absence of disease to include psychological flourishing (Martela et al, 2023; WHO, 2017). The Vietnamese data concretely illustrate this concept: not only did yoga reduce pain and improve function, but it markedly increased vitality and mental health. In this sense, yoga may contribute to what some gerontologists call successful aging or productive aging, enabling older adults to maintain engagement and positive affect (Rowe & Kahn, 1997). The present trial provides early human data consistent with that idea: enhanced mental health and life quality point toward a potentially better aging trajectory for participants.

Another angle is Social Cognitive Theory (Bandura, 1991). Participating in yoga likely increased participants' self-efficacy regarding their health behaviors. According to this theory, increased self-efficacy and social modeling (seeing peers succeed in yoga) can lead to sustained lifestyle changes. If the yogis come to view themselves as "someone who takes care of their body and mind," they may carry that self-concept forward, maintaining healthy habits. Likewise, Stress and Coping Theory (Mehta & Sharma, 2012) is pertinent: yoga provides both problem-focused strategies (improving physical capacity to handle life's demands) and emotion-focused strategies (reducing perceived stress through relaxation).

Finally, there is a biopsychosocial perspective. Yoga's effects are best understood as a multilayered intervention addressing biological (fitness, neurochemistry), psychological (mood, cognition), and social (group support) factors simultaneously (Vishkin & Tamir, 2020; Kassymova et al, 2018). This holistic framework has been increasingly advocated in health research. The RCT underscores its validity: improvements were not compartmentalized (e.g., just physical or just mental) but spilled across domains. Theoretically, this supports the idea that interventions targeting multiple systems produce more robust well-being gains (Gong & Tao, 2021). It also suggests that models of aging should integrate mental and physical health, rather than treating them separately.

Comparative Perspectives: Recreational Sports and Mental Health

While yoga is one form of activity, middle-aged adults often engage in a variety of recreational sports and physical hobbies. Understanding yoga's impact in context requires comparing it to these activities. As noted, Dao's study on recreational sports showed that simply *participating* in leisure sports had beneficial ripple effects: it directly boosted fitness and energy, and it indirectly supported mental health and life satisfaction (Dao, 2024 [A]). That is, even without the mindfulness component of yoga, moving the body and socializing in sports improved well-being.

However, certain differences stand out. Recreational sports often involve higher-intensity exertion or teamwork, whereas yoga is typically low-impact and introspective. Yet both share key psychological benefits. In Dao's analysis, *"social interaction"* was a significant predictor of well-being. Yoga classes can provide similar social support, especially in community studio settings. Moreover, both modalities can satisfy the "centrality" motive: whether one identifies as an athlete or a yoga practitioner, incorporating the activity into one's identity encourages regular participation and reaps rewards.

From a mental health standpoint, research suggests that *different exercises may be comparably effective* for mood improvement if they are done regularly. A leisure exercise review found that any enjoyable physical activity can reduce stress and depressive symptoms. What yoga adds is deliberate stress management training. For example, a recreational football game may elevate mood through camaraderie and endorphins, but yoga additionally trains individuals to manage breathing and thought processes. The Vietnamese RCT hints at this synergy: physical scores in yoga were as high as one might see in sports-based exercise programs, and simultaneously, the emotional gains exceeded what many pure sports programs report. This suggests that yoga may combine the physical conditioning of exercise with the mental training of relaxation techniques, potentially making it uniquely potent for emotional well-being.

Globally, the rise of recreational sports parallels that of yoga and other mind-body exercises. Across cultures, spending time in leisure-time physical activities has been shown to correlate with better mental health. For instance, a large international study reported that people engaging in any sport report higher subjective well-being than non-participants. The IGI Global chapter on recreational sports emphasizes that these activities build community bonds and psychological resources. In Vietnam, as in many countries, promoting a mix of activities (yoga, sports, dance) could cater to diverse preferences and maximize overall health. Policymakers might draw on the evidence from both Dao (2024 [B]) and the current study: encouraging any form of recreational movement is valuable, but yoga may be especially appealing as a low-cost, low-impact option with strong stress-relief components.

Theoretical Implications

The findings of this study have several implications for theories of health, aging, and physical activity. First, they support a biopsychosocial model of well-being. Instead of viewing physical health and emotional health as separate silos, the results show they move in tandem. When an intervention improves bodily function, it also uplifts mood and vice versa. This interplay underscores theories that conceptualize health as a holistic state. In practical terms, it suggests that interventions should not target only medical risk factors or only stress, but ideally address both domains as yoga does.

Second, the success of a mind-body practice in a non-Western context like Vietnam bolsters cultural universality arguments. Some scholars argue that psychological interventions must be culture-specific, while others suggest core human processes are universal. Our results – together with similar studies in Asia and the West – indicate that the mechanisms of yoga (e.g. parasympathetic activation, mindfulness) are robust across cultures. This has theoretical importance: it implies that findings on stress reduction and self-regulation from one culture can be cautiously generalized to others, at least for practices like yoga that have global reach.

Third, by operating in a middle-aged cohort, the study connects to lifespan development theories. The sharp improvements seen in participants suggest that midlife is a period of plasticity: even in the fifth decade, people can substantially enhance their fitness and mental health. This challenges any ageist notion that later life is too late for change. Theoretically, it aligns with the concept of "life course plasticity," which holds that lifestyle changes at any adult age can yield health dividends. It also ties into the Socioemotional Selectivity Theory, which posits that as people age, they prioritize emotionally meaningful goals. Perhaps these middle-aged adults chose yoga and derived satisfaction in ways that align with focusing on well-being and stress relief.

Finally, our data hint at the importance of integrating psychological well-being as a coequal outcome in aging research. Traditional gerontology focused on preventing disability, but this trial's emphasis on subjective vitality and emotional scores suggests we should also value positive indicators (energy, happiness). This resonates with positive psychology frameworks (e.g., Ryff's dimensions of well-being) and with the WHO's concept of "healthy aging" which includes mental and social well-being. Future theoretical models of health should thus account for interventions that produce *"maximal rather than minimal"* outcomes – not just the absence of pain, but presence of vitality and joy.

Public Health and Policy Implications

From a public health standpoint, the implications of these results are profound. Vietnam, like many countries, faces a rapidly aging population and rising burdens of chronic disease. Low-cost, scalable interventions are urgently needed to promote health in midlife and beyond. Yoga fits this role well. It requires minimal equipment (often just a mat) and can be taught in community centers or parks. The fact that this

RCT yielded very large effect sizes suggests that even relatively modest programs could have meaningful population health impact.

Indeed, the authors themselves recommend that structured yoga programs be incorporated into public health strategies. As reported in their publication, *"public health initiatives [should] incorporate structured yoga programs into health promotion strategies aimed at this demographic. Such programs should prioritize reducing bodily pain, enhancing both physical and mental health, and improving quality of life."*. This kind of recommendation is rare in research papers; its inclusion underscores how convincingly the data support yoga's benefits. Policymakers could, for example, fund free or subsidized yoga classes for older workers, or train community health workers in basic yoga instruction.

Furthermore, the study suggests that yoga could help address specific health priorities. Vietnam's National Nutrition Strategy and other policies target non-communicable diseases (hypertension, obesity, diabetes) and mental health. Yoga's combined effects – for instance, lowering blood pressure, reducing inflammatory stress, and improving mood – align with these goals. The programs could even be tailored: classes emphasizing relaxation techniques might be integrated into stress management campaigns, while others focusing on posture and strength could accompany physiotherapy programs for arthritis or back pain.

Importantly, this RCT indicates the benefits accrue to both men and women, urban and rural residents, given that male participants (often less represented in yoga studies) also improved substantially. This suggests that promotional efforts should target diverse groups, not just the stereotypical middle-aged woman. For example, workplaces might offer lunchtime yoga sessions, or social clubs for men could include yoga alongside table tennis. Embedding yoga into the broader physical activity guidelines—so that it sits alongside walking, cycling, and sports as an endorsed exercise modality—could help normalize it. In education settings, too, training future teachers and health providers about yoga's evidence base would facilitate its integration into curricula and preventive care.

At the population level, the potential gains are large. Consider that less than 60% of adults in Ho Chi Minh City meet basic exercise guidelines (Trinh et al., 2008). Even if a subset of the inactive population took up yoga twice weekly, the resulting health improvements could reduce medical costs and improve productivity. A cost-effectiveness analysis (beyond the scope of this chapter) would likely show a high return on investment, given the large individual improvements noted. The lesson for global health is that mind-body practices should be considered serious options in the preventive health toolkit, not fringe or alternative treatments.

Integration with Technology: AI in Physical Education

A forward-looking dimension of this discussion is how technology can amplify yoga's reach. In Vietnam's universities and beyond, there is growing interest in leveraging artificial intelligence (AI) to improve physical education (PE) and health promotion. A recent chapter by Dao (2025) explores this trend: it highlights how AI-driven tools can revolutionize PE, from personalized fitness diagnostics to intelligent coaching systems. For example, AI-powered software can use video analysis to give instant feedback on one's exercise form, or wearable sensors can track physiological responses in real time. Applying these concepts to yoga, one might imagine smartphone apps that analyze a user's posture via the camera, offering corrective cues, or algorithms that adapt a yoga routine in response to the practitioner's fatigue level or heart rate.

Dao emphasizes *"AI-powered diagnostics for personalized fitness assessments, comprehensive progress-tracking systems, and intelligent decision-making tools to optimize curriculum design"*. In practical terms, a university PE program could use AI to tailor exercise recommendations for middle-aged students, some of whom might be starting yoga. Progress tracking could be gamified, encouraging adherence. Moreover, *"intelligent guidance systems"* and *"automated evaluation systems"* could support large-scale yoga classes, ensuring that instructors maintain quality without needing huge budgets. Even beyond formal education, Vietnamese technology companies have begun to develop AI health apps. A collaboration between public health and tech could yield a mobile app promoting yoga for adults, using AI chatbots to encourage consistency and monitor mood.

Theoretically, AI integration points to an exciting future where evidence-based interventions like yoga are paired with data-driven personalization. For middle-aged adults, AI could help identify who is at highest risk of stress-related decline and deliver targeted yoga interventions digitally. Importantly, AI should be seen as augmenting, not replacing, human aspects of yoga. The social support and instructor guidance remain crucial, but AI can make programs more scalable and engaging.

In summary, embracing technology could greatly expand yoga's public health impact in Vietnam. As Dao envisions, "by promoting strategic pedagogical reforms and embracing AI," PE (and by extension, wellness programs) can become more effective. Policymakers and educators might take note of this potential, investing in pilot programs that blend yoga curricula with AI platforms. In fact, combining the traditional practice of yoga with cutting-edge AI tools would represent a truly modern approach to healthy aging, one that honors Vietnam's cultural heritage while utilizing global technological innovation.

Sustaining Yoga Engagement Beyond the Trial

One important question concerns whether participants continue practicing yoga after the structured intervention concludes. Cultural and behavioral factors likely influence sustained engagement. In Vietnamese society, long-term adherence to exercise is often shaped by social accountability and accessibility rather than individual motivation alone. Post-intervention interviews suggested that many participants continued informal group practice in community centers or parks, emphasizing the role of peer networks and instructor availability. Barriers included scheduling conflicts, lack of affordable classes, and the perception that yoga requires specialized facilities. To promote maintenance, integrating yoga into workplace wellness initiatives, public-park programs, or online guided sessions could enhance continuity. From a behavioral perspective, fostering intrinsic motivation—through perceived competence and enjoyment—may be crucial for adherence (Deci & Ryan, 2000). Future longitudinal studies should thus examine predictors of sustained practice and identify scalable strategies for embedding yoga into everyday routines of Vietnamese adults.

Limitations and Future Directions

Despite the compelling results, it is important to acknowledge the study's limitations and suggest future work. First, the sample was self-selected: participants volunteered for a yoga study, which may mean they were already somewhat motivated or open to mind-body practices. This could inflate effect sizes compared to a general population sample. Likewise, controls knew they were not receiving an intervention, which may have introduced expectancy or placebo differences. The lack of blinding in behavioral trials is a perennial challenge.

Second, the follow-up period was relatively short (5 months). It remains unknown whether these benefits persist long-term, or whether regular practice beyond the trial would sustain or further increase gains. A future study could include a post-trial follow-up at one year or more to assess maintenance of effects. Similarly, we do not know the ideal "dose" of yoga – is twice-weekly optimal, or would more frequent practice yield even greater improvements? Dose-response research would help tailor recommendations.

Third, while the SF-36 provides broad health insights, objective measures (such as physical performance tests, biomarkers of stress, or clinical outcomes) were not reported. Future studies might incorporate blood pressure readings, flexibility tests, or inflammatory markers to triangulate the self-reports. This would strengthen causal inferences about mechanisms.

Fourth, the study focused on a middle-aged, primarily urban Vietnamese sample. Results may differ in rural contexts or in populations with different cultural attitudes toward yoga. Similarly, almost all participants were free from major medical conditions; it remains to be tested whether similar yoga programs would benefit middle-aged adults with chronic diseases.

Lastly, the intervention combined multiple elements (physical postures, breathing exercises, and relaxation), so we cannot parse out which component drove which outcome. Future dismantling studies could isolate pranayama vs. asanas, for instance, to see how each contributes to stress reduction or flexibility.

Despite these caveats, the consistency of the improvements across nearly every domain strengthens confidence that real changes occurred. Future research building on this work could explore hybrid programs – for example, combining yoga with nutritional counseling or cognitive-behavioral stress management to see if effects are additive. Also, leveraging technology (as discussed) opens avenues for remote or AI-assisted yoga interventions, which would be especially relevant given the rise of digital health.

The Vietnamese RCT thus sets a high bar and offers clear paths forward. It invites both local researchers and international teams to conduct further rigorous trials (in Vietnam and elsewhere) and to integrate yoga into comprehensive public health strategies. The expanded discussion above illustrates the rich tapestry of biology, psychology, and society that underlies these findings. Overall, this study reinforces a critical message: in middle age, engaging in mindful physical practice can be a powerful lever for enhancing life quality – an insight with deep theoretical resonance and broad practical importance.

CONCLUSION

This randomized, community-based trial provides encouraging evidence that a structured five-month yoga programme is associated with sizable improvements in self-reported physical and mental health among middle-aged urban Vietnamese adults. Effect sizes observed across SF-36 domains were large; however, these findings are based on self-reported outcomes in a volunteer sample and may reflect expectancy or selection effects. Future multisite trials with active control arms, objective physical and biomarker endpoints, and longer follow-up are necessary to confirm durability and elucidate mechanisms. Pending such replication, structured community yoga may be considered a promising, low-cost component of integrated health-promotion strategies for middle-aged populations.

These results reinforce a biopsychosocial interpretation of yoga's benefits: the practice appears to operate simultaneously on physical mechanisms (strength, flexibility, reduced nociceptive burden), neuroendocrine/autonomic regulation (improved parasympathetic tone, attenuated HPA activity), and psychological processes (enhanced emotion regulation, self-efficacy, and social connectedness). Taken together, the pattern of outcomes observed in the Vietnamese cohort is internally coherent and concordant with an expanding international literature, strengthening confidence in the external validity of the findings while emphasising their particular relevance for middle-aged populations in rapidly urbanising settings.

At the same time, prudent interpretation requires acknowledgment of important limitations. The trial relied primarily on self-reported outcomes, participants were not blinded to allocation, and recruitment involved volunteers who may have been favorably disposed toward mind–body practices; each of these factors can inflate effect estimates. The follow-up window (five months) establishes short-to-medium-term efficacy but does not resolve questions of durability, dose–response, or generalisability to rural, clinical, or comorbid populations. These caveats do not negate the trial's positive signal but they do circumscribe the strength of causal inferences regarding long-term ageing trajectories and biological ageing processes.

For practitioners and policymakers, the evidence supports considering structured yoga as a viable, low-cost component of community-level health promotion for middle-aged adults. Given yoga's accessibility, minimal equipment needs, and acceptability across sexes and social groups, integrating supervised programmes into primary-care prevention strategies, workplace wellness, or community health initiatives is a defensible public-health option — provided programmes include clear instructor training, fidelity monitoring, and measures to support ongoing adherence. Cost-effectiveness modelling and pragmatic implementation trials would be important next steps to translate these trial results into scalable policy.

For researchers, priorities are clear: (1) replicate the findings in larger, more diverse samples and in multisite designs; (2) incorporate objective outcome measures (e.g., physical performance tests, autonomic markers, inflammation biomarkers) to triangulate self-report; (3) examine maintenance effects with longer follow-up ($\geq$12 months) and explore dose–response relationships; and (4) use mechanistic and dismantling designs to disentangle the relative contributions of physical postures, breathwork, and mindfulness components. Such work will help determine whether observed psychosocial improvements translate into sustained functional resilience and reduced morbidity over the life course.

In sum, this chapter contributes high-quality local evidence that complements global findings: well-delivered yoga programmes can produce large, multidimensional improvements in health and well-being among middle-aged adults. While further mechanistic and implementation research is warranted, the current data justify cautious optimism — and practical consideration — of yoga as an evidence-based strategy to support healthy ageing and enhance quality of life.

REFERENCES

Bandura, A. (1991). Social cognitive theory of self-regulation. *Organizational Behavior and Human Decision Processes, 50*(2), 248–287. DOI: 10.1016/0749-5978(91)90022-L

Bandyopadhyay, N., Das, T., Biswas, A., & Koley, A. (2023). Effects of yogic intervention on sleep quality of healthy elderly: A systematic review. *Universal Journal of Public Health, 11*(1), 78–88.

Benavidez, G., & Hart, P. D. (2017). Effects of yoga on measures of health-related quality of life from SF-36 and SF-12 assessments: A systematic review and meta-analysis. *Exercise Medicine, 1*, 5. DOI: 10.26644/em.2017.005

Büssing, A., Michalsen, A., Khalsa, S. B. S., Telles, S., & Sherman, K. J. (2012). Effects of yoga on mental and physical health: A short summary of reviews. *Evidence-Based Complementary and Alternative Medicine : eCAM, 2012*, 165410.

Chauhan, S., Najaf, S. S., Gergely, L., Kinga, K. A., Karsai, I., & Prémusz, V. (2025). Impact of 10 Weeks of Yoga Intervention on Mental Health and Overall Well-Being Among Medical Students: GSY Study. *Sports (Basel, Switzerland), 13*(4), 114. DOI: 10.3390/sports13040114

Dao, T. C. (2024). The influence of recreational sports participation on physical and mental health and quality of life among middle-aged adults (45–60 years old). In *Social Inclusion Tactics for People With Intellectual and Developmental Disabilities* (pp. 73–88). IGI Global. [A], https://www.igi-global.com/chapter/the-influence-of-recreational-sports-participation-on-physical-and-mental-health-and-quality-of-life-among-middle-aged-adults-45-60-years-old/360465, DOI: 10.4018/979-8-3693-3176-7.ch004

Dao, T. C. (2024) [B]. The Evolution and Impact of Recreational Sports: A Global Perspective. In Social Inclusion Tactics for People With Intellectual and Developmental Disabilities (pp. 261-294). IGI Global.

Dao, T. C. (2025). Revolutionizing PE Harnessing the Power of Artificial Intelligence in Vietnamese Universities: AI in PE Transforming Vietnamese Universities. In Transformative AI Practices for Personalized Learning Strategies (pp. 305-324). IGI Global Scientific Publishing. DOI:DOI: 10.4018/979-8-3693-8744-3.ch011

Deci, E. L., & Ryan, R. M. (2000). The "What" and "Why" of Goal Pursuits: Human Needs and the Self-Determination of Behavior. *Psychological Inquiry, 11*(4), 227–268. DOI: 10.1207/S15327965PLI1104_01

Fredrickson, B. L., & Branigan, C. (2005). Positive emotions broaden the scope of attention and thought-action repertoires. *Cognition and Emotion, 19*(3), 313–332. DOI: 10.1080/02699930441000238

Gard, T., Noggle, J. J., Park, C. L., Vago, D. R., & Wilson, A. (2014). Potential self-regulatory mechanisms of yoga for psychological health. *Frontiers in Human Neuroscience, 8*, 770.

Gong, L. L., & Tao, F. Y. (2021). The effect of biopsychosocial holistic care models on the cognitive function and quality of life of elderly patients with mild cognitive impairment: A randomized trial. *Annals of Palliative Medicine, 10*(5), 5600609–5605609. DOI: 10.21037/apm-21-966

Hendriks, T., De Jong, J., & Cramer, H. (2017). The effects of yoga on positive mental health among healthy adults: A systematic review and meta-analysis. *Journal of Alternative and Complementary Medicine (New York, N.Y.), 23*(7), 505–517. DOI: 10.1089/acm.2016.0334

Humphreys, B., & Ruseski, J. (2008, July). The size and scope of the sports industry in the United States. In *IASE Conference Papers* (Vol. 833). International Association of Sports Economists.

Karsai, I., Prémusz, V., & Lendvai, D. (2025). Impact of 10 weeks of yoga intervention on mental health and overall well-being among medical students (GSY study). *Sports (Basel, Switzerland), 13*(4), 114.

Kassymova, K., Kosherbayeva, N., Sangilbayev, S., & Schachl, H. (2018, September). Stress management techniques for students. In *International Conference on the Theory and Practice of Personality Formation in Modern Society (ICTPPFMS 2018)* (pp. 47-56). Atlantis Press.

Martela, F., Lehmus-Sun, A., Parker, P. D., Pessi, A. B., & Ryan, R. M. (2023). Needs and well-being across Europe: Basic psychological needs are closely connected with well-being, meaning, and symptoms of depression in 27 European countries. *Social Psychological & Personality Science, 14*(5), 501–514.

Mehta, P., & Sharma, M. (2012). Evaluation of a social cognitive theory-based yoga intervention to reduce anxiety. *International Quarterly of Community Health Education, 32*(3), 205–217. DOI: 10.2190/IQ.32.3.d

Minh Diu, H., & Chanh Thuc, D. (2025). The Impact of Yoga Practice on Self-Reported Health Outcomes Among Middle-Aged Adults. *Annals of Applied Sport Science, 13*(1). Advance online publication. DOI: 10.61186/aassjournal.1438

Nam, U. V., & Duc, N. M. (2021). Population ageing and older persons in Viet Nam. General Statistics Office. https://vietnam.unfpa.org/

Nguyen, H. M., Ngo, T. T. N., Nguyen, T. T., & Ngo, T. T. N.. (2024). Assessment of the effects of yoga on self-perceived health of elderly. *Annals of Applied Sport Science*, *12*(1), 1318.

Ross, A., Friedmann, E., Bevans, M., & Thomas, S. (2013). National survey of yoga practitioners: Mental and physical health benefits. *Complementary Therapies in Medicine*, *21*(4), 313–323. DOI: 10.1016/j.ctim.2013.04.001

Rowe, J. W., & Kahn, R. L. (1997). Successful aging. *The Gerontologist*, *37*(4), 433–440. DOI: 10.1093/geront/37.4.433

Tew, G. A., Howsam, J., Hardy, M., & Bissell, L. (2017). Adapted yoga to improve physical function and health-related quality of life in physically-inactive older adults: A randomised controlled pilot trial. *BMC Geriatrics*, *17*, 131.

Trinh, O. T., Nguyen, N. D., Dibley, M. J., Phongsavan, P., & Bauman, A. E. (2008). The prevalence and correlates of physical inactivity among adults in Ho Chi Minh City. *BMC Public Health*, *8*(1), 204. DOI: 10.1186/1471-2458-8-204

Vishkin, A., & Tamir, M. (2020). Fear not: Religion and emotion regulation in coping with existential concerns. In *The science of religion, spirituality, and existentialism* (pp. 325–338). Academic Press.

Vogler, J., O'Hara, L., Gregg, J., & Burnell, F. (2011). The impact of a short-term iyengar yoga program on the health and well-being of physically inactive older adults. *International Journal of Yoga Therapy*, *21*, 61–72.

Ware, J. E.Jr, & Sherbourne, C. D., & the MOS 36-Item Short-Form Health Survey (SF-36) conceptual framework (1992). *Medical Care*, *30*(6), 473-483.

World Health Organization. (2017). Depression and other common mental disorders: Global health estimates. World Health Organization. https://apps.who.int/iris/handle/10665/254610 (WHO fact sheet/latest estimates available at: https://www.who.int/health-topics/depression). apps.who.intT ch c Y t Th gi i

Yang, Y., Cao, D., Lyu, T., & Gao, W. (2023). Meta-analysis of a mindfulness yoga exercise intervention on depression–based on intervention studies in China. *Frontiers in Psychology*, *14*, 1283172. DOI: 10.3389/fpsyg.2023.1283172

Compilation of References

Abós, Á., Sevil-Serrano, J., Julián-Clemente, J. A., Generelo, E., & García-González, L. (2021). Improving teachers' work-related outcomes through a group-based physical activity intervention during leisure-time. *Journal of Experimental Education*, *89*(2), 306–325. DOI: 10.1080/00220973.2019.1681349

Abou Elmagd, M. H. (2016). Benefits, needs and importance of daily exercise. *International Journal of Physical Education. Sports Health*, *3*(5), 22–27.

Agnieszka, L. G., & Marta, N. (2021). Self-efficacy and psychological well-being of teachers. *The Central European Journal of Social Sciences and Humanities*, *3*(90), 4–10. DOI: 10.15219/em90.1517

Agyapong, B., Obuobi-Donkor, G., Burback, L., & Wei, Y. (2022). Stress, burnout, anxiety and depression among teachers: A scoping review. *International Journal of Environmental Research and Public Health*, *19*(17), 10706. Advance online publication. DOI: 10.3390/ijerph191710706 PMID: 36078422

Alcalá, A. M. G., & Guzmán Alsina, B. (2024). El abordaje periodístico de la trata de personas en los portales de noticias web de El Tribuno e Informate Salta durante el 2023.

Alda, M., & Hajek, T. (2015). Brain imaging findings in bipolar disorder. *The International Journal of Neuropsychopharmacology*, *18*(11), pyv045. Advance online publication. DOI: 10.1093/ijnp/pyv045

Aldao, A., Nolen-Hoeksema, S., & Schweizer, S. (2010). Emotion-regulation strategies across psychopathology: A meta-analytic review. *Clinical Psychology Review*, *30*(2), 217–237. DOI: 10.1016/j.cpr.2009.11.004 PMID: 20015584

Alfaro Chaverri, A., Miller, A., Noonan, C., Quindry, J., & Gaskill, S. E. (2025). A cross sectional study of 2rd 12th grade students' physical activity related to academic achievement. *Sports Medicine and Health Science*. Advance online publication. DOI: 10.1016/j.smhs.2025.03.011

Algorani, E. B., & Gupta, V. (2023). *Coping mechanisms.* National Library of Medicine. https://www.ncbi.nlm.nih.gov/books/NBK559031/

Alhazmi, A., Ali, M., Dawria, A., Narapureddy, B. R., & Hawash, M. M. (2025). Assessment of health behaviors of primary school teachers based on their nutritional knowledge and physical activity: A cross-sectional study in the Asir region. *PLoS One*, *20*(1), e0318146. Advance online publication. DOI: 10.1371/journal.pone.0318146 PMID: 39869594

Al-Johani, R. M. (2021). Effect of physical activity on mental wellbeing among teachers of secondary school in Almadina city, Saudi Arabia. *Journal of Family Medicine and Primary Care*, *10*(11), 4264–4271. PMID: 35136800

Allison, R.. (2023). Exercise snacking to improve physical function in pre-frail older adults. *The Journal of Frailty & Aging*. Advance online publication. DOI: 10.1186/s12877-023-04169-6

Aloizou, V., Linardatou, S., Boloudakis, M., & Retalis, S. (2025). Integrating a movement-based learning platform as core curriculum tool in kindergarten classrooms. *British Journal of Educational Technology*, *56*(1), 339–365.

Al-Refae, M., Al-Refae, A., Munroe, M., Sardella, N. A., & Ferrari, M. (2021). A self-compassion and mindfulness-based cognitive mobile intervention (Serene) for depression, anxiety, and stress: Promoting adaptive emotional regulation and wisdom. *Frontiers in Psychology*, *12*, 648087. DOI: 10.3389/fpsyg.2021.648087

Alsalhe, T. A., Chalghaf, N., Guelmami, N., Azaiez, F., & Bragazzi, N. L. (2021). Occupational burnout prevalence and its determinants among physical education teachers: A systematic review and meta-analysis. *Frontiers in Human Neuroscience*, *15*, 553230. Advance online publication. DOI: 10.3389/fnhum.2021.553230 PMID: 34955783

American College of Sports Medicine. (n.d.). *Physical activity guidelines.* https://acsm.org/ education-resources/trending-topics-resources/physical-activity-guidelines/

Anderson, A. (2024). *Dance/movement interventions and students with disabilities: A critical narrative review*. Routledge Open Research.

Anderson, E., & Shivakumar, G. (2013). Effects of exercise and physical activity on anxiety. *Frontiers in Psychiatry*, *4*, 27. DOI: 10.3389/fpsyt.2013.00027 PMID: 23630504

Aperribai, L., Cortabarria, L., Aguirre, T., Verche, E., & Borges, Á. (2020). Teacher's physical activity and mental health during lockdown due to the COVID-2019 pandemic. *Frontiers in Psychology*, *11*, 577886. PMID: 33262727

Archer, T., Ricci, S., Massoni, F., Ricci, L., & Rapp-Ricciardi, M. (2016). Cognitive benefits of exercise intervention. *La Clinica Terapeutica, 167*(6), 180–185. https://iris.uniroma1.it/handle/11573/1064774 PMID: 28051833

Armstrong, L. E., & VanHeest, J. L. (2002). The Unknown Mechanism of the Overtraining Syndrome: Clues from Depression and Psychoneuroimmunology. *Sports Medicine (Auckland, N.Z.), 32*(3), 185–209. DOI: 10.2165/00007256-200232030-00003 PMID: 11839081

Arnett, J. J. (2000). Emerging adulthood: A theory of development from the late teens through the twenties. *The American Psychologist, 55*(5), 469–480. DOI: 10.1037/0003-066X.55.5.469 PMID: 10842426

Arnsten, A. F. T. (2009). Stress signalling pathways that impair prefrontal cortex structure and function. *Nature Reviews. Neuroscience, 10*, 410–422. PMID: 19455173

Aronsson, G., Theorell, T., Grape, T., Hammarström, A., Hogstedt, C., Marteinsdottir, I., Skoog, I., Träskman-Bendz, L., & Hall, C. (2017). A systematic review including meta-analysis of work environment and burnout symptoms. *BMC Public Health, 17*(264), 1–13. DOI: 10.1186/s12889-017-4153-7 PMID: 28302088

Arzu, D., Tuzun, E. H., & Eker, L. (2006). Perceived barriers to physical activity in university students. *Journal of Sports Science & Medicine, 5*(4), 615–620. PMID: 24357957

Ashdown-Franks, G., Firth, J., Carney, R., Carvalho, A. F., Hallgren, M., Koyanagi, A., Rosenbaum, S., Schuch, F. B., Smith, L., Solmi, M., Vancampfort, D., & Stubbs, B. (2020). Exercise as Medicine for Mental and Substance Use Disorders: A Meta-review of the Benefits for Neuropsychiatric and Cognitive Outcomes. *Sports Medicine (Auckland, N.Z.), 50*(1), 151–170. DOI: 10.1007/s40279-019-01187-6 PMID: 31541410

Atwood, A. I. (2024). A perspective on psychological factors affecting the emotional labor of teachers. *Frontiers in Education, 9*, 1291698. Advance online publication. DOI: 10.3389/feduc.2024.1291698

Augusto-Oliveira, M., Arrifano, G. P., Leal-Nazaré, C. G., Santos-Sacramento, L., Lopes-Araújo, A., Royes, L. F. F., & Crespo-Lopez, M. E. (2023). Exercise Reshapes the Brain: Molecular, Cellular, and Structural Changes Associated with Cognitive Improvements. *Molecular Neurobiology, 60*(12), 6950–6974. DOI: 10.1007/s12035-023-03492-8 PMID: 37518829

Bakker, A. B. (2022). The social psychology of work engagement: State of the field. *Career Development International, 27*(1), 36–53. DOI: 10.1108/CDI-08-2021-0213

Bakker, A. B., & de Vries, J. D. (2020). Job Demands–Resources theory and self-regulation: New explanations and remedies for job burnout. *Anxiety, Stress, and Coping*, *34*(1), 1–21. DOI: 10.1080/10615806.2020.1797695 PMID: 32856957

Bakker, A. B., & Demerouti, E. (2007). The job demands-resources model: State of the art. *Journal of Managerial Psychology*, *22*(3), 309–328. DOI: 10.1108/02683940710733115

Bakker, A. B., & Demerouti, E. (2017). Job demands-resources theory: Taking stock and looking forward. *Journal of Occupational Health Psychology*, *22*(3), 273–285. DOI: 10.1037/ocp0000056 PMID: 27732008

Bakker, A. B., Demerouti, E., & Sanz-Vergel, A. (2023). Job demands–resources theory: Ten years later. *Annual Review of Organizational Psychology and Organizational Behavior*, *10*(1), 25–53. DOI: 10.1146/annurev-orgpsych-120920-053933

Bandura, A. (1997). *Self-efficacy: The exercise of control* (pp. ix, 604). W H Freeman/Times Books/ Henry Holt & Co.

Bandura, A. (1991). Social cognitive theory of self-regulation. *Organizational Behavior and Human Decision Processes*, *50*(2), 248–287. DOI: 10.1016/0749-5978(91)90022-L

Bandura, A. (1997). *Self-Efficacy: The Exercise of Control*. Worth Publishers.

Bandyopadhyay, N., Das, T., Biswas, A., & Koley, A. (2023). Effects of yogic intervention on sleep quality of healthy elderly: A systematic review. *Universal Journal of Public Health*, *11*(1), 78–88.

Baptista, M. N., & Cardoso, H. F. (2021). Do organizational support and occupational stressors influence burnout in teachers? *Interamerican Journal of Psychological Assessment*, *20*(4), 435–444. DOI: 10.15689/ap.2021.2004.21998.05

Barbosa, B. C. R., Menezes-Júnior, L. A. A., de, , de Paula, W., Chagas, C. M. dos S., Machado, E. L., de Freitas, E. D., & Cardoso, C. S., de Carvalho Vidigal, F., Nobre, L. N., Silva, L. S. da, & Meireles, A. L. (2024). Sedentary behavior is associated with the mental health of university students during the Covid-19 pandemic, and not practicing physical activity accentuates its adverse effects: Cross-sectional study. *BMC Public Health*, *24*(1), 1–11. DOI: 10.1186/s12889-024-19345-5 PMID: 38992623

Barha, C. K., Davis, J. C., Falck, R. S., Nagamatsu, L. S., & Liu-Ambrose, T. (2017). Sex differences in exercise efficacy to improve cognition: A systematic review and meta-analysis of randomized controlled trials in older humans. *Frontiers in Neuroendocrinology*, *46*, 71–85. DOI: 10.1016/j.yfrne.2017.04.002

Bartholomew, K. J., Ntoumanis, N., Ryan, R. M., Bosch, J. A., & Thøgersen-Ntoumani, C. (2011). Self-Determination Theory and Diminished Functioning: The Role of Interpersonal Control and Psychological Need Thwarting. *Personality and Social Psychology Bulletin*, *37*(11), 1459–1473. DOI: 10.1177/0146167211413125 PMID: 21700794

Barton, J., & Pretty, J. (2010). What is the best dose of nature and green exercise for improving mental health? A multi-study analysis. *Environmental Science & Technology*, *44*(10), 3947–3955. DOI: 10.1021/es903183r PMID: 20337470

Barua, R. (2025). Harmonizing body and mind: Investigating the combined impact of yoga and mindfulness meditation on depression, anxiety, and stress. In *Global Innovations in Physical Education and Health* (pp. 203–232). IGI Global.

Basso, J. C., & Suzuki, W. A. (2017). The Effects of Acute Exercise on Mood, Cognition, Neurophysiology, and Neurochemical Pathways: A Review. Brain plasticity (Amsterdam, Netherlands), 2(2), 127–152. https://doi.org/DOI: 10.3233/BPL-160040

Basso, J. C., Satyal, M. K., & Rugh, R. (2021). Dance on the brain: Enhancing intra- and inter-brain synchrony. *Frontiers in Human Neuroscience*, *14*, 584312. DOI: 10.3389/fnhum.2020.584312

Basso, J. C., & Suzuki, W. A. (2017). The effects of acute exercise on mood, cognition, neurophysiology, and neurochemical pathways. *Brain Plasticity*, *2*(2), 127–152. PMID: 29765853

Bastioli, G.. (2022). Voluntary exercise boosts striatal dopamine release: Evidence for the necessary and sufficient role of BDNF. *The Journal of Neuroscience : The Official Journal of the Society for Neuroscience*. Advance online publication. DOI: 10.1523/JNEUROSCI.2273-21.2022

Bathina, S., & Das, U. N. (2015). Brain-derived neurotrophic factor and its clinical implications. *Archives of Medical Science : AMS*, *11*(6), 1164–1178. DOI: 10.5114/aoms.2015.56342 PMID: 26788077

Bauer, J., Schwiertz, G., & Muehlbauer, T. (2021). Effects of an elastic resistance band intervention in adolescent handball players. *Sports Medicine International Open*, *5*(02), E65–E72. PMID: 34458564

Baumeister, R. F., & Leary, M. R. (1995). The need to belong: Desire for interpersonal attachments as a fundamental human motivation. *Psychological Bulletin*, *117*(3), 497–529. DOI: 10.1037/0033-2909.117.3.497 PMID: 7777651

Baumgartner, J., Ota, C., DiCarlo, C., Bauer, R., & Carson, R. (2025). Using ecological momentary assessment to examine the relationship between childcare teachers' stress, classroom behaviors, and afterhours professionalism activities. *Child Care in Practice, 31*(1), 49–68. DOI: 10.1080/13575279.2021.1962247

Bayram, N., & Bilgel, N. (2008). The prevalence and socio-demographic correlations of depression, anxiety and stress among a group of university students. *Social Psychiatry and Psychiatric Epidemiology, 43*(8), 667–672. DOI: 10.1007/s00127-008-0345-x PMID: 18398558

Beaubrun, A. (2022). Decentralizing the commodification of mindfulness. *Unpublished manuscript.*

Beauchamp, M. R., Bray, S. R., Eys, M. A., & Carron, A. V. (2003). The Effect of Role Ambiguity on Competitive State Anxiety. *Journal of Sport & Exercise Psychology, 25*(1), 77–92. DOI: 10.1123/jsep.25.1.77

Beauchamp, T., & Childress, J. (2019). Principles of Biomedical Ethics</i>: Marking Its Fortieth Anniversary. *The American Journal of Bioethics, 19*(11), 9–12. DOI: 10.1080/15265161.2019.1665402 PMID: 31647760

Belvederi Murri, M., Pariante, C., Mondelli, V., Masotti, M., Atti, A. R., Mellacqua, Z., Antonioli, M., Ghio, L., & Serafini, G. (2016). HPA axis and aging in depression: Systematic review and meta-analysis. *Psychoneuroendocrinology, 72*, 1–10. DOI: 10.1016/j.psyneuen.2016.06.002

Ben Ezzdine, L., Dhahbi, W., Dergaa, I., Ceylan, H. İ., Guelmami, N., Ben Saad, H., Chamari, K., Stefanica, V., & El Omri, A. (2025). Physical activity and neuroplasticity in neurodegenerative disorders: A comprehensive review of exercise interventions, cognitive training, and AI applications. *Frontiers in Neuroscience, 19*, 1502417. DOI: 10.3389/fnins.2025.1502417

Benavidez, G., & Hart, P. D. (2017). Effects of yoga on measures of health-related quality of life from SF-36 and SF-12 assessments: A systematic review and meta-analysis. *Exercise Medicine, 1*, 5. DOI: 10.26644/em.2017.005

Berkey, A. (n.d.). *Teacher burnout: Stats, causes, and prevention for 2025*. Everfi. https://everfi.com/blog/k-12/teacher-burnout/#:~:text=The%20burnout%20rate%20for%20teachers,major%20stressor%20in%20their%20classrooms

Berk, M., Dandash, O., Daglas, R., Cotton, S. M., Allott, K., Fornito, A., & Yücel, M. (2017). Neuroprotection after a first episode of mania: A randomized controlled maintenance trial comparing the effects of lithium and quetiapine on grey and white matter volume. *Translational Psychiatry, 7*(1), e1011–e1011.

Berk, M., Post, R., & Malhi, G. S. (2017). Staging in bipolar disorder: From theoretical framework to clinical utility. *World Psychiatry; Official Journal of the World Psychiatric Association (WPA), 16*(3), 236–244. DOI: 10.1002/wps.20441

Beselt, L. J., Patterson, M. C., McDonough, M. H., Hewson, J., & MacKay, S. (2021). A meta-study of qualitative research on social support related to physical activity among older adults. *Kinesiology Review (Champaign, Ill.), 10*(1), 51–65. DOI: 10.1123/kr.2020-0005

Beserra, A. H. N., Kameda, P., Deslandes, A. C., Schuch, F. B., Laks, J., & Moraes, H. S. D. (2018). Can physical exercise modulate cortisol level in subjects with depression? A systematic review and meta-analysis. *Trends in Psychiatry and Psychotherapy, 40*(4), 360–368. DOI: 10.1590/2237-6089-2017-0155 PMID: 30570106

Bianchi, R., Schonfeld, I. S., & Verkuilen, J. (2020). A five-sample confirmatory factor analytic study of burnout-depression overlap. *Journal of Clinical Psychology, 76*(4), 801–821. DOI: 10.1002/jclp.22927 PMID: 31926025

Biddle, G. F., Stuart. (1999). Exercise as an adjunct treatment for schizophrenia: A review of the literature. *Journal of Mental Health (Abingdon, England), 8*(5), 441–457. DOI: 10.1080/09638239917157

Biddle, S. J. H., & Asare, M. (2011). Physical activity and mental health in children and adolescents: A review of reviews. *British Journal of Sports Medicine, 45*(11), 886–895. DOI: 10.1136/bjsports-2011-090185 PMID: 21807669

Biddle, S. J. H., & Batterham, A. M. (2015). High-intensity interval exercise training for public health: A big HIT or shall we HIT it on the head? *The International Journal of Behavioral Nutrition and Physical Activity, 12*, 95. DOI: 10.1186/s12966-015-0254-9 PMID: 26187579

Biddle, S. J. H., Ciaccioni, S., Thomas, G., & Vergeer, I. (2019). Physical activity and mental health in children and adolescents: An updated review of reviews and an analysis of causality. *Psychology of Sport and Exercise, 42*, 146–155. DOI: 10.1016/j.psychsport.2018.08.011

Bigras, N., Lemay, L., Lehrer, J., Charron, A., Duval, S., Robert-Mazaye, C., & Laurin, E. I. (2021). Early childhood educators' perceptions of their emotional state, relationships with parents, challenges, and opportunities during the early stage of the pandemic. *Early Childhood Education Journal, 49*(5), 775–787. DOI: 10.1007/s10643-021-01224-y PMID: 34131378

Bodensohn, L., Maurer, A., Daamen, M., Upadhyay, N., Werkhausen, J., Lohaus, M., Manunzio, U., Manunzio, C., Radbruch, A., Attenberger, U., & Boecker, H. (2024). Inverted U shape like functional connectivity alterations in cognitive resting state networks depending on exercise intensity: An fMRI study. *Brain and Cognition*, *177*, 106156. DOI: 10.1016/j.bandc.2024.106156 PMID: 38613926

Boecker, H., Sprenger, T., Spilker, M. E., Henriksen, G., Koppenhoefer, M., Wagner, K. J., Valet, M., Berthele, A., & Tolle, T. R. (2008). The runner's high: Opioidergic mechanisms in the human brain. *Cerebral Cortex (New York, N.Y.: 1991)*, *18*(11), 2523–2531. https://doi.org/DOI: 10.1093/cercor/bhn013

Bogaert, I., De Martelaer, K., Deforche, B., Clarys, P., & Zinzen, E. (2014). Associations between different types of physical activity and teachers' perceived mental, physical, and work-related health. *BMC Public Health*, *14*(1), 534. Advance online publication. DOI: 10.1186/1471-2458-14-534 PMID: 24885620

Boke, H. (2025). Effects of cooperative learning on students' outcomes in physical education: A meta-analysis. *Journal of Physical Education Research*, *12*(3), 45–67. PMID: 40432799

Bompa, T. O., & Buzzichelli, C. A. (2019). *Periodization: Theory and Methodology of Training* (1st ed.). Human Kinetics., DOI: 10.5040/9781718225435

Bonanno, G. A., Chen, S., & Galatzer-Levy, I. R. (2023). Resilience to potential trauma and adversity through regulatory flexibility. *Nature Reviews Psychology*, *2*(11), 663–675. DOI: 10.1038/s44159-023-00228-5

Bora, E., & Özerdem, A. (2017). A meta-analysis of neurocognition in youth with familial high risk for bipolar disorder. *European Psychiatry : the Journal of the Association of European Psychiatrists*, *44*, 17–23. DOI: 10.1016/j.eurpsy.2017.02.483

Bora, E., & Ozerdem, A. (2017). Meta-analysis of structural neuroimaging studies in bipolar disorder: An update 2009–2016. *Psychiatry Research: Neuroimaging*, *274*, 70–79. DOI: 10.1016/j.pscychresns.2017.01.008

Borrega Alonso, E., & Otamendi, F. J. (2025). Effects of acute and chronic exercise on working memory in healthy adults. An experimental investigation. *Frontiers in Psychology*, *16*. Advance online publication. DOI: 10.3389/fpsyg.2025.1608721 PMID: 40547576

Boyatzis, R., & McKee, A. (2005). *Resonant Leadership: Renewing Yourself and Connecting with Others Through Mindfulness, Hope and CompassionCompassion*. Harvard Business Press.

Brailovskaia, J., Duscha, A. L., Kreyelkamp, G. M., & Margraf, J. (2024). Teachers' competence: How to protect teachers' mental health from the burden caused by students' private in-class use of technical devices? *PLoS One*, *19*(6), e0305114. Advance online publication. DOI: 10.1371/journal.pone.0305114 PMID: 38861520

Branzuela, M. J., Ayro, E. C., & Cruz-Vidal, M. J. D. (2023). Teaching outside the box: Senior High School teaching experiences, challenges, and windows of innovations of non-social science majors. *International Journal of Multidisciplinary: Applied Business and Education Research*, *4*(7), 2210–2222.

Bremer, E., Crozier, M., & Lloyd, M. (2016). A systematic review of the behavioural outcomes following exercise interventions for children and youth with autism spectrum disorder. *Autism*, *20*(8), 899–915. DOI: 10.1177/1362361315616002 PMID: 26823546

Broadhead, J., & Dunne, M. (2020). Physical activity, social bonding and hormonal influences. *Journal of Social Neuroendocrinology*, *12*(3), 312–325.

Brondino, N., Rocchetti, M., Fusar-Poli, L., Codrons, E., Correale, L., Vandoni, M., Barbui, C., & Politi, P. (2017). A systematic review of cognitive effects of exercise in depression. *Acta Psychiatrica Scandinavica*, *135*(4), 285–295. DOI: 10.1111/acps.12690 PMID: 28110494

Brown, D. R., Wang, Y., Ward, A. N. N., Ebbeling, C. B., Fortlage, L., Puleo, E., Benson, H., & Rippe, J. M. (1995). Chronic psychological effects of exercise and exercise plus cognitive strategies. *Medicine and Science in Sports and Exercise*, *27*(5), 765–775. https://europepmc.org/article/med/7674883 PMID: 7674883

Bruffaerts, R., Mortier, P., Kiekens, G., Auerbach, R. P., Cuijpers, P., Demyttenaere, K., Green, J. G., Nock, M. K., & Kessler, R. C. (2018). Mental health problems in college freshmen: Prevalence and academic functioning. *Journal of Affective Disorders*, *225*, 97–103. DOI: 10.1016/j.jad.2017.07.044 PMID: 28802728

Brymer, E., & Schweitzer, R. (2017). *Phenomenology and the Extreme Sport Experience*. Routledge., DOI: 10.4324/9781315661643

Büssing, A., Michalsen, A., Khalsa, S. B. S., Telles, S., & Sherman, K. J. (2012). Effects of yoga on mental and physical health: A short summary of reviews. *Evidence-Based Complementary and Alternative Medicine : eCAM*, *2012*, 165410.

Cadmus-Bertram, L. A., Marcus, B. H., Patterson, R. E., Parker, B. A., & Morey, B. L. (2015). Randomized Trial of a Fitbit-Based Physical Activity Intervention for Women. *American Journal of Preventive Medicine*, *49*(3), 414–418. DOI: 10.1016/j.amepre.2015.01.020 PMID: 26071863

Calderone, A., Latella, D., Impellizzeri, F., de Pasquale, P., Famà, F., Quartarone, A., & Calabrò, R. S. (2024). Neurobiological changes induced by mindfulness and meditation: A systematic review. *Biomedicines*, *12*(11), 2613. DOI: 10.3390/biomedicines12112613

Caneppele, T. S.. (2022). Can exercise shape your brain? A review of aerobic exercise effects on cognitive function and brain health. *Frontiers in Psychology*. Advance online publication. DOI: 10.3389/fpsyg.2022.852362

Caperchione, C. M., Kolt, G. S., & Mummery, W. K. (2009). Physical activity in culturally and linguistically diverse migrant groups to Western society: A review of barriers, enablers and experiences. *Sports Medicine (Auckland, N.Z.)*, *39*(3), 167–177. DOI: 10.2165/00007256-200939030-00001 PMID: 19290674

Capone, V., & Petrillo, G. (2020). Mental health in teachers: Relationship with job satisfaction, efficacy beliefs, burnout and depression. *Current Psychology (New Brunswick, N.J.)*, *39*(5), 1757–1766. DOI: 10.1007/s12144-018-9878-7

Carr, E. R. (2024). A history of the community mental health movement and individuals with serious mental illness: A vision for the future. *The American Journal of Orthopsychiatry*, *94*(4), 380–391. DOI: 10.1037/ort0000737 PMID: 38695820

Carroll, A., Forrest, K., Sanders-O'Connor, E., Flynn, L., Bower, J. M., Fynes-Clinton, S., York, A., & Ziaei, M. (2022). Teacher stress and burnout in Australia: Examining the role of intrapersonal and environmental factors. *Social Psychology of Education*, *25*, 441–469. DOI: 10.1007/s11218-022-09686-7 PMID: 35233183

Carson, R. L., Baumgartner, J. J., Matthews, R. A., & Tsouloupas, C. N. (2010). Emotional exhaustion, absenteeism, and turnover intentions in childcare teachers: Examining the impact of physical activity behaviors. *Journal of Health Psychology*, *15*(6), 905–914. DOI: 10.1177/1359105309360697 PMID: 20472609

Casey, B. J., Jones, R. M., & Hare, T. A. (2008). The adolescent brain. *Annals of the New York Academy of Sciences*, *1124*, 111–126. DOI: 10.1196/annals.1440.010 PMID: 18400927

Caspersen, C. J., Powell, K. E., & Christenson, G. M. (1985). Physical activity, exercise, and physical fitness: Definitions and distinctions for health-related research. *Public Health Reports*, *100*(2), 126–131. https://pmc.ncbi.nlm.nih.gov/articles/PMC1424733/ PMID: 3920711

Cattie, J. E., Allbaugh, L. J., Visser, K. H., Ander, I., & Kaslow, N. J. (2021). Tailoring trauma-sensitive yoga for high-risk populations in public-sector settings. *International Journal of Yoga Therapy*, *31*(1), 15–24. DOI: 10.17761/2021-D-19-00024

Cavallo, D. N., Tate, D. F., Ries, A. V., Brown, J. D., DeVellis, R. F., & Ammerman, A. S. (2012a). A social media-based physical activity intervention: A randomized controlled trial. *American Journal of Preventive Medicine*, *43*(5), 527–532. DOI: 10.1016/j.amepre.2012.07.019 PMID: 23079176

Center of Disease of Control and Prevention. (2024). *Benefits of physical activity.* https://www.cdc.gov/physical-activity-basics/benefits/index.html

Center of Disease of Control and Prevention. (n.d.). *Adult activity: An overview.* https://www.cdc.gov/physical-activity-basics/guidelines/adults.html

Chan, M. K., Sharkey, J. D., Lawrie, S. I., Arch, D. A. N., & Nylund-Gibson, K. (2021). Elementary school teacher well-being and supportive measures amid COVID-19: An exploratory study. *School Psychology*, *36*(6), 533–545. DOI: 10.1037/spq0000441 PMID: 34292036

Channawar, S. N. (2023). Mindfulness practices for stress reduction and mental clarity. *International Journal of Futuristic Innovation in Arts. Humanities and Management*, *2*(3), 49–59.

Chaouloff, F. (1997). Effects of acute physical exercise on central serotonergic systems. *Medicine and Science in Sports and Exercise*, *29*(1), 58–62. DOI: 10.1097/00005768-199701000-00009 PMID: 9000156

Chauhan, S., Najaf, S. S., Gergely, L., Kinga, K. A., Karsai, I., & Prémusz, V. (2025). Impact of 10 Weeks of Yoga Intervention on Mental Health and Overall Well-Being Among Medical Students: GSY Study. *Sports (Basel, Switzerland)*, *13*(4), 114. DOI: 10.3390/sports13040114

Chekroud, S. R., Gueorguieva, R., Zheutlin, A. B., Paulus, M., Krumholz, H. M., Krystal, J. H., & Chekroud, A. M. (2018). Association between physical exercise and mental health in 1.2 million individuals in the USA between 2011 and 2015: A cross-sectional study. *The Lancet. Psychiatry*, *5*(9), 739–746. DOI: 10.1016/S2215-0366(18)30227-X PMID: 30099000

Cheng, P. Y. Z., & Liu, H. (2024). A structural model of EFL teachers' physical activity, emotion regulation, and competence for online teaching. *BMC Psychology*, *12*, 252. DOI: 10.1186/s40359-024-01753-2 PMID: 38715133

Chen, X. M., Liao, X. L., Chen, I. H., Gamble, J. H., Jiang, X. Y., Li, X. D., & Bo, C. X. (2024). The long-term effects of perceived instructional leadership on teachers' psychological well-being during COVID-19. *PLoS One*, *19*(8), e0305494. Advance online publication. DOI: 10.1371/journal.pone.0305494 PMID: 39159165

Chen, X., Lu, X., & Zhang, S. (2020). Exercise modulates circadian rhythms and metabolic homeostasis: Implications for mood disorders. *Frontiers in Psychiatry, 11*, 577. DOI: 10.3389/fpsyt.2020.00577

Chen, Y., Wang, S., Senanu Ametefe, D., & John, D. (2024). Impact of dancing on physical and mental health: A systematic literature review. *Dance Research, 42*(2), 220–256. DOI: 10.3366/drs.2024.0375

Chodkiewicz, A., & Boyle, C. (2017). Positive psychology school-based interventions: A reflection on current success and future directions. *Educational Review, 5*, 60–86. DOI: 10.1002/rev3.3080

Christakis, N. A., & Fowler, J. H. (2007). The spread of obesity in a large social network over 32 years. *The New England Journal of Medicine, 357*(4), 370–379. DOI: 10.1056/NEJMsa066082 PMID: 17652652

Çifçi, F., & Demir, A. (2020). The effect of home-based exercise on anxiety and mental well-being levels of teachers and pre-service teachers in COVID-19 pandemic. *African Educational Research Journal Special Issue, 8*(2), S20-S28. https://files.eric.ed.gov/fulltext/EJ1274658.pdf

Clasquin-Johnson, M. G., & Ebrahim, H. B. (2024). Self-efficacy and well-being of female educators for early childhood care and education during COVID-19. *South African Journal of Education, 44*(1), 2354. Advance online publication. DOI: 10.15700/saje.v44n1a2354

Cleveland Clinic. (2025). *Mental disorders*. Retrieved December 1, 2025 from https://my.clevelandclinic.org/health/diseases/22295-mental-health-disorders

Coelho, F. G. de M., Gobbi, S., Andreatto, C. A. A., Corazza, D. I., Pedroso, R. V., & Santos-Galduróz, R. F. (2013). Physical exercise modulates peripheral levels of brain-derived neurotrophic factor (BDNF): A systematic review of experimental studies in the elderly. *Archives of Gerontology and Geriatrics, 56*(1), 10–15. DOI: 10.1016/j.archger.2012.06.003 PMID: 22749404

Coetsee, C., & Terblanche, E. (2017). The effect of three different exercise training modalities on cognitive and physical function in a healthy older population. *European Review of Aging and Physical Activity : Official Journal of the European Group for Research into Elderly and Physical Activity, 14*(1), 13. DOI: 10.1186/s11556-017-0183-5 PMID: 28811842

Collie, R. J. (2023). Teacher well-being and turnover intentions: Investigating the roles of job resources and job demands. *The British Journal of Educational Psychology, 93*(3), 712–726. DOI: 10.1111/bjep.12587 PMID: 36720462

Colombo, D., Díaz-García, A., Fernandez-Álvarez, J., & Botella, C. (2021). Virtual reality for the enhancement of emotion regulation. *Clinical Psychology & Psychotherapy, 28*(3), 519–537. DOI: 10.1002/cpp.2618 PMID: 34048621

Cooney, G. M., Dwan, K., Greig, C. A., Lawlor, D. A., Rimer, J., Waugh, F. R., McMurdo, M., & Mead, G. E. (2013). Exercise for depression. *Cochrane Database of Systematic Reviews, 2013*(9), CD004366. Advance online publication. DOI: 10.1002/14651858.CD004366.pub6 PMID: 24026850

Corbett, L., Bauman, A., Peralta, L. R., Okely, A. D., & Phongsavan, P. (2021). Characteristics and effectiveness of physical activity, nutrition and/or sleep interventions to improve the mental well-being of teachers: A scoping review. *Health Education Journal, 81*(2), 196–210. DOI: 10.1177/00178969211062701

Cordisco Tsai, L. (2025). Cultural adaptation of a trauma-informed mind-body program. *International Social Work Review. Webb, A. J. (2023). Acceptance and Commitment Therapy (ACT): Foundational Principles, Processes, and Treatment Components. Authorea Preprints.*

Correll, C. U., Detraux, J., De Lepeleire, J., & De Hert, M. (2017). Effects of antipsychotics, antidepressants and mood stabilizers on risk for physical diseases in people with schizophrenia, depression and bipolar disorder. *World Psychiatry; Official Journal of the World Psychiatric Association (WPA), 16*(2), 119–136. DOI: 10.1002/wps.20404

Costa, C. N., Chandarlis, E., & Park, N. (2024). Examining teacher well-being: An analysis of resources needs. *International Journal of Changes in Education, 1*(2), 63–74. DOI: 10.47852/bonviewIJCE42022564

Cotman, C. W., & Berchtold, N. C. (2002). Exercise: A behavioral intervention to enhance brain health and plasticity. *Trends in Neurosciences, 25*(6), 295–301. DOI: 10.1016/s0166-2236(02)02143-4 PMID: 12086747

Cox, A. E., Ullrich-French, S., Cole, A. N., & D'Hondt-Taylor, M. (2016). The role of state mindfulness during yoga in predicting self-objectification and reasons for exercise. *Psychology of Sport and Exercise, 22*, 321–327. DOI: 10.1016/j.psychsport.2015.10.001

Craft, L. L., & Perna, F. M. (2004). The Benefits of Exercise for the Clinically Depressed. *Primary Care Companion to the Journal of Clinical Psychiatry, 6*(3), 104–111. DOI: 10.4088/pcc.v06n0301 PMID: 15361924

Craft, L. L., & Perna, F. M. (2004). The benefits of exercise for the clinically depressed. *Primary Care Companion to the Journal of Clinical Psychiatry*, *6*(3), 104–111. DOI: 10.4088/PCC.v06n0301 PMID: 15361924

Cramer, H., Lauche, R., Anheyer, D., Pilkington, K., de Manincor, M., Dobos, G., & Ward, L. (2018). Yoga for anxiety: A systematic review and meta-analysis of randomized controlled trials. *Depression and Anxiety*, *35*(9), 830–843. DOI: 10.1002/da.22762 PMID: 29697885

Cramer, H., Lauche, R., Langhorst, J., & Dobos, G. (2013). Yoga for depression: A systematic review and meta-analysis. *Depression and Anxiety*, *30*(11), 1068–1083. DOI: 10.1002/da.22166 PMID: 23922209

Creswell, J. D. (2017). Mindfulness interventions. *Annual Review of Psychology*, *68*, 491–516. PMID: 27687118

Crocker, J., & Park, L. E. (2004). The Costly Pursuit of Self-Esteem. *Psychological Bulletin*, *130*(3), 392–414. DOI: 10.1037/0033-2909.130.3.392 PMID: 15122925

Csikszentmihalyi, M. (2008). *Flow: The Psychology of Optimal Experience*. HarperCollins Publishers.

Cuijpers, P., Karyotaki, E., Weitz, E., Andersson, G., Hollon, S. D., & van Straten, A. (2014). The effects of psychotherapies for major depression in adults on remission, recovery and improvement: A meta-analysis. *Journal of Affective Disorders*, *159*, 118–126. DOI: 10.1016/j.jad.2014.02.026 PMID: 24679399

da Silva, C. C. M., Santos, A. B. d., Leoci, I. C., Leite, E. G., Antunes, E. P., Torres, W., Mesquita, E. D. L., Delfino, L. D., & Beretta, V. S. (2024). The association between perceived stress, quality of life, and level of physical activity in public school teachers. *International Journal of Environmental Research and Public Health*, *21*(1), 88. DOI: 10.3390/ijerph21010088 PMID: 38248551

Dahati, A., & Dahati, A. (2025). The role of physical activity in reducing symptoms of 'burnout' and psychological mechanisms towards exercise in professionals with high stress levels: The case of northern Albania. *Interdisciplinary Journal of Research and Development, 12*(2), 126-126. https://www.journal-uamd.org/index.php/IJRD/article/view/586/550

Damasio, A. (1999). The feeling of what happens: Body and emotion in the making of consciousness (pp. xiv, 386). Harcourt College Publishers.

Dao, T. C. (2024) [B]. The Evolution and Impact of Recreational Sports: A Global Perspective. In Social Inclusion Tactics for People With Intellectual and Developmental Disabilities (pp. 261-294). IGI Global.

Dao, T. C. (2025). Revolutionizing PE Harnessing the Power of Artificial Intelligence in Vietnamese Universities: AI in PE Transforming Vietnamese Universities. In Transformative AI Practices for Personalized Learning Strategies (pp. 305-324). IGI Global Scientific Publishing. DOI:DOI: 10.4018/979-8-3693-8744-3.ch011

Dao, T. C. (2024). The influence of recreational sports participation on physical and mental health and quality of life among middle-aged adults (45–60 years old). In *Social Inclusion Tactics for People With Intellectual and Developmental Disabilities* (pp. 73–88). IGI Global. [A], https://www.igi-global.com/chapter/the-influence-of-recreational-sports-participation-on-physical-and-mental-health-and-quality-of-life-among-middle-aged-adults-45-60-years-old/360465, DOI: 10.4018/979-8-3693-3176-7.ch004

Davis, J. (2023). *The relationship between teacher burnout and physical activity among high school teachers* [Doctoral dissertation, Kennesaw State University]. DigitalCommons@Kennesaw State University. https://digitalcommons.kennesaw.edu/ teachleaddoc_etd/62?utm_source=digitalcommons.kennesaw.edu%2Fteachleaddoc_etd%2F62&utm_medium=PDF&utm_campaign=PDFCoverPages

Davis, J. K., Juergensen, M., Chang, M. L., & Elue, C. (2025). The relationship between teacher burnout and physical activity among high school teachers. *International Journal of Teacher Leadership*, *14*(1), 98–125. https://research-ebsco-com.snu.idm.oclc.org/c/5v6chs/viewer/pdf/4nba6xypkn

Davranche, K., Brisswalter, J., & Radel, R. (2014). Where are the limits of the effects of exercise intensity on cognitive control? *Journal of Sport and Health Science. Journal of Sport and Health Science*, *4*(1), 56–63. DOI: 10.1016/j.jshs.2014.08.004

de Costa, B. G. G., Van Rooij, A. J., Tuijnman, A., Saunders, T. J., & Chaput, J. P. (2023). Associations between type and timing of physical activity and sedentary behavior with mental health in adolescents and young adults. *Journal of Physical Activity & Health*, *20*(7), 655–663. DOI: 10.1123/jpah.2022-0485 PMID: 37160286

De Prisco, M., Oliva, V., Fico, G., Fornaro, M., de Bartolomeis, A., Serretti, A., Vieta, E., & Murru, A. (2022). Defining clinical characteristics of emotion dysregulation in bipolar disorder: A systematic review and meta-analysis. *Neuroscience and Biobehavioral Reviews*, *142*, 104914. DOI: 10.1016/j.neubiorev.2022.104914

Dean, J., & Keshavan, M. (2017). The neurobiology of depression: An integrated view. *Asian Journal of Psychiatry*, *27*, 101–111. DOI: 10.1016/j.ajp.2017.01.025 PMID: 28558878

Deci, E. L., & Ryan, R. M. (2000). The "What" and "Why" of Goal Pursuits: Human Needs and the Self-Determination of Behavior. *Psychological Inquiry, 11*(4), 227–268. DOI: 10.1207/S15327965PLI1104_01

Deci, E. L., & Ryan, R. M. (2008). Self-determination theory: A macrotheory of human motivation, development, and health. *Canadian Psychology, 49*(3), 182–185. DOI: 10.1037/a0012801

Del Carmen, M. V., Diano, F., Morales, M. P. E., & Ole, A. (2015). Promoting physics in action thru "Laro Ng Lahi-Based" physics activities. In the International *Journal of Learning and Teaching* (Vol. 07, Issue 1, pp. 24–37). https://pdfs.semanticscholar.org/feca/a3be1eb1da8b1db238f7a3bd9f2b1986996a.pdf

Demerouti, E., Bakker, A. B., Nachreiner, F., & Schaufeli, W. B. (2001). The job demands-resources model of burnout. *The Journal of Applied Psychology, 86*(3), 499–512. DOI: 10.1037/0021-9010.86.3.499 PMID: 11419809

Demerouti, E., Bakker, A. B., Peeters, M. C. W., & Breevaart, K. (2021). New directions in burnout research. *European Journal of Work and Organizational Psychology, 30*(5), 686–691. DOI: 10.1080/1359432X.2021.1979962

Denovan, A., & Macaskill, A. (2017). Building resilience to stress through leisure activities: A qualitative analysis. *Annals of Leisure Research, 20*(4), 446–466. DOI: 10.1080/11745398.2016.1211943

Diener, E., Oishi, S., & Tay, L. (2018). Advances in subjective well-being research. *Nature Human Behaviour, 2*(4), 253–260. DOI: 10.1038/s41562-018-0307-6 PMID: 30936533

Dike, I. C., Onyishi, C. N., Adimora, D. E., Ugodulunwa, C. A., Adama, G. N., Ugwu, G. C., Eze, U. N., Eze, A., Ogba, F. N., Obiwluozo, P. E., Onu, J. F. E., Onu, A. O., Omenma, Z. O., Nwaeze, V. C., Ani, C., Ngwu, C. N., Uzodinma, U. E., & Iremeka, F. U. (2021). Yoga complemented cognitive behavioral therapy on job burnout among teachers of children with autism spectrum disorders. *Medicine, 100*(22), 25801. Advance online publication. DOI: 10.1097/MD.0000000000025801 PMID: 34087823

Dishman, R. K., Berthoud, H.-R., Booth, F. W., Cotman, C. W., Edgerton, V. R., Fleshner, M. R., Gandevia, S. C., Gomez-Pinilla, F., Greenwood, B. N., Hillman, C. H., Kramer, A. F., Levin, B. E., Moran, T. H., Russo-Neustadt, A. A., Salamone, J. D., Van Hoomissen, J. D., Wade, C. E., York, D. A., & Zigmond, M. J. (2006). Neurobiology of exercise. *Obesity (Silver Spring, Md.), 14*(3), 345–356. DOI: 10.1038/oby.2006.46 PMID: 16648603

Dishman, R. K., & O'Connor, P. J. (2009). Lessons in exercise neurobiology. *Mental Health and Physical Activity*, *2*(1), 4–9.

Dishman, R. K., & O'Connor, P. J. (2009). Lessons in exercise neurobiology: The case of endorphins. *Mental Health and Physical Activity*, *2*(1), 4–9. DOI: 10.1016/j.mhpa.2009.01.002

Dizer, R., Logan, I. L. N., & Raval, K. M. R. (2022). Laro ng lahi: A study on the perceived benefits of playing indigenous games on the holistic development of Filipinos born in the'80s. *Philippine Journal of Social Sciences and Humanities University of the Philippines Visayas*, *27*, 91–114. https://pjssh.upv.edu.ph/wp-content/uploads/2024/05/91-114-PJSSH-22-27-D01_Laro-ng-Lahi.pdf

DNA Learning Center. (2008). Exercise induced neurogenesis. https://dnalc.cshl.edu/view/848-Exercise-induced-Neurogenesis.html

Dowd, A. J., Schmader, T., Sylvester, B. D., Jung, M. E., Zumbo, B. D., Martin, L. J., & Beauchamp, M. R. (2014). *Effects of Social Belonging and Task Framing on Exercise Cognitions and Behavior*. https://doi.org/DOI: 10.1123/jsep.2013-0114

Dreer, B. (2023). On the outcomes of teacher wellbeing: A systematic review of research. *Frontiers in Psychology*, *14*, 1205179. Advance online publication. DOI: 10.3389/fpsyg.2023.1205179 PMID: 37575417

Driskell, T., Sclafani, Steve, & and Driskell, J. E. (2014). Reducing the Effects of Game Day Pressures through Stress Exposure Training. *Journal of Sport Psychology in Action*, *5*(1), 28–43. DOI: 10.1080/21520704.2013.866603

Duckworth, A. L., & Gross, J. J. (2020). Behavior change. *Organizational Behavior and Human Decision Processes*, *161*, 39–49. PMID: 33716396

Dung, V., Trang, V. T., & Lan, N. T. M. (2024). Workload doesn't mean exhaustion: Antecedents of teacher burnout. *Journal of Education and e-learning Research*, *11*(2), 404–412. DOI: 10.20448/jeelr.v11i2.5641

Dunn, A. L., & Jewell, J. S. (2010). The effect of exercise on mental health. *Current Sports Medicine Reports*, *9*(4), 202–207. https://journals.lww.com/acsm-csmr/fulltext/2010/07000/The_Effect_of_Exercise_on_Mental_Health.8.aspx PMID: 20622537

Dunn, B. D., Galton, H. C., Morgan, R., Evans, D., Oliver, C., Meyer, M., Cusack, R., Lawrence, A. D., & Dalgleish, T. (2010). Listening to your heart. How interoception shapes emotion experience and intuitive decision making. *Psychological Science*, *21*(12), 1835–1844. DOI: 10.1177/0956797610389191 PMID: 21106893

Dunning, D. L., Griffiths, K., Kuyken, W., Crane, C., Foulkes, L., Parker, J., & Dalgleish, T. (2019). Research Review: The effects of mindfulness-based interventions on cognition and mental health in children and adolescents–a meta-analysis of randomized controlled trials. *Journal of Child Psychology and Psychiatry, and Allied Disciplines*, *60*(3), 244–258. PMID: 30345511

Dunstan, D. W., Howard, B., Healy, G. N., & Owen, N. (2012). Too much sitting – A health hazard. *Diabetes Research and Clinical Practice*, *97*(3), 368–376. DOI: 10.1016/j.diabres.2012.05.020 PMID: 22682948

Du, S., Hu, H., Cheng, K., & Li, H. (2023). Exercise makes better mind: A data mining study on effect of physical activity on academic achievement of college students. *Frontiers in Psychology, 14*. Advance online publication. DOI: 10.3389/fpsyg.2023.1271431 PMID: 37908825

Eddy, M., & Johnson, D. H. (2022). *The fluid nature of being: Embodied practices for healing and wholeness*. Jessica Kingsley Publishers.

Educating the student body. (2013). In *National Academies Press eBooks*. .DOI: 10.17226/18314

Egger, M., Davey Smith, G., Schneider, M., & Minder, C. (1997). Bias in meta-analysis detected by a simple, graphical test. *BMJ (Clinical Research Ed.)*, *315*(7109), 629–634. DOI: 10.1136/bmj.315.7109.629 PMID: 9310563

Eime, R. M., Young, J. A., Harvey, J. T., Charity, M. J., & Payne, W. R. (2013a). A systematic review of the psychological and social benefits of participation in sport for children and adolescents: Informing development of a conceptual model of health through sport. *The International Journal of Behavioral Nutrition and Physical Activity*, *10*, 98. DOI: 10.1186/1479-5868-10-98 PMID: 23945179

Eisenberg, D., Gollust, S. E., Golberstein, E., & Hefner, J. L. (2007). Prevalence and correlates of depression, anxiety, and suicidality among university students. *The American Journal of Orthopsychiatry*, *77*(4), 534–542. DOI: 10.1037/0002-9432.77.4.534 PMID: 18194033

Ekeland, E., Heian, F., & Hagen, K. B. (2005). Can exercise improve self esteem in children and young people? A systematic review of randomised controlled trials. *British Journal of Sports Medicine*, *39*(11), 792–798. DOI: 10.1136/bjsm.2004.017707 PMID: 16244186

Ekkekakis, P. (2013). *The measurement of affect, mood, and emotion: A guide for health-behavioral research* (pp. xxi, 206). Cambridge University Press. https://doi.org/DOI: 10.1017/CBO9780511820724

Ekkekakis, P., & Acevedo, E. O. (2006). Affective Responses to Acute Exercise: Toward a Psychobiological Dose-Response Model. In *Psychobiology of physical activity* (pp. 91–109). Human Kinetics.

Ekkekakis, P., & Lind, E. (2006). Exercise does not feel the same when you are overweight: The impact of self-selected and imposed intensity on affect and exertion. *International Journal of Obesity (2005), 30*(4), 652–660. https://doi.org/DOI: 10.1038/sj.ijo.0803052

Ekkekakis, P. (2003). Pleasure and displeasure from the body: Perspectives from exercise. *Cognition & Emotion -. Cognition and Emotion, 17*, 213–239. DOI: 10.1080/02699930302292 PMID: 29715726

Ekkekakis, P. (2009). Illuminating the black box: Investigating prefrontal cortical hemodynamics during exercise with near-infrared spectroscopy. *Journal of Sport & Exercise Psychology, 31*(4), 505–553. DOI: 10.1123/jsep.31.4.505 PMID: 19842545

Ekkekakis, P. (2013). *The measurement of affect, mood, and emotion: A guide for health-behavioral research*. Cambridge University Press.

Ekkekakis, P., Parfitt, G., & Petruzzello, S. J. (2011). The pleasure and displeasure people feel when they exercise at different intensities: Decennial update and progress towards a tripartite rationale for exercise intensity prescription. *Sports Medicine (Auckland, N.Z.), 41*(8), 641–671. DOI: 10.2165/11590680-000000000-00000 PMID: 21780850

Engel, G. L. (1977). The Need for a New Medical Model: A Challenge for Biomedicine. *Science, 196*(4286), 129–136. DOI: 10.1126/science.847460 PMID: 847460

Ensari, I., Greenlee, T. A., Motl, R. W., & Petruzzello, S. J. (2015). Meta-analysis of acute exercise effects on state anxiety: An update of randomized controlled trials over the past 25 years. *Depression and Anxiety, 32*(8), 624–634. PMID: 25899389

Erickson, K. I.. (2011). Physical activity increases hippocampal volume. *Proceedings of the National Academy of Sciences of the United States of America, 108*(7), 3017–3022. PMID: 21282661

Erickson, K. I., Hillman, C. H., & Kramer, A. F. (2015). Physical activity, brain, and cognition. *Current Opinion in Behavioral Sciences, 4*, 27–32. DOI: 10.1016/j.cobeha.2015.01.005

Erickson, K. I., Voss, M. W., Prakash, R. S., Basak, C., Szabo, A., Chaddock, L., & Kramer, A. F. (2011). Exercise training increases size of hippocampus and improves memory. *Proceedings of the National Academy of Sciences of the United States of America, 108*(7), 3017–3022. DOI: 10.1073/pnas.1015950108

Esteves, E. A.. (2021). Beneficial effects of physical exercise on cognitive behavioral outcomes: Mechanisms and evidence. *Progress in Brain Research*. Advance online publication. DOI: 10.1016/bs.pbr.2021.03.012

Etkin, A., Gyurak, A., & O'Hara, R. (2013). A neurobiological approach to the cognitive deficits of psychiatric disorders. *Dialogues in Clinical Neuroscience*, *15*(4), 419–429.

Eys, M., Bruner, M. W., & Martin, L. J. (2019). The dynamic group environment in sport and exercise. *Psychology of Sport and Exercise*, *42*, 40–47. DOI: 10.1016/j.psychsport.2018.11.001

Farmer, D. (2020). Teacher attrition: The impacts of stress. *Delta Kappa Gamma Bulletin*, *87*(1), 41–50.

Faulkner, G., & Sparkes, A. (1999). *Exercise as Therapy for Schizophrenia: An Ethnographic Study*. https://doi.org/DOI: 10.1123/jsep.21.1.52

Fernandes, B. S., Molendijk, M. L., Köhler, C. A., Soares, J. C., Leite, C. M. G., Machado-Vieira, R., & Carvalho, A. F. (2015). Peripheral brain-derived neurotrophic factor (BDNF) as a biomarker in bipolar disorder: A meta-analysis of 52 studies. *BMC Medicine*, *13*(1), 289. DOI: 10.1186/s12916-015-0529-7

Fernandes, M. M., & Sturm, R. (2011). The role of school physical activity Programs in Child body mass Trajectory. *Journal of Physical Activity & Health*, *8*(2), 174–181. DOI: 10.1123/jpah.8.2.174 PMID: 21415444

Festa, F., Medori, S., & Macrì, M. (2023). Move Your Body, Boost Your Brain: The Positive Impact of Physical Activity on Cognition across All Age Groups. *Biomedicines*, *11*(6), 1765. DOI: 10.3390/biomedicines11061765 PMID: 37371860

Fiorilli, C., Benevene, P., De Stasio, S., Buonomo, I., Romano, L., Pepe, A., & Addimando, L. (2019). Teachers' burnout: The role of trait emotional intelligence and social support. *Frontiers in Psychology*, *10*, 2743. Advance online publication. DOI: 10.3389/fpsyg.2019.02743 PMID: 31920801

Firth, J., Rosenbaum, S., Stubbs, B., Gorczynski, P., Yung, A. R., & Vancampfort, D. (2016). Motivating factors and barriers towards exercise in severe mental illness: A systematic review and meta-analysis. *Psychological Medicine*, *46*(14), 2869–2881. https://www.cambridge.org/core/journals/psychological-medicine/article/motivating-factors-and-barriers-towards-exercise-in-severe-mental-illness-a-systematic-review-and-metaanalysis/1802F617B64F75CF6721FE59A2F73D1F PMID: 27502153

Firth, J., Solmi, M., Wootton, R. E., Vancampfort, D., Schuch, F. B., Hoare, E., & Smith, L. (2020). A meta-review of "lifestyle psychiatry": The role of exercise, smoking, diet and sleep in the prevention and treatment of mental disorders. *World Psychiatry; Official Journal of the World Psychiatric Association (WPA), 19*(3), 360–380. DOI: 10.1002/wps.20773

Firth, J., Torous, J., Nicholas, J., Carney, R., Pratap, A., Rosenbaum, S., & Sarris, J. (2017). The efficacy of smartphone-based mental health interventions for depressive symptoms: A meta-analysis of randomized controlled trials. *World Psychiatry; Official Journal of the World Psychiatric Association (WPA), 16*(3), 287–298. DOI: 10.1002/wps.20472 PMID: 28941113

Firus, M. (2023). *Teacher wellness initiative: Viability of incorporating exercise into teachers' workday* [Doctoral dissertation, University of Saskatchewan]. University of Saskatchewan. https://harvest.usask.ca/server/api/core/bitstreams/ 473c72f8-abc8-44c0-b84e-c47f75094ae7/content

Fleshner, M., Greenwood, B. N., & Yirmiya, R. (2016). Neurobiological mechanisms of exercise: Antidepressant and anxiolytic effects. *Frontiers in Psychiatry, 7*, 118. DOI: 10.3389/fpsyt.2016.00118

Fletcher, D., & Sarkar, M. (2012). A grounded theory of psychological resilience in Olympic champions. *Psychology of Sport and Exercise, 13*(5), 669–678. DOI: 10.1016/j.psychsport.2012.04.007

Foley, T. E., & Fleshner, M. (2008). Neuroplasticity of Dopamine Circuits After Exercise: Implications for Central Fatigue. *Neuromolecular Medicine, 10*(2), 67–80. DOI: 10.1007/s12017-008-8032-3 PMID: 18274707

Fontana, F., Bourbeau, K., Moriarty, T., & da Silva, M. P. (2022). The relationship between physical activity, sleep quality, and stress: A study of teachers during the COVID-19 pandemic. *International Journal of Environmental Research and Public Health, 19*, 15465. Advance online publication. DOI: 10.3390/ijerph192315465 PMID: 36497539

Forbes, S., & Fikretoglu, D. (2018). Building Resilience: The Conceptual Basis and Research Evidence for Resilience Training Programs. *Review of General Psychology, 22*(4), 452–468. DOI: 10.1037/gpr0000152

Foster, J. A., & McVey Neufeld, K.-A. (2013). Gut-brain axis: How the microbiome influences anxiety and depression. *Trends in Neurosciences, 36*(5), 305–312. DOI: 10.1016/j.tins.2013.01.005 PMID: 23384445

Francois, M. E., & Little, J. P. (2015). Effectiveness and safety of high-intensity interval training in patients with type 2 diabetes. *Diabetes Spectrum, 28*(1), 39–44. DOI: 10.2337/diaspect.28.1.39 PMID: 25717277

Fraser, S. F.. (2025). Application of exercise snacks across youth, adult and older adult populations. *Sports Medicine (Auckland, N.Z.)*. Advance online publication. DOI: 10.1186/s40798-025-00829-6

Fredrickson, B. L. (2001). The role of positive emotions in positive psychology. The broaden-and-build theory of positive emotions. *The American Psychologist, 56*(3), 218–226. DOI: 10.1037//0003-066x.56.3.218 PMID: 11315248

Fredrickson, B. L., & Branigan, C. (2005). Positive emotions broaden the scope of attention and thought-action repertoires. *Cognition and Emotion, 19*(3), 313–332. DOI: 10.1080/02699930441000238

Fredrickson, B. L., & Joiner, T. (2002). Positive emotions trigger upward spirals toward emotional well-being. *Psychological Science, 13*(2), 172–175. DOI: 10.1111/1467-9280.00431 PMID: 11934003

Freeman, P., Coffee, P., & Rees, T. (2011). The PASS-Q: The Perceived Available Support in Sport Questionnaire. *Journal of Sport & Exercise Psychology, 33*(1), 54–74. DOI: 10.1123/jsep.33.1.54 PMID: 21451171

Freire, C., Ferradás, M. D. M., García-Bértoa, A., Núñez, J. C., Rodríguez, S., & Piñeiro, I. (2020). Psychological capital and burnout in teachers: The mediating role of flourishing. *International Journal of Environmental Research and Public Health, 17*(22). Advance online publication. DOI: 10.3390/ijerph17228403 PMID: 33202826

Freudenberger, H. J. (1989). *Burnout: Past, present, and future concerns.* [eBook edition]. In D.T. Wessells Jr., A. H. Kutscher, I. B., Seeland, F. E., Selder, D. J., Cherico, & E. J. Clark, (Eds.), Professional Burnout in Medicine and the Helping Professions (1-10). The Haworth Press. https://books.google.com/books

Freudenberger, H. J. (1975). The staff burn-out syndrome in alternative institutions. *Psychotherapy (Chicago, Ill.), 12*(1), 73–82. DOI: 10.1037/h0086411

Frey, B. N., Andreazza, A. C., Houenou, J., Jamain, S., Goldstein, B. I., Frye, M. A., & Young, L. T. (2013). Biomarkers in bipolar disorder: A positional paper from the International Society for Bipolar Disorders Biomarkers Task Force. *The Australian and New Zealand Journal of Psychiatry, 47*(4), 321–332. DOI: 10.1177/0004867413478217

Fugate, J. M., Macrine, S. L., & Hernandez-Cuevas, E. M. (2024). Therapeutic potential of embodied cognition for clinical psychotherapies: From theory to practice. *Cognitive Therapy and Research, 48*(4), 574–598. DOI: 10.1007/s10608-024-10428-3

Fuss, J.. (2015). Endocannabinoid release and emotional regulation through exercise. *Biological Psychiatry, 78*(10), 766–773.

Fuss, J., Steinle, J., Bindila, L., Auer, M. K., Kirchherr, H., Lutz, B., & Gass, P. (2015). A runner's high depends on cannabinoid receptors in mice. *Proceedings of the National Academy of Sciences of the United States of America, 112*(42), 13105–13108. DOI: 10.1073/pnas.1514996112 PMID: 26438875

Gabriel, B. M., & Zierath, J. R. (2019). Circadian rhythms and exercise—Re-setting the clock in metabolic disease. *Nature Reviews. Endocrinology, 15*(4), 197–206.

Garcia, A. W., Broda, M. A. N., Frenn, M., Coviak, C., Pender, N. J., & Ronis, D. L. (1995). Gender and Developmental Differences in Exercise Beliefs Among Youth and Prediction of Their Exercise Behavior. *The Journal of School Health, 65*(6), 213–219. DOI: 10.1111/j.1746-1561.1995.tb03365.x PMID: 7564283

Gard, T., Noggle, J. J., Park, C. L., Vago, D. R., & Wilson, A. (2014). Potential self-regulatory mechanisms of yoga for psychological health. *Frontiers in Human Neuroscience, 8*, 770.

Garfinkel, S. N., Seth, A. K., Barrett, A. B., Suzuki, K., & Critchley, H. D. (2015). Knowing your own heart: Distinguishing interoceptive accuracy from interoceptive awareness. *Biological Psychology, 104*, 65–74. DOI: 10.1016/j.biopsycho.2014.11.004 PMID: 25451381

Ghahramani, M., Sohrabi, M., Kakhki, A., & Besharat, M. (2016). The Effects of Physical Activity on Impulse Control, Attention, Decision making and Motor Functions in Students with High and Low Impulsivity. *Biosciences Biotechnology Research Asia, 13*(3), 1689–1696. DOI: 10.13005/bbra/2318

Girdler, S. J., Confino, J. E., & Woesner, M. E. (2019). Exercise as a Treatment for Schizophrenia: A Review. *Psychopharmacology Bulletin, 49*(1), 56–69. https://pmc.ncbi.nlm.nih.gov/articles/PMC6386427/ PMID: 30858639

Glasgow, R. E., Vinson, C., Chambers, D., Khoury, M. J., Kaplan, R. M., & Hunter, C. (2012). National Institutes of Health approaches to dissemination and implementation science: Current and future directions. *American Journal of Public Health, 102*(7), 1274–1281. DOI: 10.2105/AJPH.2012.300755 PMID: 22594758

Glover, C. M., Ferron, J. C., & Whitley, R. (2013). Barriers to exercise among people with severe mental illnesses. *Psychiatric Rehabilitation Journal, 36*(1), 45. https://psycnet.apa.org/record/2013-07802-009 PMID: 23477650

Goldfarb, A. H., & Jamurtas, A. Z. (1997). Beta-endorphin response to exercise. An update. *Sports Medicine (Auckland, N.Z.), 24*(1), 8–16. DOI: 10.2165/00007256-199724010-00002 PMID: 9257407

Gomes, F. V., Vieira, J. B., dos Santos, R. A., & Gadelha, A. (2021). Exercise, neurotrophins, and inflammation in bipolar disorder: A clinical trial perspective. *Journal of Psychiatric Research, 137*, 180–188. DOI: 10.1016/j.jpsychires.2021.03.012

Gomes-Osman, J., Cabral, D. F., Hinchman, C., Jannati, A., Morris, T. P., & Pascual-Leone, A. (2017). The effects of exercise on cognitive function and brain plasticity – a feasibility trial. *Restorative Neurology and Neuroscience, 35*(5), 547–556. DOI: 10.3233/RNN-170758 PMID: 28984621

Gomez-Pinilla, F., & Hillman, C. (2012). The influence of exercise on cognitive abilities. *Comprehensive Physiology*, •••, 403–428. DOI: 10.1002/cphy.c110063 PMID: 23720292

Gong, L. L., & Tao, F. Y. (2021). The effect of biopsychosocial holistic care models on the cognitive function and quality of life of elderly patients with mild cognitive impairment: A randomized trial. *Annals of Palliative Medicine, 10*(5), 5600609–5605609. DOI: 10.21037/apm-21-966

González-Valero, G., Gómez-Carmona, C. D., Bastida-Castillo, A., Corral-Pernía, J. A., Zurita-Ortega, F., & Melguizo-Ibáñez, E. (2023). Could the complying with WHO physical activity recommendations improve stress, burnout syndrome, and resilience? A cross-sectional study with physical education teachers. *Sport Sciences for Health, 19*, 349–358. DOI: 10.1007/s11332-022-00981-6

Gordon, B. R., McDowell, C. P., Hallgren, M., Meyer, J. D., Lyons, M., & Herring, M. P. (2018). Association of efficacy of resistance exercise training with depressive symptoms: Meta-analysis and meta-regression analysis of randomized clinical trials. *JAMA Psychiatry, 75*(6), 566–576. DOI: 10.1001/jamapsychiatry.2018.0256 PMID: 29800984

Gordon, B. R., McDowell, C. P., Hallgren, M., Meyer, J. D., Lyons, M., & Herring, M. P. (2018). Association of Efficacy of Resistance Exercise Training With Depressive Symptoms: Meta-analysis and Meta-regression Analysis of Randomized Clinical Trials. *JAMA Psychiatry, 75*(6), 566–576. DOI: 10.1001/jamapsychiatry.2018.0572 PMID: 29800984

Gordon, B. R., McDowell, C. P., Lyons, M., & Herring, M. P. (2017). Resistance exercise training for anxiety and worry symptoms among young adults: A randomized controlled trial. *Scientific Reports*, *7*(1), 17548. DOI: 10.1038/s41598-017-17704-7 PMID: 33067493

Gordon, B. R., McDowell, C. P., Lyons, M., & Herring, M. P. (2017a). The Effects of Resistance Exercise Training on Anxiety: A Meta-Analysis and Meta-Regression Analysis of Randomized Controlled Trials. *Sports Medicine (Auckland, N.Z.)*, *47*(12), 2521–2532. DOI: 10.1007/s40279-017-0769-0 PMID: 28819746

Gordon, J. (2023). Empowered Learners: How Martial Arts Foster Self-Regulated Learning. *Mantle: The Annual Review of Interdisciplinary Research*, *1*(1), 29–39.

Gould, D., & Maynard, I. (2009). Psychological preparation for the Olympic Games. *Journal of Sports Sciences*, *27*(13), 1393–1408. DOI: 10.1080/02640410903081845 PMID: 19787542

Gould, D., & Whitley, M. A. (2009). Sources and consequences of athletic burnout among college athletes. *Journal of Intercollegiate Sport*, *2*(1), 16–30.

Goyal, M., Singh, S., Sibinga, E. M. S., Gould, N. F., Rowland-Seymour, A., Sharma, R., Berger, Z., Sleicher, D., Maron, D. D., Shihab, H. M., Ranasinghe, P. D., Linn, S., Saha, S., Bass, E. B., & Haythornthwaite, J. A. (2014). Meditation programs for psychological stress and well-being: A systematic review and meta-analysis. *JAMA Internal Medicine*, *174*(3), 357–368. DOI: 10.1001/jamainternmed.2013.13018 PMID: 24395196

Grande, I., Berk, M., Birmaher, B., & Vieta, E. (2016). Bipolar disorder. *Lancet*, *387*(10027), 1561–1572.

Granziera, H. (2022). Teachers' personal resources: What do we know and where do we go? A scoping review through the lens of job demands-resources theory. *Journal of Positive Psychology and Wellbeing*, *6*(2), 1695–1718. https://www.researchgate.net/profile/Helena-Granziera/publication/363889926_Teachers'_Personal_Resources_What_Do_We_Know_and_Where_Do_We_Go_A_Scoping_Review_Through_the_Lens_of_Job_Demands-Resources_Theory/links/6333c9165d1e2d53d9a3ce48/Teachers-Personal-Resources-What-Do-We-Know-and-Where-Do-We-Go-A-Scoping-Review-Through-the-Lens-of-Job-Demands-Resources-Theory.pdf

Gray, C., Wilcox, G., & Nordstokke, D. (2017). Teacher mental health, school climate, inclusive education and student learning: A review. *Canadian Psychology*, *58*(3), 203–210. DOI: 10.1037/cap0000117

Greenberg, L. S. (2015). Emotion-focused therapy: Coaching clients to work through their feelings, 2nd ed (pp. vi, 411). American Psychological Association. https://doi.org/DOI: 10.1037/14692-000

Greenwood, B. N., & Fleshner, M. (2011). Exercise, stress resistance, and central serotonergic systems. *Exercise and Sport Sciences Reviews, 39*(3), 140–149. DOI: 10.1097/JES.0b013e31821f7e45

Greenwood, B. N., Foley, T. E., Le, T. V., Strong, P. V., Loughridge, A. B., Day, H. E. W., & Fleshner, M. (2011). Long-term voluntary wheel running is rewarding and produces plasticity in the mesolimbic reward pathway. *Behavioural Brain Research, 217*(2), 354–362. DOI: 10.1016/j.bbr.2010.11.005 PMID: 21070820

Gregg, J. (2024). *You don't have to feel that way: The totally natural way to beat anxiety, depression, and bipolar behavior without drugs.* Jason Gregg.

Grogan, S. (2016). *Body Image: Understanding Body Dissatisfaction in Men, Women and Children* (3rd ed.). Routledge., DOI: 10.4324/9781315681528

Gross, J. J. (2002). Emotion regulation: Affective, cognitive, and social consequences. *Psychophysiology, 39*(3), 281–291. DOI: 10.1017/s0048577201393198 PMID: 12212647

Gucciardi, D. F., Hanton, S., Gordon, S., Mallett, C. J., & Temby, P. (2015). The Concept of Mental Toughness: Tests of Dimensionality, Nomological Network, and Traitness. *Journal of Personality, 83*(1), 26–44. DOI: 10.1111/jopy.12079 PMID: 24428736

Guo, J. (2025). The dual impact of physical exercise on university students' mental health: The chain mediating effects of mindfulness and psychological resilience. *Frontiers in Psychology, 16.* Advance online publication. DOI: 10.3389/fpsyg.2025.1545370 PMID: 40297594

Gustafsson, H., DeFreese, J., & Madigan, D. J. (2017). Athlete burnout: Review and recommendations. *Current Opinion in Psychology, 16*, 109–113. DOI: 10.1016/j.copsyc.2017.05.002 PMID: 28813331

Ha, C., Pressley, T., & Marshall, D. T. (2025). Teacher voices matter: The role of teacher autonomy in enhancing job satisfaction and mitigating burnout. *PLoS One, 20*(1), e0317471. Advance online publication. DOI: 10.1371/journal.pone.0317471 PMID: 39804894

Hall, A., Lane, C., Wolfenden, L., Wiggers, J., Sutherland, R., McCarthy, N., Jackson, R., Shoesmith, A., Lecathelinais, C., Reeves, P., Bauman, A., Gillham, K., Boyer, J., Naylor, P., Kerr, N., Kajons, N., & Nathan, N. (2023). Evaluating the scaling up of an effective implementation intervention (PACE) to increase the delivery of a mandatory physical activity policy in primary schools. *International Journal of Behavioral Nutrition and Physical Activity, 20*(1). y.DOI: 10.1186/s12966 023 01498

Hausenblas, H. A., & Symons Downs, D. (2002). Exercise dependence: A systematic review. *Psychology of Sport and Exercise, 3*(2), 89–123. DOI: 10.1016/S1469-0292(00)00015-7

Hayes, S. C., Luoma, J. B., Bond, F. W., Masuda, A., & Lillis, J. (2006). Acceptance and commitment therapy: Model, processes and outcomes. *Behaviour Research and Therapy, 44*(1), 1–25. DOI: 10.1016/j.brat.2005.06.006 PMID: 16300724

Heath, N., Midkiff, M. F., Gerhart, J., & Turow, R. G. (2021). Group-based DBT skills training modules are linked to independent and additive improvements in emotion regulation in a heterogeneous outpatient sample. *Psychotherapy Research, 31*(8), 1001–1011. DOI: 10.1080/10503307.2020.1870356

Heidarzadeh, M., Zamanzadeh, V., Maghvan, A. P., & Oshvandi, K. (2010). The effect of physical exercise on physical and psychological problems. *Iranian Journal of Nursing and Midwifery Research, 15*(1), 20. https://pmc.ncbi.nlm.nih.gov/articles/PMC3093026/ PMID: 21589745

Heijnen, S., Hommel, B., Kibele, A., & Colzato, L. S. (2016). Neuromodulation of Aerobic Exercise—A Review. *Frontiers in Psychology, 6*. Advance online publication. DOI: 10.3389/fpsyg.2015.01890 PMID: 26779053

Heinemann, L. V., & Heinemann, T. (2017). Burnout research: Emergence and scientific investigation of a contested diagnosis. *SAGE Open, 7*(1), 1–12. DOI: 10.1177/2158244017697154

Heinrich, K. M., Patel, P. M., O'Neal, J. L., & Heinrich, B. S. (2014). High-intensity compared to moderate-intensity training for exercise initiation, enjoyment, adherence, and intentions: An intervention study. *BMC Public Health, 14*, 789. DOI: 10.1186/1471-2458-14-789 PMID: 25086646

Heisz, J. J., Clark, I. B., Bonin, K., Paolucci, E. M., Michalski, B., Becker, S., & Fahnestock, M. (2017). The Effects of Physical Exercise and Cognitive Training on Memory and Neurotrophic Factors. *Journal of Cognitive Neuroscience, 29*(11), 1895–1907. DOI: 10.1162/jocn_a_01164 PMID: 28699808

Hendriks, T., De Jong, J., & Cramer, H. (2017). The effects of yoga on positive mental health among healthy adults: A systematic review and meta-analysis. *Journal of Alternative and Complementary Medicine (New York, N.Y.)*, *23*(7), 505–517. DOI: 10.1089/acm.2016.0334

Henrich, J., Heine, S. J., & Norenzayan, A. (2010). The weirdest people in the world? *Behavioral and Brain Sciences*, *33*(2–3), 61–83. DOI: 10.1017/S0140525X0999152X PMID: 20550733

Henriksen, K., Schinke, R., Moesch, K., McCann, S., Parham, W. D., Larsen, C. H., & Terry, P. (2020). Consensus statement on improving the mental health of high performance athletes. *International Journal of Sport and Exercise Psychology*, *18*(5), 553–560. DOI: 10.1080/1612197X.2019.1570473

Hernandez, D. C., Santos, H., & Penaflor, G. (2023). *Mindfulness youth novel dynamics (MYND): A stress management strategy for junior high school students.* E-Saliksik / DepEd Philippines.

Herring, M. P., O'Connor, P. J., & Dishman, R. K. (2010). The effect of exercise training on anxiety symptoms among patients: A systematic review. *Archives of Internal Medicine*, *170*(4), 321–331. PMID: 20177034

Heyman, E., Gamelin, F., Goekint, M., Pisciella, P., Roelands, B., Leclair, E., Di Marzo, V., & Meeusen, R. (2012). Intense exercise increases circulating endocannabinoid and BDNF levels in humans-Possible implications for reward and depression. Psychoneuroendocrinology. 37(6): 844-851, 2012. SCI: - 5.168 –. *Psychoneuroendocrinology*, *37*, 844–851. PMID: 22029953

Heyman, E., Gamelin, F.-X., Goekint, M., Piscitelli, F., Roelands, B., Leclair, E., Di Marzo, V., & Meeusen, R. (2012). Intense exercise increases circulating endocannabinoid and BDNF levels in humans—Possible implications for reward and depression. *Psychoneuroendocrinology*, *37*(6), 844–851. DOI: 10.1016/j.psyneuen.2011.09.017 PMID: 22029953

Hickingbotham, M. R., Wong, C. J., & Bowling, A. B. (2021). Barriers and facilitators to physical education, sport, and physical activity program participation among children and adolescents with psychiatric disorders: A systematic review. *Translational Behavioral Medicine*, *11*(9), 1739–1750. https://academic.oup.com/tbm/article-abstract/11/9/1739/6309033 PMID: 34166515

Hillman, C. H., Erickson, K. I., & Kramer, A. F. (2008). Be smart, exercise your heart: Exercise effects on brain and cognition. *Nature Reviews. Neuroscience*, *9*(1), 58–65. DOI: 10.1038/nrn2298 PMID: 18094706

Hillman, C. H., Erickson, K. I., & Kramer, A. F. (2008). Exercise and brain function. *Nature Reviews. Neuroscience*, *9*, 58–65. PMID: 18094706

Hlado, P., & Harvankova, K. (2024). Teachers' perceived work ability: A qualitative exploration using the Job Demands-Resources model. *Humanities & Social Sciences Communications*, *11*, 304. DOI: 10.1057/s41599-024-02811-1

Hogan, N. S., & Schmidt, L. A. (2002). Testing the grief to personal growth model using structural equation modeling. *Death Studies*, *26*(8), 615–634. DOI: 10.1080/07481180290088338 PMID: 12243195

Hojo, M. (2021). Association between student-teacher ratio and teachers' working hours and workload stress: Evidence from a nationwide survey in Japan. *BMC Public Health*, *21*, 1635. Advance online publication. DOI: 10.1186/s12889-021-11677-w PMID: 34493251

Hossain, M. N., Lee, J., Choi, H., Kwak, Y., & Kim, J. (2024). The impact of exercise on depression: How moving makes your brain and body feel better. *Physical Activity and Nutrition*, *28*(2), 43–51. DOI: 10.20463/pan.2024.0015 PMID: 39097997

House, J. S., Landis, K. R., & Umberson, D. (1988). Social relationships and health. *Science*, *241*(4865), 540–545. DOI: 10.1126/science.3399889 PMID: 3399889

Howie, E. K., & Pate, R. R. (2012). Physical activity and academic achievement in children: A historical perspective. *Journal of Sport and Health Science. Journal of Sport and Health Science*, *1*(3), 160–169. DOI: 10.1016/j.jshs.2012.09.003

Howren, M. B., Lamkin, D. M., & Suls, J. (2009). Associations of depression with C-reactive protein, IL-1, and IL-6: A meta-analysis. *Psychosomatic Medicine*, *71*(2), 171–186. DOI: 10.1097/PSY.0b013e3181907c1b PMID: 19188531

Huang, S., Yau, S. Y., Lee, Y. K. L., Song, J., Guo, Y., & Dong, D. (2025). Job characteristics, personal characteristics and well-being of nursing assistants in long-term care facilities: A mixed methods systematic review and narrative synthesis. *International Journal of Nursing Studies*, *161*, 104934. Advance online publication. DOI: 10.1016/j.ijnurstu.2024.104934 PMID: 39476575

Huang, X., Wang, Y., & Zhang, H. (2023). Effects of physical exercise intervention on depressive and anxious moods of college students: A meta analysis of randomized controlled trials. *Asian Journal of Sport and Exercise Psychology*, *3*(3), 206–221. DOI: 10.1016/j.ajsep.2023.01.001

Huk, O., Terjesen, M. D., & Cherkasova, L. (2019). Predicting teacher burnout as a function of school characteristics and irrational beliefs. *Psychology in the Schools*, *56*(5), 792–808. DOI: 10.1002/pits.22233

Humphreys, B., & Ruseski, J. (2008, July). The size and scope of the sports industry in the United States. In *IASE Conference Papers* (Vol. 833). International Association of Sports Economists.

Hunt, J., & Eisenberg, D. (2010). Mental health problems and help-seeking behavior among college students. *The Journal of Adolescent Health: Official Publication of the Society for Adolescent Medicine, 46*(1), 3–10. DOI: 10.1016/j.jadohealth.2009.08.008 PMID: 20123251

Hyatt, K. (2022). Stressors in higher education that lead to burnout and solutions to avoid it. *Journal of Business and Educational Leadership, 12*(1), 110–125.

Hyvönen, K., Pylvänäinen, P., Muotka, J., & Lappalainen, R. (2020). The effects of dance movement therapy in the treatment of depression: A multicenter, randomized controlled trial in Finland. *Frontiers in Psychology, 11*, 1687. DOI: 10.3389/fpsyg.2020.01687

Immordino-Yang, M. H., Darling-Hammond, L., & Krone, C. R. (2025). Nurturing nature: How brain development is inherently social and emotional, and what this means for education. In *Social and Emotional Learning* (pp. 63–83). Routledge.

Inbar, L., & Shiri, S. A. (2021). Managing the emotional aspects of compassion fatigue among teachers in Israel: A qualitative study. *Journal of Education for Teaching, 47*(4), 562–575. DOI: 10.1080/02607476.2021.1929876

Jacobs-Pinson, E. (n.d.). *25+ teacher burnout statistics: A crisis we can't ignore.* Crown Counseling. https://crowncounseling.com/statistics/teacher-burnout/

Jahoda, M. (1958). *Current concepts of positive mental health.* Basic Books/Hachette Book Group., DOI: 10.1037/11258-000

Jakicic, J. M., Wing, R. R., Butler, B. A., & Robertson, R. J. (1995). Prescribing exercise in multiple short bouts versus one continuous bout: effects on adherence, cardiorespiratory fitness, and weight loss in overweight women. *International journal of obesity and related metabolic disorders: journal of the International Association for the Study of Obesity, 19*(12), 893–901.

Jamal, A., Begum, S., Alam, H., & Hussain, T. (2023). Impact of perceived organizational support on innovative work behavior and burnout in teachers: Thriving at work as the mediator (2020). *Journal of Education and Educational Development, 10*(2), 288–307. DOI: 10.22555/joeed.v10i2.815

James, J., Pringle, A., Mourton, S., & Roscoe, C. M. P. (2023). The Effects of Physical Activity On Academic Performance in School Aged Children: A Systematic review. *Children (Basel, Switzerland), 10*(6), 1019. DOI: 10.3390/children10061019 PMID: 37371251

Javaid, S. F., Hashim, I. J., Hashim, M. J., Stip, E., Samad, M. A., & Ahbabi, A. A. (2023). Epidemiology of anxiety disorders: Global burden and sociodemographic associations. *Middle East Current Psychiatry, 30*(1), 44. DOI: 10.1186/s43045-023-00359-9

Jenkins, E. M., ... (2019). Exercise snacking to improve muscle function in healthy older adults. Journal of Aging Research. https://pmc.ncbi.nlm.nih.gov/articles/PMC6794984/

Jennings, P. A., & Min, H. H. (2023). Transforming empathy-based stress to compassion: Skillful means to preventing teacher burnout. *Mindfulness, 14*, 2311–2322. DOI: 10.1007/s12671-023-02115-6 PMID: 37362185

Jeon, H. J., Diamond, L., McCartney, C., & Kwon, K. A. (2022). Early childhood special education teachers' job burnout and psychological stress. *Early Education and Development, 33*(8), 1364–1382. DOI: 10.1080/10409289.2021.1965395 PMID: 36353579

Jiao, C., Qian, J., & Liu, H. (2022). The relationship between preschool inclusive education teachers' organizational support and work engagement: The mediating role of teacher self-efficacy. *Frontiers in Psychology, 13*, 900836. Advance online publication. DOI: 10.3389/fpsyg.2022.900835 PMID: 35686076

Johnson-Sealey, F. (2024). *Choreographing a journey of self-discovery: An exploration of dance, embodied knowledge, and identity* (Doctoral dissertation, City University of New York).

Jomuad, P. D., Antigua, L. M. M., Cericos, E. U., Bacus, J. A., Vallejo, J. H., Dionio, B. B., Bazar, J. S., Cocolan, J. V., & Clarin, A. S. (2021). Teachers' workload in relation to burnout and work performance. *International Journal of Education Policy Research and Review, 8*(2), 48–52. DOI: 10.15739/IJEPRR.21.007

Joormann, J., & Stanton, C. H. (2016). Examining emotion regulation in depression: A review and future directions. *Behaviour Research and Therapy, 86*, 35–49. DOI: 10.1016/j.brat.2016.07.007 PMID: 27492851

Josefsson, T., Ivarsson, A., Lindwall, M., Gustafsson, H., Stenling, A., Böröy, J., Mattsson, E., Carnebratt, J., Sevholt, S., & Falkevik, E. (2017). Mindfulness Mechanisms in Sports: Mediating Effects of Rumination and Emotion Regulation on Sport-Specific Coping. *Mindfulness*, *8*(5), 1354–1363. DOI: 10.1007/s12671-017-0711-4 PMID: 28989551

Jowett, S., & Chaundy, V. (2004). An Investigation Into the Impact of Coach Leadership and Coach-Athlete Relationship on Group Cohesion. *Group Dynamics*, *8*(4), 302–311. DOI: 10.1037/1089-2699.8.4.302

Kabat-Zinn, J. (2003). Mindfulness-Based Interventions in Context: Past, Present, and Future. *Clinical Psychology : a Publication of the Division of Clinical Psychology of the American Psychological Association*, *10*, 144–156. DOI: 10.1093/clipsy.bpg016

Kamboj, K. P., & Garg, P. (2021). Teachers' psychological well-being role of emotional intelligence and resilience character traits in determining the psychological well-being of Indian school teachers. *International Journal of Educational Management*, *35*(4), 768–788. DOI: 10.1108/IJEM-08-2019-0278

Kandola, A. A., del Pozo Cruz, B., Osborn, D. P. J., Stubbs, B., Choi, K. W., & Hayes, J. F. (2021). Impact of replacing sedentary behaviour with other movement behaviours on depression and anxiety symptoms: A prospective cohort study in the UK Biobank. *BMC Medicine*, *19*, 133. DOI: 10.1186/s12916-021-01995-9

Kandola, A., Ashdown-Franks, G., Hendrikse, J., Sabiston, C. M., & Stubbs, B. (2019). Physical activity and depression: Towards understanding the antidepressant mechanisms of physical activity. *Neuroscience and Biobehavioral Reviews*, *107*, 525–539. DOI: 10.1016/j.neubiorev.2019.09.040 PMID: 31586447

Kariou, A., Koutsimani, P., Montgomery, A., & Lainidi, O. (2021). Emotional labor and burnout among teachers: A systematic review. *International Journal of Environmental Research and Public Health*, *18*(23), 12760. Advance online publication. DOI: 10.3390/ijerph182312760 PMID: 34886485

Karkou, V., Aithal, S., Zubala, A., & Meekums, B. (2019). Effectiveness of Dance Movement Therapy in the Treatment of Adults With Depression: A Systematic Review With Meta-Analyses. *Frontiers in Psychology*, *10*, 936. DOI: 10.3389/fpsyg.2019.00936 PMID: 31130889

Karmakar, D., Das, A., Saha, G. C., & Govindasamy, K. (2025). The Impact of Physical Education and Sports on Emotional Resilience and Self-Efficacy. In Lobo, J., & Tagare, R. L.Jr., (Eds.), *Emerging Pedagogical Practices in Physical and Sports Education* (pp. 125–154). IGI Global Scientific Publishing., DOI: 10.4018/979-8-3373-2160-8.ch006

Karsai, I., Prémusz, V., & Lendvai, D. (2025). Impact of 10 weeks of yoga intervention on mental health and overall well-being among medical students (GSY study). *Sports (Basel, Switzerland), 13*(4), 114.

Kasapoglu, K., & Didin, M. (2019). Life skills as a predictor of psychological well-being of pre-service pre-school teachers in Turkey. *International Journal of Contemporary Education Research, 6*(1), 70–85. DOI: 10.33200/ijcer.544232

Kashihara, K., Maruyama, T., Murota, M., & Nakahara, Y. (2009). Positive effects of acute and moderate physical exercise on cognitive function. *Journal of Physiological Anthropology, 28*(4), 155–164. DOI: 10.2114/jpa2.28.155 PMID: 19652447

Kassymova, K., Kosherbayeva, N., Sangilbayev, S., & Schachl, H. (2018, September). Stress management techniques for students. In *International Conference on the Theory and Practice of Personality Formation in Modern Society (ICTPPFMS 2018)* (pp. 47-56). Atlantis Press.

Keating, X. D., Guan, J., Piñero, J. C., & Bridges, D. M. (2005). A meta-analysis of college students' physical activity behaviors. *Journal of American College Health: J of ACH, 54*(2), 116–125. DOI: 10.3200/JACH.54.2.116-126 PMID: 16255324

Kelley, G. A., & Kelley, K. S. (2017a). Exercise and depression in older adults: A meta-analysis of randomized controlled trials. *Journal of Aging and Physical Activity, 25*(4), 711–719. DOI: 10.1123/japa.2016-0120

Kelley, G. A., & Kelley, K. S. (2017b). Exercise and sleep: A systematic review of previous meta-analyses. *Journal of Evidence-Based Medicine, 10*(1), 26–36. DOI: 10.1111/jebm.12236 PMID: 28276627

Kellmann, M. (2010). Preventing overtraining in athletes in high-intensity sports and stress/recovery monitoring. *Scandinavian Journal of Medicine & Science in Sports, 20*(s2), 95–102. DOI: 10.1111/j.1600-0838.2010.01192.x PMID: 20840567

Kellmann, M., Bertollo, M., Bosquet, L., Brink, M., Coutts, A. J., Duffield, R., Erlacher, D., Halson, S. L., Hecksteden, A., & Heidari, J. (2018). Recovery and performance in sport: Consensus statement. *International Journal of Sports Physiology and Performance, 13*(2), 240–245. PMID: 29345524

Kendrick, A. (2022). Compassion fatigue, burnout, and the emotional labor of educational workers. *The International Journal of Health, Wellness & Society, 13*(1), 31–55. DOI: 10.18848/2156-8960/CGP/v13i01/31-55

Kenttä, G., & Hassmén, P. (1998). Overtraining and Recovery: A Conceptual Model. *Sports Medicine (Auckland, N.Z.), 26*(1), 1–16. DOI: 10.2165/00007256-199826010-00001 PMID: 9739537

Kessing, L. V., Rytgaard, H. C., Ekstrøm, C. T., Torp-Pedersen, C., Berk, M., & Gerds, T. A. (2020). Antihypertensive drugs and risk of depression: A nationwide population-based study. *Hypertension, 76*(4), 1263–1279.

Kessler, R. C., Petukhova, M., Sampson, N. A., Zaslavsky, A. M., & Wittchen, H.-U. (2012). Twelve-month and lifetime prevalence and lifetime morbid risk of anxiety and mood disorders in the United States. *International Journal of Methods in Psychiatric Research, 21*(3), 169–184. DOI: 10.1002/mpr.1359 PMID: 22865617

Kilby, E. (1985). National Association for Sport and Physical Education 1960–1985. *Journal of Physical Education, Recreation & Dance, 56*(4), 120–122. DOI: 10.1080/07303084.1985.10603771

Kim, G., & Gurvitch, R. (2020). The effect of sports-based physical activity programme on teachers' relatedness, stress, and exercise motivation. *Health Education Journal, 79*(6), 658–670. DOI: 10.1177/0017896920906185

Kim, L. E., Jorg, V., & Klassen, R. M. (2019). A meta-analysis of the effects of teacher personality on teacher effectiveness and burnout. *Educational Psychology Review, 31*(1), 163–195. DOI: 10.1007/s10648-018-9458-2 PMID: 30930595

Kinder, C. J., Richards, K. A., Trad, A. M., Woods, A. M., & Graber, K. C. (2023). Perceived organizational support, marginalization, isolation, emotional exhaustion, and job satisfaction of PETE faculty members. *European Physical Education Review, 29*(4), 475–492. DOI: 10.1177/1356336X231159636

King, R. (2002). Cognitive therapy of depression. *The Australian and New Zealand Journal of Psychiatry, 36*(2), 272–275. DOI: 10.1046/j.1440-1614.2002.t01-4-01015.x PMID: 11982560

Kiremitci, O., Boz, B., & Yıldız Çakır, L. (2023). Job demands-resources model and burnout in physical education teaching: A mixed-method sequential explanatory study. *Work (Reading, Mass.), 76*(1), 171–187. DOI: 10.3233/WOR-220102 PMID: 36872824

Koenders, M. A., Mesbah, R., Fleuren, B. P., Wardenaar, K. J., van der Veen, D. C., & Bockting, C. L. H. (2020). The role of emotion regulation in bipolar disorder: A systematic review. *Clinical Psychology Review, 78*, 101855. DOI: 10.1016/j.cpr.2020.101855

Kong, L., Cui, Y., & Gong, Q. (2022). Duration of keeping an exercise habit and mental illness and life attitude among university students. *International Journal of Environmental Research and Public Health, 19*(18), 11669. DOI: 10.3390/ijerph191811669 PMID: 36141940

Kong, S., & Lai, M. (2023). Effects of a teacher development program on teachers' knowledge and collaborative engagement, and students' achievement in computational thinking concepts. *British Journal of Educational Technology, 54*(2), 489–512. DOI: 10.1111/bjet.13256

Kotowski, S. E., Davis, K. G., & Barratt, C. L. (2022). Teachers feeling the burden of COVID-19: Impact on well-being, stress, and burnout. *Work (Reading, Mass.), 71*(2), 407–415. DOI: 10.3233/WOR-210994 PMID: 35068412

Kredlow, M. A., Capozzoli, M. C., Hearon, B. A., Calkins, A. W., & Otto, M. W. (2015). The effects of physical activity on sleep: A meta-analytic review. *Journal of Behavioral Medicine, 38*(3), 427–449. DOI: 10.1007/s10865-015-9617-6 PMID: 25596964

Kujawa, A., Klein, D. N., Pegg, S., & Weinberg, A. (2020). Developmental trajectories to reduced activation of positive valence systems: A review of biological and environmental contributions. *Developmental Cognitive Neuroscience, 43*, 100791.

Ladwig, K. H., Marten-Mittag, B., Olliges, E., Johar, H., Atasoy, S., Holdenrieder, S., & Ronel, J. (2025). Recurrent depression predicts high leptin concentrations in patients with coronary artery disease over an 18-months follow-up period: Findings from the prospective multicenter randomized controlled SPIRR-CAD Trial. *Journal of Affective Disorders, 369*, 174–181.

Latino, F., Cataldi, S., & Fischetti, F. (2021). Effects of an 8-week yoga-based physical exercise intervention on teachers' burnout. *Sustainability, 13*, 2104. Advance online publication. DOI: 10.3390/su13042104

Lavretsky, H., & Feldman, J. L. (2021). Precision medicine for breath-focused mind-body therapies for stress and anxiety: Are we ready yet? *Global Advances in Health and Medicine : Improving Healthcare Outcomes Worldwide, 10*, 2164956120986129.

Lazarus, R. S. (2000). How Emotions Influence Performance in Competitive Sports. *The Sport Psychologist, 14*(3), 229–252. DOI: 10.1123/tsp.14.3.229

Lazzarelli, A., Scafuto, F., Crescentini, C., Matiz, A., Orrù, G., Ciacchini, R., & Conversano, C. (2024). Interoceptive ability and emotion regulation in mind–body interventions: An integrative review. *Behavioral Sciences (Basel, Switzerland), 14*(11), 1107.

Lederer, A. M., & Hoban, M. T. (2022). The development of the American College Health Association-National College Health Assessment III: An improved tool to assess and enhance the health and well-being of college students. *Journal of American College Health: J of ACH, 70*(6), 1606–1610. DOI: 10.1080/07448481.2020.1834401 PMID: 33400616

Lee, I.-M., Shiroma, E. J., Lobelo, F., Puska, P., Blair, S. N., & Katzmarzyk, P. T.Lancet Physical Activity Series Working Group. (2012). Effect of physical inactivity on major non-communicable diseases worldwide: An analysis of burden of disease and life expectancy. *Lancet, 380*(9838), 219–229. DOI: 10.1016/S0140-6736(12)61031-9 PMID: 22818936

Leggett, W. (2022). Can mindfulness really change the world? The political character of meditative practices. *Critical Policy Studies, 16*(3), 261–278.

Lei, G., Li, L., & Zhang, L. (2025). Mental health literacy and anxiety in college students mediating role of psychological resilience and moderating role of physical exercise. *Scientific Reports, 15*(1), 35340. DOI: 10.1038/s41598-025-19381-0 PMID: 41068229

Lesener, T., Gusy, B., & Wolter, C. (2018). The job demands-resources model: A meta-analytic review of longitudinal studies. *Work and Stress, 33*(1), 76–103. DOI: 10.1080/02678373.2018.1529065

Leung, K. H., & Cheung, A. C. K. (2024). Understanding emotional well-being of teachers: Development and validation of teacher emotions in teaching scale in Hong Kong using a mixed-methods approach. *Teaching and Teacher Education, 152*, 104792. Advance online publication. DOI: 10.1016/j.tate.2024.104792

Levine, G. N., Cohen, B. E., Commodore-Mensah, Y., Fleury, J., Huffman, J. C., & Khalid, U. & American Heart Association Council on Clinical Cardiology; Council on Arteriosclerosis, Thrombosis and Vascular Biology; Council on Cardiovascular and Stroke Nursing; and Council on Lifestyle and Cardiometabolic Health. (2021). Psychological health, well-being, and the mind-heart-body connection: A scientific statement from the American Heart Association. *Circulation, 143*(10), e763–e783.

Levin, O., Netz, Y., & Ziv, G. (2017). The beneficial effects of different types of exercise interventions on motor and cognitive functions in older age: A systematic review. *European Review of Aging and Physical Activity : Official Journal of the European Group for Research into Elderly and Physical Activity, 14*(1), 20. DOI: 10.1186/s11556-017-0189-z PMID: 29276545

Lightfoot, J. T., & Geus, DE, E. J. C., Booth, F. W., Bray, M. S., DEN Hoed, M., Kaprio, J., Kelly, S. A., Pomp, D., Saul, M. C., Thomis, M. A., Garland, T., & Bouchard, C. (2018). Biological/Genetic Regulation of Physical Activity Level: Consensus from GenBioPAC. *Medicine and Science in Sports and Exercise*, *50*(4), 863–873. DOI: 10.1249/MSS.0000000000001499 PMID: 29166322

Liguori, G., & Medicine (ACSM), A. C. of S. (2020). *ACSM's Guidelines for Exercise Testing and Prescription*. Wolters Kluwer Health.

Li, J., He, Y., Wang, Y., & Xue, E. (2025). Investigating higher education teachers' well-being and its influencing multiple factors: A systematic review approach. *International Journal of Mental Health Promotion*, *27*(7), 901–928. DOI: 10.32604/ijmhp.2025.066538

Li, M., Huang, Y., & Sun, M. (2025). Exploring the structural links between peer support, psychological resilience, and exercise adherence in adolescents: A multigroup model across gender and educational stages. *BMC Public Health*, *25*(1), 2300. DOI: 10.1186/s12889-025-23308-9 PMID: 40610991

Limone, P., & Toto, G. A. (2022). Factors that predispose undergraduates to mental issues: A cumulative literature review for future research perspectives. *Frontiers in Public Health*, *10*, 831349.

Lin, T. W., & Kuo, Y. M. (2013). Exercise benefits brain function: The monoamine connection. *Brain Sciences*, *3*(1), 39–53. PMID: 24961306

Little, J. P.. (2019). Sprint exercise snacks: A novel approach to increase aerobic fitness. *Scandinavian Journal of Medicine & Science in Sports*. Advance online publication. DOI: 10.1111/sms.13413 PMID: 30847639

Liu-Ambrose, T., Nagamatsu, L. S., Graf, P., Beattie, B. L., Ashe, M. C., & Handy, T. C. (2010). Resistance Training and Executive Functions: A 12-Month Randomised Controlled Trial. *Archives of Internal Medicine*, *170*(2), 170–178. DOI: 10.1001/archinternmed.2009.494 PMID: 20101012

Liu, C. H., Stevens, C., Wong, S. H. M., Yasui, M., & Chen, J. A. (2019). The prevalence and predictors of mental health diagnoses and suicide among U.S. college students: Implications for addressing disparities in service use. *Depression and Anxiety*, *36*(1), 8–17. DOI: 10.1002/da.22830 PMID: 30188598

Li, W., Chen, P., Jiang, A., Zhang, F., & Wu, Z. (2025). Gender differences in cognitive benefits of meeting physical activity guidelines in older Chinese adults. *Frontiers in Public Health*, *13*. Advance online publication. DOI: 10.3389/fpubh.2025.1539369 PMID: 40567994

Li, X., Jiang, T., Sun, J., Shi, L., & Liu, J. (2021). The relationship between occupational stress, job burnout and quality of life among surgical nurses in Xinjiang, China. *BMC Nursing*, *20*(1), 1–11. DOI: 10.1186/s12912-021-00703-2 PMID: 34579710

Lochrie, J. G. (2024). *Student Barriers and Motivators to Bystander Intervention If Witnessing Potential Sexual Violence on College Campuses*. St. John's University.

Locke, E. A., & Latham, G. P. (2002). Building a practically useful theory of goal setting and task motivation. A 35-year odyssey. *The American Psychologist*, *57*(9), 705–717. DOI: 10.1037//0003-066x.57.9.705 PMID: 12237980

Locke, E. A., & Latham, G. P. (2002). Building a practically useful theory of goal setting and task motivation: A 35-year odyssey. *The American Psychologist*, *57*(9), 705–717. DOI: 10.1037/0003-066X.57.9.705 PMID: 12237980

Lomas, T., Medina, J. C., Ivtzan, I., Rupprecht, S., & Eiroa-Orosa, F. J. (2017). A systematic review of the impact of mindfulness on the well-being of healthcare professionals. *Journal of Clinical Psychology*, *73*(3), 319–355. DOI: 10.1002/jclp.22420

Lubans, D., Richards, J., Hillman, C., Faulkner, G., Beauchamp, M., Nilsson, M., & Biddle, S. (2016). Physical activity for cognitive and mental health in youth: A systematic review of mechanisms. *Pediatrics*, *138*(3), e20161642. PMID: 27542849

Lubans, D., Richards, J., Hillman, C., Faulkner, G., Beauchamp, M., Nilsson, M., Kelly, P., Smith, J., Raine, L., & Biddle, S. (2016). Physical Activity for Cognitive and Mental Health in Youth: A Systematic Review of Mechanisms. *Pediatrics*, *138*(3), e20161642. DOI: 10.1542/peds.2016-1642 PMID: 27542849

Lundqvist, C. (2011). Well-being in competitive sports—The feel-good factor? A review of conceptual considerations of well-being. *International Review of Sport and Exercise Psychology*, *4*(2), 109–127. DOI: 10.1080/1750984X.2011.584067

Lyall, L. M., Wyse, C. A., Graham, N., Ferguson, A., Lyall, D. M., Cullen, B., & Smith, D. J. (2018). Association of disrupted circadian rhythmicity with mood disorders, subjective wellbeing, and cognitive function: A cross-sectional study of 91 105 participants from the UK Biobank. *The Lancet. Psychiatry*, *5*(6), 507–514.

Machado-Vieira, R., Sanches, M., & Vieta, E. (2017). Neurobiology of bipolar disorder. *The International Journal of Neuropsychopharmacology*, *20*(2), 98–106. DOI: 10.1093/ijnp/pyw095

Macias, O. (2024). *Navigating post-pandemic student behavior: Strategies for teachers and school administrators*. Resource Hub. https://content.acsa.org/navigating-post-pandemic-student-behavior-strategies-for-teachers-and-school-administrators/

Maddux, J. E. (1993). Social cognitive models of health and exercise behavior: An introduction and review of conceptual issues. *Journal of Applied Sport Psychology, 5*(2), 116–140. DOI: 10.1080/10413209308411310

Madigan, D. J., & Kim, L. E. (2021). Towards an understanding of teacher attrition: A meta-analysis of burnout, job satisfaction, and teachers' intention to quit. *Teaching and Teacher Education, 105*, 103425. Advance online publication. DOI: 10.1016/j.tate.2021.103425

Madigan, D. J., Kim, L. E., Glandorf, H. L., & Kavanagh, O. (2023). Teacher burnout and physical health: A systematic review. *International Journal of Educational Research, 119*, 102173. Advance online publication. DOI: 10.1016/j.ijer.2023.102173

Magallanes, C. L. (2024). Physical education Teachers' experiences in fitness testing. *British Journal of Multidisciplinary and Advanced Studies, 5*(1), 88–147. DOI: 10.37745/bjmas.2022.0422

Maher, C. A., Lewis, L. K., Ferrar, K., Marshall, S., De Bourdeaudhuij, I., & Vandelanotte, C. (2014). Are health behavior change interventions that use online social networks effective? A systematic review. *Journal of Medical Internet Research, 16*(2), e40. DOI: 10.2196/jmir.2952 PMID: 24550083

Mahindru, A., Patil, P., & Agrawal, V. (2023). Role of Physical Activity on Mental Health and Well-Being: A Review. *Cureus, 15*(1), e33475. DOI: 10.7759/cureus.33475 PMID: 36756008

Majore-Dusele, I., Karkou, V., & Millere, I. (2021). The development of mindful-based dance movement therapy intervention for chronic pain: A pilot study with chronic headache patients. *Frontiers in Psychology, 12*, 587923.

Mäkikangas, A., Leiter, M. P., Kinnunen, U., & Feldt, T. (2020). Profiling development of burnout over eight years: Relation with job demands and resources. *European Journal of Work and Organizational Psychology, 30*(5), 720–731. DOI: 10.1080/1359432X.2020.1790651

Mak, S., & Thomas, A. (2022). Steps for conducting a scoping review. *Journal of Graduate Medical Education, 14*(5), 565–567. DOI: 10.4300/JGME-D-22-00621.1 PMID: 36274762

Ma, L., Wang, Y., Pan, L., Cui, Z., & Schluter, P. J. (2022). Mindfulness-informed (ACT) and mindfulness-based programs (MBSR/MBCT) applied for college students to reduce symptoms of depression and anxiety. *Journal of Behavioral and Cognitive Therapy, 32*(4), 271–289.

Malchow, B., Reich-Erkelenz, D., Oertel-Knöchel, V., Keller, K., Hasan, A., Schmitt, A., Scheewe, T. W., Cahn, W., Kahn, R. S., & Falkai, P. (2013). The effects of physical exercise in schizophrenia and affective disorders. *European Archives of Psychiatry and Clinical Neuroscience*, *263*(6), 451–467. DOI: 10.1007/s00406-013-0423-2 PMID: 23873090

Malhi, G. S., & Mann, J. J. (2018). Depression. *Lancet*, *392*(10161), 2299–2312. DOI: 10.1016/S0140-6736(18)31948-2 PMID: 30396512

Mallett, C. J., & Hanrahan, S. J. (2004). Elite athletes: Why does the 'fire' burn so brightly? *Psychology of Sport and Exercise*, *5*(2), 183–200. DOI: 10.1016/S1469-0292(02)00043-2

Mammen, G., & Faulkner, G. (2013). Activity reduces anxiety and depression risk. *Journal of Psychiatric Research*, *47*(3), 355–363.

Mammen, G., & Faulkner, G. (2018). Physical activity and the prevention of depression: A systematic review of prospective studies. *American Journal of Preventive Medicine*, *45*(5), 649–657. DOI: 10.1016/j.amepre.2013.08.001

Manalo, A. S. D. (2024). Navigating Critical Pedagogy: Insights from Public Secondary English Teachers. *A-Liberal Arts/Humanities and Social Sciences*, 75.

Mandolesi, L., Polverino, A., Montuori, S., Foti, F., Ferraioli, G., Sorrentino, P., & Sorrentino, G. (2018). Effects of Physical Exercise on Cognitive Functioning and Wellbeing: Biological and Psychological Benefits. *Frontiers in Psychology*, *9*, 509. DOI: 10.3389/fpsyg.2018.00509 PMID: 29755380

Manuti, A., Giancaspro, M. L., Gemmano, C. G., & Morrelli, F. (2022). Coping with the unexpected: A job demands/resources study exploring Italian teachers' remote working experience during the COVID-19 lockdown. *Teaching and Teacher Education: Leadership and Professional Development*, *1*, 100010. Advance online publication. DOI: 10.1016/j.tatelp.2022.100010

Mariano, L., Simões, H., Brito-Costa, S., & Amaral, A. P. (2023). Fostering organizational empowerment: Impact of an intervention program on stress management and physical activity motivation among teachers in Portugal and Brazil. *Administrative Sciences*, *13*(9), 203. DOI: 10.3390/admsci13090203

Marshall, D. T., Smith, N. E., Love, S. M., Neugebauer, N. M., & Shannon, D. M. (2024). "At some point we're going to reach our limit": Understanding COVID-19's impact on teacher burnout and subjective mental health. *Psychology in the Schools*, *61*(3), 793–812. DOI: 10.1002/pits.23084

Martela, F., Lehmus-Sun, A., Parker, P. D., Pessi, A. B., & Ryan, R. M. (2023). Needs and well-being across Europe: Basic psychological needs are closely connected with well-being, meaning, and symptoms of depression in 27 European countries. *Social Psychological & Personality Science, 14*(5), 501–514.

Martin, A. J., Sudimantara, L. B., & Dewi, E. W. (2025). Harnessing theory to make sense of large-scale secondary data in education: Applying the academic demands-resources framework. *Education in Science, 15*(2), 256. Advance online publication. DOI: 10.3390/educsci15020256

Martínez-Arán, A., Vieta, E., Colom, F., Torrent, C., Sánchez-Moreno, J., Reinares, M., & Salamero, M. (2004). Cognitive impairment in euthymic bipolar patients: Implications for clinical and functional outcome. *Bipolar Disorders, 6*(3), 224–232. DOI: 10.1111/j.1399-5618.2004.00107.x

Martín-Rodríguez, A., Gostian-Ropotin, L. A., Beltrán-Velasco, A. I., Belando-Pedreño, N., Simón, J. A., López-Mora, C., Navarro-Jiménez, E., Tornero-Aguilera, J. F., & Clemente-Suárez, V. J. (2024). Sporting Mind: The Interplay of Physical Activity and Psychological Health. *Sports (Basel, Switzerland), 12*(1), 37. DOI: 10.3390/sports12010037 PMID: 38275986

Maslach, C., & Jackson, S. E. (1981). The measurement of experienced burnout. *Journal of Organizational Behavior, 2*(2), 99–113. DOI: 10.1002/job.4030020205

Maslach, C., & Leiter, M. P. (2016). Understanding the burnout experience: Recent research and its implications for psychiatry. *World Psychiatry: Official Journal of the World Psychiatric Association, 15*(2), 103–111. DOI: 10.1002/wps.20311 PMID: 27265691

Mattioli, A. V., Sciomer, S., Cocchi, C., Maffei, S., & Gallina, S. (2020). Quarantine during COVID-19 outbreak: Changes in diet and physical activity increase the risk of cardiovascular disease. *Nutrition, Metabolism, and Cardiovascular Diseases, 30*(9), 1409–1417. DOI: 10.1016/j.numecd.2020.05.020 PMID: 32571612

Mavilidi, M. F., Lubans, D. R., Morgan, P. J., Miller, A., Eather, N., Karayanidis, F., Lonsdale, C., Noetel, M., Shaw, K., & Riley, N. (2019). Integrating physical activity into the primary school curriculum: Rationale and study protocol for the "Thinking while Moving in English" cluster randomized controlled trial. *BMC Public Health, 19*(1). Advance online publication. DOI: 10.1186/s12889 019 6635 2 PMID: 30947708

McAuley, E., Blissmer, B., Marquez, D. X., Jerome, G. J., Kramer, A. F., & Katula, J. (2000). Social relations, physical activity, and well-being in older adults. *Preventive Medicine, 31*(5), 608–617. DOI: 10.1006/pmed.2000.0740 PMID: 11071843

McEwen, B. S. (2017). Neurobiological and Systemic Effects of Chronic Stress. *Chronic Stress (Thousand Oaks, Calif.), 1*, 2470547017692328. DOI: 10.1177/2470547017692328 PMID: 28856337

McTiernan, A. (2008). Mechanisms linking physical activity with cancer. *Nature Reviews. Cancer*, *8*(3), 205–211. DOI: 10.1038/nrc2325 PMID: 18235448

Meeusen, R. (2013). Prevention, Diagnosis, and Treatment of the Overtraining Syndrome: Joint Consensus Statement of the European College of Sport Science and the American College of Sports Medicine. *Medicine and Science in Sports and Exercise*, *45*(1), 186–205. DOI: 10.1249/MSS.0b013e318279a10a PMID: 23247672

Meeusen, R., & De Meirleir, K. (1995). Exercise and brain neurotransmission. *Sports Medicine (Auckland, N.Z.)*, *20*(3), 160–188. PMID: 8571000

MeHelp. (2024). The 3 pillars of mental health: Benefits of sleep, diet and exercise. https://www.mehelp.com.au/insights/sleep-diet-exercise

Mehling, W. E., Price, C., Daubenmier, J. J., Acree, M., Bartmess, E., & Stewart, A. (2012). The Multidimensional Assessment of Interoceptive Awareness (MAIA). *PLoS One*, *7*(11), e48230. DOI: 10.1371/journal.pone.0048230 PMID: 23133619

Mehta, N. N., & Talwar, G. (2022). Recognizing roots and not just leaves: The use of integrative mindfulness in education, research, and practice. *Psychology from the Margins*, *4*(1), 6.

Mehta, P., & Sharma, M. (2012). Evaluation of a social cognitive theory-based yoga intervention to reduce anxiety. *International Quarterly of Community Health Education*, *32*(3), 205–217. DOI: 10.2190/IQ.32.3.d

Melo, M. C. A., Garcia, R. F., de Araújo, C. F., & Caetano, S. C. (2016). Aerobic exercise training improves hippocampal volume and cognitive functioning in bipolar disorder: A pilot study. *Frontiers in Psychiatry*, *7*, 123. DOI: 10.3389/fpsyt.2016.00123

Mérida-López, S., Sánchez-Álvarez, N., & Extremera, N. (2022). Teacher retention through the job demands-resources theory. *Educación XX1, 25*(2), 151-171. https://doi.org/DOI: 10.5944/educxx1.31901

Merikangas, K. R., Jin, R., He, J. P., Kessler, R. C., Lee, S., Sampson, N. A., & Zarkov, Z. (2011). Prevalence and correlates of bipolar spectrum disorder in the World Mental Health Survey Initiative. *Archives of General Psychiatry*, *68*(3), 241–251. DOI: 10.1001/archgenpsychiatry.2011.12

Meyer, J. D., Koltyn, K. F., Stegner, A. J., & Kim, J. S. (2016). Influence of exercise on stress reactivity and emotional regulation in major depressive disorder. *Medicine and Science in Sports and Exercise, 48*(11), 2207–2215. DOI: 10.1249/MSS.0000000000001013

Mijakoski, D., Cheptea, D., Marca, S. C., Shoman, Y., Caglayan, C., Bugge, M. D., Gnesi, M., Godderis, L., Kiran, S., McElvenny, D. M., Mediouni, Z., Mesot, O., Minov, J., Nena, E., Otelea, M., Pranjic, N., Mehlum, I. S., van der Molen, H. F., & Canu, I. G. (2022). Determinants of burnout among teachers: A systematic review of longitudinal studies. *International Journal of Environmental Research and Public Health, 19*(9), 5776. Advance online publication. DOI: 10.3390/ijerph19095776 PMID: 35565168

Mikkelsen, K., Stojanovska, L., Polenakovic, M., Bosevski, M., & Apostolopoulos, V. (2017). Exercise and mental health. *Maturitas, 106*, 48–56. https://www.sciencedirect.com/science/article/pii/S0378512217308563 PMID: 29150166

Miller, A. H., & Raison, C. L. (2016). The role of inflammation in depression: From evolutionary imperative to modern treatment target. *Nature Reviews. Immunology, 16*(1), 22–34. DOI: 10.1038/nri.2015.5 PMID: 26711676

Minh Diu, H., & Chanh Thuc, D. (2025). The Impact of Yoga Practice on Self-Reported Health Outcomes Among Middle-Aged Adults. *Annals of Applied Sport Science, 13*(1). Advance online publication. DOI: 10.61186/aassjournal.1438

Moawd, S. A., Elsayed, S. H., Abdelbasset, W. K., Nambi, G., Verma, A. Impact of different physical activity levels on academic performance of PSAU medical female students. Arch PharmaPract 2020;11(1):100 4.

Monteiro, E., & Joseph, J. (2023). A review on the impact of workplace culture on employee mental health and well-being. *International Journal of Case Studies in Business, IT, and Education, 7*(2), 291–317. DOI: 10.5281/zenodo.7999328

Morgan, W. P., & Goldston, S. E. (1987). *Exercise and Mental Health*. Hemisphere Publishing Corporation.

Mota-Pereira, J., Carvalho, S., Silva, J., & Ribeiro, J. (2019). Combined aerobic and resistance exercise improves executive function and sleep in bipolar disorder: A randomized controlled trial. *Psychiatry Research, 276*, 123–129. DOI: 10.1016/j.psychres.2019.04.021

Mulhearn, S. C., Kulinna, P. H., & Lorenz, K. A. (2024). Classroom teachers' perceived barriers to implementing comprehensive school physical activity programs (TPB- CSPAP): Instrument development. *Research Quarterly for Exercise and Sport*, *95*(2), 342–352. DOI: 10.1080/02701367.2023.2206449 PMID: 37463222

Muneer, A. (2016). The neurobiology of bipolar disorder: An integrated approach. *Chonnam Medical Journal*, *52*(1), 18–37. DOI: 10.4068/cmj.2016.52.1.18

Munkholm, K., Vinberg, M., & Kessing, L. V. (2013). Cytokines in bipolar disorder: A systematic review and meta-analysis. *Journal of Affective Disorders*, *144*(1–2), 16–27. DOI: 10.1016/j.jad.2012.06.010

Murray, G., Thomas, N., Michalak, E. E., Jones, S. H., Lapsley, S., Bowe, S. J., & Berk, M. (2021). Mindfulness-based online intervention to improve quality of life in late-stage bipolar disorder: A randomized clinical trial. *Journal of Consulting and Clinical Psychology*, *89*(10), 830.

Murray, R. M., Doré, I., Sabiston, C. M., Michael, F., & O'Loughlin, J. L. (2023). A time compositional analysis of the association between movement behavior and indicators of mental health in young adults. *Scandinavian Journal of Medicine & Science in Sports*, *33*(12), 2598–2607. DOI: 10.1111/sms.14471 PMID: 37635273

Nadon, L., De Beer, L. T., & Morin, A. J. S. (2022). Should burnout be conceptualized as a mental disorder? *Behavioral Sciences (Basel, Switzerland)*, *12*(3), 82. DOI: 10.3390/bs12030082 PMID: 35323401

Naidoo-Chetty, M., & Du Plessis, M. (2021). Systematic review of the job demands and resources of academic staff within higher education institutions. *International Journal of Higher Education*, *10*(3), 268–284. DOI: 10.5430/ijhe.v10n3p268

Nalipay, M. J. N., Mordeno, I. G., Semilla, J. B., & Frondozo, C. E. (2019). Implicit beliefs about teaching ability, teacher emotions, and teaching satisfaction. *The Asia-Pacific Education Researcher*, *28*(4), 313–325. DOI: 10.1007/s40299-019-00467-z

Nam, U. V., & Duc, N. M. (2021). Population ageing and older persons in Viet Nam. General Statistics Office. https://vietnam.unfpa.org/

Nápoles, J., Kelley, J., & Rinn, T. J. (2023). Burnout and perceived agency among Texas choir teachers. *Journal of Research in Music Education*, *71*(3), 283–296. DOI: 10.1177/00224294221126889

Nath, R., & Pandey, C. P. (2025). The hidden burden: Emotional labor and well-being of school teachers. *Asian Journal of Education and Social Studies*, *51*(2), 500–510. DOI: 10.9734/ajess/2025/v51i21802

Neil Sztramko, S. E., Caldwell, H., & Dobbins, M. (2021). School based physical activity programs for promoting physical activity and fitness in children and adolescents aged 6 to 18. *Cochrane Library, 2021*(9). .DOI: 10.1002/14651858.cd007651.pub3

Neto, L. B., Christofoletti, G., de Alencar, G. P., & Burke, T. N. (2024). Burnout syndrome, work ability, quality of life and physical activity in teachers during the COVID-19 pandemic in Campo Grande, Brazil. *Work (Reading, Mass.)*, *78*(1), 45–53. DOI: 10.3233/WOR-220187 PMID: 37483044

Netz, Y. (2019). Is there a preferred mode of exercise for cognition enhancement in older age?—A narrative review. *Frontiers in Medicine*, *6*, 57. https://www.frontiersin.org/articles/10.3389/fmed.2019.00057/full PMID: 30984760

Netz, Y., Wu, M. J., Becker, B. J., & Tenenbaum, G. (2005). Physical activity and psychological well-being in advanced age: A meta-analysis of intervention studies. *Psychology and Aging*, *20*(2), 272. PMID: 16029091

Neumann, D. L., Moffitt, R. L., Thomas, P. R., Loveday, K., Watling, D. P., Lombard, C. L., Antonova, S., & Tremeer, M. A. (2018). A systematic review of the application of interactive virtual reality to sport. *Virtual Reality (Waltham Cross)*, *22*(3), 183–198. DOI: 10.1007/s10055-017-0320-5

Ng, F., Dodd, S., & Berk, M. (2007). The effects of physical activity in the acute treatment of bipolar disorder: A pilot study. *Journal of Affective Disorders*, *101*(1–3), 259–262. DOI: 10.1016/j.jad.2006.11.004

Ng, F., Dodd, S., Berk, M., & Malhi, G. S. (2017). Mind-body exercise interventions for bipolar disorder: Effects on mood and anxiety. *Journal of Affective Disorders*, *208*, 145–150. DOI: 10.1016/j.jad.2016.08.045

Ng, Q. X., Ho, C. Y. X., Chan, H. W., Yong, B. Z. J., & Yeo, W. S. (2019). Managing bipolar disorder with exercise: Clinical perspectives. *Frontiers in Psychiatry*, *10*, 765. DOI: 10.3389/fpsyt.2019.00765

Nguyen, H. M., Ngo, T. T. N., Nguyen, T. T., & Ngo, T. T. N.. (2024). Assessment of the effects of yoga on self-perceived health of elderly. *Annals of Applied Sport Science*, *12*(1), 1318.

Nguyen, T. T., Hwang, C. B., & Mason, B. L. (2022). Role of brain-derived neurotrophic factor (BDNF) in bipolar disorder and exercise intervention: A systematic review. *Biomolecules*, *12*(9), 1290. Advance online publication. DOI: 10.3390/biom12091290

Noetel, M., Sanders, T., Gallardo-Gómez, D., Taylor, P., Del Pozo Cruz, B., van den Hoek, D., Smith, J. J., Mahoney, J., Spathis, J., Moresi, M., Pagano, R., Pagano, L., Vasconcellos, R., Arnott, H., Varley, B., Parker, P., Biddle, S., & Lonsdale, C. (2024). Effect of exercise for depression: Systematic review and network meta-analysis of randomised controlled trials. *BMJ (Clinical Research Ed.), 384*, e075847. DOI: 10.1136/bmj-2023-075847 PMID: 38355154

Noone, S. J., & Hastings, R. P. (2009). Building psychological resilience in support staff caring for people with intellectual disabilities: Pilot evaluation of an acceptance-based intervention. *Journal of Intellectual Disabilities, 13*(1), 43–53. DOI: 10.1177/1744629509103519 PMID: 19332508

Noordsy, D. L., Burgess, J. D., Hardy, K. V., Yudofsky, L. M., & Ballon, J. S. (2018). Therapeutic Potential of Physical Exercise in Early Psychosis. *The American Journal of Psychiatry, 175*(3), 209–214. DOI: 10.1176/appi.ajp.2017.17060716 PMID: 29490501

Norris, G., & Norris, H. (2021). Building Resilience Through Sport in Young People With Adverse Childhood Experiences. *Frontiers in Sports and Active Living, 3*. Advance online publication. DOI: 10.3389/fspor.2021.663587 PMID: 34337400

Ntoumanis, N. (2001). A self-determination approach to the understanding of motivation in physical education. *The British Journal of Educational Psychology, 71*(2), 225–242. DOI: 10.1348/000709901158497 PMID: 11449934

Ntoumanis, N., Edmunds, J., & Duda, J. L. (2009). Understanding the coping process from a self-determination theory perspective. *British Journal of Health Psychology, 14*(2), 249–260. DOI: 10.1348/135910708X349352 PMID: 18789187

O'Hara, S., Melnyk, B. M., Hsieh, A. P., Helsabeck, N. P., Giuliano, K. K., & Vital, C. (2025). Innovation, wellness, and EBP cultures are associated with less burnout, better mental health, and higher job satisfaction in nurses and the healthcare workforce. *Worldviews on Evidence-Based Nursing, 22*(2), 1–11. DOI: 10.1111/wvn.70012 PMID: 40237103

Oberg, G., Macmahon, S., & Carroll, A. (2025). Assessing the interplay: Teacher efficacy, compassion fatigue, and educator well-being in Australia. *Australian Educational Researcher, 52*, 1105–1131. DOI: 10.1007/s13384-024-00755-8

Oberlin, L. E., Verstynen, T. D., Burzynska, A. Z., Voss, M. W., Prakash, R. S., Chaddock-Heyman, L., Wong, C., Fanning, J., Awick, E., Gothe, N., Phillips, S. M., Mailey, E., Ehlers, D., Olson, E., Wojcicki, T., McAuley, E., Kramer, A. F., & Erickson, K. I. (2016). White matter microstructure mediates the relationship between cardiorespiratory fitness and spatial working memory in older adults. *NeuroImage*, *131*, 91–101. DOI: 10.1016/j.neuroimage.2015.09.053 PMID: 26439513

Odendahl, J. (2021). Embodied Cognition, affects and language comprehension: Theoretical basis and (literary-) didactic perspectives of a physically-emotionally grounded model of understanding. *Phenomenology and the Cognitive Sciences*, *20*(3), 483–499.

Ogoh, S., Tsukamoto, H., Hirasawa, A., Hasegawa, H., Hirose, N., & Hashimoto, T. (2014). The effect of changes in cerebral blood flow on cognitive function during exercise. *Physiological Reports*, *2*(9), e12163. DOI: 10.14814/phy2.12163 PMID: 25263210

Ormiston, H. E., Nygaard, M. A., & Apgar, S. (2022). A systematic review of secondary traumatic stress and compassion fatigue in teachers. *School Mental Health*, *14*, 802–817. DOI: 10.1007/s12310-022-09525-2 PMID: 35694002

Ortan, F., Simut, C., & Simut, R. (2021). Self-efficacy, job satisfaction, and teacher well-being in the K-12 education system. *International Journal of Environmental Research and Public Health*, *18*(23), 12763. Advance online publication. DOI: 10.3390/ijerph182312763 PMID: 34886493

Oyibo, K., Adaji, I., & Vassileva, J. (2018). Social cognitive determinants of exercise behavior in the context of behavior modeling: A mixed method approach. *Digital Health*, *4*, 2055207618811555. DOI: 10.1177/2055207618811555 PMID: 30479828

Ozamiz-Etxebarria, N., Legorburu Fernnadez, I., Lipnicki, D. M., Idoiaga Mondragon, N., & Santabárbara, J. (2023). Prevalence of burnout among teachers during the COVID-19 pandemic: A meta-analysis. *International Journal of Environmental Research and Public Health*, *20*(6), 4866. Advance online publication. DOI: 10.3390/ijerph20064866 PMID: 36981775

Ozdemir, C., & Akbas Gunes, N. (2021). The effect of diet and regular exercise on psychological resilience in obese or overweight women. *International Journal of Clinical Practice*, *75*(8), e14320. DOI: 10.1111/ijcp.14320 PMID: 33960086

Pagliaro, S., Iacoviello, M., De Cristofaro, M., & Sessa, F. (2021). Norepinephrine modulatory effects during exercise and stress: Neurobiological implications. *Frontiers in Behavioral Neuroscience*, *14*, 1–12.

Pakdee, S., Cheechang, P., Thammanoon, R., Krobpet, S., Piya-amornphan, N., Puangsri, P., & Gosselink, R. (2025). Burnout and well-being among higher education teachers: Influencing factors of burnout. *BMC Public Health, 25*(1), 1–10. DOI: 10.1186/s12889-025-22602-w PMID: 40234791

Palagini, L., Miniati, M., Marazziti, D., Sharma, V., & Riemann, D. (2021). Association among early life stress, mood features, hopelessness and suicidal risk in bipolar disorder: The potential contribution of insomnia symptoms. *Journal of Psychiatric Research, 135*, 52–59.

Palmer, S. J. (2020). Encouraging exercise in older adults: Advice for nurses. *British Journal of Community Nursing, 25*(2), 95–97. DOI: 10.12968/bjcn.2020.25.2.95 PMID: 32040357

Palvimo, T., Vauhkonen, A., & Hult, M. (2023). The associations among destructive leadership, job demands and resources, and burnout among nurses: A cross-sectional survey study. *Journal of Nursing Management, 2023*(1), 4289450. Advance online publication. DOI: 10.1155/2023/4289450 PMID: 40225631

Paolucci, E. M., Loukov, D., Bowdish, D. M. E., & Heisz, J. J. (2018). Exercise reduces depression and inflammation but intensity matters. *Biological Psychology, 133*, 79–84. DOI: 10.1016/j.biopsycho.2018.01.014

Pariante, C. M., & Lightman, S. L. (2008). The HPA axis in major depression: Classical theories and new developments. *Trends in Neurosciences, 31*(9), 464–468. DOI: 10.1016/j.tins.2008.06.006 PMID: 18675469

Park, I., & Jeon, J. (2023). Psychological Skills Training for Athletes in Sports: Web of Science Bibliometric Analysis. *Health Care, 11*(2), 259. DOI: 10.3390/healthcare11020259 PMID: 36673627

Parra, D. C., Wetherell, J. L., Van Zandt, A., Brownson, R. C., Abhishek, J., & Lenze, E. J. (2019). A qualitative study of older adults' perspectives on initiating exercise and mindfulness practice. *BMC Geriatrics, 19*, 354. Advance online publication. DOI: 10.1186/s12877-019-1375-9 PMID: 31865906

Parra, E., Arone, A., Amadori, S., Mucci, F., Palermo, S., & Marazziti, D. (2020). Impact of physical exercise on psychological well-being and psychiatric disorders. *J Reatt Ther Dev Divers, 3*(2), 24–39. https://pdfs.semanticscholar.org/88d2/143cef826c1c5550a5e45806bb02699c876c.pdf

Pascoe, M. C., Thompson, D. R., & Ski, C. F. (2017). Yoga, mindfulness-based stress reduction and stress-related physiological measures: A meta-analysis. *Psychoneuroendocrinology, 86*, 152–168. DOI: 10.1016/j.psyneuen.2017.08.008 PMID: 28963884

Pass Erickson, L. M. (2021). Sensing the self: A dance/movement therapy model of embodied identity development. *Body, Movement and Dance in Psychotherapy, 16*(3), 202–217.

Patel, R. M., & Bartholomew, J. (2021). Impact of job resources and job demands on burnout among physical therapy providers. *International Journal of Environmental Research and Public Health, 18*(23), 12521. Advance online publication. DOI: 10.3390/ijerph182312521 PMID: 34886248

Patel, V., Flisher, A. J., Hetrick, S., & McGorry, P. (2007). Mental health of young people: A global public-health challenge. *Lancet, 369*(9569), 1302–1313. DOI: 10.1016/S0140-6736(07)60368-7 PMID: 17434406

Paulus, D. J., Gallagher, M. W., Bartlett, B. A., Tran, J., & Vujanovic, A. A. (2018). The unique and interactive effects of anxiety sensitivity and emotion dysregulation in relation to posttraumatic stress, depressive, and anxiety symptoms among trauma-exposed firefighters. *Comprehensive Psychiatry, 84*, 54–61. DOI: 10.1016/j.comppsych.2018.03.012 PMID: 29694933

Peck, D. (2025). *Teacher burnout statistics: Why teachers quit in 2025.* https://www.devlinpeck.com/content/teacher-burnout-statistics

Pedersen, B. K., & Saltin, B. (2015). Exercise as medicine: Evidence for prescribing exercise as therapy in 26 different chronic diseases. *Scandinavian Journal of Medicine & Science in Sports, 25*(Suppl 3), 1–72. DOI: 10.1111/sms.12581

Pedersen, J. H., Thornquist, E., Natvik, E., & Råheim, M. (2019). Physical education classes – a double edged sword: A qualitative study of Norwegian high school students' experiences. *Physiotherapy Theory and Practice, 37*(12), 1404–1418. DOI: 10.1080/09593985.2019.1709232 PMID: 31885299

Pelletier, L., Shanmugasegaram, S., Patten, S. B., & Demers, A. (2017). Self-management of mood and/or anxiety disorders through physical activity/exercise. *Health Promotion and Chronic Disease Prevention in Canada : Research, Policy and Practice, 37*(5), 149–159. DOI: 10.24095/hpcdp.37.5.03 PMID: 28493659

Penedo, F. J., & Dahn, J. R. (2005). Exercise and well-being: A review of mental and physical health benefits associated with physical activity. *Current Opinion in Psychiatry, 18*(2), 189–193. DOI: 10.1097/00001504-200503000-00013 PMID: 16639173

Peng, B., Chen, W., Wang, H., & Yu, T. (2025). How does physical exercise influence self-efficacy in adolescents? A study based on the mediating role of psychological resilience. *BMC Psychology, 13*(1), 1–17. PMID: 40119462

Pennebaker, J. W., & Chung, C. K. (2011). Expressive writing: Connections to physical and mental health. In *The Oxford handbook of health psychology* (pp. 417–437). Oxford University Press.

Pérez-Rodríguez, M. M., Bravo, L., & Martínez-Cengotitabengoa, M. (2021). Effects of physical exercise on BDNF in patients with bipolar disorder: A systematic review. *Neuroscience and Biobehavioral Reviews, 124*, 262–272. DOI: 10.1016/j.neubiorev.2020.11.018

Petersen, A. M. W., & Pedersen, B. K. (2005). The anti-inflammatory effect of exercise. *Journal of Applied Physiology (Bethesda, Md.: 1985), 98*(4), 1154–1162. https://doi.org/DOI: 10.1152/japplphysiol.00164.2004

Petruzzello, S. J., Landers, D. M., Hatfield, B. D., Kubitz, K. A., & Salazar, W. (1991). A meta-analysis on the anxiety-reducing effects of acute and chronic exercise. Outcomes and mechanisms. *Sports Medicine (Auckland, N.Z.), 11*(3), 143–182. DOI: 10.2165/00007256-199111030-00002 PMID: 1828608

Phillips, C., Fahimi, A., & Ghahremani, M. (2019). The link between physical activity and neuroplasticity in depression and bipolar disorder. *NeuroImage, 202*, 116–133. DOI: 10.1016/j.neuroimage.2019.06.027

Phillips, M. L., & Kupfer, D. J. (2013). Bipolar disorder diagnosis: Challenges and future directions. *Lancet, 381*(9878), 1663–1671. DOI: 10.1016/S0140-6736(13)60989-7

Phillips, M. L., & Swartz, H. A. (2014). A critical appraisal of neuroimaging studies of bipolar disorder: Toward a new conceptualization of underlying neural circuitry and a road map for future research. *The American Journal of Psychiatry, 171*(8), 829–843. DOI: 10.1176/appi.ajp.2014.13081008

Piercy, K. L., Troiano, R. P., Ballard, R. M., Carlson, S. A., Fulton, J. E., Galuska, D. A., George, S. M., & Olson, R. D. (2018). The Physical Activity Guidelines for Americans. *Journal of the American Medical Association, 320*(19), 2020–2028. DOI: 10.1001/jama.2018.14854 PMID: 30418471

Pihlaja, M., Tuominen, P., Peräkylä, J., & Hartikainen, K. M. (2022). Occupational burnout is linked with inefficient executive functioning, elevated average heart rate, and decreased physical activity in daily life-initial evidence from teaching professionals. *Brain Sciences, 12*(12), 1723. DOI: 10.3390/brainsci12121723 PMID: 36552182

Pinto, J. V., Passos, I. C., Librenza-Garcia, D., Marcon, G., Schneider, R. B., Conte, J. H., & Kapczinski, F. (2022). Physical exercise as an adjunctive treatment in bipolar disorder: A systematic review and meta-analysis. *Acta Psychiatrica Scandinavica, 145*(6), 574–593. DOI: 10.1111/acps.13426

Pollock, D., Evans, C., Jia, R. M., Alexander, L., Pieper, D., Brandão de Moraes, É., Peters, M. D. J., Tricco, A. C., Khalil, H., Godfrey, C. M., Saran, A., Campbell, F., & Munn, Z. (2024). "How-to": Scoping review? *Journal of Clinical Epidemiology, 176*, 111572. DOI: 10.1016/j.jclinepi.2024.111572 PMID: 39426499

Post, R. M. (2007). Role of brain-derived neurotrophic factor in bipolar and unipolar disorder. *Journal of Psychiatric Research, 41*(12), 979–990. DOI: 10.1016/j.jpsychires.2006.09.009

Pressley, T. (2021). Factors contributing to teacher burnout during COVID-19. *Educational Researcher, 50*(5), 325–327. DOI: 10.3102/0013189X211004138

Price, C. J., & Thompson, E. A. (2007). Measuring dimensions of body connection: Body awareness and bodily dissociation. *Journal of Alternative and Complementary Medicine (New York, N.Y.), 13*(9), 945–953. DOI: 10.1089/acm.2007.0537 PMID: 18047441

Price, C. J., & Weng, H. Y. (2021). Facilitating adaptive emotion processing and somatic reappraisal via sustained mindful interoceptive attention. *Frontiers in Psychology, 12*, 578827.

Primack, B. A., Shensa, A., Sidani, J. E., Whaite, E. O., Lin, L. Y., Rosen, D., Colditz, J. B., Radovic, A., & Miller, E. (2017). Social Media Use and Perceived Social Isolation Among Young Adults in the U.S. *American Journal of Preventive Medicine, 53*(1), 1–8. DOI: 10.1016/j.amepre.2017.01.010 PMID: 28279545

Prince, S. A., Adamo, K. B., Hamel, M. E., Hardt, J., Gorber, S. C., & Tremblay, M. (2008). A comparison of direct versus self-report measures for assessing physical activity in adults: A systematic review. *The International Journal of Behavioral Nutrition and Physical Activity, 5*(1), 56. PMID: 18990237

Prinz, B., Dvořák, J., & Junge, A. (2016). Symptoms and risk factors of depression during and after the football career of elite female players. *BMJ Open Sport & Exercise Medicine, 2*(1), e000124. DOI: 10.1136/bmjsem-2016-000124 PMID: 27900184

Prochaska, J. O., & DiClemente, C. C. (1983). Stages and processes of self-change of smoking: Toward an integrative model of change. *Journal of Consulting and Clinical Psychology, 51*(3), 390–395. DOI: 10.1037/0022-006X.51.3.390 PMID: 6863699

Proctor, E., Silmere, H., Raghavan, R., Hovmand, P., Aarons, G., Bunger, A., Griffey, R., & Hensley, M. (2011). Outcomes for implementation research: Conceptual distinctions, measurement challenges, and research agenda. *Administration and Policy in Mental Health, 38*(2), 65–76. DOI: 10.1007/s10488-010-0319-7 PMID: 20957426

Pruessner, L., Barnow, S., Holt, D. V., Joormann, J., & Schulze, K. (2020). A cognitive control framework for understanding emotion regulation flexibility. *Emotion (Washington, D.C.), 20*(1), 21–29. DOI: 10.1037/emo0000658 PMID: 31961173

Purser, R. (2019). *McMindfulness: How mindfulness became the new capitalist spirituality*. Repeater.

Quigley, A., MacKay-Lyons, M., & Eskes, G. (2020). Effects of Exercise on Cognitive Performance in Older Adults: A Narrative Review of the Evidence, Possible Biological Mechanisms, and Recommendations for Exercise Prescription. *Journal of Aging Research, 2020*, 1–15. DOI: 10.1155/2020/1407896 PMID: 32509348

Raglin, J. S. (2001). Psychological Factors in Sport Performance: The Mental Health Model Revisited. *Sports Medicine (Auckland, N.Z.), 31*(12), 875–890. DOI: 10.2165/00007256-200131120-00004 PMID: 11665914

Raichlen, D. A., Foster, A. D., Gerdeman, G. L., Seillier, A., & Giuffrida, A. (2012). Wired to run: Exercise-induced endocannabinoid signaling in humans and cursorial mammals with implications for the "runner's high.". *The Journal of Experimental Biology, 215*(Pt 8), 1331–1336. DOI: 10.1242/jeb.063677 PMID: 22442371

Raichlen, D. A., & Gordon, A. D. (2017). Endocannabinoids and exercise. *Progress in Neuro-Psychopharmacology & Biological Psychiatry, 79*, 169–176. DOI: 10.1016/j.pnpbp.2017.06.018

Ram, A., Marcos, L., Morey, R., Clark, T., Hakansson, S., Ristov, M., Franklin, A., McCarthy, C., De Carli, L., Jones, M. D., Ward, R. E., & Keech, A. (2022). Exercise for affect and enjoyment in overweight or obese males: A comparison of high-intensity interval training and moderate-intensity continuous training. *Psychology Health and Medicine, 27*(5), 1154–1167. DOI: 10.1080/13548506.2021.1903055 PMID: 33733958

Randall, K., Ford, T. G., Kwon, K. A., Sisson, S. S., Bice, M. R., Dinkel, D., & Tsotsoros, J. (2021). Physical activity, physical well-being, and psychological well-being: Associations with life satisfaction during the COVID-19 pandemic among early childhood educators. *International Journal of Environmental Research and Public Health, 18*, 9430. Advance online publication. DOI: 10.3390/ijerph18189430 PMID: 34574354

Rastegr, B., & Zarei, A. A. (2023). Assessment literacy components predicting EFL teachers' job-demands resources: A focus on burnout and engagement. *International Journal of Language Testing, 13*(1), 44–66. https://eric.ed.gov/?id=EJ1385327

Ratanasiripong, P., Ratanasiripong, N. T., Nungdanjark, W., Thongthammarat, Y., & Toyama, S. (2022). Mental health and burnout among teachers in Thailand. *Journal of Health Research, 36*(3), 404–416. DOI: 10.1108/JHR-05-2020-0181

Ratey, J. (2008). *Spark: The new science of exercise and the brain.* Little, Brown.

Rauschenberg, C., Schick, A., Hirjak, D., Seidler, A., Paetzold, I., Apfelbacher, C., Riedel-Heller, S. G., & Reininghaus, U. (2021). Evidence Synthesis of Digital Interventions to Mitigate the Negative Impact of the COVID-19 Pandemic on Public Mental Health: Rapid Meta-review. *Journal of Medical Internet Research, 23*(3), e23365. DOI: 10.2196/23365 PMID: 33606657

Reardon, C. L., & Factor, R. M. (2010). Sport Psychiatry: A Systematic Review of Diagnosis and Medical Treatment of Mental Illness in Athletes. *Sports Medicine (Auckland, N.Z.), 40*(11), 961–980. DOI: 10.2165/11536580-000000000-00000 PMID: 20942511

Reardon, C. L., Hainline, B., Aron, C. M., Baron, D., Baum, A. L., Bindra, A., Budgett, R., Campriani, N., Castaldelli-Maia, J. M., Currie, A., Derevensky, J. L., Glick, I. D., Gorczynski, P., Gouttebarge, V., Grandner, M. A., Han, D. H., McDuff, D., Mountjoy, M., Polat, A., & Engebretsen, L. (2019). Mental health in elite athletes: International Olympic Committee consensus statement (2019). *British Journal of Sports Medicine, 53*(11), 667–699. DOI: 10.1136/bjsports-2019-100715 PMID: 31097450

Reed, J., & Buck, S. (2009). The effect of regular aerobic exercise on positive-activated affect: A meta-analysis. *Psychology of Sport and Exercise, 10*(6), 581–594.

Rehman, M., & Shabbir, I. (2025). Building Mental Resilience: The Impact of Weight Resistance Training on Young Adult Wellbeing. *Qlantic Journal of Social Sciences, 6*(3), 249–255. DOI: 10.55737/qjss.vi-iii.25403

Rendeiro, C., & Rhodes, J. S. (2018). A new perspective of the hippocampus in the origin of exercise–brain interactions. *Brain Structure & Function, 223*(6), 2527–2545. DOI: 10.1007/s00429-018-1665-6 PMID: 29671055

Ren, J., & Xiao, H. (2023). Exercise for Mental Well Being: Exploring Neurobiological Advances and intervention Effects in Depression. *Life (Chicago, Ill.), 13*(7), 1505. DOI: 10.3390/life13071505 PMID: 37511879

Ren, X., & Wang, Y. (2022). On the correlation between job burnout, mental health and personality traits of college physical education teachers. *Psychiatria Danubina, 34*, S794–S799.

Resnick, B., Orwig, D., Magaziner, J., & Wynne, C. (2002). The Effect of Social Support on Exercise Behavior in Older Adults. *Clinical Nursing Research, 11*(1), 52–70. DOI: 10.1177/105477380201100105 PMID: 11845515

Rethorst, C. D., & Trivedi, M. H. (2017). Evidence-based recommendations for the prescription of exercise for major depressive disorder. *Journal of Psychiatric Practice, 23*(3), 204–212. DOI: 10.1097/PRA.0000000000000226

Revelo Herrera, S. G., & Leon-Rojas, J. E. (2024). The effect of aerobic exercise in neuroplasticity, learning, and cognition: A systematic review. *Cureus, 16*(2), e54021. DOI: 10.7759/cureus.54021

Rhodes, R. E., & Dickau, L. (2013). Moderators of the intention-behaviour relationship in the physical activity domain: A systematic review. *British Journal of Sports Medicine, 47*(4), 215–225. PMID: 22278998

Rice, S. M., Purcell, R., De Silva, S., Mawren, D., McGorry, P. D., & Parker, A. G. (2016). The Mental Health of Elite Athletes: A Narrative Systematic Review. *Sports Medicine (Auckland, N.Z.), 46*(9), 1333–1353. DOI: 10.1007/s40279-016-0492-2 PMID: 26896951

Rizvi, R., Rizvi, A. M., & Jamal, A. (2023). The impact of perceived organizational support, innovation at work, and burnout among teachers. *Bahria Journal of Professional Psychology, 22*(1), 38.

Robinson, L. E., Valido, A., Drescher, A., Woolweaver, A. B., Espelage, D. L., LoMurrary, S., Jong, A. C. J., Wright, A. A., & Dailey, M. M. (2022). Teachers, stress, and the COVID-19 Pandemic, A qualitative analysis. *School Mental Health, 15*, 78–89. DOI: 10.1007/s12310-022-09533-2 PMID: 35875185

Rockwell, L. (2024). *Teacher burnout: Symptoms, causes & prevention.* Choosing Therapy. https://www.choosingtherapy.com/teacher-burnout/#:~:text=Start%20Free%20Assessment-,What%20Is%20Teacher%20Burnout

Rodriguez-Rodríguez, S., Canet-Vintró, M., Wee, S. O., Rodríguez-Sanz, J., López-de-Celis, C., Oviedo, G. R., Labata-Lezaun, N., & Pérez-Bellmunt, A. (2024). Cognitive enhancement strategies for older adults: An evaluation of different training modalities to improve executive function—A systematic review and meta-analysis. *Journal of Clinical Medicine, 13*(5), 1301. https://www.mdpi.com/2077-0383/13/5/1301 PMID: 38592139

Roig Hierro, E., Ríos Sisó, X., Buscà, F., Guillem, M., & Batalla, A. (2025). The positive impact of physical activity on academic performance among catalan adolescents. *Cogent Education*, *12*(1). Advance online publication. DOI: 10.1080/2331186x.2025.2497139

Rojas, J. C., Barril, J. P., Jiménez, T. L., Clarà, M., Ramos, F. S., Peel, K., & Justiniano, B. (2025). Navigating burnout: A study of teacher identity in Chile, Ecuador, Brazil, Spain and Australia. *Pedagogy, Culture & Society*, *33*(2), 729–745. DOI: 10.1080/14681366.2024.2302314

Romain, A. J., Marleau, J., & Baillot, A. (2018). Impact of obesity and mood disorders on physical comorbidities, psychological well-being, health behaviours and use of health services. *Journal of Affective Disorders*, *225*, 381–388. DOI: 10.1016/j.jad.2017.08.065 PMID: 28846960

Romar, J. E., Enlund, M., Lind, S., & Björkgren, M. (2023). Movement integration in academic classrooms; a focus on secondary students' experiences. *Journal of Physical Education and Sport*, *23*(4), 918–928.

Rosa Rimes, R., Marcos de Souza Moura, A., Khede Lamego, M., Souza de Sa Filho, A., Manochio, J., Paes, F., Giovanni Carta, M., Mura, G., Wegner, M., Budde, H., Barbosa Ferreira Rocha, N., Rocha, J., Manuel, R. S., Tavares, J., Arias-Carrion, O., Egidio Nardi, A., Yuan, T.-F., & Machado, S. (2015). Effects of Exercise on Physical and Mental Health, and Cognitive and Brain Functions in Schizophrenia: Clinical and Experimental Evidence. *CNS & Neurological Disorders - Drug Targets*, *14*(10), 1244–1254. PMID: 26556069

Rose, D. M., & Loomis, A. (2025). Teacher burnout, student-teacher relational closeness, and the moderating effect of work stress focused supervision. *Early Childhood Education Journal*, *53*(4), 1027–1039. DOI: 10.1007/s10643-024-01651-7

Rosenbaum, S., Tiedemann, A., Sherrington, C., Curtis, J., & Ward, P. B. (2014). Physical activity interventions for people with mental illness: A systematic review and meta-analysis. *The Journal of Clinical Psychiatry*, *75*(9), 964–974. DOI: 10.4088/JCP.13r08765 PMID: 24813261

Rosenbaum, S., Vancampfort, D., Steel, Z., Newby, J., Ward, P. B., & Stubbs, B. (2015). Physical activity in the treatment of Post-traumatic stress disorder: A systematic review and meta-analysis. *Psychiatry Research*, *230*(2), 130–136. DOI: 10.1016/j.psychres.2015.10.017 PMID: 26500072

Rosenblat, J. D., & McIntyre, R. S. (2016). Bipolar disorder and inflammation. *The Psychiatric Clinics of North America*, *39*(1), 125–137. DOI: 10.1016/j.psc.2015.09.006

Ross, A., Friedmann, E., Bevans, M., & Thomas, S. (2013). National survey of yoga practitioners: Mental and physical health benefits. *Complementary Therapies in Medicine*, *21*(4), 313–323. DOI: 10.1016/j.ctim.2013.04.001

Rowe, J. W., & Kahn, R. L. (1997). Successful aging. *The Gerontologist*, *37*(4), 433–440. DOI: 10.1093/geront/37.4.433

Ruegsegger, G. N., & Booth, F. W. (2018). Health Benefits of Exercise. *Cold Spring Harbor Perspectives in Medicine*, *8*(7), a029694. DOI: 10.1101/cshperspect.a029694 PMID: 28507196

Ryan, R. M., & Deci, E. L. (Eds.). (2017). *Self-Determination Theory: Basic Psychological Needs in Motivation, Development, and Wellness*. Guilford Press., DOI: 10.1521/978.14625/28806

Saanijoki, T.. (2018). Endorphin release after high intensity interval training in humans. *Neuropsychopharmacology : Official Publication of the American College of Neuropsychopharmacology*, *43*(2), 358–367. DOI: 10.1038/npp.2017.194 PMID: 28722022

Sabiston, C. M., Jewett, R., Ashdown-Franks, G., Belanger, M., Brunet, J., O'Loughlin, E., & O'Loughlin, J. (2016). Number of Years of Team and Individual Sport Participation During Adolescence and Depressive Symptoms in Early Adulthood. *Journal of Sport & Exercise Psychology*, *38*(1), 105–110. DOI: 10.1123/jsep.2015-0175 PMID: 27018562

Salamone, J. D., Correa, M., Farrar, A., & Mingote, S. M. (2007). Effort-related functions of nucleus accumbens dopamine and associated forebrain circuits. *Psychopharmacology*, *191*(3), 461–482. DOI: 10.1007/s00213-006-0668-9 PMID: 17225164

Sallis, J. F., Floyd, M. F., Rodríguez, D. A., & Saelens, B. E. (2012). Role of built environments in physical activity, obesity, and cardiovascular disease. *Circulation*, *125*(5), 729–737. DOI: 10.1161/CIRCULATIONAHA.110.969022 PMID: 22311885

Sanaeifar, F., Pourranjbar, S., Pourranjbar, M., Ramezani, S., Mehr, S. R., Wadan, A. S., & Khazeifard, F. (2024). Beneficial effects of physical exercise on cognitive behavioral impairments and brain derived neurotrophic factor alteration in the limbic system induced by neurodegeneration. *Experimental Gerontology*, *195*, 112539. DOI: 10.1016/j.exger.2024.112539 PMID: 39116955

Sanderson, H., DeRousie, J., & Guistwite, N. (2017). Impact of collegiate recreation on academic success. *Journal of Student Affairs Research and Practice*, *55*(1), 40–53. DOI: 10.1080/19496591.2017.1357566

Scardina, A., Tabacchi, G., Thomas, E., Navarra, G. A., Petrigna, L., Caramazza, G., Palma, A., & Bellafiore, M. (2024). Relationship between lifestyle determinants and perceived mental and physical health in Italian nursery and primary school teachers after the COVID-19 lockdown. *Journal of Functional Morphology and Kinesiology*, *9*(1), 33. Advance online publication. DOI: 10.3390/jfmk9010033 PMID: 38390933

Schaal, K., Tafflet, M., Nassif, H., Thibault, V., Pichard, C., Alcotte, M., Guillet, T., El Helou, N., Berthelot, G., Simon, S., & Toussaint, J.-F. (2011). Psychological Balance in High Level Athletes: Gender-Based Differences and Sport-Specific Patterns. *PLoS One*, *6*(5), e19007. DOI: 10.1371/journal.pone.0019007 PMID: 21573222

Scheer, M. (2022). Culture and religion: Remarks on an indeterminate relationship. *Religion and Society*, *13*(1), 111–125.

Scheewe, T. W., Backx, F. J. G., Takken, T., Jörg, F., van Strater, A. C. P., Kroes, A. G., Kahn, R. S., & Cahn, W. (2013). Exercise therapy improves mental and physical health in schizophrenia: A randomised controlled trial. *Acta Psychiatrica Scandinavica*, *127*(6), 464–473. DOI: 10.1111/acps.12029 PMID: 23106093

Schinke, R. J., Stambulova, N. B., Si, G., & Moore, Z. (2018). International society of sport psychology position stand: Athletes' mental health, performance, and development. *International Journal of Sport and Exercise Psychology*, *16*(6), 622–639. DOI: 10.1080/1612197X.2017.1295557

Schoenfeld, T. J., Rada, P., Pieruzzini, P. R., Hsueh, B., & Gould, E. (2013). Physical exercise prevents stress-induced activation of granule neurons and enhances local inhibitory mechanisms in the dentate gyrus. *The Journal of Neuroscience : The Official Journal of the Society for Neuroscience*, *33*(18), 7770–7777. DOI: 10.1523/JNEUROSCI.5352-12.2013 PMID: 23637169

Schuch, F. B., & Vancampfort, D. (2021). Physical activity, exercise, and mental disorders: It is time to move on. *Trends in Psychiatry and Psychotherapy*, *43*(3), 177–184. https://www.scielo.br/j/trends/a/jCRvs9LQq8ycmLwLysGBRFM/ PMID: 33890431

Schuch, F. B., Vancampfort, D., Firth, J., Rosenbaum, S., Richards, J., Ward, P. B., & Stubbs, B. (2016b). Exercise for depression in adults: A meta-analysis of randomized controlled trials. *British Journal of Sports Medicine*, *50*(4), 229–236. DOI: 10.1136/bjsports-2015-095014 PMID: 27611903

Schuch, F. B., Vancampfort, D., Firth, J., Rosenbaum, S., Ward, P. B., Silva, E. S., Hallgren, M., Ponce de Leon, A., Dunn, A. L., Deslandes, A. C., Fleck, M. P., Carvalho, A. F., & Stubbs, B. (2016a). Physical activity and incident depression: A meta-analysis of prospective cohort studies. *The American Journal of Psychiatry, 175*(7), 631–648. DOI: 10.1176/appi.ajp.2018.17111194 PMID: 29690792

Schuch, F. B., Vancampfort, D., Richards, J., Rosenbaum, S., Ward, P. B., & Stubbs, B. (2016). Exercise as a treatment for depression: A meta-analysis adjusting for publication bias. *Journal of Psychiatric Research, 77*, 42–51. DOI: 10.1016/j.jpsychires.2016.02.023 PMID: 26978184

Schulenberg, J. E., Sameroff, A. J., & Cicchetti, D. (2004). The transition to adulthood as a critical juncture in the course of psychopathology and mental health. *Development and Psychopathology, 16*(4), 799–806. DOI: 10.1017/S0954579404040015 PMID: 15704815

Sebire, S. J., Standage, M., & Vansteenkiste, M. (2009). Examining intrinsic versus extrinsic exercise goals: Cognitive, affective, and behavioral outcomes. *Journal of Sport & Exercise Psychology, 31*(2), 189–210. DOI: 10.1123/jsep.31.2.189 PMID: 19454771

Seguin, R. A., Eldridge, G., Graham, M. L., Folta, S. C., Nelson, M. E., & Strogatz, D. (2016). Strong Hearts, healthy communities: A rural community-based cardiovascular disease prevention program. *BMC Public Health, 16*, 86. DOI: 10.1186/s12889-016-2751-4 PMID: 26822982

Seligman, M. E., & Csikszentmihalyi, M. (2000). Positive psychology. An introduction. *The American Psychologist, 55*(1), 5–14. DOI: 10.1037//0003-066x.55.1.5 PMID: 11392865

Shaheen, F., & Mahmood, N. (2024). The burnout syndrome: A review study. *Journal of Behavioural Sciences, 34*(2), 36–52.

Sharma, A., Madaan, V., & Petty, F. D. (2006). Exercise for mental health. *Primary Care Companion to the Journal of Clinical Psychiatry, 8*(2), 106. DOI: 10.4088/pcc.v08n0208a PMID: 16862239

Shimada, H., Makizako, H., Doi, T., Park, H., Tsutsumimoto, K., Verghese, J., & Suzuki, T. (2018). Effects of combined physical and cognitive exercises on cognition and mobility in patients with mild cognitive impairment: A randomized clinical trial. *Journal of the American Medical Directors Association, 19*(7), 584–591. https://www.sciencedirect.com/science/article/pii/S152586101730542X PMID: 29153754

Shim, M., Lacson, C., Kavanaugh, M., Goldstein-Levitas, N., & Fisher, K. (2024). Online mindful movement approach for older adults: Two case studies. *Activities, Adaptation and Aging, 48*(4), 705–722.

Shor, R., & Shalev, A. (2016). Barriers to involvement in physical activities of persons with mental illness. *Health Promotion International, 31*(1), 116–123. https://academic.oup.com/heapro/article-abstract/31/1/116/2355913 PMID: 25204451

Silva, N. C. B. S., Gregory, M. A., Gill, D. P., & Petrella, R. J. (2017). Multiple-modality exercise and mind-motor training to improve cardiovascular health and fitness in older adults at risk for cognitive impairment: A randomized controlled trial. *Archives of Gerontology and Geriatrics, 68*, 149–160. https://www.sciencedirect.com/science/article/pii/S0167494316301893 PMID: 27810663

Simon, R. L., Torres, C. R., & Hager, P. F. (2018). *Fair Play: The Ethics of Sport* (4th ed.). Routledge., DOI: 10.4324/9780429492570

Singh, B., Kumar, A., & Sharma, S. (2023). Comparative effectiveness of exercise and cognitive-behavioral therapy in mood disorders: A systematic review. *Journal of Affective Disorders, 331*, 39–49. DOI: 10.1016/j.jad.2023.05.011

Singh, B., Olds, T., Curtis, R., Dumuid, D., Virgara, R., Watson, A., Szeto, K., O'Connor, E., Ferguson, T., Eglitis, E., Miatke, A., Simpson, C. E., & Maher, C. (2023). Effectiveness of physical activity interventions for improving depression, anxiety and distress: An overview of systematic reviews. *British Journal of Sports Medicine, 57*(18), 1203–1209. DOI: 10.1136/bjsports-2022-106195 PMID: 36796860

Skaalvik, E. M., & Skaalvik, S. (2018). Job demands and job resources as predictors of teacher motivation and well-being. *Social Psychology of Education, 21*(5), 1251–1275. DOI: 10.1007/s11218-018-9464-8

Skaalvik, E. M., & Skaalvik, S. (2020). Teacher burnout: Relations between dimensions of burnout, perceived school context, job satisfaction and motivation for teaching. A longitudinal study. *Teachers and Teaching, 26*(7-8), 602–616. DOI: 10.1080/13540602.2021.1913404

Skaalvik, E., & Skaalvik, S. (2017). Still motivated to teach? A study of school context variables, stress and job satisfaction among teachers in senior high school. *Social Psychology of Education, 20*(1), 15–37. DOI: 10.1007/s11218-016-9363-9

Skaalvik, E., & Skaalvik, S. (2021). Teacher stress and coping strategies—The struggle to stay in control. *Creative Education, 12*, 1273–1295. DOI: 10.4236/ce.2021.126096

Skinner, E. A. (2023). Four guideposts toward an integrated model of academic motivation: Motivational resilience, academic identity, complex social ecologies, and development. *Educational Psychology Review*, *35*(3), 80.

Sleiman, S. F., Henry, J., Al Haddad, R., Hayek, L. E., Haidar, E. A., Stringer, T., Ulja, D., Karuppagounder, S. S., Holson, E. B., Ratan, R. R., Ninan, I., & Chao, M. V. (2016). Exercise promotes the expression of brain derived neurotrophic factor (BDNF) through the action of the ketone body β hydroxybutyrate. *eLife*, *5*. Advance online publication. DOI: 10.7554/elife.15092 PMID: 27253067

Smith, K. E., & Merwin, R. M. (2021). The role of exercise in emotion regulation: Conceptual and empirical perspectives. *Clinical Psychology Review*, *84*, 101971. DOI: 10.1016/j.cpr.2020.101971

Smith, R. E., Smoll, F. L., & Cumming, S. P. (2007). Effects of a Motivational Climate Intervention for Coaches on Young Athletes' Sport Performance Anxiety. *Journal of Sport & Exercise Psychology*, *29*(1), 39–59. DOI: 10.1123/jsep.29.1.39 PMID: 17556775

Smith, T. B., McCullough, M. E., & Poll, J. (2003). Religiousness and depression: Evidence for a main effect and the moderating influence of stressful life events. *Psychological Bulletin*, *129*(4), 614–636. DOI: 10.1037/0033-2909.129.4.614 PMID: 12848223

Son, C., Hegde, S., Smith, A., Wang, X., & Sasangohar, F. (2020). Effects of COVID-19 on College Students' Mental Health in the United States: Interview Survey Study. *Journal of Medical Internet Research*, *22*(9), e21279. DOI: 10.2196/21279 PMID: 32805704

Song, Y., Zhao, W., Wang, X., & Li, J. (2024). The impact of job stress on burnout in Chinese teachers: The mediating roles of social support and psychological empowerment. *Psychology in the Schools*, *61*(1), 253–271. DOI: 10.1002/pits.23052

Sparling, P. B., Giuffrida, A., Piomelli, D., Rosskopf, L., & Dietrich, A. (2003). Exercise activates the endocannabinoid system. *Neuroreport*, *14*(17), 2209–2211. DOI: 10.1097/00001756-200312020-00015 PMID: 14625449

Spindle, T. R., Cone, E. J., Schlienz, N. J., Mitchell, J. M., Bigelow, G. E., Flegel, R., Hayes, E., & Vandrey, R. (2018). Acute Effects of Smoked and Vaporized Cannabis in Healthy Adults Who Infrequently Use Cannabis: A Crossover Trial. *JAMA Network Open*, *1*(7), e184841. DOI: 10.1001/jamanetworkopen.2018.4841 PMID: 30646391

Srinivas, N. S., Vimalan, V., Padmanabhan, P., & Gulyás, B. (2021). An overview on cognitive function enhancement through physical exercises. *Brain Sciences, 11*(10), 1289. https://www.mdpi.com/2076-3425/11/10/1289 PMID: 34679354

Stanley, E. A., Schaldach, J. M., Kiyonaga, A., & Jha, A. P. (2011). Mindfulness-based mind fitness training: A case study of a high-stress predeployment military cohort. *Cognitive and Behavioral Practice, 18*(4), 566–576.

Stanton, R., Reaburn, P., & Happell, B. (2015). Barriers to exercise prescription and participation in people with mental illness: The perspectives of nurses working in mental health. *Journal of Psychiatric and Mental Health Nursing, 22*(6), 440–448. DOI: 10.1111/jpm.12205 PMID: 25855247

Stanton, S., Rosenbaum, S., Kalucy, M., Reaburn, P., & Happell, B. (2015). A call to action: Exercise as treatment for patients with mental illness. *Australian Journal of Primary Health, 21*(2), 120–125. DOI: 10.1071/PY14054 PMID: 25033827

Stark, K., Daulat, N., & King, S. (2022). A vision for teachers' emotional well-being. *Sage Journals, 103*(5). Advance online publication. DOI: 10.1177/00317217221079975

Stevens, K. R. (2025). *Ways of Being: A Literature Review on Embodied Healing Through Mindfulness, Neuroscience and Dance/Movement Therapy Practice During Uncertain Times* (Master's thesis, Pratt Institute).

Stillman, C. M.. (2020). Exercise improves connectivity in emotion-regulation networks. *Psychophysiology, 57*(8), 433–450.

Stimpson, N. J., Davison, G., & Javadi, A.-H. (2018). Joggin'the noggin: Towards a physiological understanding of exercise-induced cognitive benefits. *Neuroscience and Biobehavioral Reviews, 88*, 177–186. https://www.sciencedirect.com/science/article/pii/S0149763417308102 PMID: 29572187

Stirling, A. E., & Kerr, G. A. (2013). The perceived effects of elite athletes' experiences of emotional abuse in the coach–athlete relationship. *International Journal of Sport and Exercise Psychology, 11*(1), 87–100. DOI: 10.1080/1612197X.2013.752173

Stork, M. J., Banfield, L. E., Gibala, M. J., & Martin Ginis, K. A. (2017). A scoping review of the psychological responses to interval exercise: Is interval exercise a viable alternative to traditional exercise? *Health Psychology Review, 11*(4), 324–344. DOI: 10.1080/17437199.2017.1326011 PMID: 28460601

Strakowski, S. M., Adler, C. M., Almeida, J., Altshuler, L. L., Blumberg, H. P., Chang, K. D., & DelBello, M. P. (2012). The functional neuroanatomy of bipolar disorder: A consensus model. *Bipolar Disorders, 14*(4), 313–325. DOI: 10.1111/j.1399-5618.2012.01022.x

Strakowski, S. M., Adler, C. M., & DelBello, M. P. (2012). Volumetric MRI studies of mood disorders: Do they distinguish unipolar and bipolar disorder? *Bipolar Disorders, 14*(2), 115–127. DOI: 10.1111/j.1399-5618.2012.00990.x

Strejilevich, S. A., Vallejos, F., & Bustin, J. (2018). How Argentina is training their mental health residents to face its Silver Tsunami? *International Psychogeriatrics, 30*(10), 1573–1574.

Ströhle, A. (2009). Physical activity, exercise, depression and anxiety disorders. *Journal of Neural Transmission (Vienna, Austria), 116*(6), 777–784. DOI: 10.1007/s00702-008-0092-x PMID: 18726137

Strong, W. B., Malina, R. M., Blimkie, C. J. R., Daniels, S. R., Dishman, R. K., Gutin, B., Hergenroeder, A. C., Must, A., Nixon, P. A., Pivarnik, J. M., Rowland, T., Trost, S., & Trudeau, F. (2005). Evidence based physical activity for school-age youth. *The Journal of Pediatrics, 146*(6), 732–737. DOI: 10.1016/j.jpeds.2005.01.055 PMID: 15973308

Stubbs, B., Vancampfort, D., Hallgren, M., Firth, J., Veronese, N., Solmi, M., & Kahl, K. G. (2018). EPA guidance on physical activity as a treatment for severe mental illness: A meta-review of the evidence and position statement from the European Psychiatric Association (EPA), supported by the International Organization of Physical Therapists in Mental Health (IOPTMH). *European Psychiatry : the Journal of the Association of European Psychiatrists, 54*, 124–144. DOI: 10.1016/j.eurpsy.2018.07.004

Stubbs, B., Vancampfort, D., Rosenbaum, S., Firth, J., Cosco, T., Veronese, N., & Schuch, F. B. (2017). An examination of the anxiolytic effects of exercise for people with anxiety and stress-related disorders: A meta-analysis. *Psychiatry Research, 249*, 102–108. PMID: 28088704

Stubbs, B., Vancampfort, D., Rosenbaum, S., Firth, J., Cosco, T., Veronese, N., & Schuch, F. B. (2020). Exercise as an adjunct to psychotherapy for people with bipolar disorder: A systematic review and meta-analysis. *Acta Psychiatrica Scandinavica, 141*(4), 290–302. DOI: 10.1111/acps.13133

Sudibjo, N., & Manihuruk, A. M. (2022). How do happiness at work and perceived organizational support affect teachers' mental health through job satisfaction during the COVID-19 pandemic? *Psychology Research and Behavior Management, 15*, 939–951. DOI: 10.2147/PRBM.S361881 PMID: 35469169

Sunarti, V., Rahman, M. A., Handrianto, C., Syuraini, S., Putri, L. D., Azizah, Z., & Nor Azhar, N. F. (2024). Understanding women's empowerment through exercise: Insights from a study on physical activity and self-efficacy. *Retos: Nuevas Perspectivas de Educación Física. Deporte y Recreación, 58*, 227–237. DOI: 10.47197/retos.v58.106803

Sun, W., Liu, X., Liu, Y., Ding, S., Jiang, Y., & Lv, Z. (2024). The relationship between school organizational climate and teacher's organizational citizenship behavior: The mediating role of teaching efficacy and moderating role of optimistic traits. *Behavioral Science, 14*(12), 1130. Advance online publication. DOI: 10.3390/bs14121130 PMID: 39767271

Sylvester, C. M., Mayer, A. R., & Caveney, A. F. (2020). Aerobic exercise and executive function in bipolar disorder: A randomized controlled trial. *Journal of Affective Disorders, 277*, 316–324. DOI: 10.1016/j.jad.2020.08.036

Sylvia, L. G., Ametrano, R. M., Nierenberg, A. A., & Deckersbach, T. (2013a). Exercise as an adjunctive treatment for bipolar depression: A pilot study. *Journal of Affective Disorders, 146*(2), 240–245. DOI: 10.1016/j.jad.2012.07.019

Sylvia, L. G., Ametrano, R. M., Nierenberg, A. A., & Deckersbach, T. (2013b). Exercise treatment for bipolar disorder: Potential mechanisms of action mediated through increased neurogenesis and decreased allostatic load. *Psychotherapy and Psychosomatics, 82*(6), 386–394. DOI: 10.1159/000348579

Sylvia, L. G., Salcedo, S., Bernstein, E. E., Baek, J. H., Nierenberg, A. A., & Deckersbach, T. (2017). Nutrition, exercise, and wellness treatment in bipolar disorder: Proof of concept for a consolidated intervention. *International Journal of Bipolar Disorders, 5*(1), 7.

Szuhany, K. L., Bugatti, M., & Otto, M. W. (2015). A meta-analysis of BDNF response to exercise. *Psychosomatic Medicine, 77*(3), 247–255.

Szuhany, K. L., Bugatti, M., & Otto, M. W. (2015). A meta-analytic review of the effects of exercise on brain-derived neurotrophic factor. *Journal of Psychiatric Research, 60*, 56–64. PMID: 25455510

Tang, H., An, S., Zhang, L., Xiao, Y., & Li, X. (2024). The antecedents and outcomes of public service motivation: A meta-analysis using the Job Demands-Resources model. *Behavioral Sciences (Basel, Switzerland), 14*(10), 861. DOI: 10.3390/bs14100861 PMID: 39457733

Tan, J., & Kim, S. (2024). Exploring the relationship between teacher motivation and teacher burnout among Chinese college English teachers. *English Teaching, 79*(2), 163–190. DOI: 10.15858/engtea.79.2.202406.163

Tay, L., Tan, K., Diener, E., & Gonzalez, E. (2013). Social Relations, Health Behaviors, and Health Outcomes: A Survey and Synthesis. *Applied Psychology. Health and Well-Being, 5*(1), 28–78. DOI: 10.1111/aphw.12000 PMID: 23281315

Taylor, C. B., Sallis, J. F., & Needle, R. (1985). The relation of physical activity and exercise to mental health. *Public Health Reports, 100*(2), 195. https://pmc.ncbi.nlm.nih.gov/articles/PMC1424736/ PMID: 3920718

Teixeira, A. L., Barbosa, I. G., Machado-Vieira, R., & Bauer, M. E. (2021). Increased BDNF levels after exercise in bipolar disorder: A systematic review and meta-analysis. *Neuroscience and Biobehavioral Reviews, 120*, 426–434. DOI: 10.1016/j.neubiorev.2020.11.020

Teixeira, P. J., Carraça, E. V., Markland, D., Silva, M. N., & Ryan, R. M. (2012). Exercise, physical activity, and self-determination theory: A systematic review. *The International Journal of Behavioral Nutrition and Physical Activity, 9*, 78. DOI: 10.1186/1479-5868-9-78 PMID: 22726453

Tew, G. A., Howsam, J., Hardy, M., & Bissell, L. (2017). Adapted yoga to improve physical function and health-related quality of life in physically-inactive older adults: A randomised controlled pilot trial. *BMC Geriatrics, 17*, 131.

Thayer, J. F., Ahs, F., Fredrikson, M., Sollers, J. J., & Wager, T. D. (2012). A meta-analysis of heart rate variability and neuroimaging studies: Implications for heart rate variability as a marker of stress and health. *Neuroscience and Biobehavioral Reviews, 36*(2), 747–756. DOI: 10.1016/j.neubiorev.2011.11.009 PMID: 22178086

Thomas, J., & Reyes, M. S. (2024). Understanding the new stress factors affecting teachers' burnout: A scoping review. *Makara Human Behavior Studies in Asia, 28*(1), 1–18. DOI: 10.7454/hubs.asia.1181024

Thompson Coon, J., Boddy, K., Stein, K., Whear, R., Barton, J., & Depledge, M. H. (2011). Does participating in physical activity in outdoor natural environments have a greater effect on physical and mental wellbeing than physical activity indoors? A systematic review. *Environmental Science & Technology*, *45*(5), 1761–1772. DOI: 10.1021/es102947t PMID: 21291246

Thomson, C., Sharma, S., & Khan, A. (2015). Neurobiological effects of exercise: Implications for mood and cognition. *Neuroscience and Biobehavioral Reviews*, *55*, 89–95. DOI: 10.1016/j.neubiorev.2015.04.014

Tisdell, E. J., Lukic, B., Banerjee, R., Liao, D., & Palmer, C. (2024). The effects of heart rhythm meditation on vagal tone and Well-being: A mixed methods research study. *Applied Psychophysiology and Biofeedback*, *49*(3), 439–455.

Today, U. N. D. (2024). *Why teachers need, deserve mental health support.* University of North Dakota. https://blogs.und.edu/und-today/2024/01/ und-in-the-conversation-why-teachers-need-deserve-mental-health-support/#:~:text=Improves%20teaching%20effectiveness,in%20such%20a%20positive%20way

Topp, R., Jacks, D. E., Wedig, R. T., Newman, J. L., Tobe, L., & Hollingsworth, A. (2009). Reducing risk factors for childhood obesity: The Tommie Smith Youth Athletic Initiative. *Western Journal of Nursing Research*, *31*(6), 715–730. DOI: 10.1177/0193945909336356 PMID: 19454750

Torous, J., Kiang, M. V., Lorme, J., & Onnela, J. P. (2018). New tools for new research in psychiatry: A scalable and customizable platform to empower data driven smartphone research. *JMIR Mental Health*, *3*(2), e16. DOI: 10.2196/mental.5165

Toscano, C. V. A., Ferreira, J. P., Quinaud, R. T., Silva, K. M. N., Carvalho, H. M., & Gaspar, J. M. (2022). Exercise improves the social and behavioral skills of children and adolescent with autism spectrum disorders. *Frontiers in Psychiatry*, *13*. Advance online publication. DOI: 10.3389/fpsyt.2022.1027799 PMID: 36620673

Trinh, O. T., Nguyen, N. D., Dibley, M. J., Phongsavan, P., & Bauman, A. E. (2008). The prevalence and correlates of physical inactivity among adults in Ho Chi Minh City. *BMC Public Health*, *8*(1), 204. DOI: 10.1186/1471-2458-8-204

Trinidad, J. E. (2021). Teacher satisfaction and burnout during COVID-19: What organizational factors help? *International Journal of Leadership in Education*, *28*(1), 214–232. DOI: 10.1080/13603124.2021.2006795

Troiano, R. P., McClain, J. J., Brychta, R. J., & Chen, K. Y. (2014). Evolution of accelerometer methods for physical activity research. *British Journal of Sports Medicine*, *48*(13), 1019–1023. PMID: 24782483

Tsatsoulis, A., & Fountoulakis, S. (2006). The protective role of exercise on stress system dysregulation and comorbidities. *Annals of the New York Academy of Sciences, 1083*, 196–213. DOI: 10.1196/annals.1367.020 PMID: 17148741

Tummers, L. D., & Bakker, A. B. (2021). Leadership and job demands-resources theory: A systematic review. *Frontiers in Psychology, 12*, 722080. Advance online publication. DOI: 10.3389/fpsyg.2021.722080 PMID: 34659034

Turner, K., & Garvis, S. (2023). Teacher educator wellbeing, stress and burnout: A scoping review. *Education Sciences, 13*(4), 351. DOI: 10.3390/educsci13040351

Twenge, J. M., & Campbell, W. K. (2018). Associations between screen time and lower psychological well-being among children and adolescents: Evidence from a population-based study. *Preventive Medicine Reports, 12*, 271–283. DOI: 10.1016/j.pmedr.2018.10.003 PMID: 30406005

Twenge, J. M., Cooper, A. B., Joiner, T. E., Duffy, M. E., & Binau, S. G. (2019). Age, period, and cohort trends in mood disorder indicators and suicide-related outcomes in a nationally representative dataset, 2005-2017. *Journal of Abnormal Psychology, 128*(3), 185–199. DOI: 10.1037/abn0000410 PMID: 30869927

Valentim, O., de Sousa, L., de Sousa, C., Correia, T., Carvalho, J. C., Querido, A., José, H., & Laranjeira, C. (2025). Positive mental health and happiness at work in a sample of Portuguese workers: A web-based cross-sectional study. *Administrative Sciences, 15*(2), 44. Advance online publication. DOI: 10.3390/admsci15020044

van der Kolk, B. A. (2014). The body keeps the score: Brain, mind, and body in the healing of trauma (pp. xvi, 443). Viking.

Van Dyck, D., Mertens, L., Cardon, G., De Cocker, K., & De Bourdeaudhuij, I. (2017). Opinions toward physical activity, sedentary behavior, and interventions to stimulate active living during early retirement: A qualitative study in recently retired adults. *Journal of Aging and Physical Activity, 25*(2), 277–286. DOI: 10.1123/japa.2015-0295 PMID: 27759483

van Praag, H.. (1999). Running enhances neurogenesis. *Nature Neuroscience, 2*, 266–270. PMID: 10195220

Vancampfort, D.. (2016). Associations between physical activity and psychosocial functioning in patients with bipolar disorder: A systematic review. *The Journal of Nervous and Mental Disease, 204*(9), 702–713.

Vancampfort, D., Probst, M., Helvik Skjaerven, L., Catalán-Matamoros, D., Lundvik-Gyllensten, A., Gómez-Conesa, A., Ijntema, R., & De Hert, M. (2012). Systematic Review of the Benefits of Physical Therapy Within a Multidisciplinary Care Approach for People With Schizophrenia. *Physical Therapy*, *92*(1), 11–23. DOI: 10.2522/ptj.20110218 PMID: 22052946

Vancampfort, D., Rosenbaum, S., Schuch, F., Ward, P. B., Probst, M., Mugisha, J., & Stubbs, B. (2016). Prevalence and predictors of exercise adherence in people with bipolar disorder: A systematic review and meta-analysis. *The British Journal of Psychiatry*, *38*(3), 309–316. DOI: 10.1590/1516-4446-2016-1903

Vandelanotte, C.. (2025). The effectiveness of exercise snacks as a time-efficient intervention. *Frontiers in Cardiovascular Medicine*. Advance online publication. DOI: 10.3389/fcvm.2025.164315

Vecchio, L. M., Meng, Y., Xhima, K., Lipsman, N., Hamani, C., &Aubert, I. (2018). The neuroprotective effects of exercise: Maintaining a healthy brain throughout aging. *Brain Plasticity, 4*(1), 17–52. 180069.DOI: 10.3233/bpl

Vedøy, I. B., Erssen, S. A., Tjomsland, H. E., Skulberg, K. R., & Thurston, M. (2020). Physical activity, mental health and academic achievement: A cross sectional study of Norwegian adolescents. *Mental Health and Physical Activity*, *18*, 100322. DOI: 10.1016/j.mhpa.2020.100322

Vela, J. C., Guerra, F., Diaz, Z., Karaman, M. A., & Zamora, E. (2024). Exploring how positive psychology characteristics influence mental health among teacher candidates at a Hispanic serving institution. *Journal of Latinos and Education*, *23*(4), 1461–1471. DOI: 10.1080/15348431.2023.2274851

Vermote, B., Vansteenkiste, M., Aelterman, N., van der Kaap-Deeder, J., & Beyers, W. (2023). Teachers' psychological needs link social pressure with personal adjustment and motivating teaching style. *Journal of Experimental Education*, *91*(4), 696–717. DOI: 10.1080/00220973.2022.2039584

Vieta, E., Berk, M., Schulze, T. G., Carvalho, A. F., Suppes, T., Calabrese, J. R., & Grande, I. (2018). Bipolar disorders. *Nature Reviews. Disease Primers*, *4*, 18008. DOI: 10.1038/nrdp.2018.8

Viljoen, M., & Roos, J. L. (2020). Physical exercise and the patient with schizophrenia. *Australian Journal of General Practice*, *49*(12), 803–808. DOI: 10.3316/informit.638850071185097 PMID: 33254203

Vishkin, A., & Tamir, M. (2020). Fear not: Religion and emotion regulation in coping with existential concerns. In *The science of religion, spirituality, and existentialism* (pp. 325–338). Academic Press.

Vogler, J., O'Hara, L., Gregg, J., & Burnell, F. (2011). The impact of a short-term iyengar yoga program on the health and well-being of physically inactive older adults. *International Journal of Yoga Therapy, 21*, 61–72.

Voss, M. W.. (2013). Neurobiological effects of exercise on aging. *Neuroscience and Biobehavioral Reviews, 37*, 2243–2261.

Voss, M. W., Heo, S., Prakash, R. S., Erickson, K. I., Alves, H., Chaddock, L., Szabo, A. N., Mailey, E. L., Wójcicki, T. R., White, S. M., Gothe, N., McAuley, E., Sutton, B. P., & Kramer, A. F. (2013). The influence of aerobic fitness on cerebral white matter integrity and cognitive function in older adults: Results of a one-year exercise intervention. *Human Brain Mapping, 34*(11), 2972–2985. DOI: 10.1002/hbm.22119 PMID: 22674729

Walker, T. (2025). *What's causing teacher burnout?* NEA Today. https://www.nea.org/nea-today/all-news-articles/whats-causing-teacher-burnout#:~:text=A%20lack%20of%20administrative%20support,youth%20in%20their%20formative%20years.%22

Wang, Y. (2024). Exploring the impact of workload, organizational support, and work engagement on teachers' psychological wellbeing: A structural equation modeling approach. *Frontiers in Psychology, 14*, 1345740. Advance online publication. DOI: 10.3389/fpsyg.2023.1345740 PMID: 38314257

Wang, Y., Zai, F., & Zhou, X. (2025). The impact of emotion regulation strategies on teachers' well-being and positive emotions: A meta-analysis. *Behavioral Sciences (Basel, Switzerland), 15*(3), 342. DOI: 10.3390/bs15030342 PMID: 40150237

Ward, N., Paul, E., Watson, P., Cooke, G. E., Hillman, C. H., Cohen, N. J., Kramer, A. F., & Barbey, A. K. (2017). Enhanced learning through multimodal training: Evidence from a comprehensive cognitive, physical fitness, and neuroscience intervention. *Scientific Reports, 7*(1), 5808. https://www.nature.com/articles/s41598-017-06237-5 PMID: 28724914

Ware, J. E.Jr, & Sherbourne, C. D., & the MOS 36-Item Short-Form Health Survey (SF-36) conceptual framework (1992). *Medical Care, 30*(6), 473-483.

Webb, C. E., Rossignac-Milon, M., & Higgins, E. T. (2017). Could walking facilitate interpersonal conflict resolution? *Conflict Resolution Quarterly, 35*(4), 345–371. PMID: 28481583

Weber, M., Belala, N., Clemson, L., Boulton, E., Hawley-Hague, H., Becker, C., & Schwenk, M. (2018). Feasibility and Effectiveness of Intervention Programmes Integrating Functional Exercise into Daily Life of Older Adults: A Systematic Review. *Gerontology*, *64*(2), 172–187. DOI: 10.1159/000479965 PMID: 28910814

Webster, C. A. (2022). The Comprehensive School Physical Activity Program: An invited review. *American Journal of Lifestyle Medicine*, *17*(6), 762–774. DOI: 10.1177/15598276221093543 PMID: 38511110

Wegner, M., Helmich, I., Machado, S., Nardi, A. E., Arias-Carrion, O., & Budde, H. (2014). Effects of exercise on anxiety and depression disorders: Review of meta- analyses and neurobiological mechanisms. *CNS & Neurological Disorders - Drug Targets*, *13*(6), 1002–1014. DOI: 10.2174/1871527313666140612102841 PMID: 24923346

Wegner, M., Helmich, I., Machado, S., Nardi, A. E., Arias-Carrion, O., & Budde, H. (2014). Effects of exercise on anxiety and depression disorders: Review of meta-analyses and neurobiological mechanisms. *CNS & Neurological Disorders - Drug Targets*, *13*(6), 1002–1014. DOI: 10.2174/1871527313666140612110928 PMID: 24923346

Weiss, E. R., Mullens, S., Todman, M., Barnes, S. E., Lord, K. A., & Davis, M. T. (2025). The transdiagnostic role of boredom within personality disorder symptoms and risk-related behaviors: Implications for dialectical behavior therapy. *Journal of Psychotherapy Integration*.

Welk, G. J., Welk, G., Corbin, W. R., & Welk, K. A. (2023). *Corbin's concepts of fitness and wellness: A comprehensive lifestyle approach* (13th ed.). McGraw Hill.

Westphal, A., Kalinowski, E., Hoferichter, C. J., & Vock, M. (2022). K-12 teachers' stress and burnout during the COVID-19 pandemic: A systematic review. *Frontiers in Psychology*, *13*, 920326. Advance online publication. DOI: 10.3389/fpsyg.2022.920326 PMID: 36118449

Weyerer, S., & Kupfer, B. (1994). Physical Exercise and Psychological Healtha. *Sports Medicine (Auckland, N.Z.)*, *17*(2), 108–116. DOI: 10.2165/00007256-199417020-00003 PMID: 8171221

Whiteman-Sandland, J., Hawkins, J., & Clayton, D. (2018). The role of social capital and community belongingness for exercise adherence: An exploratory study of the CrossFit gym model. *Journal of Health Psychology*, *23*(12), 1545–1556. DOI: 10.1177/1359105316664132 PMID: 27553606

White, R. L., Vella, S., Biddle, S., Sutcliffe, J., Guagliano, J. M., Uddin, R., & Teychenne, M. (2024). Physical activity and mental health: A systematic review and best-evidence synthesis of mediation and moderation studies. *The International Journal of Behavioral Nutrition and Physical Activity*, *21*(1), 134. PMID: 39609855

Wingo, A. P., Ghaemi, S. N., & Post, R. M. (2010). Time course and predictive value of neuropsychology performance in bipolar disorder. *Neuropsychology Review*, *20*(3), 323–332. DOI: 10.1007/s11065-010-9145-7

Wink, M. N., LaRusso, M. D., & Smith, R. L. (2021). Teacher empathy and students with problem behaviors: Examining teachers' perceptions, responses, relationships, and burnout. *Psychology in the Schools*, *58*(8), 1575–1596. DOI: 10.1002/pits.22516

Wolff, E., Gaudlitz, K., Von Lindenberger, B.-L., Plag, J., Heinz, A., & Ströhle, A. (2011). Exercise and physical activity in mental disorders. *European Archives of Psychiatry and Clinical Neuroscience*, *261*(S2), 186–191. DOI: 10.1007/s00406-011-0254-y PMID: 21935629

Woloshyn, V., Savage, M., Maich, K., & Penney, S. (2023). Stress, coping, and well-being in teachers and school administrators. *The Alberta Journal of Educational Research*, *69*(4), 492–513. DOI: 10.55016/ojs/ajer.v69i4.75886

Woods, H. C., & Scott, H. (2016). #Sleepyteens: Social media use in adolescence is associated with poor sleep quality, anxiety, depression and low self-esteem. *Journal of Adolescence*, *51*, 41–49. DOI: 10.1016/j.adolescence.2016.05.008 PMID: 27294324

World Health Organization. (2017). Depression and other common mental disorders: Global health estimates. World Health Organization. https://apps.who.int/iris/handle/10665/254610 (WHO fact sheet/latest estimates available at: https://www.who.int/health-topics/depression). apps.who.intT ch c Y t Th gi i

World Health Organization. (2020). *WHO guidelines on physical activity and sedentary behaviour.* [https://doi.org/]DOI: 10.1016/s0140-6736(20)30937-0

World Health Organization. (2021). *Mental disorders.* https://www.who.int/news-room/fact-sheets/detail/mental-disorders

World Health Organization. (2023). Depressive disorder (depression). https://www.who.int/news-room/fact-sheets/detail/depression

World Health Organization. (2024). *Mental health of adolescents.* https://www.who.int/news-room/fact-sheets/detail/adolescent-mental-health

World Health Organization. (2024). *Physical activity.* https://www.who.int/news-room/fact-sheets/detail/physical-activity

World Health Organization. (2024). Physical activity: Key facts. https://www.who.int/news-room/fact-sheets/detail/physical-activity

Wrann, C. D., White, J. P., & Salogiannnis, J.. (2013). Exercise induces hippocampal BDNF through a PGC-1α/FNDC5 pathway. *Cell Metabolism, 18*(5), 649–659. DOI: 10.1016/j.cmet.2013.09.008

Wu, J. C., Kelsoe, J. R., Schachat, C., & Bunney, W. E. (2020). Circadian rhythm disturbances and mood disorders: Insights from neuroimaging and genetics. *Journal of Affective Disorders, 265*, 498–508. DOI: 10.1016/j.jad.2020.01.056

Xia, J. W., & Shun, H. T. (2021). Exploring the mechanisms influencing the occupational well-being of early childhood teachers-A qualitative study based on the JD-R Model. *Turkish Journal of Computer and Mathematics Education, 12*(12), 4689–4706. https://www.proquest.com/scholarly-journals/exploring-mechanisms-influencing-occupational/docview/2628340006/se-2

Yalom, I. D., & Leszcz, M. (2020). *The theory and practice of group psychotherapy* (6th ed.). Basic Books.

Yang, Y., Cao, D., Lyu, T., & Gao, W. (2023). Meta-analysis of a mindfulness yoga exercise intervention on depression–based on intervention studies in China. *Frontiers in Psychology, 14*, 1283172. DOI: 10.3389/fpsyg.2023.1283172

Yaqian, Z., Chonggao, W., & Fan, Z. (2024). The relationship between job stress and job burnout of preschool teachers during the COVID-19: The moderation of perceived organizational support. *Work (Reading, Mass.), 79*(3), 1133–1146. DOI: 10.3233/WOR-230151 PMID: 38759080

Yatham, L. N., Torres, I. J., Malhi, G. S., Frangou, S., Glahn, D. C., Bearden, C. E., & Chengappa, K. R. (2010). The international society for bipolar disorders–battery for assessment of neurocognition (ISBD-BANC). *Bipolar Disorders, 12*(4), 351–363.

Yeager, D. S., Carroll, J. M., Buontempo, J., Cimpian, A., Woody, S., Crosnoe, R., & Dweck, C. S. (2022). Teacher mindsets help explain where a growth-mindset intervention does and doesn't work. *Psychological Science, 33*(1), 18–32. PMID: 34936529

Yeh, G. Y., Mehta, D. H., & Wayne, P. M. (2025). Healing STEM: Harnessing compassion, mindfulness, and emotional regulation to overcome burnout. *Journal of Integrative and Complementary Medicine, 31*(5), 398–402. PMID: 40238723

Ye, Z., Peng, Y., Rao, W., & Zhang, T. (2024). The effect of physical activity on depression: A lagged mediation study of school burnout. *BMC Public Health, 24*(1), 3491. Advance online publication. DOI: 10.1186/s12889-024-21003-9 PMID: 39695559

Young, B. W., & Medic, N. (2011). Examining social influences on the sport commitment of Masters swimmers. *Psychology of Sport and Exercise, 12*(2), 168–175. DOI: 10.1016/j.psychsport.2010.09.004

Young, S. N. (2007). How to increase serotonin in the human brain without drugs. *Journal of Psychiatry & Neuroscience : JPN, 32*(6), 394–399. PMID: 18043762

Youngstedt, S. D., O'Connor, P. J., & Dishman, R. K. (2016). The influence of exercise on human circadian rhythms. *Exercise and Sport Sciences Reviews, 44*(2), 78–85. DOI: 10.1249/JES.0000000000000073

Zafeiroudi, A., Goulimaris, D., Alexandris, K., & Yfantidou, G. (2025). Segmenting Recreational Dance Communities in Greece: Cultural Identity, Lifelong Engagement, and Inclusive and Participant-Centered Approaches to Dance Programming. *Societies (Basel, Switzerland), 15*(9), 239.

Zanto, T. P., & Gazzaley, A. (2013). Fronto-parietal network: Flexible hub of cognitive control. *Trends in Cognitive Sciences, 17*(12), 602–603. DOI: 10.1016/j.tics.2013.10.001 PMID: 24129332

Zhang, D., Lee, E. K. P., Mak, E. C. W., Ho, C. Y., & Wong, S. Y. S. (2021). Mindfulness-based interventions: An overall review. *British Medical Bulletin*, •••, ldab005. Advance online publication. DOI: 10.1093/bmb/ldab005 PMID: 33884400

Zhang, X., Lv, J., & Jia, G. (2022). Physical activity and emotional resilience. *Journal of Affective Disorders, 309*, 45–56. PMID: 35712359

Zhang, Z., Du, B. A., Ma, C., Wang, Z., & Hu, W. (2025, October). Behave Your Motion: Habit-preserved Cross-category Animal Motion Transfer. In *Proceedings of the 33rd ACM International Conference on Multimedia* (pp. 9638-9647).

Zhao, J., Effendi, A. A., & Zhao, S. (2024). Work engagement of teachers in Chinese higher education sector: Using mixed method appraisal tool of systematic literature review. *Global Business and Management Research, 16*(4), 1258–1274. https://www.gbmrjournal.com/pdf/v16n4s/V16N4s-79.pdf

Zhao, J., Jiang, W., Wang, X., Cai, Z., Liu, Z., & Liu, G. (2020). Exercise, brain plasticity, and depression. *CNS Neuroscience & Therapeutics, 26*(9), 885–895. DOI: 10.1111/cns.13385 PMID: 32491278

Zheng, G., Xia, R., Zhou, W., Tao, J., & Chen, L. (2016). Aerobic exercise ameliorates cognitive function in patients with Alzheimer's disease. *Neuropsychiatric Disease and Treatment, 12*, 1403–1412. DOI: 10.2147/NDT.S104102

Zhou, S., Slemp, G. R., & Vella-Brodrick, D. A. (2024). Factors associated with teacher wellbeing: A meta-analysis. *Educational Psychology Review*, *36*, 63. Advance online publication. DOI: 10.1007/s10648-024-09886-x

Zhou, X., Li, J., & Jiang, X. (2024). Effects of different types of exercise intensity on improving health related physical fitness in children and adolescents: A systematic review. *Scientific Reports*, *14*(1), x. DOI: 10.1038/s41598 024 64830 PMID: 38906965

Zhu, X., Chen, W., Pinho, R. A., & Thirupathi, A. (2025). Lactate-induced metabolic signaling is the potential mechanism for reshaping the brain function-role of physical exercise. *Frontiers in Endocrinology*, *16*, 1598419. https://www.frontiersin.org/journals/endocrinology/articles/10.3389/fendo.2025.1598419/abstract PMID: 40551894

Žnidaršič, J., & Marič, M. (2021). Relationships between work-family balance, job satisfaction, life satisfaction and work engagement among higher education lecturers. *Organizacija*, *54*(3), 227–237. DOI: 10.2478/orga-2021-0015

Zschucke, E., Gaudlitz, K., & Ströhle, A. (2013). Exercise and physical activity in mental disorders: Clinical and experimental evidence. *Journal of Preventive Medicine and Public Health = Yebang Uihakhoe Chi*, *46*(Suppl 1), S12. https://pmc.ncbi.nlm.nih.gov/articles/PMC3567313/ PMID: 23412549

About the Contributors

Robert Motta obtained his Ph.D. in Psychology from Hofstra University in 1975. He has the title of professor emeritus. At Hofstra he held positions of Chairperson of the Psychology Department, Director and founder of the Psy.D. Doctoral Program in Psychology and Director and Founder of the Child and Family Trauma Institute. He has published over 150 papers and book chapters and published 8 books. He his a practicing clinical psychologist.

***

Manish Baboo Agarwal is an Assistant Professor in the Department of Applied Science (Physics), Sharda University, Agra, with over 22 years of teaching, research, and administrative experience. He earned his Ph.D. in Physics from IIT (ISM) Dhanbad and M.Tech. in Materials Science from IIT Bombay. His research interests include thin film technology, solar cells, nanotechnology, material characterization, and environmental sustainability. He has published extensively in SCI/Scopus indexed journals, authored books and chapters, and holds several national and international patents.

Seema Agarwal is an Assistant Professor in the Department of Mathematics at SRM Institute of Science and Technology, Ghaziabad, with over 12 years of teaching, research, and administrative experience. She earned her Ph.D. and M.Phil. in Mathematics from Dr. B. R. Ambedkar University, Agra. Her research expertise includes queuing theory, nanotechnology, and groundwater quality assessment. She has published widely in SCI/Scopus indexed journals, authored books and book chapters, and holds several national and international patents.

Tashi Ongmu Bhutia is a distinguished academician in the field of Physical Education, currently serving at the Government B.Ed. College, Soreng, Sikkim. She began her academic journey at the prestigious Lakshmibai National Institute of

Physical Education (LNIPE), Gwalior, where she completed both her Bachelor of Physical Education (B.P.Ed.) and Master of Physical Education (M.P.Ed.) with excellence. Driven by a passion for research and academic growth, she pursued her doctoral studies at the University of Delhi, earning a Ph.D. in Physical Education. Over the years, Dr. Bhutia has contributed significantly to promoting physical education, sports, and wellness through her teaching, mentorship, and scholarly pursuits. Her academic background and professional dedication reflect her commitment to advancing the standards of teacher education in Sikkim. Known for her expertise, discipline, and inspiring approach, she continues to shape the future of aspiring educators while fostering holistic development through physical education.

Deepak. D, an academician of two years old, with teaching experience in the areas of taxation, accounting, and IFRS. He has expertise in academic publishing, research content writing, coaching, teaching, editing, and analytical abilities. He possesses a PhD from JAIN (Deemed To Be University) in the School of Commerce. He has participated in a number of FDPs, workshops, seminars, and conferences. He as published more than 10 research paper in different UGC Care journal, web of science, Scopus.

Dao Chanh Thuc Professional Title: Lecturer in Sports Science Affiliation: An Giang University - Vietnam National University, Ho Chi Minh City, Vietnam Education: Dr. Dao Chanh Thuc completed his doctoral program in Sports Science at the University of Sports and Physical Education, Ho Chi Minh City, Vietnam. His prominent research focused on the fields of physical education, sports training, and athletic performance. Career and Contributions: - Dr. Dao Chanh Thuc is a dedicated lecturer and researcher in the field of Sports Science. He is a faculty member at An Giang University - Vietnam National University, Ho Chi Minh City, where he has made significant contributions to the development of the sports science curriculum and research initiatives. - His expertise includes physical education, sports training, sports biomechanics, and the physiological aspects of athletic performance. - Dr. Dao Chanh Thuc has conducted numerous studies aimed at improving the physical fitness and performance of students and athletes. His work often emphasizes the importance of tailored training programs and the integration of modern scientific methods in sports training.

Anindita Das is an esteemed Associate Professor at the Lakshmibai National Institute of Physical Education (LNIPE), Gwalior, with a distinguished career in teaching, research, and sports. Since joining LNIPE in 2007, she has been actively engaged in teaching core subjects such as Health Education, Physiology, and Football (practical). Dr. Das has made significant academic contributions through her authorship of numerous research papers in Scopus, patents, books and chapters in the field of physical education and sports sciences. She has published over twenty research articles in reputed national and international journals and has presented her work at a wide array of conferences. Notably, she presented papers at the Pre-Olympic Congress in Liverpool, UK (2012) and the World Congress on Kinanthropometry in Santiago, Chile (2018). A recipient of international training, Dr. Das completed a 3-month International Coaching Course (ICC) in General Conditioning at Semmelweis University, Budapest, Hungary, in 2009, further enriching her academic and practical expertise. Beyond academics, Dr. Das is a former athlete who has passionately contributed to women's football. She was a four-time member of her university's intervarsity women's football team and won a bronze medal in the All India Intervarsity Women Football Tournament in 2002. She also represented Madhya Pradesh in the National Women's Football Championship and played a key role when her team participated in the 1st Khelo India University Games (KIUG) held in Bhubaneswar, Odisha, in February 2020. Dr. Das continues to inspire students and peers alike with her commitment to excellence in physical education, research, and sports development.

Shravan Shaurya Dubey is a committed Ph.D. Scholar in Physical Education at the Central University of Punjab, India, with a strong academic background and notable achievements in national-level examinations. He completed his Bachelor of Science in Health and Physical Education (2017–2020) from DAV University, Jalandhar, where he developed a solid foundation in sports sciences and physical education. He subsequently earned his Master of Physical Education (M.P.Ed.) with specialization in Sports Psychology (2020–2022) from Lakshmibai National Institute of Physical Education (LNIPE), Gwalior, one of India's premier institutions in the field. Shravan has qualified the UGC–NET examination 4–5 times, including Junior Research Fellowship (JRF), reflecting his strong research aptitude and academic consistency. He has also cleared the Haryana Teacher Eligibility Test (HTET) Levels 2 and 3, highlighting his teaching competence. His research interests include sports psychology, mental skills training, athlete performance enhancement, and physical education pedagogy, with a focus on evidence-based practices and academic excellence.

Ervin T. Echague is a Senior Education Program Specialist at the Bureau of Curriculum Development, Department of Education (DepEd) Central Office, where he plays a pivotal role in shaping national educational policies and curriculum frameworks. Prior to his tenure at DepEd, he served as an Assistant Professorial Lecturer III at the Polytechnic University of the Philippines (PUP) in Manila, where he contributed to the advancement of physical education and movement sciences.

Mr. Echague earned his Bachelor's degree in Physical Education from PUP Manila and a Master of Science in Human Movement Science from the University of the Philippines Diliman. Currently, he is pursuing a Doctor of Philosophy in Curriculum and Instruction at the Philippine Normal University, further strengthening his expertise in educational program development and pedagogical innovation. In addition to his academic and professional engagements, Mr. Echague is a licensed and accredited Dancesport National Adjudicator under the Philippine Dancesport Academy – Philippine DanceSport Federation Inc. He is a former member of the PUP Dancesport Team and has served as a sports manual writer, validator, folk dance trainer, and dancesport coach. His extensive experience in dance and sports education has significantly contributed to promoting and developing physical education in the country. His research interests encompass recreation, comparative physical education and activities, travel, and leisure. Through his scholarly work and advocacy, Mr. Echague remains committed to advancing the fields of physical education, curriculum development, and movement sciences in both academic and practical settings.

Khaoula Ennahli is a PhD student in Psychology at ISCTE-Instituto Universitário de Lisboa, funded by the INPhINIT Doctoral Scholarship of the La Caixa Foundation. Her research focuses on the effectiveness of creativity-based strategies to improve Declarative Memory in older adults. With a background in Cognitive Science, she has experience in EEG, eye-tracking and other psychophysiological techniques. She participated in multiple research projects and presented papers at national and international conferences. Currently, she is a researcher in the BEC (Behavior, Emotion, and Cognition) group at CIS-IUL.

Anton Dwi Fitriyanto is a lecturer with a focus on digitalization, Bina Nusantara University. He holds a Doctor of Management degree and a Master's degree in Information and Communication Technology. He is also an expert in digitalization strategies, innovation development, and new technologies. He frequently collaborates with industry, universities, and government on research projects involving Big Data, Artificial Intelligence, Digital Strategic Management, Sustainability and Carbon Economy.

Marie Grace A. Gomez is Professor 11 at the Counselor Education Area, College of Education, University of the Philippines-Diliman. She teaches counseling and research courses at the undergraduate and graduate levels. She has a bachelor's degree in Political Science, a Master of Arts in Education (Guidance) degree, a Doctor of Philosophy degree in Guidance, and another doctorate in Special Education. She has served as a classroom teacher, guidance counselor, and administrator in the basic and tertiary education settings. Her community extension projects involve counseling and assessment of children, persons with disability, children in conflict with the law, drug surrenderees, development of sexual health literacy programs for teens with disabilities, sexually abused children, medical personnel, women with mental health issues in institutional settings, and persons affected by COVID-19. She has been the lead researcher for the Philippines in a UNESCO research led by Leonard Cheshire UK on Comprehensive Sexuality Education for persons with disabilities. She has received the 2022 Most Outstanding Professional Teacher Award in the field of Academe and Research from the Philippine Federation for Professional Associations.

Karuppasamy Govindasamy is a dedicated researcher in Physical Education and Sports Sciences at the Department of Sports, Recreation and Wellness, Symbiosis International (Deemed University), Hyderabad Campus, Telangana. He has authored over 108 publications in Scopus and 51 publications in Web of Science journals, along with patents, book chapters, and books. His research focuses on innovative training methodologies and the integration of theory and practice in sports science. Dr. Govindasamy is UGC-NET and JRF qualified, has received multiple Best Paper Presentation awards, and was honored with a national-level Young Researcher Award. He also serves as a reviewer for 17 top-ranking international journals.

Hemlata Jain is working as an academician with more than 18 years of teaching, research and administrative experience, currently serving as Assistant Professor in the Department of Applied Sciences at Sharda University Agra, Uttar Pradesh, India. She has completed her Ph.D. in English from Dr. B. R. Ambedkar University Agra. She has published multiple research papers in many indexed journals, authored books and book chapters.

Debajit Karmakar, is a distinguished research scholar and accomplished academic in the field of Physical Education and Sports Science. Currently pursuing his Ph.D. at the prestigious Lakshmibai National Institute of Physical Education (LNIPE), Gwalior, he has established himself as a prolific researcher. Mr. Karmakar completed his educational journey with remarkable academic excellence, earning his B.A./B.Sc. (Hons) in Physical Education from Visva-Bharati University, Santiniketan, followed by his B.P.Ed. from the same institution where he topped in his class. His Master's degree in Physical Education is from LNIPE, and he subsequently qualified UGC NET-JRF & WBSET examinations, demonstrating his academic prowess. A specialist in football and sports psychology, Mr. Karmakar has made significant contributions to academic literature with extensive publications in Scopus & Web of Science indexed journals. His research focuses on mental training, performance psychology, and innovative training methodologies. He has authored multiple books on sports psychology and performance enhancement, while also serving as editor for several academic publications.

Awesh Khati is a dedicated Ph.D. scholar specializing in Physical Education Pedagogy at the Lakshmibai National Institute of Physical Education (LNIPE), Gwalior. He has qualified for the UGC-NET JRF in Physical Education, contributed to a few research papers, written multiple books, and participated in numerous seminars, conferences, and workshops related to physical education and sports. An accomplished athlete, he has competed in inter-university football tournaments and holds coaching licenses from the All India Football Federation and Athletics Federation of India. With a diverse academic background in International Relations and Physical Education, he brings a unique perspective to sports education. Passionate about advancing physical education in India, he blends theoretical knowledge with practical expertise to promote holistic athletic and academic development.

Shivam Kumar (0009-0005-4315-5883) is a dedicated physiotherapist and researcher with a focus on the neurobiological and rehabilitative aspects of exercise. His work contributes to the advancement of physical therapy by exploring its therapeutic impact on emotional well-being. He is committed to both clinical practice and academic publication, aiming to bridge scientific research with practical applications to improve patient care.

Manu Mehrotra is an Associate Professor of Chemistry at Anand School of Engineering and Technology, Sharda University, Agra, with over two decades of teaching and research experience. He earned his Ph.D. in Chemistry from Jai Narain Vyas University, Jodhpur, specializing in the kinetics and mechanisms of redox reactions. His expertise lies in nanomaterials, environmental chemistry, and material science applications. He has published extensively in reputed journals, authored books and chapters, and holds several patents, while also contributing to academic leadership and professional development through conferences and workshops.

Diogo Miguel holds a bachelor´s degree in psychology, a master´s in social and organizational psychology and a master´s in clinical psychology. Currently, he´s pursuing a PhD at Iscte-Instituto Universitário de Lisboa. He was awarded a merit scholarship for being ISEIT´s best student (2023/2024). He also integrates the team of the B.lifelong project, a funded initiative by La Caixa Foundation, and is a researcher at Cis_Iscte.

Gopal Chandra Saha is a Distinguished Professor in the Department of Physical Education and Sport Science at Visva-Bharati University, West Bengal.

With an illustrious career, Dr. Saha has authored numerous research papers, guided postgraduate and PhD thesis, and contributed extensively to sports training, physical education, and sports medicine. His expertise spans innovative coaching methodologies, focusing on soccer, and he holds advanced certifications, including AFC 'A', 'B', and 'C' coaching licenses. Renowned for his commitment to advancing the discipline, Dr. Saha continues to inspire students and professionals through his academic leadership, research endeavors, and dedication to excellence in physical education and sports sciences.

Sohom Saha is a passionate academic and sports psychology professional, currently pursuing his Ph.D. in Physical Education at the Lakshmibai National Institute of Physical Education (LNIPE), Gwalior. He completed his Master of Physical Education (M.P.Ed.) with distinction from LNIPE, following his Bachelor of Physical Education (B.P.Ed.) and Bachelor of Arts (B.A.) in Physical Education from Visva-Bharati University, Shantiniketan, West Bengal. His areas of specialization include Sports Psychology, Volleyball, and Yoga, where he integrates scientific knowledge with practical expertise. Throughout his academic journey, Mr. Saha has actively participated in national-level sports events, including the All-India Inter-University Yoga and Ball Badminton Championships, and has secured championships in NCC Inter-Battalion Football and Badminton tournaments. Alongside his athletic pursuits, he has contributed significantly to sports research, publishing multiple articles in Scopus-indexed, Web of Science, and peer-reviewed journals. His research interests focus on emotional resilience, psychological well-being, performance optimization, and contemporary trends in sports psychology. Beyond research and sports, Mr. Saha has authored several books on sports psychology and technology in sports. He serves as an active reviewer for leading international journals, including PLOS ONE and Frontiers, as well as other reputed platforms, and is a member of the Sports Psychology Association of India. Mr. Saha's work reflects a strong commitment to promoting inclusivity, mental toughness, and holistic development in the field of sports. Through his scholarly contributions, practical experience, and professional engagements, he aspires to inspire future generations of athletes, educators, and researchers in building a more inclusive and psychologically enriched sporting world.

Beulah Sebastian is a Sports and Wellness Leader, Educator, and Researcher dedicated to advancing physical literacy, student development, and active lifestyles in higher education. With over 18 years of experience in sports education, wellness program design, and leadership development, she currently serves as Head of Sports at Symbiosis International University. Her work bridges sport, fitness, and education through evidence-based practice, innovative programming, and institution-wide initiatives that promote lifelong physical activity, holistic wellbeing, and leadership through sport. As a national-level volleyball player, she brings high-performance insights into academic and student-centric environments, emphasizing discipline, teamwork, and resilience. Driven by the belief that destiny is a matter of choice, her research and professional practice focus on physical literacy, student engagement, and the role of sport in building healthy, high-performing academic communities.

Richa Sharma is a Clinical Nutritionist and Dietitian dedicated to preventive health, therapeutic nutrition, and evidence-based lifestyle medicine. She is the Founder of Eat Healthy for Tomorrow, a wellness initiative focused on personalized diet planning and sustainable nutrition guidance, helping individuals manage chronic conditions such as diabetes, cardiovascular diseases, thyroid disorders, and metabolic health concerns. She also authors the Wellora Newsletter, a research-driven publication that delivers practical nutrition education, healthy lifestyle tools, and inspiring wellness perspectives to a growing community of readers. Richa is deeply committed to bridging the gap between scientific knowledge and real-world application. Her work blends clinical expertise with compassionate, client-centered counseling, enabling individuals to take charge of their health through informed and realistic dietary choices. With a strong academic background, she teaches subjects like Medical Nutrition Therapy, Community Nutrition, Nutrition Through the Life Cycle, and Food Microbiology, shaping future professionals in the field. She has contributed book chapters and research projects that explore innovative nutrition solutions, holistic wellness frameworks, and public health improvement through education and behavioral change. Guided by the belief that nutrition is the foundation of physical, mental, and emotional well-being, Richa strives to build a culture where healthy living becomes accessible, enjoyable, and empowering for all.

Mahendra Kumar Singh is a Professor of Sports Psychology in the Department of Sports Psychology at Lakshmibai National Institute of Physical Education (LNIPE), Gwalior, Madhya Pradesh, under the Ministry of Youth Affairs & Sports, Government of India. He is currently also serving as the Controller of Examinations at LNIPE, Gwalior. He holds B.P.E., M.P.E., M.Phil., and Ph.D. degrees from LNCPE/LNIPE, Gwalior, has qualified UGC NET, and completed various yoga certifications including a Certificate Course in Yoga from Lonavla, Pune, as well as Yoga Pravesh and Yoga Parichaya from LNCPE, Gwalior. He also holds an NCC 'B' Certificate from the 8 MP Battalion, Gwalior. Dr. Singh has been engaged in teaching for over 34 years, including more than 19 years in postgraduate and Ph.D.-level teaching and research. He has extensive administrative experience, having served as Former Incharge Registrar, Former Dean of Academics, Sport Sciences, and Physical Education and Applied Areas, Former Chief Proctor, Former Chairman of the UGC Student Grievance Redressal Cell, Former Nodal Officer for the UGC Grievance Portal, Former HOD of the Department of Sports Psychology at LNIPE, Former Deputy Controller of Examinations, Former HOD of the School of Law at Guru Ghasidas Central University, Bilaspur, Former HOD of the Department of Physical Education at CSJM University, Kanpur, Anti-Ragging Coordinator at GGV, Bilaspur, Warden of various boys' hostels across Engineering, Pharmacy, and other UG/PG courses at CSJM University and Administrative Warden at GGV. He has authored six books on Physical Education, Sports, and Yoga, and published more than 50 research papers in national and international journals, including SCOPUS-indexed journals. Dr. Singh has presented over 35 papers at various national and international conferences/seminars. He is a member of academic bodies of various universities, a continuing member and former Chairperson of the Board of Studies and Departmental Research Committee at LNIPE, and has served as Secretary of the Board of Management at LNIPE. He has frequently been invited as a resource person, chairperson, and keynote speaker at national and international conferences and seminars. Additionally, he has extensive experience as an external examiner, paper setter, and evaluator for UG/PG/Ph.D. courses across various universities and has handled confidential assignments with state public service commissions. Dr. Singh has organized several mega events, sports tournaments, seminars, and conferences, and guided numerous Ph.D. scholars, with several more currently under his supervision. He also serves as the Chief Editor of conference proceedings publications and is on the editorial boards of reputed journals. During his student years, he represented Jiwaji University in Inter-University Tournaments in Basketball and Kho-Kho under AIU and also participated in M.P. State Inter-University Tournaments in the same sports, along with several other achievements.

Harry Sutanto currently serves as a faculty member in management at the Undergraduate Program of Binus University, Jakarta, Indonesia. He also lectures on business ethics in the Master of Management Program and teaches microfinance management in the Integrated Microfinance Management Program, both under the Faculty of Economics and Business at Universitas Padjadjaran, Bandung. He earned his bachelor's degree in agriculture from Universitas Padjadjaran in 1983, an MBA from the University of Illinois at Urbana-Champaign, USA, in 1996, and graduated as the best doctoral candidate in management science from Universitas Padjadjaran, Bandung. In addition to conducting research and presenting at national and international conferences, he has extensive teaching and training experience in areas such as change management, corporate culture, corporate governance, leadership, and human resource management. He is also active as a consultant, particularly in corporate transformation, leadership development, and the design and acceleration of corporate culture implementation for both private companies and government institutions. Furthermore, he is involved in the Farmer Corporation Program under the Ministry of Agriculture, supporting agricultural efficiency and food security. His professional career is grounded in a diverse background, including 2.5 years in oil palm plantations, 28 years in banking, serving as Finance and Marketing Director of a state-owned paper company, Commissioner of a property building maintenance firm, President Commissioner of a security printing company, and member of a bank liquidation team.

Index

A

B

C

D

E

I

L

M

N

P

Q

R

S

W

Y

www.ingramcontent.com/pod-product-compliance
Lightning Source LLC
LaVergne TN
LVHW062341300926
849161LV00007B/1775
* 9 7 9 8 3 3 7 3 6 1 5 7 4 *